Study Guide

Today's Medical Assistant

Study Guide

Today's Medical Assistant: Clinical and Administrative Procedures

Second Edition

Kathy Bonewit-West, BS, MEd
Coordinator and Instructor
Medical Assistant Technology
Hocking College
Nelsonville, Ohio
Former Member, Curriculum Review Board of the American Association of Medical Assistants

Sue A. Hunt, MA, RN, CMA (AAMA)
Professor Emeritus
Medical Assisting Program
Middlesex Community College
Lowell, Massachusetts

Edith Applegate, MS
Professor of Biological Sciences
Kettering College of Medical Arts
Kettering, Ohio

SAUNDERS

3251 Riverport Lane
St. Louis, Missouri 63043

STUDY GUIDE FOR TODAY'S MEDICAL ASSISTANT: CLINICAL
AND ADMINISTRATIVE PROCEDURES, SECOND EDITION

ISBN: 978-1-4557-0151-3

Notice

Knowledge and best practice in this field are constantly changing. As new research and experience broaden
our understanding, changes in research methods, professional practices, or medical treatment may become
necessary.

Practitioners and researchers must always rely on their own experience and knowledge in evaluating and
using any information, methods, compounds, or experiments described herein. In using such information or
methods they should be mindful of their own safety and the safety of others, including parties for whom they
have a professional responsibility.

With respect to any drug or pharmaceutical products identified, readers are advised to check the most
current information provided (i) on procedures featured or (ii) by the manufacturer of each product to be
administered, to verify the recommended dose or formula, the method and duration of administration, and
contraindications. It is the responsibility of practitioners, relying on their own experience and knowledge of
their patients, to make diagnoses, to determine dosages and the best treatment for each individual patient, and
to take all appropriate safety precautions.

To the fullest extent of the law, neither the Publisher nor the authors, contributors, or editors, assume any
liability for any injury and/or damage to persons or property as a matter of products liability, negligence or
otherwise, or from any use or operation of any methods, products, instructions, or ideas contained in the
material herein.

Executive Content Strategist: John Dolan
Senior Content Development Specialist: Jennifer Bertucci
Project Manager: Maria Bernard
Designer: Jessica Williams

Printed in the United States of America.

Last digit is the print number: 9   8   7   6   5   4   3   2   1

Preface

Outcome-based education prepares individuals to perform the prespecified tasks of an occupation under real-world conditions at a level of accuracy and speed required of the entry-level practitioner of that profession. Outcome-based education plays an important role in medical assisting programs in preparing qualified individuals for careers in medical offices, clinics, and related health care facilities. *The Study Guide for Today's Medical Assistant* has been developed using a thorough outcome-based approach. It meets the criteria stipulated by the Commission on Accreditation of Allied Health Education (CAAHEP)* Standards and Guidelines for the Medical Assisting Educational Programs and the Accrediting Bureau of Health Education Schools (ABHES)† Programmatic Evaluation Standards for Medical Assisting. Instructors should find this Study Guide a valuable teaching aid for training students who are able to think critically and to perform competently in the clinical setting.

Each study guide chapter is organized into the following sections:

1. **ASSIGNMENT SHEETS:** The textbook and Study Guide Assignment Sheets indicate the assignments for each chapter, along with a space provided for the student to document the following: the date each assignment is due, completion of the assignment, and points earned for each assignment. The Laboratory Assignment Sheet indicates the procedures required in each chapter, along with the textbook and Study Guide reference pages, the number of practices required to attain competency, and a space for documenting the score earned on the Performance Evaluation Checklist.

2. **PRETEST AND POSTTEST:** These tests have been included for each chapter using true or false questions, which allow the student to test his or her acquisition of knowledge before and after completing the chapter. These tests can be used as a study guide to prepare for chapter tests.

3. **KEY TERM ASSESSMENT:** This section provides the student with an assessment of his or her knowledge of the medical terms covered in each chapter. This section also includes an assessment of the word parts of the medical terms (prefixes, suffixes, and combining forms) to evaluate the student's knowledge of the meaning of the medical term through its parts.

4. **EVALUATION OF LEARNING:** These questions help the student evaluate his or her progress throughout each chapter. After the student has completed these questions and checked them for accuracy, they provide an ongoing review of the textbook material. Individuals preparing for a certification examination will find the completed Evaluation of Learning sections a useful study aid for the clinical aspect of the examination.

5. **CRITICAL THINKING ACTIVITIES:** In this section, the student performs activities that enhance his or her ability to think critically. Some situations require the student to become involved in a game or play a role; others require the student to use independent study to answer questions posed by a patient. Independent study helps the student become familiar with resources available to acquire additional knowledge and skills outside the classroom. By learning techniques of self-development, the medical assisting student may become aware of the necessity for continuing education after graduation and entrance into the medical assisting profession.

6. **PRACTICE FOR COMPETENCY:** This section consists of worksheets that provide the student with a guide for the practice of each clinical skill presented in the textbook.

7. **EVALUATION OF COMPETENCY:** This section has two parts. The first part is the Performance Objective, which provides an exact description of what the learner must be able to demonstrate to attain competency and has been developed to correspond with the procedures presented in the textbook. A performance objective consists of the (1) outcome, (2) conditions, and (3) standards. The second part is the Performance Evaluation Checklist, which provides quality control by comparing the student's performance against an established set of performance standards.

8. **SUPPLEMENTAL EDUCATION:** Several medical assisting content areas are more difficult than the others for the student to comprehend and perform. Because students have a particular difficulty in noting patients' symptoms and in calculating drug dosage, two supplemental education sections have been incorporated into this manual. The section "Taking Patients' Symptoms" provides supplemental education for Chapter 36 (The Medical Record) in the

---

*CAAHEP competencies used on the "Evaluation of Competency" checklists are from the American Association of Medical Assistants, Chicago, Illinois, and the Commission on Accreditation of Allied Health Education Programs, Clearwater, Florida.
†ABHES competencies used on the "Evaluation of Competency" checklists are from the Accrediting Bureau of Health Education Schools, Falls Church, Virginia.

textbook; the section "Drug Dosage Calculation" provides supplemental education for Chapter 26 (Administration of Medication). In these two sections, a step-by-step, self-directed approach has been used, beginning with basic concepts and advancing to more difficult ones. The student should find that this type of approach facilitates the process of becoming proficient in these areas.

9. **EVOLVE SITE:** The Evolve site (http://evolve.elsevier.com/Bonewit/today/) offers many opportunities for students to apply the theory and skills learned throughout the textbook. Organized by chapter, the Evolve site includes several games (e.g., Quiz Show, Road to Recovery) and question sets (e.g., Apply Your Knowledge and Prepare for Certification) to provide entertainment while learning important concepts related to selected chapters, matching exercises, labeling exercises, identification exercises, multiple choice and drag-and-drop questions, and other helpful activities for the student. Also, there are helpful supplemental resources like Practicum Activities (which assist the student in relating classroom knowledge to the real-world setting of the medical office) and Video Evaluations (which assess the student's knowledge of key points in the procedural DVDs that accompany the textbook).

We would like to thank the staff at Elsevier for their assistance and support in preparing this Study Guide. We would also like to express our appreciation to the following individuals who provided encouragement and friendship throughout this endeavor: Dave Brennan, Marlene Donovan, Dawn Shingler, Deborah Murray, Rob Bonewit, Hollie Bonewit-Cron, Tristen West, and Caitlin Brennan.

Kathy Bonewit-West, BS, MEd
Sue A. Hunt, MA, RN, CMA (AAMA)
Edith Applegate, MS

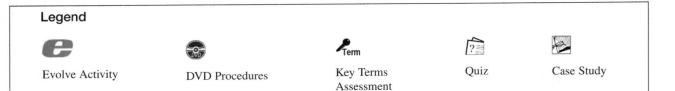

Legend				
Evolve Activity	DVD Procedures	Key Terms Assessment	Quiz	Case Study

Message to the Student

This Study Guide has been designed to facilitate the attainment of competency in the clinical theory and procedures in your textbook. Each chapter of the manual has been organized into the following 9 components. By completing each component, it is hoped that your ability to assimilate the theory and perform the clinical skills will be greatly enhanced.

1. **TEXTBOOK AND STUDY GUIDE ASSIGNMENT SHEETS**
   A. Each time your instructor makes an assignment from the textbook, Study Guide, or Evolve site, document the date due in the appropriate space on the Textbook or Study Guide Assignment Sheet.
   B. Complete each assignment by the due date. Place a checkmark in the appropriate space on the Textbook or Study Guide Assignment Sheet after completing each assignment.
   C. Grade the assignment according to the directions stipulated by your instructor.
   D. Record your points earned in the appropriate space on the Textbook or Study Guide Assignment sheet.

2. **LABORATORY ASSIGNMENT SHEET**
   A. Your instructor will assign the procedures to be completed for each laboratory practice session. Check the assigned procedures in the appropriate space on the Laboratory Assignment Sheet.
   B. Refer to the page numbers on the Laboratory Assignment Sheet for the Practice for Competency and Evaluation of Competency worksheets required for each procedure your instructor assigned.
   C. Locate and tear out the worksheets required for each procedure, and bring them to your lab.
   D. Record the score you earned on the Evaluation of Competency Performance Evaluation Checklist in the appropriate space on the Laboratory Assignment Sheet. This will provide you with a record of your progress.

3. **PRETEST AND POSTTEST**
   A. Complete the Pretest before beginning a study of each chapter. Complete the Posttest after completing the study of the chapter. Place a checkmark in the appropriate space on the Study Guide Assignment Sheet after completing each test.
   B. Check your work for accuracy against the textbook, and correct any errors.
   C. Grade the tests according to the directions stipulated by your instructor.
   D. Record the points you earned in the appropriate space on the Study Guide Assignment Sheet.
   E. Review the Pretest and Posttest before taking your chapter test.

4. **KEY TERM ASSESSMENT**
   A. Study the Terminology Review section located at the end of each chapter in the textbook.
   B. Match the medical terms with the definitions and complete the word parts table. Place a checkmark in the appropriate space on the Study Guide Assignment Sheet after completing the exercise.
   C. Check your work for accuracy against the textbook, and correct any errors.
   D. Grade the exercise according to the directions stipulated by your instructor.
   E. Record the points you earned in the appropriate space on the Study Guide Assignment Sheet.
   F. Review the Key Term Assessment before taking your chapter test.

5. **EVALUATION OF LEARNING QUESTIONS**
   A. Read the textbook chapter.
   B. Complete the Evaluation of Learning questions. Place a checkmark in the appropriate space on the Study Guide Assignment Sheet after completing the questions.
   C. Check your work for accuracy against the textbook, and correct any errors.
   D. Grade the questions according to the directions stipulated by your instructor.
   E. Record the points you earned in the appropriate space on the Textbook Assignment Sheet.
   F. Review the Evaluation of Learning questions before taking your chapter test.

6. **CRITICAL THINKING ACTIVITIES**
   A. Review the information required to complete the Critical Thinking Activities.
   B. Obtain any additional materials or resources required.

C. Complete each Critical Thinking Activity. Place a checkmark in the appropriate space on the Study Guide Assignment Sheet after completing each assigned activity.

D. Grade each Critical Thinking Activity according to the directions stipulated by your instructor.

E. Record the points you earned in the appropriate space on the Textbook Assignment Sheet.

7. **EVOLVE SITE ACTIVITIES**

A. Review the information required to complete the Evolve site activities.

B. Using the Evolve site, complete the activities.

C. Place a checkmark in the appropriate section on the Study Guide Assignment Sheet after completing each Evolve site activity.

D. Record the points you earned in the appropriate space on the Study Guide Assignment Sheet.

8. **PRACTICE FOR COMPETENCY**

A. Your instructor will assign the procedure(s) to be completed for each laboratory practice session. For each procedure assigned, place a checkmark in the appropriate space on the Laboratory Assignment Sheet.

B. Refer to the page numbers on the Laboratory Assignment Sheet for the Practice for Competency and Evaluation of Competency sheets required for each procedure your instructor assigned. Locate and tear out the sheets required for each procedure to be performed, and bring them to your laboratory practice session.

C. Practice each assigned procedure the required number of times indicated on the Laboratory Assignment Sheet or as designated by your instructor. Use the following guidelines when practicing the procedure to attain competency:

   1. Information indicated on the Practice for Competency sheet
      - Record your practices in the chart provided.

   2. Procedure as presented in your textbook

   3. Video of the procedure (on companion DVDs accompanying your textbook, or on the Evolve site)
      - View each procedure several times to make sure you understand the correct technique and theory.

   4. Evaluation of Competency Performance Checklist
      - Make sure that you can perform each procedure according to the criteria stipulated under conditions and standards.

   5. Peer evaluation
      - If directed by your instructor, obtain a peer evaluation using the Performance Evaluation Checklist.

D. Bring the completed Practice for Competency sheet to your laboratory testing session, and present it to your instructor for his or her review before taking the procedure test .

9. **EVALUATION OF COMPETENCY PERFORMANCE CHECKLIST**

A. Write your name and date in the space indicated on the Evaluation of Competency Performance Evaluation Checklist.

   1. Do not chart the procedure (in advance) on the Evaluation of Competency sheet. You do this after you have been tested on the procedure.

B. For each procedure being evaluated, bring the following to your laboratory testing session, and present them to your instructor:

   1. Completed Practice for Competency sheet

   2. Evaluation of Competency Performance Checklist

   3. Outcome Assessment Record

C. Demonstrate the proper procedure for performing the clinical skill for your instructor.

D. Record results (if required) in the chart provided on the Evaluation of Competency Checklist.

E. Obtain your instructor's initials on your Outcome Assessment Record indicating you have performed the procedure with competency.

F. Record the score you earned in the appropriate space on your Laboratory Assignment Sheet.

After you have completed each chapter in this Study Guide, it is suggested that you place the perforated sheet into a three-ring notebook. This will provide an ongoing record of your academic progress. In addition, the notebook will be useful both as a classroom reference and as a certification examination review resource. We hope that this Study Guide will assist your attainment of competency in medical assisting procedures and will facilitate your transition from the classroom to the workplace.

Kathy Bonewit-West, BS, MEd
Sue A. Hunt, MA, RN, CMA (AAMA)
Edith Applegate, MS

Outcome Assessment Record

This list of outcomes is used to maintain an ongoing record of classroom and practicum outcome assessments. Your instructor should initial each outcome when you have performed it competently in the classroom. When you have performed the outcome with competency at your practicum facility, it should be initialed by your practicum supervisor. Space is provided for three practicum experiences in the event that you extern at more than one practicum site.

Name_____	Classroom Performance	Practicum	Practicum	Practicum
MEDICAL ASEPSIS AND THE OSHA STANDARD				
Wash hands.				
Apply an alcohol-based hand rub.				
Apply and remove clean disposable gloves.				
Adhere to the OSHA Standard.				
STERILIZATION AND DISINFECTION				
Sanitize instruments.				
Wrap instruments using paper or muslin.				
Wrap instruments using a pouch.				
Sterilize articles in the autoclave.				
VITAL SIGNS				
Measure oral body temperature.				
Measure axillary body temperature.				
Measure rectal body temperature.				
Measure aural body temperature.				
Measure temporal artery body temperature.				
Measure pulse and respiration.				
Measure apical pulse.				
Perform pulse oximetry.				
Measure blood pressure.				

Name_____	Classroom Performance	Practicum	Practicum	Practicum
THE PHYSICAL EXAMINATION				
Measure weight and height.				
Demonstrate proper body mechanics.				
Position and drape an individual.				
Transfer a patient to and from a wheelchair.				
Prepare a patient for a physical examination.				
Assist the physician with the physical examination.				
EYE AND EAR PROCEDURES				
Assess distance visual acuity.				
Assess color vision.				
Perform an eye irrigation.				
Perform an eye instillation.				
Perform an ear irrigation.				
Perform an ear instillation.				
PHYSICAL AGENTS TO PROMOTE TISSUE HEALING				
Apply a heating pad.				
Apply a hot soak.				
Apply a hot compress.				
Apply an ice bag.				
Apply a cold compress.				
Apply a chemical pack.				
Measure a patient for axillary crutches.				
Instruct a patient in mastering crutch gaits.				
Instruct a patient in the use of a cane.				
Instruct a patient in the use of a walker.				
THE GYNECOLOGIC EXAMINATION AND PRENATAL CARE				
Provide instructions for a breast self-examination.				
Prepare the patient for a gynecologic examination.				

x

Outcome Assessment Record

Name_____	Classroom Performance	Practicum	Practicum	Practicum
Assist with a gynecologic examination.				
Prepare the patient for a prenatal examination.				
Assist with a return prenatal examination.				
THE PEDIATRIC EXAMINATION				
Carry an infant in the following positions: cradle and upright.				
Measure the weight and length of an infant.				
Measure the head and chest circumference of an infant.				
Plot pediatric measurements on a growth chart.				
Apply a pediatric urine collector.				
MINOR OFFICE SURGERY				
Apply and remove sterile gloves.				
Open a sterile package.				
Add a sterile article to a sterile field using a peelapart package.				
Pour a sterile solution into a container on a sterile field.				
Change a sterile dressing.				
Remove sutures.				
Remove staples.				
Apply and remove adhesive skin closures.				
Set up a surgical tray for minor office surgery.				
Assist with minor office surgery.				
Apply the following bandage turns: circular, spiral, spiral-reverse, figure-eight, and recurrent.				

Outcome Assessment Record

Name_____	Classroom Performance	Practicum	Practicum	Practicum
ADMINISTRATION OF MEDICATION AND INTRAVENOUS THERAPY				
Administer oral medication.				
Prepare an injection from a vial.				
Prepare an injection from an ampule.				
Reconstitute a powdered drug.				
Administer a subcutaneous injection.				
Locate the following intramuscular injection sites: dorsogluteal, deltoid, vastus lateralis, and ventrogluteal.				
Administer an intramuscular injection.				
Administer an injection using the Z-track method.				
Administer an intradermal injection.				
Administer a Mantoux test.				
Read and interpret Mantoux test results.				
CARDIOPULMONARY PROCEDURES				
Record a 12-lead, three-channel electrocardiogram (ECG).				
Perform a spirometry test.				
Measure peak flow rate.				
COLON PROCEDURES AND MALE REPRODUCTIVE HEALTH				
Instruct a patient in the specimen collection procedure for a fecal occult blood test.				
Develop the hemoccult slide test.				
Provide instructions for a testicular self-examination.				
RADIOLOGY AND DIAGNOSTIC IMAGING				
Instruct a patient in the proper preparation required for each of the following x-ray examinations: mammogram, bone density scan, upper GI, lower GI, and intravenous pyelogram.				

Outcome Assessment Record

Name_____	Classroom Performance	Practicum	Practicum	Practicum
Instruct a patient in the proper preparation required for each of the following: ultrasonography, computed tomography, magnetic resonance imaging, and nuclear medicine.				
INTRODUCTION TO THE CLINICAL LABORATORY				
Use a laboratory directory.				
Complete a laboratory request form.				
Prepare a laboratory report for review by the physician.				
Instruct the patient in advance on preparation requirements for a laboratory test.				
Collect a specimen.				
Properly handle and store a specimen.				
Review a laboratory report.				
URINALYSIS				
Instruct a patient in clean-catch midstream urine specimen collection.				
Assess the color and appearance of a urine specimen.				
Perform a chemical assessment of a urine specimen.				
Prepare a urine specimen for microscopic examination.				
Perform a urine pregnancy test.				
PHLEBOTOMY				
Perform a venipuncture using the vacuum tube method.				
Perform a venipuncture using the butterfly method.				
Perform a skin puncture using a disposable semiautomatic lancet device.				
Obtain a capillary blood specimen.				

Name_____	Classroom Performance	Practicum	Practicum	Practicum
HEMATOLOGY				
Perform a hemoglobin determination.				
Perform a hematocrit determination.				
Prepare a blood smear for a differential cell count.				
BLOOD CHEMISTRY AND IMMUNOLOGY				
Perform blood chemistry testing.				
Perform a fasting blood glucose test using a glucose monitor.				
Perform a rapid mononu-cleosis test.				
MEDICAL MICROBIOLOGY				
Use a microscope.				
Collect a throat specimen.				
Obtain a specimen using a collection and transport system.				
Perform a rapid strep test.				
Prepare a wet-mount slide.				
Prepare a microbiologic smear.				
THE MEDICAL RECORD				
Prepare a medical record for a new patient.				
Complete a consent form for treatment.				
Assist a patient in the completion of a consent to release medical information form.				
Release information according to a completed release of medical information form.				
Complete or assist the patient in completing a health history form.				
Obtain and record a patient's symptoms.				

Name_____	Classroom Performance	Practicum	Practicum	Practicum
PATIENT RECEPTION				
Open the medical office.				
Close the medical office.				
Obtain new patient information.				
Explain office policies and procedures.				
TELEPHONE TECHNIQUES				
Perform a telephone screening.				
Take a telephone message.				
Take requests for medication or prescription refills.				
Telephone a patient for followup.				
SCHEDULING APPOINTMENTS				
Set up the appointment schedule.				
Make an appointment.				
Manage the appointment schedule.				
Schedule inpatient or outpatient diagnostic tests or procedures.				
Schedule inpatient or outpatient admission.				
MEDICAL RECORDS MANAGEMENT				
File patient records alphabetically.				
File patient records numerically.				
File reports.				
WRITTEN COMMUNICATIONS				
Compose a business letter.				
Send a fax.				
Prepare copies of multiple-page documents.				
MAIL				
Process incoming mail.				
Look up a ZIP code.				
Prepare envelopes for mailing.				

Outcome Assessment Record

Name_____	Classroom Performance	Practicum	Practicum	Practicum
MANAGING PRACTICE FINANCES				
Complete a patient charge slip.				
Post charges.				
Post payments and/or adjustments.				
Record a patient's visit on the day sheet.				
Use a computerized office billing system.				
Write a check.				
Prepare a bank deposit.				
Reconcile a bank statement.				
Create and maintain a petty cash log.				
MEDICAL CODING				
Perform CPT coding.				
Perform HCPCS coding.				
Perform ICDM coding.				
MEDICAL INSURANCE				
Apply managed care policies and procedures.				
Obtain insurance preauthorization (precertification).				
Complete/review the CMS-1500 insurance claim form.				
BILLING AND COLLECTIONS				
Process patient bills.				
Post an NSF check.				
Process a credit balance.				
Process a refund.				
Create an accounts receivable aging record.				
Write a collection letter.				
Post a collection agency payment.				

Name_____	Classroom Performance	Practicum	Practicum	Practicum
THE MEDICAL ASSISTANT AS OFFICE MANAGER				
Create an environmental checklist and perform a safety inspection.				
Perform routine maintenance of equipment.				
Take a supply or equipment inventory.				
Locate community resources.				
Complete an incident report.				
EMERGENCY PROTECTIVE PRACTICES FOR THE MEDICAL OFFICE				
Demonstrate proper use of a fire extinguisher.				
Participate in a mock environmental exposure event.				
Maintain a list of community resources for emergency preparedness.				
ADDITIONAL OUTCOMES (List)				

Outcome Assessment Record

Contents

1 The Health Care System

CHAPTER ASSIGNMENTS

√ After Completing	Date Due	Textbook Page(s)	TEXTBOOK ASSIGNMENTS	Possible Points	Points You Earned
		1-17	Read Chapter 1: The Health Care System		
		9 16	Read Case Study 1 Case Study questions	5	
		12 16	Read Case Study 2 Case Study questions	5	
		15 16	Read Case Study 3 Case Study question	5	
			TOTAL POINTS		
√ After Completing	**Date Due**	**Study Guide Page(s)**	**STUDY GUIDE ASSIGNMENTS** **(CTA: Critical Thinking Activity)**	**Possible Points**	**Points You Earned**
		3	Pretest	10	
		4	Term Key Term Assessment A. Definitions B. Word Parts (Add 1 point for each medical term)	13 6	
		4-7	Evaluation of Learning questions	24	
		7	CTA A: Allied Health Professionals	10	
		8	CTA B: The Medical Office	10	
		8	CTA C: Medical Specialties	10	
			Evolve Site: Flashcards: Historical Figures in Medicine (Record points earned)		
			Evolve Site: Apply Your Knowledge questions	10	
		3	Posttest	10	
			ADDITIONAL ASSIGNMENTS		
			TOTAL POINTS		

Notes

Name _____   Date _____

True or False

_____ 1. Palliative treatment attempts to reduce the effects of a disease or condition but does not cure disease.

_____ 2. In the past 30 years there has been a trend to avoid admitting patients to the hospital if possible.

_____ 3. The first health insurance plans in the United States were provided by the federal government.

_____ 4. The managed care movement has put pressure on physicians to limit time spent with individual patients.

_____ 5. After graduating from medical school, a physician spends 2 to 5 years in postgraduate training called an internship.

_____ 6. If laboratory tests are done in the medical office, there is a specific room or area set aside for this.

_____ 7. Some medical offices use paper medical records, but other offices store patient records electronically.

_____ 8. The physician who provides general medical care to an adult is usually an internist or a family practitioner.

_____ 9. A group practice often consists of three or four physicians in the same specialty.

_____ 10. Only a few patients, in addition to receiving standard medical treatment, also receive treatments that can be called complementary medicine.

?≣ POSTTEST

True or False

_____ 1. In order to be hospitalized, a patient's condition must be very unstable or require regulation of therapy.

_____ 2. Managed care insurance is another name for fee-for-service insurance.

_____ 3. A nurse practitioner manages routine patient care and can write prescriptions in most states.

_____ 4. When a patient enters the office, he or she is immediately taken to a treatment room.

_____ 5. The government agency that provides for health and safety in the workplace is CLIA.

_____ 6. Medical records for all patients who have been seen in the past 10 years are kept in the medical office.

_____ 7. The medical office may have a special room just for treatments or procedures.

_____ 8. An osteopathic physician (DO) provides primary care and has the same legal status as a physician with an MD degree.

_____ 9. The physician who specializes in diseases of the nervous system is a neurologist.

_____ 10. Acupuncture is considered to be a standard medical treatment.

Directions: Match each medical term with its definition.

_____ 1. Ambulatory care

_____ 2. Capitation

_____ 3. Curative

_____ 4. Empirical

_____ 5. Fee-for-service

_____ 6. Formulary

_____ 7. Health insurance

_____ 8. Holistic

_____ 9. Managed care

_____ 10. Palliative treatment

_____ 11. Residency

_____ 12. Symptomatic treatment

_____ 13. Utilization review

A. A system that manages the delivery of health care with the intention of controlling costs

B. A set payment provided by managed care insurance per patient per month regardless of the amount of service the patient receives

C. Considering the whole; in medicine, considering the entire person when providing health care

D. Therapy that reduces the effects of disease or condition but does not remove the disease itself

E. A program to provide training in a medical specialty to a physician who has finished medical school

F. Medical care that is provided on an outpatient basis

G. Therapy for symptoms of a disease or condition

H. Purchase of protection for covered services related to health care

I. Assessing medical services to determine whether they are appropriate, necessary, and of high quality

J. A means of payment for health care in which each service provided is reimbursed in full or in part

K. Learned from observation or experiment

L. A list of prescription drugs covered or preferred by a managed care insurance company

M. Treatment that cures disease

B. Word Parts

Directions: Indicate the meaning of each word part in the space provided. List as many medical terms as possible that incorporate the word part in the space provided.

Word Part	Meaning of Word Part	Medical Terms That Incorporate Word Part
1. -al		
2. ambul/o		
3. empiric/o		
4. hol/o		
5. -ic		
6. -ory		

EVALUATION OF LEARNING

Directions: Fill in each blank with the correct answer.

1. What is the World Health Organization's definition of health?

_____

_____

_____

2. What historical figure is considered to be the first to see illness as a result of physical and environmental factors? When did he live?

_____

3. What three trends in modern medicine have increased the importance of ambulatory care?

_____

_____

_____

4. What is fee-for-service health insurance?

_____

_____

5. List and give a short description of three government insurance plans that were introduced starting in the 1960s.

_____

_____

_____

6. Briefly describe what managed care is.

_____

_____

_____

7. If a managed care insurance plan uses capitation to pay for health care, what does this mean?

_____

_____

_____

8. How do managed care plans attempt to reduce the cost of prescription medications?

_____

_____

_____

9. List the six steps of an ordinary patient visit to a medical office.

_____

_____

_____

10. Identify at least six other health professionals beside the physician and the medical assistant who may work in the medical office.

_____

_____

_____

11. Describe briefly how physicians are educated.

_____

_____

_____

12. What examination does a physician take to obtain a state license to practice medicine? How does a physician become "board certified?"

_____

_____

_____

13. Describe the education and training of a physician assistant (PA) and a nurse practitioner (NP).

_____

_____

_____

_____

14. What is teamwork? Identify at least four components of effective teamwork.

_____

_____

_____

15. Identify the major areas of a typical medical office and their functions.

_____

_____

_____

_____

16. Identify four other areas that can be found in larger offices.

_____

_____

_____

17. Identify three types of primary care physicians.

_____

_____

18. Describe osteopathy. Are osteopaths licensed to practice medicine?

_____

_____

19. What is podiatry, and what kinds of patients might be referred to a podiatrist?

   _____

20. What is chiropractic, and what kinds of patients seek care from a chiropractor?

   _____

21. What is the difference between a solo practice and a group practice?

   _____

   _____

22. What type of medical facility was traditionally called a clinic?

   _____

   _____

23. What is acupuncture?

   _____

   _____

   _____

24. What is the role of complementary medicine in the United States today?

   _____

   _____

CRITICAL THINKING ACTIVITIES

A. Allied Health Professionals

Refer to Table 1-2 and select the allied health professionals, other than a medical assistant, who are most qualified to perform each of the following tasks.

1. Take an x-ray of the lower leg: _____

2. Create a meal plan for a patient with a gastrointestinal disease: _____

3. Supervise laboratory operations: _____

4. Pass instruments during surgery to repair a hernia: _____

5. Plan an exercise program for a patient after replacement of a hip: _____

6. Help a patient learn how to get dressed after a stroke: _____

7. Provide respiratory treatments to a patient with pneumonia: _____

8. Perform an ultrasound of the gallbladder: _____

9. Assign codes to office surgical procedures for billing: _____

10. Set up a medical record filing system: _____

B. The Medical Office

Where in the medical office shown in Figure 1-3 would the following activities probably take place?

1. Put a patient's medical record after use: _____

2. Physical examination by the physician: _____

3. Patient telephones for an appointment: _____

4. Patient is weighed: _____

5. Test urine specimens: _____

6. Physician meeting with patient and family: _____

7. Prepare patient bills for mailing: _____

8. Suture a laceration: _____

9. Patient checks in: _____

10. Patient charges posted to patient accounts: _____

C. Medical Specialties

Look up each of the following conditions as needed and refer to Box 1-1 in the textbook to identify which medical specialist would treat an adult patient with the following problems:

1. Recurrent urinary tract infections: _____

2. Tumor of the colon: _____

3. Acne: _____

4. Brain tumor: _____

5. Ovarian cyst: _____

6. Cataract: _____

7. Hip fracture: _____

8. Growth on the vocal cords: _____

9. Stroke with paralysis: _____

10. Repair of fractured cheek bone: _____

2 The Professional Medical Assistant

CHAPTER ASSIGNMENTS

√ After Completing	Date Due	Textbook Page(s)	TEXTBOOK ASSIGNMENTS	Possible Points	Points You Earned
		18-31	Read Chapter 2: The Professional Medical Assistant		
		21 29	Read Case Study 1 Case Study questions	5	
		23 29-30	Read Case Study 2 Case Study questions	5	
		24 30	Read Case Study 3 Case Study questions	5	
			TOTAL POINTS		
√ After Completing	Date Due	Study Guide Page(s)	STUDY GUIDE ASSIGNMENTS (CTA: Critical Thinking Activity)	Possible Points	Points You Earned
		11	Pretest	10	
		12	Term Key Term Assessment	7	
		12-14	Evaluation of Learning questions	26	
		14	CTA A: Professional Appearance	20	
		14-15	CTA B: Professional Behavior for Physicians	6	
		15	CTA C: Professional Organizations	6	
		16	CTA D: Scope of Practice	7	
			Evolve Site: Apply Your Knowledge questions	10	
		11	Posttest	10	
			ADDITIONAL ASSIGNMENTS		
			TOTAL POINTS		

Notes

Name _____ Date _____

True or False

_____ 1. The American Medical Technologists was the first professional organization for medical assistants.

_____ 2. A medical assistant who accepts that patients often have different beliefs is displaying dependability.

_____ 3. Being well organized helps the medical assistant respond to sudden changes in schedule or plans.

_____ 4. A medical assistant should always wait for instructions before beginning a new task.

_____ 5. Professionalism is based on both scientific knowledge and a code of ethical behavior.

_____ 6. If a physician engages in unprofessional behavior, the state may suspend or revoke his or her license to practice medicine.

_____ 7. A registered medical assistant has passed a national examination given by the American Association of Medical Assistants (AAMA).

_____ 8. Continuing education is required if a medical assistant wants to maintain certification as a certified medical assistant (CMA [AAMA]) or registered medical assistant (RMA).

_____ 9. Professional organizations for medical assistants publish journals to help medical assistants stay current.

_____ 10. Billing is performed by a specialist in the medical office, not the medical assistant.

True or False

_____ 1. Medical assisting programs seek accreditation from the American Association of Medical Assistants or the American Medical Technologists.

_____ 2. To be suited for the profession of medical assisting, an individual must be able to put the needs of a patient first.

_____ 3. In almost all offices, the medical assistant wears professional street clothes for both clinical and administrative tasks.

_____ 4. A medical assistant can demonstrate initiative by restocking examination rooms without having to be told to do so.

_____ 5. A professional medical assistant may have to report a colleague who breaks patient confidentiality.

_____ 6. If a medical assistant is certified, he or she has a state license to be a medical assistant.

_____ 7. To become a certified medical assistant, an individual must have graduated from an accredited medical assisting program.

_____ 8. Professional organizations provide programs that carry continuing education credit so that medical assistants can maintain certification.

_____ 9. State, local, and national meetings are held by professional organizations to help medical assistants meet their professional needs.

_____ 10. Risk management is a term used specifically for measures to prevent the spread of infection in a health care setting.

A. Definitions

Directions: Match each medical term (numbers) with its definition (letters).

_____ 1. Accreditation

_____ 2. Continuing education unit (CEU)

_____ 3. Externship/practicum

_____ 4. Fee splitting

_____ 5. Initiative

_____ 6. Risk management

_____ 7. Time management

A. A work experience that is required in an educational program and usually unpaid

B. Processes to protect a health care facility from the risk of legal action

C. The ability to begin or carry through on a plan of action independently

D. Credit or recognition for maintaining certain standards by a regional or national organization

E. Skills and techniques used to accomplish tasks and meet goals

F. The unethical practice of sharing fees with colleagues, especially for making referrals

G. A standard unit of continuing education for professionals

EVALUATION OF LEARNING

Directions: Fill in each blank with the correct answer.

1. Identify five changes in medical care over the past 25 years that have affected the profession of medical assisting.

_____

_____

2. List two organizations that have worked to define professionalism for medical assistants.

_____

3. What are four important character traits of a professional medical assistant?

_____

4. How is caring expressed by a medical assistant?

_____

5. Identify three reasons why neatness and good grooming are important for the medical assistant.

_____

_____

_____

6. What does the medical assistant usually wear when performing clinical tasks? Administrative tasks?

_____

7. Give two specific examples of how the medical assistant can demonstrate initiative.

_____

8. List three general principles of effective time management.

_____

_____

_____

9. List four tools that facilitate effective use of time.

_____

_____

10. Identify four sources of information about professional practice for physicians.

_____

_____

11. Who is thought to be the author of the oath that served as a guide for good conduct for ancient physicians?

_____

12. What are five ethical responsibilities of a professional medical assistant?

_____

_____

_____

13. Identify two written sets of standards that provide guidance for professional medical assistants.

_____

_____

14. What is the difference between certification and licensure?

_____

_____

15. Describe how an individual becomes a certified medical assistant.

_____

_____

16. Describe how an individual becomes a registered medical assistant.

_____

_____

17. Describe three credentials, other than certification, that a medical assistant may need to obtain.

_____

_____

_____

18. What are the continuing education requirements for a certified medical assistant to recertify?

_____

_____

19. What are the continuing education requirements for a registered medical assistant to recertify?

_____

_____

20. Describe the medical assistant's role related to making appointments and medical records.

_____

_____

_____

21. Describe the medical assistant's role in billing, accepting payments, and recording payments.

_____

_____

22. Describe any six areas of clinical responsibility for the medical assistant.

_____

_____

_____

23. Describe the medical assistant's responsibility if an emergency occurs in the medical office.

_____

24. Explain the medical assistant's responsibility related to supplies and equipment.

_____

_____

25. Give examples of three different types of instruction that a medical assistant might give to patients.

_____

_____

26. Discuss three common types of health care facilities where medical assistants often find employment.

_____

_____

CRITICAL THINKING ACTIVITIES

A. Professional Appearance

Create a poster with pictures and comments to show the proper clothing, hairstyle, and jewelry (if any) for a medical assistant assigned to various areas in the medical office. If you are female, illustrate female attire. If you are male, illustrate male attire. After your poster is completed, discuss your choices in class with a partner and/or the entire class.

1. Using items cut from a magazine (such as a uniform supply company) and items printed from the Internet, colored pencils, and markers, illustrate professional attire for the clinical or laboratory area on one half of your poster. Illustrate both short-sleeve and long-sleeve options. Write comments on the poster to describe appropriate hairstyle, jewelry, fingernail appearance, and footwear as needed.

2. Using items cut from a magazine and items printed from the Internet, colored pencils, and markers, illustrate professional attire for the administrative area of the medical office using business casual attire. Write comments on the poster to describe appropriate hairstyle, jewelry, fingernail appearance, and footwear as needed.

B. Professional Behavior For Physicians

Give reasons why each of the following behaviors by a physician would be considered professional or unprofessional.

1. Requiring a payment from any physician to whom a patient is referred

_____

_____

2. Sending prescriptions automatically to a pharmacy in which the physician owns stock without asking the patient if that is his or her preferred pharmacy

_____

_____

3. Meeting with pharmacy representatives during the lunch hour and accepting samples of new medications

_____

_____

4. Allowing the medical assistant to obtain blood specimens and perform blood tests

_____

_____

5. Dating a former patient who now obtains care from another primary care physician

_____

_____

6. Treating a patient outside the physician's specialty (e.g., a gynecologist treating a patient for diabetes mellitus)

_____

_____

C. Professional Organizations

Find information about local/state/regional chapters of the American Association of Medical Assistants (AAMA) and the American Medical Technologists (AMT). The websites of the national organizations have links to state associations.

1. What is the location of the nearest chapter of the AAMA to your school? _____

2. What is the location of the nearest chapter of the AMT to your school? _____

3. Is your medical assisting program accredited? _____ If so, by whom? _____

4. When is the next state meeting of the AAMA in your state? _____ AMT? _____

5. Are students and nonmembers welcome to attend state meetings? _____

6. From your research, identify five reasons to attend the state meeting of one or more of these organizations:

_____

_____

_____

_____

_____

D. Scope of Practice

Based on the description of the medical assistant's role in Chapter 2, investigate and discuss whether each of the following is within the medical assistant's scope of practice in your state.

1. The medical assistant obtains and tests urine specimens.

   _____

   _____

2. The medical assistant performs routine physical examinations on children and adults.

   _____

   _____

3. The medical assistant administers immunizations to infants, children, and adults.

   _____

   _____

4. The medical assistant authorizes prescription refills for patients on long-term medication therapy.

   _____

   _____

5. The medical assistant obtains specimens of venous blood by finger-stick and phlebotomy and performs diagnostic tests using the blood specimens.

   _____

   _____

6. Discuss what a medical assistant should do if he or she notices that another medical assistant in the practice has performed a sterile procedure, such as catherization or starting an intravenous infusion, with no previous training in the procedure.

   _____

   _____

   _____

7. Look up the term "scope of practice" and provide a complete definition.

   _____

   _____

3 Ethics and Law for the Medical Office

CHAPTER ASSIGNMENTS

√ After Completing	Date Due	Textbook Page(s)	TEXTBOOK ASSIGNMENTS	Possible Points	Points You Earned
		32-55	Read Chapter 3: Ethics and Law for the Medical Office		
		36 52-53	Read Case Study 1 Case Study questions	5	
		45 53	Read Case Study 2 Case Study questions	5	
		47 53	Read Case Study 3 Case Study questions	5	
			TOTAL POINTS		

√ After Completing	Date Due	Study Guide Page(s)	STUDY GUIDE ASSIGNMENTS (CTA: Critical Thinking Activity)	Possible Points	Points You Earned
		19	Pretest	10	
		20 20-21	Key Term Assessment A. Ethics B. Law	16 36	
		21-26	Evaluation of Learning questions	54	
		26	CTA A: Ethical Issues	20	
		27	CTA B: Patient Advocate	2	
		27	CTA C: Personal and Professional Ethics	14	
		28	CTA D: Patient Bill of Rights	5	
		28	CTA E: Negligence	4	
			Evolve Site: Apply Your Knowledge questions	10	
			Evolve Site: Quiz Show (Record points earned)		
		19	Posttest	10	
			ADDITIONAL ASSIGNMENTS		
			TOTAL POINTS		

Notes

Name _____ Date _____

True or False

_____ 1. Patients have the right to autonomy, which includes the right to refuse treatment.

_____ 2. Legal abortions and confidentiality are manifestations of the individual's right to privacy.

_____ 3. The branch of law that regulates interactions between individuals and groups is called criminal law.

_____ 4. To be enforceable, a contract must be written.

_____ 5. A physician cannot refuse to accept patients who seek treatment.

_____ 6. Written consent forms are usually used for surgery and other invasive procedures.

_____ 7. A wound infection after surgery is caused by negligence on the part of the physician.

_____ 8. If a patient is injured through the negligence of a medical assistant, a patient can sue the medical assistant and his or her physician employer.

_____ 9. If a trial is held for malpractice, it is only necessary to provide photocopies of the medical record.

_____ 10. A patient may begin a lawsuit for malpractice any time after an injury occurs.

?≡ **POSTTEST**

True or False

_____ 1. Physician-assisted suicide is illegal in all states because a federal law prohibits it.

_____ 2. Health professionals are considered to have a duty to be faithful to reasonable expectations of patients.

_____ 3. A serious crime committed with the intent to cause harm is called a felony.

_____ 4. For a contract to be valid, there must be a mutual agreement between the parties.

_____ 5. A physician can end a relationship with a patient, provided that the patient is notified in writing.

_____ 6. To give informed consent, a patient must understand the risks and benefits of a procedure.

_____ 7. When a physician fails to care for a patient correctly, causing injury to the patient, it is called professional negligence or malpractice.

_____ 8. Professional liability insurance only covers a physician for his or her own actions.

_____ 9. Most malpractice lawsuits are settled out of court, and no trial occurs.

_____ 10. The physician is not liable for injury to a patient if the patient refuses to follow medical advice.

Directions: Match each term with its definition.

_____ 1. Advocate

_____ 2. Autonomy

_____ 3. Beneficence

_____ 4. Cloning

_____ 5. DNR (do not resuscitate)

_____ 6. Duty

_____ 7. Etiquette

_____ 8. Fidelity

_____ 9. Gene therapy

_____ 10. Genetic engineering

_____ 11. Health care proxy

_____ 12. Living will

_____ 13. Nonmalfeasance

_____ 14. Stem cells

_____ 15. Right

_____ 16. Veracity

A. Making, altering, or repairing genetic material

B. Cells that have the capacity to develop into various types of body tissue

C. Ability to make independent decisions without constraint or coercion from others

D. Truthfulness

E. Faithfulness

F. Ethical concept requiring that an action do no harm, or do less harm than good

G. Giving patients new genes or parts of genes to treat a disease or condition

H. A legal document that names an agent to make decisions about a person's medical care if he or she becomes unable to make wishes known

I. Rules of socially acceptable behavior; manners

J. Commitment to act in a certain way

K. Acting in the best possible way; performing good deeds

L. Producing genetically identical cells or individuals artificially

M. A legal document that specifies the kind of medical treatment a patient wants or does not want if he or she becomes incapacitated

N. A medical order signed by a physician that relieves health care personnel from the obligation to resuscitate a patient who stops breathing or whose heart stops

O. A claim that is expected to be honored

P. A person who intercedes on another person's behalf

🔑Term **KEY TERM ASSESSMENT: LAW**

Directions: Match each term with its definition.

_____ 1. Abandonment

_____ 2. Act

_____ 3. Arbitration

_____ 4. Assumption of risk

_____ 5. Case law

_____ 6. Common law

_____ 7. Contingency

_____ 8. Controlled substance

_____ 9. Defendant

_____ 10. Drug Enforcement Administration (DEA)

_____ 11. Embezzlement

_____ 12. Felony

_____ 13. Fraud

_____ 14. Informed consent

_____ 15. Larceny

_____ 16. Liability

_____ 17. License

_____ 18. Litigation

A. A formal process in which the parties to a dispute agree to submit to the decision of a neutral party

B. Law established by decisions of previous court cases

C. Law enacted by a legislative body

D. Agreement to a medical procedure based on understanding of the procedure and its possible consequences and effects

E. Unwritten body of law based on general custom

F. Stealing another person's property or money without violence

G. Intentional deception resulting in injury or loss

H. A legal doctrine making an employer liable for the negligent acts of employees

I. The person or group against whom an action is brought in a court of law

J. Failing to perform an act that should have been performed

K. The person or group that makes the complaint in a lawsuit

L. Failure to continue to provide medical care to a patient without proper notification

M. Fraudulent appropriation of funds or property of an employer or client

N. Failure to act (or refrain from acting) as a reasonably prudent person would in similar circumstances

O. Performing a legal act in an improper way

P. A law limiting the time period for beginning a lawsuit

Q. A person under the age of 18 with the rights of an adult including the ability to consent to medical care

R. The federal agency that enforces the Controlled Substances Act of 1970

_____ 19. Malfeasance

_____ 20. Malpractice

_____ 21. Mediation

_____ 22. Misdemeanor

_____ 23. Misfeasance

_____ 24. Negligence

_____ 25. Nonfeasance

_____ 26. Plaintiff

_____ 27. Prescription

_____ 28. Privilege

_____ 29. Prudent

_____ 30. Reciprocity

_____ 31. *Respondeat superior*

_____ 32. Standard of care

_____ 33. Statute of limitations

_____ 34. Statutory law

_____ 35. Subpoena *duces tecum*

_____ 36. Emancipated minor

S. A defense to a lawsuit that establishes the plaintiff assumed the risk of whatever caused the injury

T. A less serious crime, punishable by a fine or imprisonment for less than 1 year

U. A court order to produce documents or records

V. A drug that has the potential for addiction or abuse

W. A bill or measure that has become law, often referring to legislation with several parts

X. Negotiation by a third party to help two parties resolve a dispute

Y. The process of taking a lawsuit through the courts

Z. A special immunity that protects against legal liability

AA. Using care or common sense

BB. Automatic issuing of a license in one state to the holder of a license in another state

CC. A crime or wrongdoing that is illegal or contrary to official obligation

DD. Legal responsibility

EE. A condition that must be met before a contract is binding

FF. Level of appropriate care required of a health professional

GG. Official permission to perform an activity or practice a profession

HH. A serious crime punishable by death or imprisonment

II. Negligence by a professional

JJ. An order to a pharmacist to dispense a supply of a medication

EVALUATION OF LEARNING

Directions: Fill in each blank with the correct answer.

1. Identify four reasons that medical assisting students can benefit from studying about ethics and bioethics.

   _____

   _____

2. Identify three sources of beliefs about the rights and duties of individuals and society as a whole.

   _____

   _____

   _____

3. Describe briefly what is included in each of the following ethical rights:

   a. Right to life _____

   b. Right to privacy _____

   c. Right to autonomy _____

   d. Right to the means to sustain life _____

4. Identify five duties of a health professional.

   _____

5. How does the medical assistant function as a patient advocate?

_____

_____

6. Why and how should a medical assistant report the illegal or unsafe behavior of another health professional?

_____

_____

_____

7. Most states have a process to file a complaint against physicians whose illegal or unsafe activities threaten the health and safety of patients or others. What is the process in your state?

_____

_____

_____

_____

8. When does ethical conflict arise?

_____

9. What are two issues that create conflict within society related to reproductive issues?

_____

10. What is the current legal position with respect to stem cell research related to federal legislation?

_____

_____

11. Define the following terms:
   a. Stem cell research _____
   b. Genetic engineering _____
   c. Cloning _____
   d. Gene therapy _____

12. What are the general provisions of the Patient Self-Determination Act of 1990?

_____

13. What is the difference between physician-assisted suicide and euthanasia? Is either legal in the United States?

_____

_____

14. Describe the difference between personal ethics and professional ethics, and explain which should take priority.

_____

_____

_____

15. What are five recommended steps to make ethical decisions?

_____

_____

16. Describe the medical assistant's ethical responsibility related to patient care in the medical office.

_____

17. What is a DNR order?

_____

18. What is the difference between a living will and a health care proxy? Which is preferable?

_____

_____

19. What is the relationship between law and ethics?

_____

20. Briefly describe the following three types of law:

    a. Criminal law _____

    b. Civil law _____

    c. Contract law _____

21. Explain how an injury can result in both civil and criminal lawsuits.

_____

22. Describe two classifications of crimes.

_____

23. Describe each of the following crimes and identify how each might occur in a medical office:

    a. Manslaughter or criminal negligence _____

    b. Embezzlement _____

    c. Fraud _____

24. What three elements are necessary for a legal contract?

_____

_____

25. Differentiate between an intentional tort and an unintentional tort.

_____

26. Differentiate among a malfeasance, a misfeasance, and a nonfeasance.

_____

_____

27. Identify how the physician–patient relationship meets the definition of a contract.

_____

_____

_____

28. Give examples of each of the following types of contracts:

    a. Implied _____

    _____

    b. Verbal _____

    _____

    c. Written _____

    _____

29. Identify four groups of people who cannot legally be party to a contract or give informed consent.

_____

_____

30. When can an individual who is not yet 18 consent to medical treatment?

_____

_____

31. When can a physician terminate care to a patient?

_____

_____

32. How should the physician notify the patient that he or she is terminating care? Why?

_____

_____

33. What does the term standard of care mean?

_____

34. Why is informed consent usually verified by having the patient sign a consent form?

_____

_____

35. What is the medical assistant's role in obtaining a signature on a consent form?

_____

36. What four elements must be proved in order to prove liability for professional negligence (malpractice)?

_____

_____

37. What does the doctrine of *res ipsa loquitur* refer to?

_____

38. What are two reasons for physicians to purchase professional liability insurance?

_____

39. If a physician believes that a patient is going to initiate a lawsuit, how should he or she respond?

_____

40. What is a subpoena and a subpoena *duces tecum*?

_____

41. Differentiate between mediation and arbitration.

_____

42. Describe the following tort defenses:

   a. Privilege _____

   b. Consent _____

   c. Self-defense _____

   d. Expiration of the statute of limitations _____

   e. Contributory negligence _____

   f. Comparative negligence _____

   g. Assumption of risk _____

43. What are controlled substances, and what law regulates their use?

_____

_____

44. What are five measures to prevent misuse of prescription forms and tampering with prescriptions?

_____

_____

45. What organization was created by the Health and Safety Act of 1970 to protect employees in the workplace?

_____

46. What are two examples of measures to protect the health of employees in the medical office?

_____

_____

47. What employee rights are protected by the following laws?

   a. Equal Opportunity Employment laws

_____

   b. Americans with Disabilities Act

_____

c. Family and Medical Leave Act

_____

d. Fair Labor Standards Act

_____

e. Employee Retirement Income Security Act

_____

48. What is the purpose of the Privacy Rule of the Health Insurance Portability and Accountability Act (HIPAA) of 1996?

_____

49. What are four other rules included in HIPAA?

_____

_____

50. Describe what a mandated report is and give five examples of mandatory reporting for physicians.

_____

_____

51. What are the four basic requirements for a physician to be licensed in most states?

_____

_____

_____

52. What are grounds for suspending or revoking a license to practice medicine?

_____

53. Which types of health care facilities usually require a state license?

_____

54. Name two organizations that provide voluntary accreditation for physician's offices.

_____

CRITICAL THINKING ACTIVITIES

A. Ethical Issues

Select one of the following topics for investigation. Do research about the topic to obtain information. Write a short paper giving information to describe the topic and demonstrate why it is controversial. Be sure to give credit for ideas and/or statistics that you have obtained from a book, journal article, or Internet article.

1. Genetically modified food products

2. Partial birth abortion

3. Federal funding for stem cell research

4. Physician-assisted suicide

5. Gene therapy

B. Patient Advocate

1. Describe the role of a medical assistant as a patient advocate.

_____

_____

_____

2. Explain how a medical assistant might help a patient who has difficulty walking obtain a handicap placard in your state.

_____

_____

_____

C. Personal and Professional Ethics

1. Write a one- to two-page plan for separation of personal and professional ethics (10 points).

2. Identify the conflicting values in each of the following situations, choose an action, and justify your action. Identify if you are guided by personal ethics, professional ethics, or both types of ethics.

   a. You find your brother, who is 12 years old, smoking a cigarette in the backyard.

   _____

   _____

   _____

   _____

   b. A patient tells you that she thinks she may be dependent on the narcotic analgesics she has been taking. Then she asks you not to tell the physician, because she still wants to get a refill for the prescription.

   _____

   _____

   _____

   _____

   c. An elderly relative whom you are extremely close to has a chronic condition causing muscle weakness. She begs you to help her "end everything."

   _____

   _____

   _____

   _____

   d. An expensive medication has been prescribed for a male relative by his personal physician. You mention that there are samples of that medication in your office. The relative asks you if you can get some for him.

   _____

   _____

   _____

   _____

D. Patient Bill of Rights

Using the summary of the Patient Bill of Rights in your textbook, give five examples of policies and procedures that a medical office might institute to protect patient rights.

a. _____

b. _____

c. _____

d. _____

e. _____

f. _____

E. Negligence

Discuss with your classmates what a "reasonably prudent person" would be expected to do in the following situations.

1. Your elderly neighbor slips and falls on a patch of ice in your driveway. She appears unable to get up and complains of pain in her left hip.

   _____

   _____

2. You are in the washroom at work and you notice that the handle on the hot water tap is not working properly so that very hot water is constantly dripping into the sink.

   _____

   _____

3. You spill some coffee on a tile floor at your school.

   _____

   _____

4. You are in a restaurant, and you see another patron who appears to be starting to choke. The person is not coughing audibly, but he is clutching his throat and trying to cough.

   _____

   _____

4 Interacting With Patients

CHAPTER ASSIGNMENTS

√ After Completing	Date Due	Textbook Page(s)	TEXTBOOK ASSIGNMENTS	Possible Points	Points You Earned
		56-72	Read Chapter 4: Interacting with Patients		
		59 70	Read Case Study 1 Case Study questions	5	
		63 70-71	Read Case Study 2 Case Study questions	5	
		67 71	Read Case Study 3 Case Study questions	5	
			TOTAL POINTS		

√ After Completing	Date Due	Study Guide Page(s)	STUDY GUIDE ASSIGNMENTS (CTA: Critical Thinking Activity)	Possible Points	Points You Earned
		31	Pretest	10	
		32	Key Term Assessment A. Definitions B. Word Parts (Add 1 point for each medical term)	25 7	
		33-36	Evaluation of Learning questions	31	
		36-38	CTA A: Nonverbal Cues	4	
		38-39	CTA B: Using Effective Communication Techniques	6	
		39	CTA C: Responses That Inhibit Communication	6	
		39	CTA D: Community Resources for Individuals With Terminal Illness	5	
			Evolve Site: Apply Your Knowledge questions	10	

√ After Completing	Date Due	Study Guide Page(s)	STUDY GUIDE ASSIGNMENTS (CTA: Critical Thinking Activity)	Possible Points	Points You Earned
		31	[?≣] Posttest	10	
			ADDITIONAL ASSIGNMENTS		
			TOTAL POINTS		

Name _____   Date _____

True or False

_____ 1. The medical assistant communicates nonverbally using tone of voice and facial gestures.

_____ 2. A closed question expects a yes/no or very short answer.

_____ 3. Silence is an effective technique to encourage a patient to continue speaking.

_____ 4. A patient who is legally blind will be unable to distinguish light and shadow.

_____ 5. If a patient is not comfortable using English, translation must be done by a native speaker in person.

_____ 6. In Maslow's hierarchy of needs, the needs for safety and security are lower than the needs for esteem and recognition.

_____ 7. A patient experiencing moderate anxiety will have difficulty learning new information.

_____ 8. The patient is aware when he or she is relying on ego defense mechanisms like denial.

_____ 9. The medical assistant should remember that anger is often displaced from the true cause to another target.

_____ 10. If a patient believes that disease has a supernatural cause, the medical assistant should tell the patient tactfully that this is impossible.

📋 **POSTTEST**

True or False

_____ 1. Internal factors that interfere with communication include excessive noise and lack of privacy.

_____ 2. Open questions encourage a patient to explain symptoms in his or her own way.

_____ 3. Paraphrasing is giving a short summary of a verbal communication.

_____ 4. The medical assistant uses both touch and words to guide a patient who is totally blind.

_____ 5. Both telephone and video translation services are available when patients are uncomfortable with English.

_____ 6. The needs depicted on the highest level of Maslow's hierarchy include oxygen, sleep, and adequate nutrition.

_____ 7. Hyperventilation may be a symptom of a full-blown anxiety attack.

_____ 8. Projection is an unconscious ego defense mechanism where an individual ascribes his or her own feelings to another.

_____ 9. If a patient is using denial as an ego defense mechanism, it is important to correct the patient as soon as possible.

_____ 10. A patient from a different culture may believe that changes in diet will help treat certain diseases.

A. Definitions

Directions: Match each medical term with its definition.

_____ 1. Acting out

_____ 2. Active listening

_____ 3. Anxiety

_____ 4. Body language

_____ 5. Chronic

_____ 6. Closed questions

_____ 7. Denial

_____ 8. Ego defense mechanism

_____ 9. Empathy

_____ 10. Hierarchy

_____ 11. Hospice

_____ 12. Judgmental

_____ 13. Nonverbal

_____ 14. Open questions

_____ 15. Oral

_____ 16. Paraphrasing

_____ 17. Physiologic

_____ 18. Projection

_____ 19. Reflecting

_____ 20. Self-actualization

_____ 21. Summarizing

_____ 22. Sympathy

_____ 23. Terminal

_____ 24. Verbal

_____ 25. Webcam

A. Existing over a long period of time

B. Expressing the meaning and emotion of another's words back to the person

C. Spoken; pertaining to the mouth

D. Unconscious mental process that offers psychological protection

E. The fulfillment of each individual's potential

F. Feeling the same emotions as another

G. Failure to acknowledge the reality of a situation

H. Making judgments about what is good or bad based on personal opinion

I. Using words to communicate

J. Translating unconscious emotions into inappropriate behavior

K. Objective awareness and sensitivity to the feelings and emotions of others

L. Questions that anticipate a yes/no or short answer

M. Pertaining to body processes

N. Small video camera attached to a computer that allows video to be transmitted on the Internet

O. Communication that occurs without words, such as through body posture or facial expression

P. Paying close attention to a speaker without thinking of anything else

Q. Classified according to rank or importance

R. Expressing the most important points of a conversation or written document

S. Communication that is expressed through facial expressions, body position, muscle activity, and other nonverbal means

T. Experiencing one's own emotions as those of another

U. A vague, unpleasant emotion of fear or dread often accompanied by restlessness or nervousness

V. A restatement of the words of another, often to clarify meaning

W. Questions that could have a variety of answers and encourage a personal response

X. The last stage of illness when death is expected to occur within 6 months

Y. An organization that manages care for dying patients

B. Word Parts

Directions: Indicate the meaning of each word part in the space provided. List as many medical terms as possible that incorporate the word part in the space provided.

Word Part	Meaning of Word Part	Medical Terms That Incorporate Word Part
1. non-		
2. verb/o		
3. -al		
4. os; or/o		
5. physi/o		
6. log/o; -logy		
7. -ic		

Directions: Fill in each blank with the correct answer.

1. Give four examples of different types of verbal communication.

   _____

2. Give four examples of nonverbal communication.

   _____

   _____

3. Identify and describe three examples of outside interference with effective communication.

   _____

   _____

4. Identify and describe three examples of inside interference with communication.

   _____

   _____

5. Describe active listening.

   _____

   _____

6. What are four listening techniques that facilitate good communication between medical assistants and patients?

   _____

   _____

7. How can the medical assistant use eye contact and body posture to facilitate communication?

   _____

   _____

8. Give two examples of how nonverbal communication is different in different cultures.

   _____

   _____

9. When is it appropriate to use closed questions during an interview?

   _____

10. When are open-ended questions more useful than closed questions?

   _____

   _____

11. Identify and describe six communication techniques that draw patients out and encourage them to keep talking.

    a. _____

    b. _____

    c. _____

    d. _____

    e. _____

    f. _____

12. What are three types of responses that inhibit communication or make the patient defensive?

_____

_____

13. How can the medical assistant improve communication with a patient whose understanding is impaired?

_____

_____

14. Differentiate between a patient who is totally blind and one who is legally blind.

_____

15. How do patients who are totally blind usually prefer to be assisted in an unknown setting?

_____

_____

16. Differentiate between a patient who is deaf and a patient who is hearing impaired.

_____

17. What measures will improve communication with a patient who is hearing impaired?

_____

_____

18. What measures should be implemented to communicate with a deaf patient?

_____

_____

19. What are three ways to provide translation services for a patient who is not comfortable communicating in English?

_____

_____

20. What are three things that patients often expect when they seek health care?

_____

_____

21. Identify the needs on each level of Maslow's hierarchy of needs.

    a. Level 1 (lowest level): _____

    b. Level 2: _____

    c. Level 3: _____

    d. Level 4: _____

    e. Level 5 (highest level): _____

22. How do unmet needs affect a patient during illness?

_____

_____

23. Why is it important for medical assistants to identify the unmet needs of patients?

_____

_____

_____

24. What are personal (self) boundaries?

_____

_____

25. Give examples of appropriate ways for a medical assistant to maintain self-boundaries when a patient or other staff member appears to assume that a closer relationship exists than the medical assistant is comfortable with.

_____

_____

_____

26. Differentiate between empathy and sympathy.

_____

_____

27. How can a medical assistant communicate caring to a patient?

_____

_____

28. Describe three ways to support a terminally ill patient in the grieving process.

_____

_____

_____

29. What do individuals from other cultures sometimes believe is a cause of illness other than physiologic factors?

_____

_____

30. What is a general rule about accepting traditional medical practices that patients may use?

_____

_____

31. Identify and discuss two different cultural practices related to behavioral requirements for women and men.

_____

_____

CRITICAL THINKING ACTIVITIES

A. Nonverbal Cues

In any interaction, a significant part of communication is nonverbal and includes individual interpretation of nonverbal cues. Examine each of the following photographs and summarize your assumptions about each person in the photograph. Who is each person? What is he or she feeling? What might be happening between the two people in the photograph? How does the person's appearance affect your assessment? Distinguish between assumptions that you are sure of and those you would need more information to confirm.

1.

_____

_____

_____

_____

2.

_____

_____

_____

_____

3.

_____

_____

_____

_____

4.

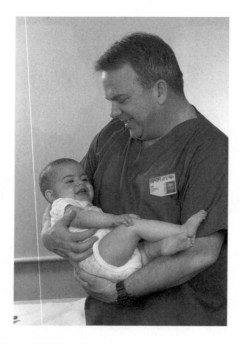

_____

_____

_____

_____

B. Using Effective Communication Techniques

After you have taken the vital signs of Valerie Hoffman, a 34-year-old teacher, she says, "I don't know if I'm sick or not. I mean, I hope that Dr. Hughes finds something wrong with me to explain why I feel so bad. I don't have any energy, you know. I get up in the morning, when I can finally get myself up, and in about 10 minutes I'm ready to go back to bed for a nap. Everything just seems like it takes so much effort."

Give an example of a response you could make that demonstrates each of the following communication techniques:

1. Paraphrasing

_____

_____

2. Translating a nonverbal message into words

_____

_____

3. Reflecting

_____

_____

4. Summarizing

_____

_____

5. Repeating or restating

_____

_____

6. Asking for clarification

_____

_____

C. Responses That Inhibit Communication

Refer to Table 4-2 in your textbook and identify how each response inhibits communication.

1. How do you know that bad spirits cause disease? Have you ever seen one?

_____

2. The physician is very busy, you know, because some patients are very ill.

_____

3. You are making a big fuss over a very small problem.

_____

4. After your chemotherapy, you will feel fine in a few hours.

_____

5. Why did you forget to take your blood pressure medication?

_____

6. Your blood sugar is very high because you are not testing it often enough.

_____

D. Community Resources for Individuals With Terminal Illness

1. What are the five steps of the grieving process as defined by Elizabeth Kübler-Ross?

_____

_____

2. List the names, addresses, and telephone numbers of at least five organizations in your community that can help patients and families struggling with a terminal illness.

_____

_____

_____

_____

_____

_____

_____

Notes

5 Introduction to Anatomy and Physiology

CHAPTER ASSIGNMENTS

√ After Completing	Date Due	Textbook Page(s)	TEXTBOOK ASSIGNMENT	Possible Points	Points You Earned
		73-99	Read Chapter 5: Introduction to Anatomy and Physiology		
√ After Completing	**Date Due**	**Study Guide Page(s)**	**STUDY GUIDE ASSIGNMENTS (CTA: Critical Thinking Activity)**	**Possible Points**	**Points You Earned**
		43	?▤ Pretest	10	
		44 44-45	✎Term Key Term Assessment: A. Definitions B. Word Parts (Add 1 point for each medical term)	26 17	
		45-58	▦ Evaluation of Learning questions The Human Body Cell Structure and Function Tissue and Membranes	19 32 68	
		58	CTA A: Planes of the Body	3	
		59	CTA B: Cavities of the Body	8	
		59	CTA C: Abdominopelvic Quadrants	4	
		60	CTA D: Abdominopelvic Regions	9	
		60	*e* Evolve Site: CTA E: Road to Recovery: Body Area Terms (Record points earned)		
		60	*e* Evolve Site: CTA F: Body Spectrum: General Human Cell	10	
		61	CTA G: Cell Structure and Function	40	
		62	*e* Evolve Site: CTA H: Animations	32	
		63	CTA I: Crossword Puzzle	25	
		43	?▤ Posttest	10	

√ After Completing	Date Due	Study Guide Page(s)	STUDY GUIDE ASSIGNMENTS (CTA: Critical Thinking Activity)	Possible Points	Points You Earned
			ADDITIONAL ASSIGNMENTS		
			TOTAL POINTS		

Name _____ Date _____

True or False

_____ 1. The study of the shape and structure of the human body is known as human anatomy.

_____ 2. The integumentary system protects underlying tissue from injury.

_____ 3. The lungs are located in the pelvic cavity.

_____ 4. The nucleolus is the control center that directs the activities of the cell.

_____ 5. The function of lysosomes is to destroy cellular debris and foreign particles.

_____ 6. A human cell has 23 pairs of chromosomes.

_____ 7. Cytology is the microscopic study of tissues.

_____ 8. Fibroblasts secrete mucus.

_____ 9. Adipose tissue protects the body from invasion by pathogens.

_____ 10. Platelets initiate the blood clotting mechanism.

? POSTTEST

True or False

_____ 1. An organ is made up of a group of tissues with a similar structure and function.

_____ 2. A frontal plane divides the body into right and left portions.

_____ 3. The plasma membrane determines what can enter or leave a cell.

_____ 4. Ribosomes are responsible for protein synthesis.

_____ 5. Microvilli are hairlike processes that move substances across the surface of a cell.

_____ 6. A red blood cell will hemolyze if it is placed in a hypertonic solution.

_____ 7. Capillary walls are made up of simple squamous epithelial tissue.

_____ 8. An endocrine gland secretes its product onto a free surface through a duct.

_____ 9. Skeletal muscle tissue is under involuntary control.

_____ 10. A mucous membrane lines a body cavity that opens to the outside.

A. Definitions

Directions: Match each medical term with its definition.

_____ 1. Active transport	A. Division of the cell at the end of mitosis to form two separate daughter cells
_____ 2. Anatomic position	B. Connective tissue cell that produces fibers
_____ 3. Chondrocyte	C. The type of nuclear division in which the number of chromosomes is reduced to half the number found in a body cell; results in the formation of an egg or sperm
_____ 4. Collagenous fibers	
_____ 5. Cytokinesis	
_____ 6. Diffusion	D. A response mechanism of the body in which a stimulus initiates reactions that reduces the stimulus
_____ 7. Elastic fibers	E. The diffusion of water through a selectively permeable membrane
_____ 8. Fibroblast	F. The standard reference position for the body
_____ 9. Histology	G. The movement of substances from a region of high concentration to a region of low concentration
_____ 10. Homeostasis	
_____ 11. Human anatomy	H. Fibers composed of elastin that have a stretching quality
_____ 12. Human physiology	I. The study of the shape and structure of the human body and the relationship of its parts
_____ 13. Macrophage	
_____ 14. Mast cell	J. Cells located in nervous tissue that provide support for neurons
_____ 15. Meiosis	K. A group of cells with a similar structure that are specialized to form a certain function
_____ 16. Metabolism	
_____ 17. Mitosis	L. Strong and flexible connective tissue fibers that contain collagen
_____ 18. Negative feedback	M. The process that moves substances across or through a membrane and requires cellular energy
_____ 19. Neuroglia	
_____ 20. Neuron	N. The microscopic study of tissues
_____ 21. Osmosis	O. The engulfing and destruction of foreign particles such as bacteria
_____ 22. Osteocyte	P. The scientific study of the functions of the human body and its parts
_____ 23. Passive transport	Q. A nerve cell
_____ 24. Phagocytosis	R. The formation of vesicles to transfer fluid droplets into a cell; cell drinking
_____ 25. Pinocytosis	S. A normal stable condition in which the body's internal environment remains the same
_____ 26. Tissue	T. A cartilage cell
	U. A large phagocytic cell that cleans up cellular debris and foreign particles from the tissues
	V. A connective tissue cell that produces heparin and histamine
	W. The process by which the nucleus of a body cell divides to form two new (daughter) cells, each identical to the parent cell
	X. A mature bone cell
	Y. The total of all biochemical reactions that take place in the body
	Z. The process that moves substances across or through a membrane and does not require cellular energy

B. Word Parts

Directions: Indicate the meaning of each word part in the space provided. List as many medical terms as possible that incorporate the word part in the space provided.

Word Part	Meaning of Word Part	Medical Terms That Incorporate Word Part
1. chondr/o		
2. -cyte		
3. -kinesis		
4. fibr/o		
5. -blast		

6. hist/o		
7. -ology		
8. home/o		
9. -stasis		
10. physi/o		
11. macro-		
12. phag/o		
13. neur/o		
14. -glia		
15. oste/o		
16. -osis		
17. pin/o		

EVALUATION OF LEARNING

Directions: Fill in each blank with the correct answer.

The Human Body

1. What is the difference between gross human anatomy and microscopic human anatomy?

   _____

   _____

2. What is the relationship between human anatomy and physiology?

   _____

   _____

3. What are the six levels of organization of the body?

   _____

   _____

4. What are the four main types of tissue found in the body?

   _____

   _____

5. What makes up an organ? List examples of organs.

   _____

   _____

6. What makes up a body system? List examples of body systems.

   _____

   _____

7. What makes up a total human organism?

_____

8. What is the function of the following systems?

   a. Integumentary: _____

   _____

   b. Skeletal: _____

   _____

   c. Muscular: _____

   _____

   d. Nervous: _____

   _____

   e. Endocrine: _____

   _____

   f. Cardiovascular: _____

   _____

   g. Lymphatic: _____

   _____

   _____

   h. Digestive: _____

   _____

   i. Respiratory: _____

   _____

   j. Urinary: _____

   _____

   k. Reproductive: _____

   _____

9. What is homeostasis? Why is it important to the body?

_____

_____

_____

10. How does the body maintain normal blood pressure using a negative feedback mechanism?

_____

_____

_____

11. Describe the body in anatomic position.

_____

_____

12. Define the following body directions and provide an example of each:

a. Superior: _____

_____

b. Inferior: _____

_____

c. Anterior: _____

_____

d. Posterior: _____

_____

e. Medial: _____

_____

f. Lateral: _____

_____

g. Proximal: _____

_____

h. Distal: _____

_____

i. Superficial: _____

_____

j. Deep: _____

_____

k. Visceral: _____

_____

l. Parietal: _____

_____

13. Define the following planes and sections of the body:

a. Sagittal plane: _____

_____

b. Midsagittal plane: _____

_____

Chapter **5** **Introduction to Anatomy and Physiology**

c. Transverse plane: _____

_____

d. Frontal plane: _____

_____

14. What are the subdivisions of the dorsal cavity? _____

_____

15. What are the subdivisions of the ventral cavity? _____

_____

16. What structures are located in the thoracic cavity? _____

_____

17. What structures are located in the abdominal cavity? _____

_____

18. What structures are located in the pelvic cavity? _____

_____

19. What structures are located in the following regions of the body?

a. Axial: _____

b. Appendicular: _____

Cell Structure and Function

1. What is the function of the plasma membrane?

_____

_____

2. What is cytoplasm?

_____

3. What are organelles?

_____

4. What substances are dissolved in the intracellular fluid of the cytoplasm?

_____

_____

5. What is the function of the nucleus?

_____

_____

6. Where is the nucleolus located?

_____

7. What is the function of the nucleolus?

_____

_____

8. What is the function of mitochondria?

_____

_____

9. What is the function of ribosomes?

_____

10. What is the function of the endoplasmic reticulum?

_____

_____

11. What is the function of the Golgi apparatus?

_____

_____

12. What is the function of lysosomes?

_____

_____

13. What are cilia, and what is their function?

_____

_____

14. What is simple diffusion?

_____

_____

15. How does diffusion result in the exchange of oxygen and carbon dioxide in the lungs?

_____

_____

_____

16. What is osmosis?

_____

_____

17. What occurs when a red blood cell is placed in an isotonic solution?

_____

_____

18. What occurs when a red blood cell is placed in a hypertonic solution? Explain the reason for your answer.

_____

_____

19. What occurs when a red blood cell is placed in a hypotonic solution? Explain the reason for your answer.

_____

_____

20. What process in the body relies on filtration?

_____

21. What is active transport?

_____

_____

22. What process in the body relies on active transport?

_____

_____

23. What is endocytosis?

_____

_____

24. What occurs during phagocytosis?

_____

_____

25. What is exocytosis?

_____

_____

26. List two examples of exocytosis.

_____

_____

27. What is a somatic cell?

_____

28. What is a gamete?

_____

29. How many pairs of chromosomes are present in a human cell?

_____

30. What are the two methods the body uses to reproduce cells?

_____

_____

31. What occurs during the following stages of mitosis?

   a. Interphase: _____

_____

   b. Prophase: _____

_____

   c. Metaphase: _____

_____

   d. Anaphase: _____

_____

   e. Telophase: _____

_____

32. What is meiosis?

_____

_____

_____

Tissues and Membranes

1. What is histology?

_____

2. What is the intercellular matrix?

_____

_____

3. What are the four main tissues of the body?

_____

4. Where is epithelial tissue located?

_____

_____

5. What is the name of the structure that attaches epithelial cells to underlying connective tissue?

_____

6. Describe the shape of the cell and its nucleus for each of the following types of epithelial cells:

   a. Squamous: _____

_____

b. Cuboidal: _____

_____

c. Columnar: _____

_____

7. What is the difference between simple epithelium and stratified epithelium?

_____

_____

8. Describe the appearance of simple squamous epithelium. In the margin of this page, draw a sketch of simple squamous epithelium.

_____

_____

9. Where is simple squamous epithelium located in the body?

_____

_____

10. Describe the appearance of simple cuboidal epithelium. In the margin of this page, draw a sketch of simple cuboidal epithelium.

_____

11. Where is simple cuboidal epithelium located in the body?

_____

_____

12. Describe the appearance of simple columnar epithelium. In the margin of this page, draw a sketch of simple columnar epithelium.

_____

_____

13. Where is simple columnar epithelium located in the body?

_____

14. What are microvilli? What is their purpose?

_____

_____

15. What is the purpose of goblet cells?

_____

16. What is the appearance of pseudostratified columnar epithelium? In the margin of this page, draw a sketch of pseudostratified columnar epithelium.

_____

_____

17. Where is pseudostratified columnar epithelium located in the body?

_____

_____

18. What is the appearance of stratified squamous epithelium? In the margin of this page, draw a sketch of stratified squamous epithelium.

_____

_____

19. Where is stratified squamous epithelium located in the body?

_____

_____

20. What special quality is present in transitional epithelium?

_____

_____

21. Where is transitional epithelium located in the body?

_____

22. What is glandular epithelium?

_____

_____

23. What is the difference between an exocrine gland and an endocrine gland?

_____

_____

24. What are examples of exocrine glands?

_____

25. What is the function of connective tissue?

_____

_____

26. What are the characteristics of collagenous fibers?

_____

_____

27. What structures are composed of collagenous fibers?

_____

28. What are the characteristics of elastic fibers?

_____

29. What three cells are most commonly found in connective tissue? List the function of each of these cells.

Cell	Function

30. What is the function of loose connective tissue?

_____

_____

31. What is the function of adipose tissue?

_____

_____

32. Describe the characteristics of dense fibrous connective tissue.

_____

_____

33. What is the function of tendons?

_____

_____

34. What is the function of ligaments?

_____

_____

35. What body structures are composed of elastic connective tissue?

_____

_____

36. What is the function of cartilage?

_____

_____

37. Describe the following components of cartilage:

Chondrocyte: _____

Perichondrium: _____

38. Where is hyaline cartilage located?

_____

_____

39. Where is fibrocartilage located in the body?

_____

_____

40. Where is elastic cartilage located in the body?

_____

41. What is the function of bone?

_____

_____

42. Describe the following components of bone:

Osteons (haversian systems): _____

Osteonic canal (haversian canal): _____

Osteocyte: _____

Canaliculi: _____

43. What qualities do the following give to bone?

Collagenous fibers: _____

Calcium: _____

44. What is the function of the following blood components?

Erythrocytes: _____

_____

Leukocytes: _____

_____

Thrombocytes: _____

_____

Plasma: _____

_____

45. What is the function of muscle tissue?

_____

_____

46. Describe the appearance of skeletal muscle cells. In the margin of this page, draw a sketch of skeletal muscle cells.

_____

_____

55

47. What is the function of skeletal muscle in the body?

_____

48. Describe the appearance of smooth muscle cells. In the margin of this page, draw a sketch of smooth muscle cells.

_____

_____

49. Where is smooth muscle located in the body?

_____

50. What is the function of smooth muscle?

_____

_____

51. Describe the appearance of cardiac muscle cells. In the margin of this page, draw a sketch of cardiac muscle cells.

_____

52. Where is cardiac muscle located in the body?

_____

53. What is the function of cardiac muscle?

_____

_____

54. Where is nervous tissue located in the body?

_____

55. What is the function of nervous tissue?

_____

_____

56. Describe the following components of nervous tissue:

Neuron: _____

Nerve cell body: _____

Dendrites: _____

Axons: _____

Neuroglia: _____

57. What is a mucous membrane?

_____

_____

58. Where are mucous membranes located in the body?

_____

_____

59. What is the function of mucus secreted by a mucous membrane?

_____

60. What is a serous membrane?

_____

_____

61. What is the function of serous fluid?

_____

_____

62. Where are serous membranes located in the body?

_____

_____

63. What are synovial membranes?

_____

_____

64. Where are synovial membranes located in the body?

_____

65. What is the function of synovial fluid?

_____

_____

66. What are the meninges?

_____

_____

67. What is the function of the meninges?

_____

_____

68. List and describe the three layers that make up the meninges.

Name	Description

CRITICAL THINKING ACTIVITIES

A. Planes of the Body

Using Figure 5-3 in your textbook as a reference, label each of the planes of the body on the following diagram.

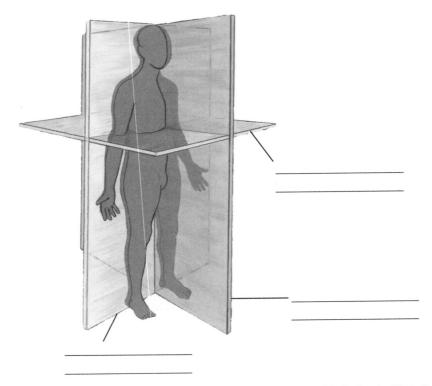

(Modified from Applegate E: *The anatomy and physiology learning system,* ed 4, St. Louis, 2011, Saunders.)

B. Cavities of the Body

Using Figure 5-4 in your textbook as a reference, label each of the cavities of the body on the following diagram.

(Modified from Applegate E: *The anatomy and physiology learning system,* ed 4, St. Louis, 2011, Saunders.)

C. Abdominopelvic Quadrants

Using Figure 5-5 in your textbook as a reference, label each of the quadrants of the body on the following diagram.

(Modified from Applegate E: *The anatomy and physiology learning system,* ed 4, St. Louis, 2011, Saunders.)

Chapter **5**   **Introduction to Anatomy and Physiology**

D. Abdominopelvic Regions

Using Figure 5-6 in your textbook as a reference, label each of the abdominopelvic regions of the body on the following diagram.

(Modified from Applegate E: *The anatomy and physiology learning system,* ed 4, St. Louis, 2011, Saunders.)

E. Evolve Site: Road to Recovery

Body Area Terms

Directions:

1. Review the body area terms presented in Table 5-2 of your textbook.
2. Access the Evolve site.
3. Play the Road to Recovery Game presented in Chapter 5.
4. Record your points on your assignment sheet.

F. Evolve Site: Body Spectrum

Cell Structure: General Human Cell

Body Spectrum directions:

1. Access the Body Spectrum on the Evolve site.
2. If necessary, access the HELP screen for directions on using the Body Spectrum program.
3. Go to the Contents screen.
4. Select the following category from the Contents screen:
   Cell Structure
5. Select the following anatomic diagram:
   General Human Cell
6. Identify the structures on the diagram.
7. Print out the diagram.

G. Cell Structure and Function

You are an oxygen molecule that has just entered a body cell. In the space provided below, describe all of the structures you see in the cell. Also describe what function each structure is performing in the cell. Each of the following structures should be included in your discussion:

a. Plasma membrane
b. Cytoplasm
c. Nucleus
d. Nuclear membrane
e. Nucleolus
f. Mitochondria
g. Ribosomes
h. Rough endoplasmic reticulum
i. Smooth endoplasmic reticulum
j. Golgi apparatus
k. Lysosomes
l. Centrioles
m. Chromatin
n. Secretory vesicle

_____

_____

_____

_____

_____

_____

_____

_____

_____

_____

_____

_____

_____

_____

_____

_____

_____

_____

_____

_____

_____

_____

_____

_____

H. Evolve Site: Chapter 5 Animations

Directions:

1. View the Chapter 5 Animations on the Evolve site.
2. For each animation, write two true or false questions in the space provided below.
3. In the classroom, find a partner.
4. For each animation, read your two questions to your partner.
5. For each correct answer, your partner is awarded two points.
6. Next, have your partner read his or her two questions to you. Award yourself two points for each question answered correctly.
7. Continue in this manner until all the questions have been answered.
8. Record your points on your Study Guide Assignment sheet.

True or False Questions

a. Directions of the Body

    1. _____

    2. _____

b. Parts of the Cell

    1. _____

    2. _____

c. Cells

    1. _____

    2. _____

d. Cell Reproduction

    1. _____

    2. _____

e. Hereditary Traits

    1. _____

    2. _____

f. Mucous Membrane

    1. _____

    2. _____

g. Serous Membrane

    1. _____

    2. _____

h. Synovial Membrane

    1. _____

    2. _____

I. Crossword Puzzle: Introduction to Anatomy and Physiology

Directions: Complete the crossword puzzle using the clues provided.

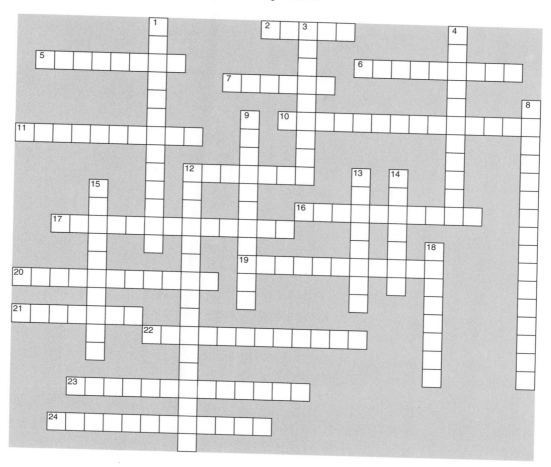

Across

2 Little hairs on cell membrane
5 Number of chromosomes in human cell
6 Synthesizes proteins
7 Connects muscle to bone
10 Packaging and shipping plant
11 Secretes mucus
12 Produces two daughter cells
16 Helps distribute chromosomes to daughter cells
17 Brain, spinal cord, and nerves
19 On or near the surface
20 Everything is A-OK
21 Cell's control center
22 Cell eating
23 Houses the brain
24 Power plant of cell

Down

1 Contains fat cells
3 Destroys cellular debris
4 Cartilage cell
8 Has same concentration as RBCs
9 Cell drinking
12 Divides body into right and left halves
13 Toward the front
14 Cell division that produces eggs and sperm
15 Lines abdominopelvic cavity
18 Sperm tail

Notes

6 Integumentary System

CHAPTER ASSIGNMENTS

√ After Completing	Date Due	Textbook Page(s)	TEXTBOOK ASSIGNMENT	Possible Points	Points You Earned
		100-105	Read Chapter 6: Integumentary System		
√ After Completing	**Date Due**	**Study Guide Page(s)**	**STUDY GUIDE ASSIGNMENTS (CTA: Critical Thinking Activity)**		
		67	🗎 Pretest	10	
		68	🔑 Term Key Term Assessment: A. Definitions B. Word Parts (Add 1 point for each medical term)	9 9	
		69-72	Evaluation of Learning questions	43	
		72	Evolve Site: CTA A: Body Spectrum: Skin Structure	10	
		72	Evolve Site: CTA B: Body Spectrum: Glands of the Skin	10	
		72	Evolve Site: CTA C: Body Spectrum: Skin and Hypodermis	10	
		73	Evolve Site: CTA D: Body Spectrum: Hair Follicle	10	
		73	Evolve Site: CTA E: Body Spectrum: Hair Follicle Enlarged	10	
		73-74	CTA F: Inquiring Patients Want to Know	20	
		75	CTA G: Crossword Puzzle	24	
		67	🗎 Posttest	10	
			ADDITIONAL ASSIGNMENTS		
			TOTAL POINTS		

Notes

Name _____ Date _____

True or False

_____ 1. The nails are part of the integumentary system.

_____ 2. The thickest layer of the epidermis is the stratum corneum.

_____ 3. Cerumen provides waterproofing for the skin.

_____ 4. Sensory receptors allow the body to detect changes in the environment.

_____ 5. The subcutaneous layer cushions underlying organs.

_____ 6. The ultraviolet rays of the sun increase melanocyte activity.

_____ 7. The face does not contain hair.

_____ 8. Hair is produced by hair follicles.

_____ 9. The neck and chest have the most sweat glands.

_____ 10. Vitamin A is necessary for the absorption of calcium in the body.

?≣ **POSTTEST**

True or False

_____ 1. The epidermis consists of simple squamous epithelial tissue.

_____ 2. Skin cells grow and multiply in the stratum basale layer of the epidermis.

_____ 3. Melanocytes produce a yellow pigment.

_____ 4. Sebaceous glands are embedded in the dermis.

_____ 5. An individual with a large number of melanin granules in his or her skin will have dry skin.

_____ 6. The part of the hair that is visible is known as the shaft.

_____ 7. The outermost covering of the hair is known as the cuticle.

_____ 8. Shivering is caused by contraction of the arrector pili muscles.

_____ 9. Sebum keeps hair and skin soft and pliable.

_____ 10. Cerumen traps foreign material.

A. Definitions

Directions: Match each medical term with its definition.

_____ 1. Arrector pili

_____ 2. Ceruminous gland

_____ 3. Dermis

_____ 4. Epidermis

_____ 5. Keratinization

_____ 6. Melanin

_____ 7. Sebaceous gland

_____ 8. Subcutaneous layer

_____ 9. Sudoriferous gland

A. A dark brown or black pigment found in parts of the body, especially skin and hair

B. A gland in the ear canal that produces cerumen or earwax

C. A gland in the skin that produces perspiration; also called *sweat gland*

D. An oil gland of the skin that produces sebum or body oil

E. Below the skin; a sheet of areolar connective tissue and adipose tissue beneath the dermis of the skin; also called *hypodermis or superficial fascia*

F. Inner layer of the skin that contains the blood vessels, nerves, glands, and hair follicles

G. Muscle associated with hair follicles

H. Outermost layer of the skin

I. Process by which the cells of the epidermis become filled with keratin and move to the surface, where they are sloughed off

B. Word Parts

Directions: Indicate the meaning of each word part in the space provided. List as many medical terms as possible that incorporate the word part in the space provided.

Word Part	Meaning of Word Part	Medical Terms That Incorporate Word Part
1. epi-		
2. kerat/o		
3. -ation		
4. melan/o		
5. seb/o		
6. -ous		
7. sub-		
8. cutane/o		
9. sud-		

Directions: Fill in each blank with the correct answer.

1. What structures make up the integumentary system?

   _____

2. What is another name for the skin?

   _____

3. What occurs during keratinization?

   _____

   _____

4. Why do cells in the epidermis flatten out and die as they reach the surface of the skin?

   _____

   _____

5. What occurs in the stratum basale?

   _____

   _____

6. What are melanocytes?

   _____

   _____

7. What makes up the stratum corneum?

   _____

   _____

8. What is the function of keratin?

   _____

   _____

9. What is another name for the dermis?

   _____

10. What structures are embedded in the dermis?

    _____

11. What happens if the dermis is overstretched?

    _____

    _____

12. What is the function of sensory receptors?

_____

_____

13. What causes fingerprints and footprints?

_____

_____

14. What are two other terms for the subcutaneous layer?

_____

15. What type of tissue is located in the subcutaneous layer?

_____

16. What is the function of subcutaneous tissue?

_____

_____

17. What controls the activity of melanocytes?

_____

_____

18. What occurs when the body is unable to produce melanin?

_____

19. What is the name of the pigment that results in a yellow tint of the skin?

_____

20. What effect does ultraviolet light have on melanocyte activity?

_____

21. What parts of the body do not grow hair?

_____

22. What is the name given to the part of the hair that is visible?

_____

23. Where is the root of the hair located?

_____

24. What is the name of the outer covering of a hair? What makes up this covering?

_____

_____

25. What is the function of a hair follicle?

_____

26. How is hair color determined?

_____

_____

27. What occurs when the arrector pili muscles contract?

_____

_____

28. What can cause the arrector pili muscles to contract?

_____

29. What makes up a nail?

_____

_____

30. What is the name given to the visible portion of a nail?

_____

31. What is another name for the cuticle of a nail?

_____

32. Why do nails appear pink?

_____

_____

33. What is the function of sebum?

_____

_____

34. What parts of the body have the most sweat glands?

_____

35. What is a sweat pore?

_____

36. What causes perspiration to occur?

_____

37. What is the function of cerumen?

_____

38. List four ways in which the skin protects the body.

_____

_____

39. How does the skin regulate body temperature?

_____

40. Vitamin D assists in the absorption of what minerals?

_____

41. What are the functions of calcium and phosphorus in the body?

_____

42. How does the skin produce vitamin D?

_____

_____

43. How do each of the following changes due to aging affect the skin?

    a. Decrease in elastic fibers and adipose tissue: _____

    b. Loss of collagen fibers:_____

    c. Slower mitotic activity in the stratum basale: _____

    d. Reduced sebaceous gland activity: _____

    e. Reduction in melanocyte activity: _____

CRITICAL THINKING ACTIVITIES

A. Evolve Site: Body Spectrum

Integumentary: Skin Structure

Body Spectrum directions:

1. Access the Body Spectrum on the Evolve site.

2. If necessary, access the HELP screen for directions on using the Body Spectrum program.

3. Go to the Contents screen.

4. Select the following category from the Contents screen:
   Integumentary

5. Select the following anatomic diagram:
   Skin Structure

6. Identify the structures on the diagram.

7. Print out the diagram.

B. Evolve Site: Body Spectrum

Integumentary: Glands of the Skin

Directions: Identify the structures on this diagram following the Body Spectrum directions outlined under CTA A.

C. Evolve Site: Body Spectrum

Integumentary: Skin And Hypodermis

Directions: Identify the structures on this diagram following the Body Spectrum directions outlined under CTA A.

D. Evolve Site: Body Spectrum

Integumentary: Hair Follicle

Directions: Identify the structures on this diagram following the Body Spectrum directions outlined under CTA A.

E. Evolve Site: Body Spectrum

Integumentary: Hair Follicle Enlarged

Directions: Identify the structures on this diagram following the Body Spectrum directions outlined under CTA A.

F. Inquiring Patients Want to Know

You are working in a general practice medical office. Your patients ask you the following questions. In the space provided, indicate how you would respond to each question in terms the patient would understand.

1. What makes skin waterproof?

   _____

   _____

2. What causes a blister?

   _____

   _____

3. What causes blushing?

   _____

   _____

4. What causes curly hair?

   _____

   _____

5. Why does it not hurt when my hair is cut?

   _____

   _____

6. What causes split ends?

   _____

   _____

7. How does hair grow?

   _____

   _____

8. What causes freckles?

   _____

   _____

9. Why do I have red hair?

   _____

   _____

10. Why does my skinny friend get cold all the time?

_____

_____

11. What causes age spots?

_____

_____

12. What causes wrinkles?

_____

_____

13. What causes a person to tan?

_____

_____

14. What causes "goose bumps?"

_____

_____

15. What causes pimples?

_____

_____

16. What causes baldness?

_____

_____

17. What causes warts?

_____

_____

18. What causes itching?

_____

_____

19. What causes hair to turn white?

_____

_____

20. How does sunshine cause the body to produce vitamin D?

_____

_____

G. Crossword Puzzle: Integumentary System

Directions: Complete the crossword puzzle using the clues provided.

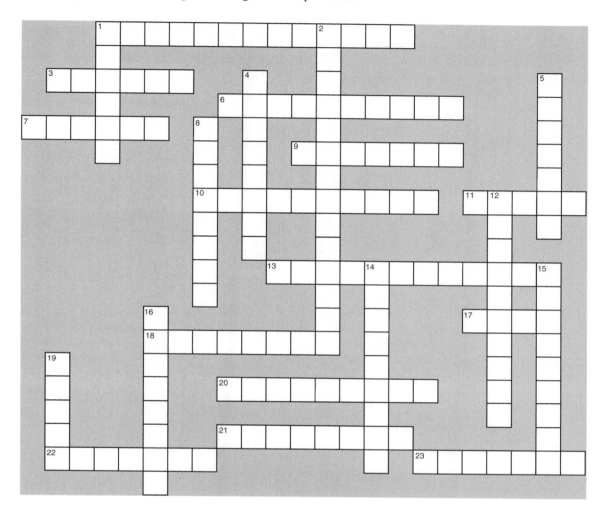

Across

1 Melanocytes live here
3 Inner skin layer
6 Inflammation of the skin
7 Converts precursor in skin to vitamin D
9 Outermost covering of hair
10 Function of skin
11 Mole
13 Caused by papillae
17 Teenager skin problem
18 Cannot produce melanin
20 Hives
21 Itching
22 Responsible for skin color
23 Earwax

Down

1 Stretch marks
2 Outermost layer of epidermis
4 Cancerous skin growth
5 Needed for vitamin D absorption
8 Baldness
12 Cuticle
14 Outer layer of skin
15 Skin opening of sweat gland
16 Yellowish pigment
19 Oily secretion

Notes

7 Skeletal System

CHAPTER ASSIGNMENTS

√ After Completing	Date Due	Textbook Page(s)	TEXTBOOK ASSIGNMENT	Possible Points	Points You Earned
		106-122	Read Chapter 7: Skeletal System		

√ After Completing	Date Due	Study Guide Page(s)	STUDY GUIDE ASSIGNMENTS (CTA: Critical Thinking Activity)	Possible Points	Points You Earned
		79	📝 Pretest	10	
		80	🔑 Key Term Assessment A. Definitions B. Word Parts (Add 1 point for each medical term)	10 10	
		81-86	📖 Evaluation of Learning questions	64	
		86	*e* Evolve Site: CTA A: Body Spectrum: Structure of Bone	10	
		87	CTA B: Long Bone	12	
		87	*e* Evolve Site: CTA C: Body Spectrum: Skeleton Anterior	10	
		87	*e* Evolve Site: CTA D: Body Spectrum: Skeleton Posterior	10	
		87	*e* Evolve Site: CTA E: Body Spectrum: Skull Anterior	10	
		87	*e* Evolve Site: CTA F: Body Spectrum: Skull Right Lateral	10	
		87	*e* Evolve Site: CTA G: Body Spectrum: Paranasal Sinuses	40	
		87	*e* Evolve Site: CTA H: Body Spectrum: Cranial Vault	10	
		88	*e* Evolve Site: CTA I: Body Spectrum: Skull Inferior	10	
		88	*e* Evolve Site: CTA J: Body Spectrum: Vertebral Column	10	
		88	*e* Evolve Site: CTA K: Body Spectrum: Individual Vertebrae	10	
		88	*e* Evolve Site: CTA L: Body Spectrum: Thorax and Ribs	10	

√ After Completing	Date Due	Study Guide Page(s)	STUDY GUIDE ASSIGNMENTS (CTA: Critical Thinking Activity)	Possible Points	Points You Earned
		88	*e* Evolve Site: CTA M: Body Spectrum: Right Wrist and Hand	10	
		88	*e* Evolve Site: CTA N: Body Spectrum: Male Pelvis	10	
		88	*e* Evolve Site: CTA O: Body Spectrum: Female Pelvis	10	
		88	*e* Evolve Site: CTA P: Body Spectrum: Right Foot	10	
		88	CTA Q: Synovial Joint	5	
		89	CTA R: Inquiring Patients Want to Know	10	
		90	CTA S: Crossword Puzzle	23	
		79	[?] Posttest	10	
			ADDITIONAL ASSIGNMENTS		
			TOTAL POINTS		

Name _____ Date _____

True or False

_____ 1. The skeletal system provides a rigid framework for the body.

_____ 2. Blood cell formation takes place in the spleen.

_____ 3. Vertebrae are made up of flat bones.

_____ 4. Articular cartilage covers the ends of long bones.

_____ 5. Long bones grow in length at the epiphyseal line.

_____ 6. The maxillary bones form the upper jaw.

_____ 7. The sacrum makes up the small of the back.

_____ 8. The shoulder is an example of a hinge joint.

_____ 9. The patella is the kneecap.

_____ 10. The humerus makes up the thigh.

📄 **POSTTEST**

True or False

_____ 1. The formation of blood cells is known as hemogenesis.

_____ 2. Osteons are the microscopic units of compact bone.

_____ 3. Calcium is located in an osteonic canal.

_____ 4. The shaft of a long bone is the diaphysis.

_____ 5. The endosteum is the tough fibrous connective tissue that covers a long bone.

_____ 6. A mature bone cell is an osteoblast.

_____ 7. The central indentation of the sternum is the jugular (suprasternal) notch.

_____ 8. The clavicle and scapula make up the pelvic girdle.

_____ 9. The ileum, ischium, and pubis make up the coxal bones.

_____ 10. The ulna is located on the lateral side of the forearm.

A. Definitions

Directions: Match each medical term with its definition.

_____ 1. Amphiarthrosis

_____ 2. Diaphysis

_____ 3. Diarthrosis

_____ 4. Epiphyseal plate

_____ 5. Epiphysis

_____ 6. Osteoblast

_____ 7. Osteoclast

_____ 8. Osteocyte

_____ 9. Osteon

_____ 10. Synarthrosis

A. A slightly movable joint
B. An immovable joint
C. Bone-forming cell
D. Cell that destroys or resorbs bone tissue
E. Freely movable joint characterized by a joint cavity; also called a *synovial joint*
F. Mature bone cell
G. Structural unit of bone; haversian system
H. The cartilaginous plate between the epiphysis and diaphysis of a bone; responsible for the lengthwise growth of a long bone
I. The end of a long bone
J. The long, straight shaft of a long bone

B. Word Parts

Directions: Indicate the meaning of each word part in the space provided. List as many medical terms as possible that incorporate the word part in the space provided.

Word Part	Meaning of Word Part	Medical Terms That Incorporate Word Part
1. arthr/o		
2. -osis		
3. dia-		
4. epi-		
5. -phys		
6. oste/o		
7. -blast		
8. -clast		
9. -cyte		
10. syn-		

Chapter **7**   *Skeletal System*

Directions: Fill in each blank with the correct answer.

1. What structures make up the skeletal system?

   _____

   _____

2. What are the five functions of the skeletal system?

   _____

   _____

3. How is the blood calcium level maintained in the body?

   _____

   _____

4. What is the function of red bone marrow?

   _____

5. Where is red bone marrow found in the adult?

   _____

   _____

6. What is an osteon?

   _____

7. Describe the following structures that make up an osteon:

   a. Osteonic canal (haversian canal): _____

   _____

   b. Lamella: _____

   _____

   c. Osteocytes: _____

   d. Lacunae: _____

   _____

   e. Canaliculi: _____

   _____

8. What is the difference between spongy bone and compact bone?

   _____

   _____

9. List examples of each of the following classifications of bone:

    a. Long bones: _____

    b. Short bones: _____

    c. Flat bones: _____

    d. Irregular bones: _____

10. Describe each of the following structures that make up a long bone:

    a. Diaphysis: _____

    b. Medullary cavity: _____

    c. Epiphysis: _____

    d. Articular cartilage: _____

    e. Periosteum: _____

    f. Nutrient foramina: _____

    g. Endosteum: _____

11. What is ossification?

_____

12. What is the function of each of the following types of bone cells?

    a. Osteoblast: _____

    b. Osteocyte: _____

    c. Osteoclast:_____

13. Where is the epiphyseal plate located in a long bone?

_____

14. What type of cartilage is found in the epiphyseal plate?

_____

15. How do long bones grow in length?

_____

_____

16. When does an individual stop growing in length?

_____

17. What happens to the epiphyseal plate when long bones stop growing?

_____

18. What influences bone growth in the body?

_____

_____

19. How many bones make up the skeleton of an adult?

_____

20. What are the two divisions of the skeleton? What structures are included in each division?

_____

_____

21. How many bones make up the skull?

_____

22. What is the function of the cranium?

_____

23. What are sinuses and what is their function?

_____

24. What bones make up the cranium?

_____

_____

25. What is the function of the facial bones?

_____

_____

26. What are the names of the three small bones located in the middle ear?

_____

27. What is the function of the hyoid bone?

_____

_____

28. How many vertebrae make up the vertebral column?

_____

29. What are the functions of the intervertebral disks?

_____

_____

30. What structures make up the vertebrae?

_____

_____

31. How many vertebrae are included in each of the following divisions of the vertebral column?

    a. Cervical: _____

    b. Thoracic: _____

    c. Lumbar: _____

32. Describe the following:

a. Sacrum: _____

_____

b. Coccyx: _____

_____

33. What are the functions of the thoracic cage?

_____

_____

_____

34. What is the name of the central indentation in the superior margin of the sternum?

_____

35. How many pairs of ribs are present in the human skeleton?

_____

36. What is the difference between true ribs and false ribs?

_____

_____

37. What are floating ribs?

_____

38. What is the function of the appendicular skeleton?

_____

39. What two bones make up the pectoral girdle?

_____

40. What is another name for the clavicle?

_____

41. What is the name of the shallow depression on the scapula where the head of the humerus connects to the scapula?

_____

42. What bone is located in the upper arm?

_____

43. What bones are located in the forearm?

_____

44. State the location of the following bones making up the hand:

a. Carpal bones: _____

b. Metacarpal bones: _____

c. Phalanges: _____

45. What are the functions of the pelvic girdle?

_____

_____

46. What three bones fuse to form a coxal bone?

_____

47. What is the symphysis pubis?

_____

48. What bone is located in the thigh?

_____

49. What is the patella?

_____

50. What is the function of the patella?

_____

51. What bones are located in the leg?

_____

52. What does the lateral malleolus do?

_____

53. Describe the location of the following bones making up the foot:

    a. Tarsal bones: _____

    b. Calcaneus bone: _____

    c. Metatarsal bones: _____

    d. Phalanges: _____

54. What is an articulation?

_____

55. What is a synarthrosis?

_____

56. What is an example of a synarthrosis?

_____

57. What is an amphiarthrosis?

_____

58. What is an example of an amphiarthrosis?

_____

59. What is a diarthrosis?

_____

60. Describe the following parts of a diarthrosis:

    a. Articular cartilage: _____

    b. Joint cavity: _____

    c. Joint capsule: _____

    d. Synovial membrane: _____

    e. Synovial fluid: _____

61. What is the function of fibrocartilaginous pads located in the knee?

_____

_____

62. What are bursae?

_____

63. What are the functions of bursae?

_____

_____

64. List examples of the following types of joints. What range of movement is possible with each of the following joints?

Joint	Examples	Range of Movement
a. Ball-and-socket		
b. Condyloid		
c. Saddle		
d. Pivot		
e. Hinge		
f. Gliding		

CRITICAL THINKING ACTIVITIES

A. Evolve Site: Body Spectrum

Skeletal: Structure of Bone

Body Spectrum directions:

1. Access the Body Spectrum program on the Evolve site.
2. If necessary, access the HELP screen for directions on using the Body Spectrum program.
3. Go to the Contents screen.
4. Select the following category from the Contents screen:
   Skeletal
5. Select the following anatomic diagram:
   Structure of Bone
6. Identify the structures on the diagram.
7. Print out the diagram.

B. Long Bone

Using Figure 7-2 in your textbook as a reference, label each of the parts of a long bone on the following diagram.

(Modified from Applegate E: *The anatomy and physiology learning system,* ed 4, St. Louis, 2011, Saunders.)

C. Evolve Site: Body Spectrum
Skeletal: Skeleton Anterior

Directions: Identify the structures on this diagram following the Body Spectrum directions outlined under CTA A.

D. Evolve Site: Body Spectrum
Skeletal: Skeleton Posterior

Directions: Identify the structures on this diagram following the Body Spectrum directions outlined under CTA A.

E. Evolve Site: Body Spectrum
Skeletal: Skull Anterior

Directions: Identify the structures on this diagram following the Body Spectrum directions outlined under CTA A.

F. Evolve Site: Body Spectrum
Skeletal: Skull Right Lateral

Directions: Identify the structures on this diagram following the Body Spectrum directions outlined under CTA A.

G. Evolve Site: Body Spectrum
Skeletal: Paranasal Sinuses

Directions: Identify the structures on this diagram following the Body Spectrum directions outlined under CTA A.

H. Evolve Site: Body Spectrum
Skeletal: Cranial Vault

Directions: Identify the structures on this diagram following the Body Spectrum directions outlined under CTA A.

I. Evolve Site: Body Spectrum

Skeletal: Skull Inferior

Directions: Identify the structures on this diagram following the Body Spectrum directions outlined under CTA A.

J. Evolve Site: Body Spectrum

Skeletal: Vertebral Column

Directions: Identify the structures on this diagram following the Body Spectrum directions outlined under CTA A.

K. Evolve Site: Body Spectrum

Skeletal: Individual Vertebrae

Directions: Identify the structures on this diagram following the Body Spectrum directions outlined under CTA A.

L. Evolve Site: Body Spectrum

Skeletal: Thorax and Ribs

Directions: Identify the structures on this diagram following the Body Spectrum directions outlined under CTA A.

M. Evolve Site: Body Spectrum

Skeletal: Right Wrist and Hand

Directions: Identify the structures on this diagram following the Body Spectrum directions outlined under CTA A.

N. Evolve Site: Body Spectrum

Skeletal: Male Pelvis

Directions: Identify the structures on this diagram following the Body Spectrum directions outlined under CTA A.

O. Evolve Site: Body Spectrum

Skeletal: Female Pelvis

Directions: Identify the structures on this diagram following the Body Spectrum directions outlined under CTA A.

P. Evolve Site: Body Spectrum

Skeletal: Right Foot

Directions: Identify the structures on this diagram following the Body Spectrum directions outlined under CTA A.

Q. Synovial Joint

Using Figure 7-17 in your textbook as a reference, label each of the parts of a synovial joint on the following diagram.

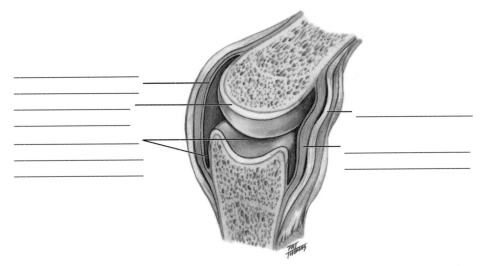

(Modified from Applegate E: *The anatomy and physiology learning system,* ed 4, St. Louis, 2011, Saunders.)

R. Inquiring Patients Want to Know

You are working in a general practice medical office. Your patients ask you the following questions. In the space provided, indicate how you would respond to each question in terms the patient would understand. Use your textbook and Internet resources to develop your responses.

1. What causes osteoporosis?

   _____

   _____

2. What causes my sinus headaches?

   _____

   _____

3. How does a baby get through the bones of the pelvis during childbirth?

   _____

   _____

4. What causes older people to break their hips?

   _____

   _____

5. What causes gout?

   _____

   _____

6. Why do people get shorter when they get older?

   _____

   _____

7. Why do babies have "soft spots" on their heads?

   _____

   _____

8. What is the difference between osteoarthritis and rheumatoid arthritis?

   _____

   _____

9. What happens when someone cracks his or her knuckles?

   _____

   _____

10. What is the difference between a strain and a sprain?

    _____

    _____

S. Crossword Puzzle: Skeletal System

Directions: Complete the crossword puzzle using the clues provided.

Across

1 Abnormal side-to-side spinal curvature
2 Bones that protect brain
4 Freely movable joint
6 Upper arm bone
7 Shaft of a long bone
9 Softening of bones
11 Collarbone
14 Bone cell
15 Air-filled cavity in the skull
17 Shoulder blade
18 Spinal cord passes through this part of the skull
19 Bones of the upper jaw
20 Lower jaw bones

Down

1 Immovable joint
3 Tailbone
5 Ankle
8 Finger bones
10 Where bones grow in length
12 Breastbone
13 Outer surface of a long bone
14 Process of bone formation
16 Kneecap
18 Thigh bone

8 Muscular System

√ After Completing	Date Due	Textbook Page(s)	TEXTBOOK ASSIGNMENT	Possible Points	Points You Earned
		123-135	Read Chapter 8: Muscular System		

√ After Completing	Date Due	Study Guide Page(s)	STUDY GUIDE ASSIGNMENTS (CTA: Critical Thinking Activity)	Possible Points	Points You Earned
		93	Pretest	10	
		93	Term Key Term Assessment	8	
		94-97	Evaluation of Learning questions	46	
		98	Evolve Site: CTA A: Body Spectrum: Face—Lateral	10	
		98	Evolve Site: CTA B: Body Spectrum: Face—Anterior	10	
		98	Evolve Site: CTA C: Body Spectrum: Anterior Abdominal	10	
		98	Evolve Site: CTA D: Body Spectrum: Musculature—Anterior	10	
		98	Evolve Site: CTA E: Body Spectrum: Upper Chest—Superficial	10	
		98	Evolve Site: CTA F: Body Spectrum: Right Arm—Lateral	10	
		98	Evolve Site: CTA G: Body Spectrum: Musculature—Posterior	10	
		98-99	CTA H: Inquiring Patients Want to Know	10	
		99-100	Evolve Site: CTA I: Animations	20	
		101	CTA J: Crossword Puzzle	25	
		93	Posttest	10	
			ADDITIONAL ASSIGNMENTS		
			TOTAL POINTS		

Notes

Name _____   Date _____

True or False

_____ 1. Skeletal muscle is under involuntary control.

_____ 2. A ligament indirectly attaches skeletal muscle to bone.

_____ 3. The cytoplasm of a muscle fiber is the sarcolemma.

_____ 4. Calcium is a neurotransmitter responsible for muscle contractions.

_____ 5. Oxygen must be present for aerobic respiration to occur.

_____ 6. Bending the elbow is an example of flexion.

_____ 7. The orbicularis oculus is used to wink, blink, and squint.

_____ 8. The diaphragm forms a partition between the thorax and abdomen.

_____ 9. The deltoid muscle moves the shoulder and upper arm.

_____ 10. Another name for the calcaneal tendon is the ankle.

📄 **POSTTEST**

True or False

_____ 1. Most of the heat produced in the body is through visceral muscle contractions.

_____ 2. The epimysium is a connective tissue sheath that surrounds a muscle.

_____ 3. The insertion is the end of a muscle that is attached to a relatively movable part.

_____ 4. An axon terminal meets a muscle fiber at the neuromuscular junction.

_____ 5. The products of anaerobic respiration are amino acids and carbon dioxide.

_____ 6. Moving the arm away from the body is an example of adduction.

_____ 7. The sternocleidomastoid muscle is located in the neck.

_____ 8. The internal intercostal muscles assist with inspiration.

_____ 9. The gluteus maximus muscle is used when an intramuscular injection is administered.

_____ 10. The quadriceps femoris muscle is used to extend the leg.

🔑Term **KEY TERM ASSESSMENT**

Directions: Match each medical term with its definition.

_____ 1. Antagonist

_____ 2. Insertion

_____ 3. Motor unit

_____ 4. Neuromuscular junction

_____ 5. Neurotransmitter

_____ 6. Origin

_____ 7. Prime mover

_____ 8. Synergist

A. A chemical substance that is released at the axon terminals to stimulate a muscle fiber contraction or an impulse in another neuron

B. A muscle that assists a prime mover but is not capable of producing the movement by itself

C. A muscle that has an action opposite to the prime mover

D. A single neuron and all the muscle fibers it stimulates

E. The area of communication between the axon terminal of a motor neuron and the sarcolemma of a muscle fiber; also called a myoneural junction

F. The end of a muscle that is attached to a relatively immovable part; the end opposite the insertion

G. The end of a muscle that is attached to a relatively movable part; the end opposite the origin

H. The muscle that is mainly responsible for a particular body movement; also called agonist

Directions: Fill in each blank with the correct answer.

1. What are the three types of muscle tissue?

   _____

   _____

2. How many skeletal muscles are found in the human body?

   _____

3. List and describe the four characteristics of skeletal muscle.

   _____

   _____

4. What four functions are provided to the body by muscle contractions?

   _____

   _____

5. What is the epimysium?

   _____

6. Describe the following parts of a muscle cell:

   a. Sarcolemma:_____

   _____

   b. Sarcoplasm: _____

7. Why does a muscle cell have numerous mitochondria?

   _____

   _____

8. List and describe the two ways in which skeletal muscle is attached to bone.

   a. _____

   _____

   b. _____

   _____

9. What is the name of the nerve cell that stimulates a skeletal muscle to contract?

   _____

10. What is a motor unit?

   _____

   _____

11. What is the neuromuscular junction?

_____

_____

12. What is a synaptic cleft?

_____

_____

13. What is the name of the neurotransmitter responsible for muscle contractions? Where is this neurotransmitter housed before being released?

_____

_____

14. Draw and label a diagram to illustrate what happens when a nerve impulse reaches its axon terminal.

_____

_____

15. What inactivates acetylcholine?

_____

16. What is the function of ATP?

_____

17. What is creatine phosphate?

_____

18. What are the primary energy sources for muscles that are actively contracting for extended periods of time?

_____

19. What must be available for aerobic respiration to occur?

_____

20. What are the products of aerobic respiration?

_____

21. What occurs when the muscles are contracting vigorously for long periods of time?

_____

_____

_____

22. How does the body produce energy when it runs out of oxygen?

_____

23. What happens when there is a buildup of lactic acid in the muscles?

_____

24. What is oxygen debt? How is oxygen debt paid back?

_____

_____

_____

25. Describe each of the following types of body movements, and give an example of each:

Type	Definition	Example
Flexion		
Extension		
Hyperextension		
Dorsiflexion		
Plantar flexion		
Abduction		
Adduction		
Rotation		
Supination		
Pronation		
Circumduction		
Inversion		
Eversion		

26. State the function of each of the following muscles involved with facial expressions:

a. Frontalis: _____

b. Orbicularis oris: _____

c. Orbicularis oculi: _____

d. Buccinator: _____

e. Zygomaticus: _____

27. What are the names of the muscles responsible for chewing?

_____

28. What is the function of the following neck muscles?

a. Sternocleidomastoid: _____

b. Trapezius: _____

29. What muscles located in the trunk are responsible for maintaining posture?

_____

30. What is the function of the intercostal muscles?

_____

31. Where is the diaphragm located?

_____

32. What is the function of the diaphragm?

_____

33. What are the four muscle pairs that make up the wall of the abdomen?

_____

_____

34. What muscles allow an individual to shrug his or her shoulders?

_____

35. Where is the pectoralis major muscle located?

_____

36. Where is the latissimus dorsi muscle located?

_____

37. What is the name of the muscle in the arm that is used for administering an intramuscular injection?

_____

38. What muscle is responsible for extending the forearm?

_____

39. What muscle is responsible for flexing the forearm?

_____

40. What thigh muscle is used to administer an intramuscular injection?

_____

41. What muscles make up the quadriceps femoris?

_____

_____

42. What is the function of the quadriceps femoris?

_____

43. What muscles are used to flex the leg?

_____

44. What muscles allow an individual to stand on his or her tiptoes?

_____

45. What is another name for the calcaneal tendon?

_____

46. What are the best deterrents to prevent the loss of muscle mass and strength as an individual ages?

_____

CRITICAL THINKING ACTIVITIES

A. Evolve Site: Body Spectrum

Muscular: Face—Lateral

Body Spectrum directions:
1. Access the Body Spectrum program on the Evolve site.
2. If necessary, access the HELP screen for directions on using the Body Spectrum program.
3. Go to the Contents screen.
4. Select the following category from the Contents screen:
   Muscular
5. Select the following anatomic diagram:
   Face—Lateral
6. Identify the structures on the diagram.
7. Print out the diagram.

B. Evolve Site: Body Spectrum

Muscular: Face—Anterior

Directions: Identify the structures on this diagram following the Body Spectrum directions outlined under CTA A.

C. Evolve Site: Body Spectrum

Muscular: Anterior Abdominal

Directions: Identify the structures on this diagram following the Body Spectrum directions outlined under CTA A.

D. Evolve Site: Body Spectrum

Muscular: Musculature—Anterior

Directions: Identify the structures on this diagram following the Body Spectrum directions outlined under CTA A.

E. Evolve Site: Body Spectrum

Muscular: Upper Chest—Superficial

Directions: Identify the structures on this diagram following the Body Spectrum directions outlined under CTA A.

F. Evolve Site: Body Spectrum

Muscular: Right Arm—Lateral

Directions: Identify the structures on this diagram following the Body Spectrum directions outlined under CTA A.

G. Evolve Site: Body Spectrum

Muscular: Musculature—Posterior

Directions: Identify the structures on this diagram following the Body Spectrum directions outlined under CTA A.

H. Inquiring Patients Want to Know

You are working in a general practice medical office. Your patients ask you the following questions. In the space provided, indicate how you would respond to each question in terms the patient would understand. Use your textbook and Internet resources to develop your responses.

1. What causes hiccups?

   _____

   _____

2. What causes menstrual cramps?

   _____

   _____

3. Why does someone get stiff and rigid after he or she dies?

_____

_____

4. What causes shin splints?

_____

_____

5. What causes an eye tic?

_____

_____

6. Why do my leg muscles burn when I run a 3-mile race?

_____

_____

7. Why do my muscles ache when I have the flu?

_____

_____

8. How does lifting weights make muscles bigger?

_____

_____

9. What causes shivering?

_____

_____

10. What happens to a muscle when it is torn?

_____

_____

I. Evolve Site: Chapter 8 Animations

Directions:

1. View the Chapter 8 Animations on the Evolve site.
2. For each animation, write two true or false questions in the space provided below.
3. In the classroom, find a partner.
4. For each animation, read your two questions to your partner.
5. For each correct answer, your partner is awarded two points.
6. Next, have your partner read his or her two questions to you. Award yourself two points for each question answered correctly.
7. Continue in this manner until all the questions have been answered.
8. Record your points on your Study Guide Assignment sheet.

True or False Questions

a. Microscopic Structure of Skeletal Muscle

    1. _____

    2. _____

b. The Motor Unit and Muscle Stimulus

    1. _____

    2. _____

c. Types of Skeletal Muscle Contractions

    1. _____

    2. _____

d. Cellular Respiration

    1. _____

    2. _____

e. Carbohydrate Metabolism: Glycolysis

    1. _____

    2. _____

J. Crossword Puzzle: Muscular System

Directions: Complete the crossword puzzle using the clues provided.

Across

- **4** Eyebrow-raising muscle
- **5** Muscle's fleshy part
- **8** Muscle that opposes a movement
- **9** Movement away from midline
- **13** Muscle-contraction neurotransmitter
- **15** Where an axon meets a muscle fiber
- **17** Movement toward midline
- **18** Winking muscle
- **19** Energy source for muscle contractions
- **21** Where ACh lives
- **22** Stimulates contraction of skeletal muscle
- **24** Kissing muscle
- **25** Chest muscle

Down

- **1** Abducts arm
- **2** Longest muscle in the body
- **3** Muscle fiber cytoplasm
- **6** Muscle fiber cell membrane
- **7** Cheek muscle
- **10** Smiling muscle
- **11** Extends vertebral column
- **12** Flexes forearm
- **14** Muscle group that extends leg
- **16** Sheath that surrounds a muscle
- **20** Shrugging shoulders muscle
- **23** Attaches muscle to bone

Notes

9 Nervous System

CHAPTER ASSIGNMENTS

√ After Completing	Date Due	Textbook Page(s)	TEXTBOOK ASSIGNMENT	Possible Points	Points You Earned
		136-154	Read Chapter 9: Nervous System		

√ After Completing	Date Due	Study Guide Page(s)	STUDY GUIDE ASSIGNMENTS (CTA: Critical Thinking Activity)	Possible Points	Points You Earned
		105	Pretest	10	
		106	Term Key Term Assessment A. Definitions B. Word Parts (Add 1 point for each medical term)	10 8	
		107-112	Evaluation of Learning questions	54	
		112	Evolve Site: CTA A: Body Spectrum: Structure of a Neuron	10	
		112	CTA B: Synapse	7	
		113	Evolve Site: CTA C: Body Spectrum: Brain—Meningeal Coverings	10	
		113	CTA D: Cerebrum	18	
		113	Evolve Site: CTA E: Body Spectrum: Spinal Cord	10	
		113	Evolve Site: CTA F: Body Spectrum: Brain—Inferior	10	
		113-114	CTA G: Inquiring Patients Want to Know	10	
		114-116	Evolve Site: CTA H: Animations	52	
		117	CTA I: Crossword Puzzle	27	
		105	Posttest	10	
			ADDITIONAL ASSIGNMENTS		
			TOTAL POINTS		

Notes

Name _____ Date _____

True or False

———————— 1. The function of a neuron is to transmit nerve impulses.

———————— 2. Neuroglia support and protect neurons.

———————— 3. Myelin is a white, fatty substance that surrounds nerve fibers.

———————— 4. Sneezing is an example of a reflex.

———————— 5. The central sulcus divides the cerebrum into two hemispheres.

———————— 6. The hypothalamus functions in the regulation of body temperature.

———————— 7. The pons functions in body coordination, posture, and balance.

———————— 8. The peripheral nervous system provides a communication network between the central nervous system (CNS) and the body.

———————— 9. Sensory nerves contain only efferent fibers.

——————— 10. The body has 12 pairs of cranial nerves.

?≣ POSTTEST

True or False

———————— 1. An axon transmits impulses toward a neuron cell body.

———————— 2. Gray matter is made up of myelinated fibers.

———————— 3. A myelin sheath is formed around axons within the CNS by Schwann cells.

———————— 4. Synapse is the name of the region of communication between two neurons.

———————— 5. The CNS is made up of cranial nerves and spinal nerves.

———————— 6. The cerebral cortex consists of gray matter.

———————— 7. The spinal cord extends from the base of the skull to the fourth lumbar vertebra.

———————— 8. The autonomic nervous system supplies motor impulses to visceral organs.

———————— 9. Nerves that carry both sensory and motor fibers are known as mixed nerves.

——————— 10. The sympathetic division of the autonomic nervous system prepares the body for fight or flight.

A. Definitions

Directions: Match each medical term with its definition.

_____ 1. Action potential

_____ 2. Brain stem

_____ 3. Cerebellum

_____ 4. Cerebrum

_____ 5. Diencephalon

_____ 6. Myelin

_____ 7. Neurilemma

_____ 8. Saltatory conduction

_____ 9. Synapse

_____ 10. Threshold stimulus

A. A nerve impulse; a rapid change in membrane potential that involves depolarization and repolarization

B. Minimum level of stimulation that is required to start a nerve impulse or muscle contraction; also called liminal stimulus

C. Part of the brain between the cerebral hemispheres and the midbrain; includes the thalamus, hypothalamus, and epithalamus

D. Process in which a nerve impulse travels along a myelinated nerve fiber by jumping from one node of Ranvier to the next

E. Second largest part of the human brain, located posterior to the pons and medulla oblongata, and involved in the coordination of muscular movements

F. The largest and uppermost part of the human brain; concerned with consciousness, learning, memory, sensations, and voluntary movements

G. The layer of cells that surrounds a nerve fiber in the peripheral nervous system and, in some cases, produces myelin

H. The portion of the brain between the diencephalon and spinal cord that contains the midbrain, pons, and medulla oblongata

I. The region of communication between two neurons

J. White, fatty substance that surrounds many nerve fibers

B. Word Parts

Directions: Indicate the meaning of each word part in the space provided. List as many medical terms as possible that incorporate the word part in the space provided.

Word Part	Meaning of Word Part	Medical Terms That Incorporate Word Part
1. act-		
2. cerebell/o		
3. cerebr/o		
4. cephal/o		
5. neur/o		
6. -lemma		
7. -tion		
8. syn-		

Directions: Fill in each blank with the correct answer.

1. What makes up the nervous system?

   _____

2. Describe the following three general functions of the nervous system:

   a. Sensory functions: _____

   b. Integrative functions: _____

   c. Motor functions: _____

3. What is an effector? What are two types of effectors?

   _____

   _____

4. What are the two main subdivisions of the nervous system?

   _____

5. What is the function of the following subdivisions of the peripheral nervous system?

   a. Afferent (sensory) division: _____

   b. Efferent (motor) division: _____

6. What function is performed by the following subdivisions of the efferent (motor) division?

   a. Somatic nervous system: _____

   b. Autonomic nervous system: _____

7. What are the two subdivisions of the autonomic nervous system?

   _____

8. What are the three basic parts of a neuron?

   _____

9. What is the function of a dendrite?

   _____

10. What is the function of an axon?

   _____

11. What is a myelin sheath?

   _____

12. What makes up the white matter in the central nervous system?

   _____

13. What makes up the gray matter in the central nervous system?

_____

14. Describe the appearance of a node of Ranvier.

_____

15. What is the neurilemma, and what is its function?

_____

_____

_____

16. What is the function of oligodendrocytes?

_____

17. Why can't nerve fibers in the central nervous system regenerate?

_____

18. Describe the structure and function of the three types of neurons:

    a. Afferent (sensory) neurons: _____

    _____

    b. Efferent (motor) neurons: _____

    _____

    c. Interneurons: _____

    _____

19. What is the function of neuroglia?

_____

20. What is a resting membrane?

_____

21. What happens to sodium ions when a neuron receives a stimulus?

_____

22. Describe how a nerve impulse is propagated along the length of a neuron through an action potential.

_____

_____

_____

_____

23. What is a synapse?

_____

108

Chapter **9** Nervous System

24. How is a nerve impulse transmitted across a synapse?

_____

_____

_____

25. What is a reflex?

_____

_____

26. What are some examples of reflexes that take place in the body?

_____

27. What makes up the central nervous system?

_____

28. What bones surround and protect the brain?

_____

29. What three layers make up the meninges, starting with the outer layer?

_____

30. What are the four parts of the human brain?

_____

31. What is the function of the corpus callosum?

_____

32. What five lobes make up the cerebral hemisphere?

_____

_____

33. Where is the cerebral cortex located? What makes up the cerebral cortex?

_____

_____

34. What functions are controlled by the cerebral cortex?

_____

_____

35. What is the function of the following structures making up the diencephalons?

a. Thalamus: _____

_____

b. Hypothalamus: _____

_____

109

c. Epithalamus: _____

_____

36. What structures make up the brain stem?_____

_____

37. List and explain the functions of the three control centers located in the medulla.

Control Center	Function
a.	
b.	
c.	

38. What is the function of the cerebellum?

_____

_____

39. What are ventricles?

_____

40. What is the function of cerebrospinal fluid?

_____

_____

_____

41. What is the starting point and ending point of the spinal cord?

_____

42. How long is the spinal cord?

_____

43. What surrounds the spinal cord?

_____

44. How many pairs of spinal nerves are present in the human body?

_____

45. What are the functions of the spinal cord?

_____

_____

46. What is the difference between ascending tracts and descending tracts of the spinal cord?

_____

_____

47. What makes up the peripheral nervous system?

_____

_____

48. What is the makeup and function of the somatic nervous system?

_____

_____

49. What is the makeup and function of the autonomic nervous system?

_____

_____

50. What type of nerve fibers make up each of the following?

   a. Sensory nerves: _____

   b. Motor nerves: _____

   c. Mixed nerves: _____

51. What are the names of the 12 cranial nerves, and what is the function of each?

Cranial Nerve	Name	Function
I		
II		
III		
IV		
V		
VI		
VII		
VIII		
IX		
X		
XI		
XII		

52. What are some examples of body functions controlled by the autonomic nervous system?

_____

53. What are the functions of the following two divisions of the autonomic nervous system?

a. Sympathetic: _____

_____

b. Parasympathetic: _____

54. How is memory affected as the nervous system ages?

_____

CRITICAL THINKING ACTIVITES

A. Evolve Site: Body Spectrum
Nervous: Structure of a Neuron
Body Spectrum directions:
1. Access the Body Spectrum program on the Evolve site.
2. If necessary, access the HELP screen for directions on using the Body Spectrum program.
3. Go to the Contents screen.
4. Select the following category from the Contents screen:
   Nervous
5. Select the following anatomic diagram:
   Structure of a Neuron
6. Identify the structures on the diagram.
7. Print out the diagram.

B. Synapse
Using Figure 9-4 in your textbook as a reference, label each of the components of a synapse on the following diagram.

(Modified from Applegate E: *The anatomy and physiology learning system,* ed 4, St. Louis, 2011, Saunders.)

C. Evolve Site: Body Spectrum
Nervous: Brain—Meningeal Coverings
Directions: Identify the structures on this diagram following the Body Spectrum directions outlined under CTA A.

D. Cerebrum
Using Figure 9-8 in your textbook as a reference, label each of the lobes and functional areas of the cerebrum on the following diagram.

(Modified from Applegate E: *The anatomy and physiology learning system,* ed 4, St. Louis, 2011, Saunders.)

E. Evolve Site: Body Spectrum
Nervous: Spinal Cord
Directions: Identify the structures on this diagram following the Body Spectrum directions outlined under CTA A.

F. Evolve Site: Body Spectrum
Nervous: Brain—Inferior
Directions: Identify the structures on this diagram following the Body Spectrum directions outlined under CTA A.

G. Inquiring Patients Want to Know
You are working in a general practice medical office. Your patients ask you the following questions. In the space provided, indicate how you would respond to each question in terms the patient would understand. Use your textbook and Internet resources to develop your responses.

1. What causes cerebral palsy?

_____

_____

2. What sometimes causes a "brain freeze" when you eat ice cream?

_____

_____

3. What does it mean if someone is right-brained or left-brained?

_____

_____

4. What happens in the brain when someone has a migraine headache?

_____

_____

5. Why do you become permanently paralyzed from a spinal cord injury?

_____

_____

6. What makes someone left-handed?

_____

_____

7. How do antidepressants like Prozac work?

_____

_____

8. Is it possible to improve your memory?

_____

_____

9. Why does your knee jerk when the doctor hits it with a rubber hammer?

_____

_____

10. What happens in the brain of a person with Alzheimer's disease?

_____

_____

H. Evolve Site: Chapter 9 Animations

Directions:

1. View the Chapter 9 Animations on the Evolve site.
2. For each animation, write two true or false questions in the space provided below.
3. In the classroom, find a partner.
4. For each animation, read your two questions to your partner.
5. For each correct answer, your partner is awarded two points.
6. Next, have your partner read his or her two questions to you. Award yourself two points for each question answered correctly.
7. Continue in this manner until all the questions have been answered.
8. Record your points on your Study Guide Assignment sheet.

True or False Questions

a. Divisions of the Nervous System

    1. _____

    2. _____

b. Neurons

    1. _____

    2. _____

c. Nerve Impulses

    1. _____

    2. _____

d. The Synapse

    1. _____

    2. _____

e. Reflex Arcs

    1. _____

    2. _____

f. Physiology of the Brain

    1. _____

    2. _____

g. Cranial Nerves

    1. _____

    2. _____

h. Comparison of Anatomic and Somatic Conduction Pathways

    1. _____

    2. _____

i. The Autonomic Nervous System as a Whole

    1. _____

    2. _____

j. Sympathetic Nervous System

   1. _____

   2. _____

k. Parasympathetic Nervous System

   1. _____

   2. _____

l. Autonomic Neurotransmitters

   1. _____

   2. _____

m. Spinal Tap

   1. _____

   2. _____

I. Crossword Puzzle: Nervous System

Directions: Complete the crossword puzzle using the clues provided.

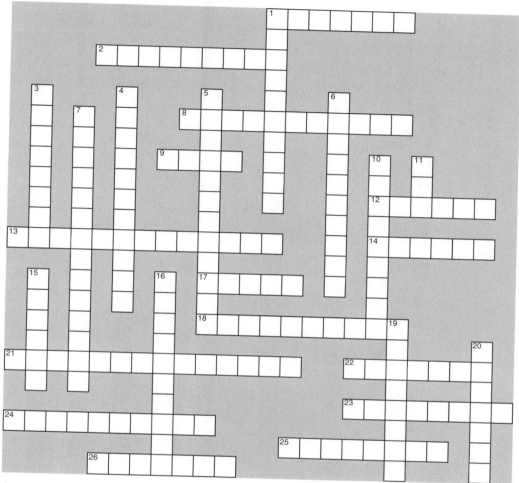

Across

1 Group of nerve cell bodies outside CNS
2 Support system for neurons
8 "Fight or flight" NS division
9 Carries impulses away from cell body
12 Automatic involuntary response
13 Space between neurons
14 White substance surrounding nerve fibers
17 Nerves that carry impulses away from CNS
18 Protected by vertebral column
21 Gaps in myelin
22 Communication region between neurons
23 Largest part of the brain
24 In charge of coordination, posture, and balance
25 Inner layer of meninges
26 Nerves that carry impulses toward CNS

Down

1 Cell bodies and unmyelinated fibers
3 Main part of neuron
4 Consists of myelinated nerve fibers
5 Regulates body temperature
6 Produces myelin in PNS
7 Outermost part of the cerebrum
10 Outer layer of meninges
11 Brain and spinal cord fluid
15 Nerve cell
16 Fluid-filled brain cavities
19 Transmits impulses to cell body
20 Respiratory center lives here

Notes

10 The Senses

CHAPTER ASSIGNMENTS

√ After Completing	Date Due	Textbook Page(s)	TEXTBOOK ASSIGNMENT	Possible Points	Points You Earned
		155-165	Read Chapter 10: The Senses		

√ After Completing	Date Due	Study Guide Page(s)	STUDY GUIDE ASSIGNMENTS (CTA: Critical Thinking Activity)	Possible Points	Points You Earned
		121	🗒 Pretest	10	
		122	🔑 Term Key Term Assessment A. Definitions B. Word Parts (Add 1 point for each medical term)	8 7	
		122-128	📝 Evaluation of Learning questions	65	
		128	*e* Evolve Site: CTA A: Body Spectrum: Right Eye—Cross Section	10	
		128	*e* Evolve Site: CTA B: Body Spectrum: Normal Structure of the Eye	10	
		128	*e* Evolve Site: CTA C: Eye-Dentify (Record points earned)		
		128-129	CTA D: Light Ray	40	
		129	*e* Evolve Site: CTA E: Body Spectrum: Ear—Cross Section	10	
		129	*e* Evolve Site: CTA F: Body Spectrum: Muscles of the Middle Ear	10	
		129	*e* Evolve Site: CTA G: Can You Hear Me Now? (Record points earned)		
		130	CTA H: Sound Wave	40	
		131	CTA I: Inquiring Patients Want to Know	10	

√ After Completing	Date Due	Study Guide Page(s)	STUDY GUIDE ASSIGNMENTS (CTA: Critical Thinking Activity)	Possible Points	Points You Earned
		132	Evolve Site: CTA J: Animations	20	
		133	CTA K: Crossword Puzzle	28	
		121	Posttest	10	
			ADDITIONAL ASSIGNMENTS		
			TOTAL POINTS		

Name _____   Date _____

True or False

_____ 1. Special senses have receptors that are localized in a particular area.

_____ 2. Thermoreceptors are located in subcutaneous tissue.

_____ 3. There are more cold receptors in a given area than heat receptors.

_____ 4. The olfactory cortex interprets smell sensations.

_____ 5. The inner layer of the eye that contains rods and cones is the retina.

_____ 6. The region of the retina that produces the sharpest image is the optic disk.

_____ 7. Visual impulses are interpreted in the occipital lobe.

_____ 8. Cerumen helps prevent foreign substances from reaching the eardrum.

_____ 9. The range of frequencies for normal speech is 300 to 4000 vibrations per second.

_____ 10. The cochlea is a coiled structure in the inner ear that functions in hearing.

? POSTTEST

True or False

_____ 1. Meissner corpuscles are stimulated by heavy pressure.

_____ 2. The sense of position or orientation is known as proprioception.

_____ 3. A nociceptor is stimulated by tissue damage.

_____ 4. Taste receptors are stimulated by the pressure of food on the tongue.

_____ 5. The white part of the eye is the choroid.

_____ 6. When the ciliary muscle contracts, the lens bulges for close vision.

_____ 7. Rhodopsin allows the eye to adapt to dim light.

_____ 8. Receptors for hearing are chemoreceptors.

_____ 9. The oval window equalizes the pressure between the outside and the middle ear.

_____ 10. The semicircular canals contain the sense organs for static equilibrium.

A. Definitions

Directions: Match each medical term with its definition.

_____ 1. Accommodation

_____ 2. Chemoreceptor

_____ 3. Mechanoreceptor

_____ 4. Nociceptor

_____ 5. Photoreceptor

_____ 6. Proprioception

_____ 7. Sensory adaptation

_____ 8. Thermoreceptor

A. A sensory receptor that detects changes in temperature
B. A sensory receptor that detects light; located in the retina of the eye
C. A sensory receptor that detects the presence of chemicals; responsible for taste, smell, and monitoring the concentration of certain chemicals in body fluids
D. A sensory receptor that responds to a bending or deformation of the cell; examples include receptors for touch, pressure, hearing, and equilibrium
E. A sensory receptor that responds to tissue damage; pain receptor
F. Mechanism that allows the eye to focus at various distances, primarily achieved by changing the curvature of the lens
G. Phenomenon in which some receptors respond when a stimulus is first applied but decrease their response if the stimulus is maintained; receptor sensitivity decreases with prolonged stimulation
H. The sense of body position and movements

B. Word Parts

Directions: Indicate the meaning of each word part in the space provided. List as many medical terms as possible that incorporate the word part in the space provided.

Word Part	Meaning of Word Part	Medical Terms That Incorporate Word Part
1. chem/o		
2. mechan/o		
3. noci-		
4. -ceptor		
5. phot/o		
6. propri/o		
7. therm/o		

EVALUATION OF LEARNING

Directions: Fill in each blank with the correct answer.

1. What is the difference between the general senses and the special senses?

_____

_____

2. What are the five types of sense receptors? Provide an example of each.

Type of Receptor	Example

3. What are the steps involved in perceiving sensation?

_____

_____

_____

4. What is sensory adaptation?

_____

_____

5. What senses are classified as the general senses?

_____

_____

6. What type of stimulus activates a mechanoreceptor?

_____

7. What is the function of each of the following mechanoreceptors involved with touch and pressure?

a. Free nerve endings: _____

_____

b. Meissner corpuscles: _____

_____

c. Pacinian corpuscles: _____

_____

8. What is proprioception?

_____

9. What mechanoreceptors are involved with proprioception?

_____

10. Where are thermoreceptors located?

_____

11. In which part of the body are thermoreceptors the most numerous? Where are they the least numerous?

_____

_____

12. How do the number of cold receptors compare with the number of heat receptors?

_____

13. What type of receptors do extreme temperatures stimulate?

_____

14. Describe the sensory adaptation that occurs with thermoreceptors.

_____

_____

15. What stimulates a nociceptor?

_____

16. Where are nociceptors located?

_____

_____

17. How do nociceptors provide a protective function in the body?

_____

_____

18. What senses are classified as special senses?

_____

19. What are the organs of taste?

_____

20. What stimulates the receptors that determine taste?

_____

21. What are the four different taste sensations?

_____

22. What happens when taste hairs are stimulated?

_____

_____

23. What is olfaction?

_____

24. What stimulates the receptors that distinguish smell?

_____

25. What area of the brain interprets smell impulses?

_____

26. What is the function of the following eye structures?

    a. Eyebrows: _____

b. Eyelids: _____

c. Eyelashes: _____

d. Sebaceous glands: _____

27. What eye muscle performs the following?

a. Closes the eye: _____

b. Opens the eye: _____

28. Describe the location of the conjunctiva.

_____

_____

29. What is the purpose of mucus secreted by the eye?

_____

30. What is a stye?

_____

31. What structure produces tears?

_____

32. What is the function of tears?

_____

_____

33. Describe the appearance of the sclera.

_____

_____

34. What are two functions of the choroid?

_____

_____

35. What effect does contraction of the ciliary muscle have on the lens of the eye?

_____

_____

36. How does the iris control the size of the pupil?

_____

37. Where are the receptor cells of the eye located?

_____

38. What is the optic disk, and why is it known as the "blind spot" of the eye?

_____

_____

39. Describe the location and appearance of the macula lutea.

_____

40. What is the name of the eye structure that produces the sharpest image?

_____

41. Where is the anterior cavity of the eye located?

_____

42. What is the function of aqueous humor?

_____

_____

43. Where is the posterior cavity of the eye located?

_____

44. What is the function of vitreous humor?

_____

45. What is refraction?

_____

46. What four structures of the eye function in refraction?

_____

47. Describe the image that forms when light rays are refracted onto the retina.

_____

48. What occurs in each of these structures during distance and close vision?

Vision	Ciliary Muscle	Suspensory Ligaments	Lens
a. Distance vision			
b. Close vision			

49. What is the function of rods?

_____

50. What is the function of cones?

_____

51. What is the function of rhodopsin?

_____

52. What part of the brain interprets visual impulses?

_____

53. What two functions are performed by the ear?

_____

54. What is the function of the auricle?

_____

_____

55. What is the function of cerumen?

_____

56. What effect do sound waves have on the tympanic membrane?

_____

57. What is the function of the eustachian tube?

_____

_____

58. What are the names of the three auditory ossicles?

_____

59. What structures in the inner ear function in equilibrium?

_____

60. What structure in the inner ear functions in hearing?

_____

61. What structure in the cochlea houses the sound receptors?

_____

62. What is the range of frequencies of normal speech?

_____

63. What nerve carries auditory impulses to the brain?

_____

64. What is static equilibrium?

_____

_____

65. What is dynamic equilibrium?

_____

_____

CRITICAL THINKING ACTIVITIES

A. Evolve Site: Body Spectrum
Senses: Right Eye—Cross Section
Body Spectrum directions:
1. Access the Body Spectrum program on the Evolve site.
2. If necessary, access the HELP screen for directions on using the Body Spectrum program.
3. Go to the Contents screen.
4. Select the following category from the Contents screen:
   Senses
5. Select the following anatomic diagram:
   Right Eye—Cross Section
6. Identify the structures on the diagram.
7. Print out the diagram.

B. Evolve Site: Body Spectrum
Senses: Normal Structure of the Eye
Directions: Identify the structures on this diagram following the Body Spectrum directions outlined under CTA A.

C. Evolve Site: Eye-Dentify
Access the Evolve site to complete this activity. Record your points earned on your assignment sheet.

D. Light Ray
You are a ray of light that is getting ready to enter the eye where you will be converted into a nerve impulse and then travel to the brain for interpretation. In the space provided below, describe all of the structures you encounter on your way to the brain. Also describe what function each structure is performing in the eye. Each of the following structures should be included in your discussion:
  a. Lacrimal apparatus
  b. Conjunctiva
  c. Sclera
  d. Iris and pupil
  e. Anterior cavity
  f. Lens and suspensory ligaments
  g. Ciliary muscle
  h. Posterior cavity
  i. Retina
  j. Macula lutea

k. Rods and cones
l. Optic nerve
m. Optic chiasma
n. Thalamus
o. Occipital lobe

_____

_____

_____

_____

_____

_____

_____

_____

_____

_____

_____

_____

_____

_____

_____

_____

_____

_____

_____

_____

E. Evolve Site: Body Spectrum

Senses: Ear—Cross Section

Directions: Identify the structures on this diagram following the Body Spectrum directions outlined under CTA A.

F. Evolve Site: Body Spectrum

Senses: Muscles of the Middle Ear

Directions: Identify the structures on this diagram following the Body Spectrum directions outlined under CTA A.

G. Evolve Site: Can You Hear Me Now?

Access the Evolve site to complete this activity. Record your points earned on your assignment sheet.

H. Sound Wave

You are a sound wave that is getting ready to enter the ear where you will be converted into a nerve impulse and then travel to the brain for interpretation. In the space provided below, describe all of the structures you encounter on your way to the brain. Also describe what function each structure is performing in the ear. Each of the following structures should be included in your discussion:

   a. Auricle
   b. External auditory canal
   c. Ceruminous glands
   d. Tympanic membrane
   e. Eustachian tube
   f. Auditory ossicles
   g. Oval window
   h. Cochlea
   i. Temporal lobe

I. Inquiring Patients Want to Know

You are working in a general practice medical office. Your patients ask you the following questions. In the space provided, indicate how you would respond to each question in terms the patient would understand. Use your textbook and Internet resources to develop your responses.

1. What causes an optical illusion?

   _____

   _____

2. How does LASIK surgery improve vision?

   _____

   _____

3. How does loud music damage hearing?

   _____

   _____

4. What is the reason for putting tubes in the eardrum?

   _____

   _____

5. What causes eye floaters?

   _____

   _____

6. Why do my ears get plugged when I am on an airplane?

   _____

   _____

7. What can cause an eardrum to rupture?

   _____

   _____

8. Why does a dog have a better sense of smell than a human?

   _____

   _____

9. Why can you not taste food when you have a bad cold?

   _____

   _____

10. Why do you feel dizzy when you spin around?

   _____

   _____

J. Evolve Site: Chapter 10 Animations

Directions:

1. View the Chapter 10 Animations on the Evolve site.
2. For each animation, write two true or false questions in the space provided below.
3. In the classroom, find a partner.
4. For each animation, read your two questions to your partner.
5. For each correct answer, your partner is awarded two points.
6. Next, have your partner read his or her two questions to you. Award yourself two points for each question answered correctly.
7. Continue in this manner until all the questions have been answered.
8. Record your points on your Study Guide Assignment sheet.

True or False Questions

a. Smell

   1. _____

   2. _____

b. Eye Anatomy

   1. _____

   2. _____

c. Eye: Aqueous Humor and Vitreous Humor

   1. _____

   2. _____

d. Visual Pathway

   1. _____

   2. _____

e. Pathway of Sound Waves

   1. _____

   2. _____

K. Crossword Puzzle: The Senses

Directions: Complete the crossword puzzle using the clues provided.

Across

1 Organs of taste
5 Produces tears
6 Visual purple
12 Blind spot
13 Colored part of eye
14 Earwax
15 White of the eye
16 Space between cornea and lens
21 Bending of light rays
22 This bulges for close vision
23 Receptors for color vision
24 Sense of smell
25 Where visual impulses are interpreted
26 Connects middle ear with throat
27 Stimulated by heat and cold

Down

1 Eardrum
2 Absorbs excess light rays
3 Covers front of eyeball except for cornea
4 Sense of position
7 Stimulated by heavy pressure
8 Sensitive to dim light
9 Contains vitreous humor
10 Yellow spot on retina
11 Muscle that closes the eye
17 Pain receptors
18 Auditory ossicle
19 Where taste impulses are interpreted
20 Collects sound waves

Notes

11 Endocrine System

CHAPTER ASSIGNMENTS

√ After Completing	Date Due	Textbook Page(s)	TEXTBOOK ASSIGNMENT	Possible Points	Points You Earned
		166-174	Read Chapter 11: Endocrine System		

√ After Completing	Date Due	Study Guide Page(s)	STUDY GUIDE ASSIGNMENTS (CTA: Critical Thinking Activity)	Possible Points	Points You Earned
		137	📋 Pretest	10	
		137 138	🔑 Key Term Assessment A. Definitions B. Word Parts (Add 1 point for each medical term)	6 8	
		138-141	📑 Evaluation of Learning questions	36	
		142	CTA A: Location of Endocrine Glands	20	
		143	CTA B: Pituitary Gland	20	
		143-144	CTA C: Inquiring Patients Want to Know	10	
		145	*e* Evolve Site: CTA D: Animations	8	
		146	CTA E: Crossword Puzzle	24	
		137	📋 Posttest	10	
			ADDITIONAL ASSIGNMENTS		
			TOTAL POINTS		

Notes

Name _____ Date _____

True or False

_____ 1. Endocrine glands have ducts that empty their secretions onto a surface.

_____ 2. Sex hormones are made up of proteins.

_____ 3. A target tissue is a tissue that has receptor sites for a particular hormone.

_____ 4. In an adult, an excess secretion of growth hormone can cause Down syndrome.

_____ 5. Oxytocin causes contraction of smooth muscle in the wall of the uterus.

_____ 6. Goiter results when there is a lack of iodine in the body.

_____ 7. Calcitonin functions by reducing the calcium level in the blood.

_____ 8. The adrenal glands are located above the kidneys.

_____ 9. Insulin is secreted by the beta cells of the pancreas.

_____ 10. Progesterone stimulates the production of milk in the lactating breast.

📋 **POSTTEST**

True or False

_____ 1. Sebaceous glands are exocrine glands.

_____ 2. Luteinizing hormone is produced by the anterior pituitary gland.

_____ 3. Follicle-stimulating hormone stimulates development of eggs in the ovaries and sperm in the testes.

_____ 4. Diabetes mellitus results when there is not enough antidiuretic hormone secreted by the body.

_____ 5. The thyroid gland consists of two lobes located on each side of the trachea.

_____ 6. Aldosterone reduces the calcium level in the body.

_____ 7. The parathyroid glands are located on the anterior surface of the thyroid gland.

_____ 8. The function of insulin is to decrease the blood glucose concentration.

_____ 9. The function of glucagon is to raise blood glucose levels.

_____ 10. Melatonin is a hormone that regulates the sleep/wake cycle.

🔑 **KEY TERM ASSESSMENT**

A. Definitions

Directions: Match each medical term with its definition.

_____ 1. Adenohypophysis

_____ 2. Endocrine gland

_____ 3. Exocrine gland

_____ 4. Hormone

_____ 5. Neurohypophysis

_____ 6. Target tissue

A. A substance secreted by an endocrine gland
B. A tissue (cells) that responds to a particular hormone because it has receptor sites for that hormone
C. Anterior portion of the pituitary gland
D. Gland that secretes its product directly into the blood
E. Gland that secretes its product to a surface or cavity through ducts
F. Posterior portion of the pituitary gland

B. Word Parts

Directions: Indicate the meaning of each word part in the space provided. List as many medical terms as possible that incorporate the word part in the space provided.

Word Part	Meaning of Word Part	Medical Terms That Incorporate Word Part
1. aden/o		
2. hypo-		
3. -physis		
4. endo-		
5. -crine		
6. exo-		
7. hormon/o		
8. neur/o		

EVALUATION OF LEARNING

Directions: Fill in each blank with the correct answer.

1. How do the following systems regulate body activities?

   a. Nervous system: _____

   b. Endocrine system: _____

2. What are exocrine glands?

   _____

   _____

3. What are four examples of exocrine glands?

   _____

   _____

4. How does an endocrine gland function?

   _____

   _____

5. Why must insulin be administered by injection?

   _____

   _____

6. What hormones consist of steroids?

   _____

7. How do hormones exert their action on the body?

   _____

   _____

8. What is the function of the following hormones secreted by the anterior lobe of the pituitary gland?

a. Growth hormone: _____

b. Thyroid stimulating hormone: _____

_____

c. ACTH: _____

_____

d. Follicle-stimulating hormone (FSH): _____

e. Luteinizing hormone:

Female: _____

Male: _____

f. Prolactin: _____

_____

9. What is the function of the following hormones secreted by the posterior lobe of the pituitary gland?

a. Antidiuretic hormone: _____

_____

b. Oxytocin: _____

_____

10. What makes up the thyroid hormone?

_____

11. Why does the adult thyroid gland enlarge when there is a lack of iodine in the body?

_____

_____

12. What effect do thyroid hormones have on the body?

_____

_____

13. What is the function of calcitonin?

_____

_____

14. Where are the parathyroid glands located?

_____

15. What is the function of the parathyroid hormone?

_____

_____

16. Where are the adrenal glands located?

_____

17. What is the function of mineralocorticoids secreted by the adrenal glands?

_____

_____

18. What is the name of the principal mineralocorticoid?

_____

_____

19. What is the function of glucocorticoids secreted by the adrenal cortex?

_____

_____

20. What is the principal glucocorticoid?

_____

21. What is the name given to the sex hormones secreted by the adrenal cortex?

_____

22. What causes the secretion of epinephrine and norepinephrine by the adrenal medulla?

_____

23. What effect does the secretion of epinephrine and norepinephrine have on the body?

_____

_____

24. What is the location of the pancreas in relation to the stomach?

_____

25. What are the names of the cells in the pancreas that secrete the following hormones?

    a. Glucagon: _____

    b. Insulin: _____

26. Why is it important for the body to maintain blood glucose levels within a normal range?

_____

27. What is the function of glucagon?

_____

28. What causes insulin to be secreted?

_____

29. What is the function of insulin?

_____

30. What are three factors that cause hypoactivity of insulin?

_____

_____

31. What are androgens?

_____

32. What structure secretes testosterone?

_____

33. What is the function of testosterone at the onset of puberty?

_____

_____

_____

34. What are the functions of estrogen and progesterone at the onset of puberty?

_____

_____

_____

35. What is the function of melatonin secreted by the pineal gland?

_____

_____

_____

36. What is the function of the thymus gland?

_____

_____

_____

A. Location of Endocrine Glands

Using Figure 11-2 as a reference, sketch an outline of the human body. Draw, color, and label the major endocrine glands on your sketch.

B. Pituitary Gland

You are a pituitary gland and have control over your target tissues. In the chart provided, indicate what hormone you would secrete to stimulate each of the following target tissues. Also indicate what effect each hormone would have on its target tissue.

Target Tissue	What Hormone Would You Secrete to Stimulate This Target Tissue?	What Effect Would This Hormone Have on the Target Tissue?
Thyroid gland		
Adrenal cortex		
Ovarian follicles		
Seminiferous tubules		
Ovaries		
Testes		
Mammary glands		
Kidneys		
Uterus and mammary glands		
Most body tissues		

C. Inquiring Patients Want to Know

You are working in a general practice medical office. Your patients ask you the following questions. In the space provided, indicate how you would respond to each question in terms the patient would understand. Use your textbook and Internet resources to develop your responses.

1. Why does an adolescent girl with anorexia not have a menstrual period?

_____

_____

2. How is the insulin used for insulin injections made?

_____

_____

3. Why do some diabetics take medication orally?

_____

_____

4. How does an insulin pump work?

_____

_____

5. What are anabolic steroids, and why are they sometimes abused by athletes?

_____

_____

6. What side effects can occur from taking anabolic steroids?

_____

_____

7. What is an adrenaline rush?

_____

_____

8. Why do I feel so irritable when I am having trouble with hypoglycemia?

_____

_____

9. What is the best diet to follow for hypoglycemia?

_____

_____

10. Can hypoglycemia be cured?

_____

_____

D. Evolve Site: Chapter 11 Animations

Directions:

1. View the Chapter 11 Animations on the Evolve site.
2. For each animation, write two true or false questions in the space provided below.
3. In the classroom, find a partner.
4. For each animation, read your two questions to your partner.
5. For each correct answer, your partner is awarded two points.
6. Next, have your partner read his or her two questions to you. Award yourself two points for each question answered correctly.
7. Continue in this manner until all the questions have been answered.
8. Record your points on your Study Guide Assignment sheet.

True or False Questions

a. Thyroid Gland

    1. _____

    2. _____

b. Function of Insulin

    1. _____

    2. _____

E. Crossword Puzzle: Endocrine System

Directions: Complete the crossword puzzle using the clues provided.

Across

- **2** Responsible for development of male reproductive structures
- **4** Thyroid hormone deficiency
- **7** Stimulates milk production by mammary gland
- **8** Reduces blood calcium level
- **10** Fight-or-flight hormone
- **13** Stimulates growth of bones and muscles
- **14** Glucocorticoid that counteracts inflammatory response
- **16** Glands with ducts
- **18** Causes uterus to contract
- **21** Sex hormones
- **22** Regulates circadian rhythms
- **24** Causes ovulation to occur

Down

- **1** Stimulates development of eggs and sperm
- **3** Glands that secrete hormones
- **5** Located on top of kidneys
- **6** Protruding eyes
- **9** Causes uterus to thicken
- **11** Increases blood calcium levels
- **12** Raises blood glucose level
- **15** Decreases blood glucose level
- **17** Dwarfism with mental retardation
- **19** Stimulates adrenal gland to secrete cortisol
- **20** Promotes reabsorption of water by kidneys
- **23** Stimulates thyroid to secrete thyroid hormone

12 Circulatory System

CHAPTER ASSIGNMENTS

√ After Completing	Date Due	Textbook Page(s)	TEXTBOOK ASSIGNMENT	Possible Points	Points You Earned
		175-193	Read Chapter 12: Circulatory System		

√ After Completing	Date Due	Study Guide Page(s)	STUDY GUIDE ASSIGNMENTS (CTA: Critical Thinking Activity)	Possible Points	Points You Earned
		149	Pretest	10	
		150	Key Term Assessment A. Definitions B. Word Parts (Add 1 point for each medical term)	15 15	
		151-156	Evaluation of Learning questions	72	
		157	Evolve Site: CTA A: Body Spectrum: Heart—Cross Section	10	
		157	Evolve Site: CTA B: Body Spectrum: Heart Circulation	10	
		157	Evolve Site: CTA C: Body Spectrum: Coronary Vessels	10	
		157	Evolve Site: CTA D: Name That Blood Cell (Record points earned)		
		157-158	CTA E: Blood Clotting	20	
		158-159	CTA F: Inquiring Patients Want to Know	10	
		159-160	CTA G: Evolve Site: Animations	56	
		161	CTA H: Crossword Puzzle	30	
		149	Posttest	10	

√ After Completing	Date Due	Study Guide Page(s)	STUDY GUIDE ASSIGNMENTS (CTA: Critical Thinking Activity)	Possible Points	Points You Earned
			ADDITIONAL ASSIGNMENTS		
			TOTAL POINTS		

Name _____   Date _____

True or False

_____ 1. The pointed end of the heart is the apex.

_____ 2. The myocardium forms the bulk of the heart wall.

_____ 3. The coronary arteries branch off the aorta to supply the heart with oxygen and nutrients.

_____ 4. The SA node is located in the right atrium.

_____ 5. The adult male has 5 to 6 L of blood.

_____ 6. Erythrocytes lack a nucleus.

_____ 7. Vitamin K is necessary for the absorption of vitamin B_{12} from the intestines.

_____ 8. Leukocytes defend the body against disease.

_____ 9. Thrombocytes develop from large cells known as macrophages.

_____ 10. Veins carry blood toward the heart.

? POSTTEST

True or False

_____ 1. The peritoneum is the loose-fitting sac that encloses the heart.

_____ 2. The superior vena cava returns blood to the heart from the lower extremities.

_____ 3. The mitral valve is located between the right atrium and right ventricle.

_____ 4. When the ventricles are contracting, the atrioventricular (AV) valves are open.

_____ 5. The buffy coat is made up of white blood cells and platelets.

_____ 6. Neutrophils are the first leukocytes to respond to tissue damage.

_____ 7. Bile is the yellow pigment that results from the breakdown of red blood cells.

_____ 8. Acute infections cause an increase in the number of neutrophils.

_____ 9. Thrombin converts fibrinogen to fibrin.

_____ 10. Microscopic arteries are known as arterioles.

A. Definitions

Directions: Match each medical term with its definition.

_____ 1. Atrioventricular valve

_____ 2. Cardiac cycle

_____ 3. Coagulation

_____ 4. Conduction myofibers

_____ 5. Diapedesis

_____ 6. Diastole

_____ 7. Erythrocyte

_____ 8. Erythropoiesis

_____ 9. Erythropoietin

_____ 10. Hemocytoblast

_____ 11. Hematopoiesis

_____ 12. Leukocyte

_____ 13. Semilunar valve

_____ 14. Systole

_____ 15. Thrombocyte

A. A complete heartbeat consisting of contraction and relaxation of both atria and both ventricles

B. A hormone released by the kidneys that stimulates red blood cell production

C. A stem cell in the bone marrow from which the blood cells arise

D. Blood cell production, which occurs in the red bone marrow

E. Cardiac muscle cells specialized for conducting action potentials to the myocardium; part of the conduction system of the heart; also called Purkinje fibers

F. Contraction phase of the cardiac cycle

G. One of the formed elements of the blood; functions in blood clotting

H. Red blood cell

I. Relaxation phase of the cardiac cycle

J. The process by which white blood cells squeeze between the cells in a vessel wall to enter the tissue spaces outside the blood vessel

K. The process of blood clotting

L. The process of red blood cell formation

M. Valve between a ventricle of the heart and the vessel that carries blood away from the ventricle

N. Valve between an atrium and a ventricle in the heart

O. White blood cell

B. Word Parts

Directions: Indicate the meaning of each word part in the space provided. List as many medical terms as possible that incorporate the word part in the space provided.

Word Part	Meaning of Word Part	Medical Terms That Incorporate Word Part
atri/o		
ventricul/o		
coagul/o		
-tion		
dia-		
erythr/o		
-cyt		
-poieses		
-poietin		
hem/o		
-blast		
hemat/o		
leuk/o		
thromb/o		
oste/o		

Directions: Fill in each blank with the correct answer.

1. What is the function of the heart?

_____

_____

2. How large is the average human heart?

_____

3. Describe the following layers of the pericardium:
   a. Fibrous pericardium: _____
   b. Parietal pericardium: _____
   c. Visceral pericardium: _____

4. What is the function of the epicardium?

_____

_____

5. What makes up the myocardium?

_____

6. Why does the endocardium have a smooth surface?

_____

7. What type of blood enters the right atrium?

_____

8. The superior vena cava returns blood to the heart from what parts of the body?

_____

9. The inferior vena cava returns blood to the heart from what parts of the body?

_____

10. What is the interarterial septum?

_____

11. What is the function of the right ventricle?

_____

12. What is the function of the left ventricle?

_____

13. Why does the left ventricle have a thicker myocardium than the right ventricle?

_____

_____

14. What is the interventricular septum?

_____

_____

15. Describe the location and function of each of the following valves:

Valve	Location	Function
a. Tricuspid valve		
b. Bicuspid valve		
c. Pulmonary semilunar valve		
d. Aortic semilunar valve		

16. Starting with the right atrium, trace the path of the blood through the heart.

_____

_____

_____

_____

17. What are the names of the vessels that supply the heart with oxygen?

_____

18. What is the function of the SA node?

_____

_____

19. What is the function of the AV node?

_____

_____

20. What structures transmit the heart's impulse from the AV node to the ventricles?

_____

21. What occurs with each of the following during atrial systole?

   a. AV valves: _____

   b. Atria: _____

   c. Ventricles: _____

   d. Semilunar valves: _____

22. What are each of the following structures doing during ventricular systole?

   a. AV valves: _____

   b. Atria: _____

   c. Ventricles: _____

   d. Semilunar valves: _____

23. What causes each of the following heart sounds?

a. Lubb:_____

b. Dupp:_____

24. What causes a heart murmur?

_____

25. How does blood function as transportation in the body?

_____

_____

_____

26. How does blood function to regulate the body?

_____

_____

_____

27. How does blood function as protection for the body?

_____

_____

_____

28. What percentage of the blood is made up of the following?

a. Plasma:_____

b. Red blood cells: _____

29. What makes up the buffy coat?

_____

30. What is the function of the following plasma proteins?

a. Albumins: _____

_____

b. Globulins: _____

_____

c. Fibrinogen: _____

31. What are the waste products of protein and nucleic acid catabolism? How are these waste products excreted?

_____

32. What seven cells develop from a hemocytoblast?

_____

_____

33. What is the normal range for a red blood count for the following?

    a. Adult male: _____

    b. Adult female: _____

34. Describe the appearance of a mature red blood cell.

_____

35. What is the function of erythrocytes?

_____

36. What is the name of the hormone that stimulates the red bone marrow to produce erythrocytes?

_____

37. What vitamins and minerals are necessary for the production of red blood cells?

_____

38. What is the function of the intrinsic factor?

_____

39. What condition results when there is a lack of the intrinsic factor?

_____

40. What is the life span of a red blood cell?

_____

41. What happens when a red blood cell is worn out?

_____

_____

42. What is bilirubin?

_____

43. What is the normal range for a white blood count?

_____

44. Where do leukocytes do their work?

_____

45. What is diapedesis?

_____

46. What is the function of neutrophils?

_____

47. What causes an increase in eosinophils?

_____

48. What is the function of the following substances secreted by a basophil?

   a. Histamine: _____

   b. Heparin: _____

49. What are macrophages, and what is their function?

   _____

   _____

50. What is another name for a thrombocyte?

   _____

51. What is a megakaryocyte?

   _____

52. What is the normal range for a platelet count?

   _____

53. What is the function of thrombocytes?

   _____

54. What is the term for the stoppage of bleeding?

   _____

55. What is the function of serotonin secreted by platelets when a blood vessel is torn or cut?

   _____

   _____

56. What is the function of a platelet plug?

   _____

57. What are procoagulants?

   _____

58. How does blood stay in a liquid form in the blood vessels?

   _____

   _____

59. What is necessary to convert inactive prothrombin to active thrombin?

   _____

60. What is the function of thrombin?

   _____

61. Why does a blood clot retract after it forms?

   _____

   _____

62. What antigens and antibodies occur with each of the following blood types?

Blood Type	Blood Antigens	Blood Antibodies
Type A		
Type B		
Type AB		
Type O		

63. What does it mean if someone is Rh positive? What does it mean if he or she is Rh negative?

_____

_____

64. What is the function of arteries?

_____

65. What are the three layers that make up the wall of an artery?

_____

66. What makes up the wall of a capillary?

_____

67. What is the function of veins?

_____

68. Why can veins hold more blood than arteries?

_____

69. What is the function of venous valves?

_____

_____

70. What is the function of the pulmonary circuit?

_____

_____

71. What is the function of the systemic circuit?

_____

72. What changes occur to the following parts of the circulatory system as an individual ages?

a. Left ventricle: _____

b. Endocardium: _____

c. Valves of the heart: _____

d. Dysrhythmias: _____

_____

CRITICAL THINKING ACTIVITIES

A. Evolve Site: Body Spectrum
Circulatory: Heart—Cross Section

Body Spectrum directions:

1. Access the Body Spectrum program on the Evolve site.
2. If necessary, access the HELP screen for directions on using the Body Spectrum program.
3. Go to the Contents screen.
4. Select the following category from the Contents screen:
   Circulatory
5. Select the following anatomic diagram:
   Heart—Cross Section
6. Identify the structures on the diagram.
7. Print out the diagram.

B. Evolve Site: Body Spectrum
Circulatory: Heart Circulation

Directions: Identify the structures on this diagram following the Body Spectrum directions outlined under CTA A.

C. Evolve Site: Body Spectrum
Circulatory: Coronary Vessels

Directions: Identify the structures on this diagram following the Body Spectrum directions outlined under CTA A.

D. Evolve Site: Name That Blood Cell
Access the Evolve site to complete this activity. Record your points earned on your assignment sheet.

E. Blood Clotting
You are a blood vessel located in the finger of a human. Your human is cutting up vegetables and accidentally severs you with a knife. Describe what tasks are performed to heal you during each of the hemostatic processes listed below.

a. Vascular Constriction:

_____

_____

_____

_____

_____

_____

_____

b. Platelet Plug Formation:

_____

_____

_____

_____

_____

_____

_____

_____

157

c. Coagulation:

_____

_____

_____

_____

_____

_____

F. Inquiring Patients Want to Know

You are working in a general practice medical office. Your patients ask you the following questions. In the space provided, indicate how you would respond to each question in terms the patient would understand. Use your textbook and Internet resources to develop your responses.

1. Why is blood red?

_____

_____

2. Why does a bruise eventually turn yellow?

_____

_____

3. What causes varicose veins?

_____

_____

4. What is the difference between iron-deficiency anemia and pernicious anemia?

_____

_____

5. How does a pacemaker work?

_____

_____

6. What happens in the body during carbon monoxide poisoning?

_____

_____

7. What is done with the plasma that is collected at plasma donor centers?

_____

_____

8. What happens to the heart when it is defibrillated?

_____

_____

9. How can poor circulation cause gangrene?

_____

_____

10. Why does the physician look at the blood vessels in my eye?

_____

_____

G. Evolve Site: Chapter 12 Animations

Directions:
1. View the Chapter 12 Animations on the Evolve site.
2. For each animation, write two true or false questions in the space provided below.
3. In the classroom, find a partner.
4. For each animation, read your two questions to your partner.
5. For each correct answer, your partner is awarded two points.
6. Next, have your partner read his or her two questions to you. Award yourself two points for each question answered correctly.
7. Continue in this manner until all the questions have been answered.
8. Record your points on your Study Guide Assignment sheet.

True or False Questions

a. Location of the Heart

1. _____

2. _____

b. Chambers of the Heart

1. _____

2. _____

c. Heart Valves and Sounds

1. _____

2. _____

d. Conduction of Heart Impulses

1. _____

2. _____

e. The Cardiac Cycle

1. _____

2. _____

f. Red Blood Cells

   1. _____

   2. _____

g. White Blood Cells

   1. _____

   2. _____

h. Phagocytes

   1. _____

   2. _____

i. Platelets and Blood Clotting

   1. _____

   2. _____

j. Blood Grouping

   1. _____

   2. _____

k. Rh Compatibility

   1. _____

   2. _____

l. Pulmonary Circulation

   1. _____

   2. _____

m. Systemic Circulation

   1. _____

   2. _____

n. Physiology of Blood Pressure

   1. _____

   2. _____

H. Crossword Puzzle: Circulatory System

Directions: Complete the crossword puzzle using the clues provided.

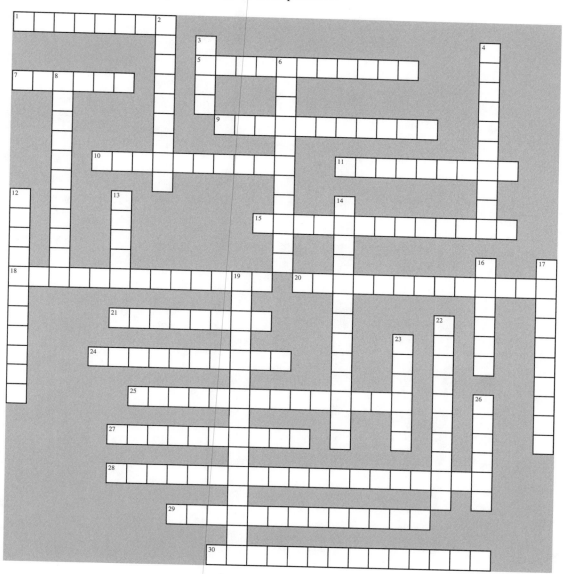

Across

1 Secretes histamine and heparin
5 Inner lining of heart wall
7 Abnormal heart sound
9 Sac that encloses the heart
10 Engulfs bacteria by phagocytosis
11 Consists of white blood cells and platelets
15 Shape of RBC
18 Production of blood cells
20 Between left atrium and left ventricle
21 Largest WBC
24 Forms bulk of heart wall
25 Between right atrium and right ventricle
27 Produces antibodies
28 Also known as the epicardium
29 Chamber that pumps blood to entire body
30 Stimulates RBC production

Down

2 White blood cell
3 Carries blood toward heart
4 Stoppage of bleeding
6 Tiny blood vessels
8 Receives deoxygenated blood
12 Red blood cell
13 No antigen blood
14 Inhibits clotting
16 Pacemaker of the heart
17 Receives oxygenated blood
19 Needed for absorption of vitamin B_{12}
22 Transports oxygen
23 Carries blood away from heart
26 Liquid part of blood

Notes

13 Respiratory System

CHAPTER ASSIGNMENTS

√ After Completing	Date Due	Textbook Page(s)	TEXTBOOK ASSIGNMENT	Possible Points	Points You Earned
		194-201	Read Chapter 13: Respiratory System		

√ After Completing	Date Due	Study Guide Page(s)	STUDY GUIDE ASSIGNMENTS (CTA: Critical Thinking Activity)	Possible Points	Points You Earned
		165	Pretest	10	
		165	Term Key Term Assessment	7	
		166-168	Evaluation of Learning questions	34	
		169	Evolve Site: CTA A: Body Spectrum: Respiratory System	10	
		169	Evolve Site: CTA B: Body Spectrum: Nasal Cavity and Pharynx	10	
		169	Evolve Site: CTA C: Body Spectrum: Larynx and Upper Trachea	10	
		169-170	CTA D: Inquiring Patients Want to Know	10	
		170-171	Evolve Site: CTA E: Animations	32	
		172	CTA F: Crossword Puzzle	23	
		165	Posttest	10	
			ADDITIONAL ASSIGNMENTS		
			TOTAL POINTS		

Name _____   Date _____

True or False

_____ 1. The lungs are located in the lower respiratory tract.

_____ 2. The function of mucus in the respiratory tract is to destroy microorganisms.

_____ 3. The nasal septum divides the nose into two parts.

_____ 4. The auditory (eustachian) tubes open into the oropharynx.

_____ 5. The uvula is the posterior portion of the soft palate that helps direct food into the oropharynx.

_____ 6. The glottis prevents food and water from entering the trachea.

_____ 7. The vocal cords are made up of ligaments.

_____ 8. The right lung is divided into two lobes.

_____ 9. The process of taking air into the lungs is known as inhalation.

_____ 10. Sneezing is a nonrespiratory air movement.

?≣ **POSTTEST**

True or False

_____ 1. The exchange of gases between the blood and tissue cells is known as external respiration.

_____ 2. The paranasal sinuses are lined by a serous membrane.

_____ 3. Cilia propel mucus toward the pharynx.

_____ 4. The nasal conchae separate the nasal cavity from the oral cavity.

_____ 5. The oropharynx receives air, food, and water from the oral cavity.

_____ 6. The thyroid cartilage located in the larynx is commonly called the Adam's apple.

_____ 7. The larynx is supported by 15 to 20 C-shaped pieces of hyaline cartilage.

_____ 8. The pleura is a double-layered serous membrane that encloses the lungs.

_____ 9. Internal respiration is the exchange of gases between the tissue cells and the blood.

_____ 10. The respiratory center is located in the hypothalamus.

🔑Term **KEY TERM ASSESSMENT**

Directions: Match each medical term with its definition.

_____ 1. Alveoli

_____ 2. Bronchial tree

_____ 3. External respiration

_____ 4. Internal respiration

_____ 5. Respiratory membrane

_____ 6. Surfactant

_____ 7. Ventilation

A. A substance, produced by certain cells in lung tissue, that reduces surface tension between fluid molecules that line the respiratory membrane and helps keep the alveolus from collapsing

B. Any surface in the lungs where diffusion occurs; consists of the layers that the gases must pass through to get into or out of the alveoli

C. Exchange of gases between the blood and tissue cells

D. Exchange of gases between the lungs and the blood

E. Microscopic dilations of terminal bronchioles in the lungs, where diffusion of gases occurs

F. Movement of air into and out of the lungs; breathing

G. The bronchi and all their branches that function as passageways between the trachea and the alveoli

Directions: Fill in each blank with the correct answer.

1. What are the functions of the respiratory system?

   _____

   _____

2. What is external respiration?

   _____

3. What is internal respiration?

   _____

4. What structures are located in the upper respiratory tract?

   _____

5. What structures are located in the lower respiratory tract?

   _____

6. Describe the following parts of the nose:

   a. Nasal cavity: _____

   b. Nasal septum: _____

   c. Nostrils: _____

   d. Internal nares: _____

   e. Palate: _____

   f. Uvula: _____

7. What is the difference between the hard palate and soft palate?

   _____

   _____

8. What are the functions of the nasal conchae?

   _____

   _____

9. What are the paranasal sinuses?

   _____

   _____

10. What are three functions of the paranasal sinuses?

   _____

   _____

11. What is the function of the mucus secreted by the mucous membrane of the nose?

_____

12. What is the function of the cilia in the nasal cavity?

_____

_____

13. What is the nasopharynx?

_____

_____

14. What is the function of the eustachian tubes?

_____

_____

15. What is the oropharynx?

_____

_____

16. What is the laryngopharynx?

_____

17. What is the layman's term for the thyroid cartilage?

_____

18. What is the function of the epiglottis?

_____

_____

19. What are the functions of the following?

a. False vocal cords: _____

b. True vocal cords: _____

20. What is the glottis?

_____

21. What holds the trachea open?

_____

22. Describe the components of the bronchial tree.

_____

_____

_____

23. Why do the walls of the alveolar ducts and alveoli consist of simple squamous epithelium?

_____

24. Why are the lungs soft and spongy?

_____

_____

25. How does the right lung differ in appearance from the left lung?

_____

_____

26. What is the pleura?

_____

_____

27. What is another name for breathing?

_____

28. What is included in one breath?

_____

29. How does air move into the lungs during inhalation?

_____

_____

30. How does air move out of the lungs during exhalation?

_____

_____

31. Where is the respiratory center located?

_____

32. What happens if there is an increase in carbon dioxide in the blood?

_____

_____

33. What are examples of nonrespiratory air movements?

_____

_____

34. What changes occur to the following parts of the respiratory system because of aging?

    a. Cartilage in the walls of the trachea and bronchi: _____

    b. Bronchioles: _____

    c. Alveoli: _____

CRITICAL THINKING ACTIVITIES

A. Evolve Site: Body Spectrum
Respiratory: Respiratory System

Body Spectrum directions:
1. Access the Body Spectrum program on the Evolve site.
2. If necessary, access the HELP screen for directions on using the Body Spectrum program.
3. Go to the Contents screen.
4. Select the following category from the Contents screen:
   Respiratory
5. Select the following anatomic diagram:
   Respiratory System
6. Identify the structures on the diagram.
7. Print out the diagram.

B. Evolve Site: Body Spectrum
Respiratory: Nasal Cavity and Pharynx

Directions: Identify the structures on this diagram following the Body Spectrum directions outlined under CTA A.

C. Evolve Site: Body Spectrum
Respiratory: Larynx and Upper Trachea

Directions: Identify the structures on this diagram following the Body Spectrum directions outlined under CTA A.

D. Inquiring Patients Want to Know
You are working in a general practice medical office. Your patients ask you the following questions. In the space provided, indicate how you would respond to each question in terms the patient would understand. Use your textbook and Internet resources to develop your responses.

1. What happens in the body when you sneeze?

_____

_____

2. Why do men have a deeper voice than women?

_____

_____

3. What do your tonsils do?

_____

_____

4. What damage does smoking do to the respiratory tract?

_____

_____

5. What do sinuses do?

_____

_____

6. Can you die from holding your breath?

_____

_____

7. What makes you yawn when someone else yawns?

_____

_____

8. Is it bad for you if you're drinking water and it goes down the wrong tube?

_____

_____

9. Why does your nose run when you have allergies?

_____

_____

10. Can you permanently lose your voice from laryngitis?

_____

_____

E. Evolve Site: Chapter 13 Animations

Directions:

1. View the Chapter 13 Animations on the Evolve site.
2. For each animation, write two true or false questions in the space provided below.
3. In the classroom, find a partner.
4. For each animation, read your two questions to your partner.
5. For each correct answer, your partner is awarded two points.
6. Next, have your partner read his or her two questions to you. Award yourself two points for each question answered correctly.
7. Continue in this manner until all the questions have been answered.
8. Record your points on your Study Guide Assignment sheet.

True or False Questions

a. Air Distribution through the Upper Respiratory Tract

1. _____

2. _____

b. Air Distribution through the Lower Respiratory Tract

1. _____

2. _____

c. Respiratory Mucosa

1. _____

2. _____

d. Bronchi and Bronchioles

　　1. _____

　　2. _____

e. Respiration

　　1. _____

　　2. _____

f. External Respiration

　　1. _____

　　2. _____

g. Internal Respiration

　　1. _____

　　2. _____

h. Respiratory Membrane

　　1. _____

　　2. _____

F. Crossword Puzzle: Respiratory System

Directions: Complete the crossword puzzle using the clues provided.

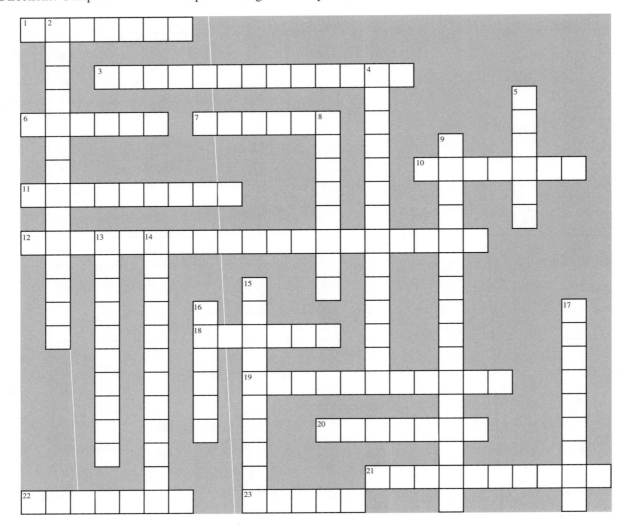

Across

1 Respiratory center
3 Contains serous fluid produced by the pleura
6 Separates nasal cavity from oral cavity
7 Opening between oral cavity and oropharynx
10 Throat
11 Has three lobes
12 Exchange of gases between tissues and blood
18 Voice box
19 Divides nose into two parts
20 Tiny air sacs
21 Prevents food from entering trachea
22 Windpipe
23 Air-filled cavity in skull

Down

2 Equalizes air pressure
4 Produces sound
5 Common cold
8 Nonrespiratory air movement
9 Adam's apple
13 Expelling air from the lungs
14 Bony ridges that warm air
15 Inflammation of the vocal cords
16 Membrane around the lungs
17 Whooping cough

14 Digestive System

CHAPTER ASSIGNMENTS

√ After Completing	Date Due	Textbook Page(s)	TEXTBOOK ASSIGNMENT	Possible Points	Points You Earned
		202-216	Read Chapter 14: Digestive System		
√ After Completing	**Date Due**	**Study Guide Page(s)**	**STUDY GUIDE ASSIGNMENTS (CTA: Critical Thinking Activity)**	**Possible Points**	**Points You Earned**
		175	Pretest	10	
		175	Key Term Assessment	6	
		176-181	Evaluation of Learning questions	66	
		182	Evolve Site: CTA A: Body Spectrum: Digestive System	10	
		182	Evolve Site: CTA B: Body Spectrum: Teeth	10	
		182	CTA C: Structure of a Tooth	11	
		182	Evolve Site: CTA D: Body Spectrum: Salivary Glands	10	
		182	Evolve Site: CTA E: Body Spectrum: Anatomy of Large Intestine	10	
		182	Evolve Site: CTA F: Body Spectrum: Intestinal Secretion Sources	10	
		183	CTA G: Pizza Digestion	20	
		183-184	CTA H: Inquiring Patients Want to Know	10	
		184-185	Evolve Site: CTA I: Animations	16	
		186	CTA J: Crossword Puzzle	38	
		175	Posttest	10	
			ADDITIONAL ASSIGNMENTS		
			TOTAL POINTS		

Notes

Name _____ Date _____

True or False

_____ 1. The pancreas is an accessory organ of the digestive system.

_____ 2. Peristalsis consists of rhythmic waves of contractions that propel food particles through the digestive tract.

_____ 3. The buccinator muscle connects the tongue anteriorly to the floor of the mouth.

_____ 4. The total number of primary teeth is 32.

_____ 5. Saliva moistens and lubricates the food.

_____ 6. The esophagus provides a passageway for food between the pharynx and stomach.

_____ 7. The first part of the small intestine is the duodenum.

_____ 8. Hepatocytes are liver cells.

_____ 9. Iron is stored in the liver.

_____ 10. The function of the gallbladder is to produce bile.

? POSTTEST

True or False

_____ 1. The taking in of food is known as mastication.

_____ 2. Mechanical digestion breaks down food into smaller particles through the mixing actions of the stomach.

_____ 3. The hard palate and uvula direct food away from the nasal cavity and into the oropharynx during swallowing.

_____ 4. Cuspids are teeth that have sharp edges used for biting food.

_____ 5. The cardiac sphincter acts as a valve between the stomach and small intestine.

_____ 6. The intrinsic factor aids in the absorption of vitamin B_{12} from the digestive tract.

_____ 7. Chyme is a semifluid that results when food is broken down in the stomach.

_____ 8. The large intestine functions in the absorption of nutrients.

_____ 9. Bile salts act as emulsifying agents to break down fat into small fat droplets.

_____ 10. The end product of protein digestion is glucose.

Term KEY TERM ASSESSMENT

Directions: Match each medical term with its definition.

_____ 1. Absorption

_____ 2. Chyme

_____ 3. Mesentery

_____ 4. Peristalsis

_____ 5. Plicae circulares

_____ 6. Rugae

A. Circular folds in the mucosa and submucosa of the small intestine
B. Extensions of peritoneum that are associated with the intestine
C. Longitudinal folds in the mucosa of the stomach
D. Rhythmic contractions of the intestine that move food along the digestive tract
E. The passage of digestive end products from the gastrointestinal tract into the blood or lymph
F. The semifluid mixture of food and gastric juice that leaves the stomach through the pyloric sphincter

Directions: Fill in each blank with the correct answer.

1. What are two other names for the digestive tract?

   _____

2. What structures make up the digestive tract?

   _____

   _____

3. What are the accessory organs of digestion?

   _____

   _____

4. What is ingestion?

   _____

5. What occurs during mechanical digestion?

   _____

   _____

6. What occurs during chemical digestion?

   _____

   _____

7. What is deglutition?

   _____

8. What is peristalsis?

   _____

   _____

9. What are the four layers of the digestive tract?

   _____

10. What are the functions of the sensory receptors located in the lips?

    _____

11. What muscle makes up the cheeks?

    _____

12. Describe the difference between the hard palate and soft palate.

    _____

    _____

    _____

13. What is the function of the uvula?

_____

_____

14. What is the lingual frenulum?

_____

15. What are two functions of the papillae located on the tongue?

_____

_____

16. What is the function of the lingual tonsils?

_____

17. What is the function of the tongue?

_____

_____

18. How many teeth make up the following?

a. Primary teeth: _____

b. Secondary teeth: _____

19. What are the functions of the following teeth?

a. Incisors: _____

b. Cuspids: _____

c. Bicuspids and molars: _____

20. Describe the following three main parts of a tooth:

a. Crown: _____

b. Root: _____

c. Neck: _____

21. Describe the following structures that make up a tooth:

a. Pulp cavity: _____

b. Pulp: _____

c. Root canal: _____

d. Apical foramen: _____

e. Dentin: _____

f. Cementum: _____

g. Periodontal ligaments: _____

h. Enamel: _____

22. What are the names and locations of the three salivary glands?

Name	Location

23. What is the function of saliva?

_____

_____

_____

24. What are the three regions of the pharynx?

_____

25. What is the function of the esophagus?

_____

26. What is the function of the esophageal sphincter?

_____

27. Describe the following structures that make up the stomach:

a. Cardiac region: _____

b. Fundus: _____

c. Body: _____

d. Lesser curvature: _____

e. Greater curvature: _____

f. Pyloric region: _____

g. Pyloric sphincter: _____

28. What are rugae, and what is their function?

_____

_____

29. Indicate the type of gastric gland cells that produce the following gastric secretions and the function of each secretion.

Gastric Gland Secretion	Secreted by	Function
a. Thick and alkaline mucus		
b. Thin and watery mucus		
c. Hydrochloric acid		
d. Intrinsic factor		
e. Pepsinogen		

30. What is the function of pepsin?

_____

31. How is inactive pepsinogen converted to active pepsin?

_____

32. What is chyme?

_____

33. What causes gastric juice to be released during the cephalic phase?

_____

34. What causes gastric juice to be released during the gastric phase?

_____

35. What triggers the intestinal phase of gastric secretion regulation?

_____

36. What is the function of the small intestine?

_____

_____

37. What is the function of the plicae circulares?

_____

38. Describe the appearance of the villi. What is the function of villi?

_____

_____

39. What are the three regions of the small intestine?

_____

40. What is the function of the mesentery?

_____

41. What are the functions of the following enzymes?
    a. Peptidase: _____
    b. Maltase, sucrose, and lactase: _____
    c. Intestinal lipase: _____

42. What is the ileocecal junction?

_____

43. What are the four regions of the large intestine?

_____

44. What are the four parts of the colon?

_____

_____

45. What is the function of the large intestine?

_____

_____

46. What is the function of the mucus secreted by the large intestine?

_____

_____

47. What is the function of the falciform ligament of the liver?

_____

_____

48. What are hepatocytes?

_____

49. What substances are stored in the liver?

_____

_____

50. What is the function of Kupffer cells?

_____

_____

51. What makes up bile?

_____

52. What are the functions of bile salts?

_____

_____

53. How are bile pigments produced?

_____

_____

54. What is the name of the principal bile pigment?

_____

55. What is the function of the gallbladder?

_____

56. What causes the release of cholecystokinin?

_____

57. What is the function of cholecystokinin?

_____

_____

58. What is the function of the islets of Langerhans?

_____

59. What is the function of pancreatic acinar cells?

_____

_____

60. What is the function of the pancreatic duct?

_____

_____

61. What digestive enzymes are found in pancreatic juice?

_____

62. What effect does cholecystokinin have on the pancreas?

_____

_____

63. What are the end products of carbohydrate digestion?

_____

64. What are the end products of protein digestion?

_____

65. What are the end products of lipid digestion?

_____

66. In what part of the small intestine does most absorption take place?

_____

CRITICAL THINKING ACTIVITIES

A. Evolve Site: Body Spectrum

Digestive: Digestive System

Body Spectrum directions:

1. Access the Body Spectrum program on the Evolve site.

2. If necessary, access the HELP screen for directions on using the Body Spectrum program.

3. Go to the Contents screen.

4. Select the following category from the Contents screen:
   Digestive

5. Select the following anatomic diagram:
   Digestive System

6. Identify the structures on the diagram.

7. Print out the diagram.

B. Evolve Site: Body Spectrum

Digestive: Teeth

Directions: Identify the structures on this diagram following the Body Spectrum directions outlined under CTA A.

C. Structure of a Tooth

Using Figure 14-4 in your textbook as a reference, label each of the structures of a tooth on the following diagram.

(Modified from Applegate E: *The anatomy and physiology learning system,* ed 4, St. Louis, 2011, Saunders.)

D. Evolve Site: Body Spectrum

Digestive: Salivary Glands

Directions: Identify the structures on this diagram following the Body Spectrum directions outlined under CTA A.

E. Evolve Site: Body Spectrum

Digestive: Anatomy of Large Intestine

Directions: Identify the structures on this diagram following the Body Spectrum directions outlined under CTA A.

F. Evolve Site: Body Spectrum

Digestive: Intestinal Secretion Sources

Directions: Identify the structures on this diagram following the Body Spectrum directions outlined under CTA A.

G. Pizza Digestion

You are a slice of pizza that has just been eaten by a human. Starting at the mouth, describe what you will go through during the digestive process.

_____
_____
_____
_____
_____
_____
_____
_____
_____
_____
_____
_____
_____
_____
_____
_____
_____
_____
_____
_____
_____
_____

H. Inquiring Patients Want to Know

You are working in a general practice medical office. Your patients ask you the following questions. In the space provided, indicate how you would respond to each question in terms the patient would understand. Use your textbook and Internet resources to develop your responses.

1. What is a cleft palate?

_____
_____

2. What causes cavities?

_____
_____

3. How does fluoride make your teeth stronger?

_____
_____

4. What causes heartburn?

_____

_____

5. What causes vomiting?

_____

_____

6. What causes someone to be lactose intolerant?

_____

_____

7. What is an ulcer?

_____

_____

8. What causes a hiatal hernia?

_____

_____

9. What causes gallstones?

_____

_____

10. How does drinking cause cirrhosis of the liver?

_____

_____

I. Evolve Site: Chapter 14 Animations

Directions:

1. View the Chapter 14 Animations on the Evolve site.
2. For each animation, write two true or false questions in the space provided below.
3. In the classroom, find a partner.
4. For each animation, read your two questions to your partner.
5. For each correct answer, your partner is awarded two points.
6. Next, have your partner read his or her two questions to you. Award yourself two points for each question answered correctly.
7. Continue in this manner until all the questions have been answered.
8. Record your points on your Study Guide Assignment sheet.

True or False Questions

a. Esophagus

    1. _____

    2. _____

b. Stomach

    1. _____

    2. _____

c. Small Intestine

    1. _____

    2. _____

d. Large Intestine

    1. _____

    2. _____

J. Crossword Puzzle: Digestive System

Directions: Complete the crossword puzzle using the clues provided.

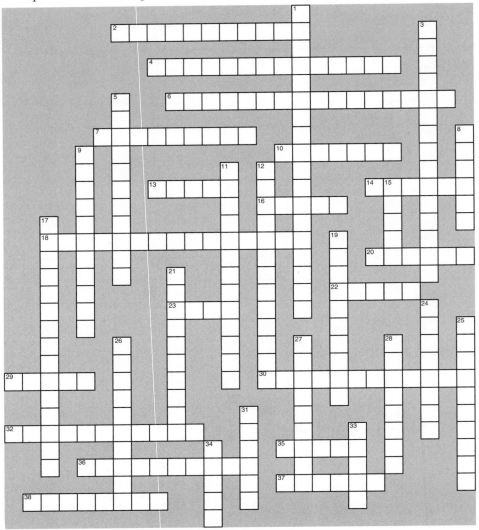

Across

2 Propels food through GI tract
4 Most food absorption occurs here
6 Valve between stomach and small intestine
7 Food tube
10 End product of carbohydrate digestion
13 Semifluid mixture of food and gastric juice
14 Innermost layer of GI tract
16 Allow stomach to expand
18 Aids in absorption of vitamin B_{12}
20 Moistens and lubricates food
22 Visible part of the tooth
23 Part of tooth that contains nerves and blood vessels
29 Last part of small intestine
30 S-shaped curve of large intestine
32 Stores bile
35 Increase surface area for food absorption
36 Length of GI tract
37 Hardest substance in the body
38 First part of small intestine

Down

1 Secrete insulin and glucagon
3 Causes gallbladder to contract
5 Chewing
8 Teeth used to crush and grind food
9 Swallowing
11 Triggered by seeing and smelling food
12 Largest salivary glands
15 Soft palate projection
17 Connects tongue to floor of mouth
19 Cheek muscle
21 Liver cell
24 Tongue projections that contain taste buds
25 End products of protein digestion
26 Removal of wastes through anus
27 Taking in of food
28 Teeth used to bite food
31 Forms bulk of tooth
33 Produces and secretes bile
34 Blind pouch in large intestine

15 Urinary System

CHAPTER ASSIGNMENTS

√ After Completing	Date Due	Textbook Page(s)	TEXTBOOK ASSIGNMENT	Possible Points	Points You Earned
		217-224	Read Chapter 15: Urinary System		

√ After Completing	Date Due	Study Guide Page(s)	STUDY GUIDE ASSIGNMENTS (CTA: Critical Thinking Activity)	Possible Points	Points You Earned
		189	Pretest	10	
		189	Term Key Term Assessment	4	
		190-193	Evaluation of Learning questions	42	
		193	Evolve Site: CTA A: Body Spectrum: Urinary Tract	10	
		193	Evolve Site: CTA B: Body Spectrum: Kidney	10	
		194	CTA C: Nephron	9	
		194-195	CTA D: Inquiring Patients Want to Know	10	
		195	Evolve Site: CTA E: Animations	8	
		196	CTA F: Crossword Puzzle	31	
		189	Posttest	10	
			ADDITIONAL ASSIGNMENTS		
			TOTAL POINTS		

Notes

Name _____   Date _____

PRETEST

True or False

_____ 1. The functional unit of the kidney is the nephron.

_____ 2. The outer portion of the kidney is known as the renal medulla.

_____ 3. The indentation in the kidney is known as the hilum.

_____ 4. The glomerulus is made up of loose connective tissue.

_____ 5. The glomerular capsule is also known as the Bowman's capsule.

_____ 6. The ureters transport urine from the urinary bladder to the outside.

_____ 7. Rugae located in the wall of the urinary bladder allow the bladder to expand.

_____ 8. The urethra in a male functions only in the transport of urine.

_____ 9. Glucose is reabsorbed into the body in the renal tubule.

_____ 10. Micturition is the act of expelling urine.

POSTTEST

True or False

_____ 1. The urinary system helps to regulate the blood pressure.

_____ 2. The renal pelvis collects urine as it is produced.

_____ 3. The nephron is made up of the glomerulus and Bowman's capsule.

_____ 4. Blood enters the glomerulus through the efferent arteriole.

_____ 5. The renal tubule carries fluid away from the Bowman's capsule toward a collecting duct.

_____ 6. Urine is expelled from the urinary bladder through contraction of the detrusor muscle.

_____ 7. The calyx is made up of three openings and is located in the floor of the urinary bladder.

_____ 8. The urethral orifice controls the passage of urine through the urethra.

_____ 9. Erythropoietin increases reabsorption of sodium and reduces urine output.

_____ 10. In the absence of ADH, the urine is more dilute.

Term KEY TERM ASSESSMENT

Directions: Match each medical term with its definition.

_____ 1. Glomerular capsule

_____ 2. Juxtaglomerular apparatus

_____ 3. Nephron

_____ 4. Renal tubule

A. Complex of modified cells in the afferent arteriole and the ascending limb/distal tubule in the kidney; helps regulate blood pressure by secreting renin; consists of the macula densa and juxtaglomerular cells

B. Double-layered epithelial cup that surrounds the glomerulus in a nephron; also called Bowman capsule

C. Functional unit of the kidney consisting of a renal corpuscle and a renal tubule

D. Tubular portion of the nephron that carries the filtrate away from the glomerular capsule; site where tubular reabsorption and secretion occur

Directions: Fill in each blank with the correct answer.

1. What are the functions of the urinary system?

_____

_____

2. What are the functions of the kidneys?

_____

_____

3. What is renal fascia, and what is its function?

_____

_____

4. What is the renal capsule, and what is its function?

_____

_____

5. Describe each of the following parts of the kidney:

   a. Hilum: _____

   b. Renal sinus: _____

   c. Renal cortex: _____

6. What makes up the renal medulla?

_____

7. What do renal pyramids contain?

_____

8. What are renal columns?

_____

_____

9. What is the function of the renal pelvis?

_____

10. What is the function of a minor calyx?

_____

11. What is a nephron?

_____

12. What are the two parts of a nephron?

_____

13. What makes up the glomerulus?

_____

14. What is the name of the vessel that delivers blood to the glomerulus?

_____

15. What vessel carries blood away from the glomerulus?

_____

16. What is the function of the renal tubule?

_____

17. What are the three regions of a renal tubule?

_____

_____

18. What is the function of renin?

_____

19. What is the function of the ureters?

_____

20. Where do the ureters enter the urinary bladder?

_____

21. What is the function of the muscular layer of the ureter?

_____

22. What is the function of the urinary bladder?

_____

23. What is the function of the rugae located in the wall of the urinary bladder?

_____

24. What is the function of the detrusor muscle?

_____

25. What three openings are located in the trigone of the urinary bladder?

_____

_____

26. Where is the trigone located?

_____

27. What is the function of the urethra?

_____

28. What are the names of the sphincters that control the flow of urine through the urethra?

_____

29. What is the external urethral orifice?

_____

30. What two functions are served by the urethra in the male?

_____

31. What are the three parts of the male urethra?

_____

32. What are the three steps involved in the formation of urine?

_____

_____

33. What occurs during glomerular filtration?

_____

_____

34. What is tubular reabsorption?

_____

_____

35. What are examples of substances that are reabsorbed into the blood?

_____

36. What is tubular secretion?

_____

_____

37. How do the following hormones influence urine concentration and volume?

    a. Aldosterone: _____

    _____

    b. Presence of antidiuretic hormone: _____

    _____

c. Absence of antidiuretic hormone: _____

_____

d. Atrial natriuretic hormone: _____

_____

38. What causes renin to be produced?

_____

39. What effect does angiotensin II have on the blood pressure?

_____

40. What is micturition?

_____

41. What stimulates the micturition reflex?

_____

_____

42. What effect does aging have on the following parts of the urinary system?

A. Muscles in the wall of the urinary structures: _____

B. Urinary bladder: _____

C. Awareness of the need to urinate: _____

CRITICAL THINKING ACTIVITIES

A. Evolve Site: Body Spectrum

Urinary: Urinary Tract

Body Spectrum directions:
1. Access the Body Spectrum program on the Evolve site.
2. If necessary, access the HELP screen for directions on using the Body Spectrum program.
3. Go to the Contents screen.
4. Select the following category from the Contents screen:
   Urinary
5. Select the following anatomic diagram:
   Urinary Tract
6. Identify the structures on the diagram.
7. Print out the diagram.

B. Evolve Site: Body Spectrum

Urinary: Kidney

Directions: Identify the structures on this diagram following the Body Spectrum directions outlined under CTA A.

C. Nephron

Using Figure 15-4 in your textbook as a reference, label each of the structures making up a nephron.

(Modified from Applegate E: *The anatomy and physiology learning system,* ed 4, St. Louis, 2011, Saunders.)

D. Inquiring Patients Want to Know

You are working in a general practice medical office. Your patients ask you the following questions. In the space provided, indicate how you would respond to each question in terms the patient would understand. Use your textbook and Internet resources to develop your responses.

1. Why is urine yellow?

_____

_____

2. Why do women have more urinary tract infections (UTIs) than men?

_____

_____

3. Is it safer to drink bottled water than tap water?

_____

_____

4. What causes kidney stones?

_____

_____

5. How are kidney stones removed?

_____

_____

6. Why is urine a darker yellow color in the morning?

_____

_____

7. What causes some older people to be incontinent?

_____

_____

8. Why should someone with a UTI drink cranberry juice?

_____

_____

9. What happens during kidney dialysis?

_____

_____

10. Do dialysis patients still urinate?

_____

_____

E. Evolve Site: Chapter 15 Animations

Directions:

1. View the Chapter 15 Animations on the Evolve site.
2. For each animation, write two true or false questions in the space provided below.
3. In the classroom, find a partner.
4. For each animation, read your two questions to your partner.
5. For each correct answer, your partner is awarded two points.
6. Next, have your partner read his or her two questions to you. Award yourself two points for each question answered correctly.
7. Continue in this manner until all the questions have been answered.
8. Record your points on your Study Guide Assignment sheet.

True or False Questions

a. The Kidneys

   1. _____

   2. _____

b. Aldosterone Regulation Mechanism

   1. _____

   2. _____

F. Crossword Puzzle: Urinary System

Directions: Complete the crossword puzzle using the clues provided.

Across

1 How urine moves through ureter
4 Formed by three openings in urinary bladder
8 Act of expelling urine
10 Cluster of capillaries in nephron
12 Cuplike projections of renal pelvis
13 Transports urine from urinary bladder to outside
15 Functional unit of kidney
16 Stores urine
17 Outer region of kidney
20 Controls RBC production
22 Helps maintain normal BP
23 Hold kidney in place
25 Opening of urethra
26 Kidney indentation
27 Expels urine from bladder by contracting
28 Takes blood to glomerulus
29 Transports urine from nephron to minor calyces

Down

1 Where most of tubular reabsorption occurs
2 Substance that is reabsorbed by the kidney
3 Connective tissue that encases the kidney
5 Filters blood and removes wastes
6 Allows bladder to expand
7 Urinary bladder capacity in milliliters
9 Takes blood away from glomerulus
11 Epithelial cup that surrounds glomerulus
13 Transports urine from renal pelvis to urinary bladder
14 Inner region of kidney
18 Adipose tissue surrounding kidney
19 Hormone that increases reabsorption of sodium
21 Collects urine
24 Hormone that increases reabsorption of water

16 Reproductive System

CHAPTER ASSIGNMENTS

√ After Completing	Date Due	Textbook Page(s)	TEXTBOOK ASSIGNMENT	Possible Points	Points You Earned
		225-238	Read Chapter 16: Reproductive System		

√ After Completing	Date Due	Study Guide Page(s)	STUDY GUIDE ASSIGNMENTS (CTA: Critical Thinking Activity)	Possible Points	Points You Earned
		199	📰 Pretest	10	
		200	🔑 Term Key Term Assessment A. Definitions B. Word Parts (1 point for each medical term)	8 7	
		200-207	📋 Evaluation of Learning questions: Male Reproductive System Female Reproductive System	44 38	
		207	*e* Evolve Site: CTA A: Body Spectrum: Male Reproductive System	10	
		208	*e* Evolve Site: CTA B: Body Spectrum: Female Reproductive System	10	
		208	*e* Evolve Site: CTA C: Body Spectrum: Fertilization to Implantation	10	
		208	CTA D: Inquiring Patients Want to Know	10	
		209-210	*e* Evolve Site: CTA E: Animations	64	
		211	CTA F: Crossword Puzzle	34	
		199	📰 Posttest	10	
			ADDITIONAL ASSIGNMENTS		
			TOTAL POINTS		

Notes

Medical Asepsis and the OSHA Standard

CHAPTER ASSIGNMENTS

√ After Completing	Date Due	Textbook Pages	TEXTBOOK ASSIGNMENTS	Possible Points	Points You Earned
		239-266	Read Chapter 17: Medical Asepsis and the OSHA Standard		
		249 264	Read Case Study 1 Case Study 1 questions	5	
		256 264	Read Case Study 2 Case Study 2 questions	5	
		259 264	Read Case Study 3 Case Study 3 questions	5	
			TOTAL POINTS		
√ After Completing	**Date Due**	**Study Guide Pages**	**STUDY GUIDE ASSIGNMENTS** **(CTA = Critical Thinking Activity)**	**Possible Points**	**Points You Earned**
		217	Pretest	10	
		218-219	Term Key Term Assessment A. Definitions B. Word Parts (Add 1 point for each medical term)	23 15	
		219-223	Evaluation of Learning questions	41	
		223	CTA A: Infection Process Cycle	5	
		224	CTA B: Handwashing	8	
		225	CTA C: Personal Protective Equipment: Gloves	8	
		225	CTA D: Personal Protective Equipment	30	
		225-227	CTA E: OSHA Standard	10	
		227	CTA F: Discarding Medical Waste	20	
			Evolve Site: Discard It! (Record points earned)		
		228	CTA G: Crossword Puzzle	25	
			Evolve Site: Quiz Show (Record points earned)		

√ After Completing	Date Due	Study Guide Pages	STUDY GUIDE ASSIGNMENTS (CTA = Critical Thinking Activity)	Possible Points	Points You Earned
			Evolve Site: Apply Your Knowledge questions (Record points earned)	10	
			Evolve Site: Video Evaluation	56	
		217	Posttest	10	
			ADDITIONAL ASSIGNMENTS		
			TOTAL POINTS		

√ When Assigned By Your Instructor	Study Guide Pages	Practices Required	LABORATORY ASSIGNMENTS (Procedure Number and Name)	Score*
	229	5	**Practice for Competency** 17-1: Handwashing Textbook reference: pp. 244-245	
	231-232		**Evaluation of Competency** 17-1: Handwashing	*
	229	4	**Practice for Competency** 17-2: Applying an Alcohol-Based Hand Rub Textbook reference: p. 246	
	233-234		**Evaluation of Competency** 17-2: Applying an Alcohol-Based Hand Rub	*
	229	5	**Practice for Competency** 17-3: Application and Removal of Clean Disposable Gloves Textbook reference: pp. 247-248	
	235-236		**Evaluation of Competency** 17-3: Application and Removal of Clean Disposable Gloves	*
			ADDITIONAL ASSIGNMENTS	

Notes

Name _____ Date _____

True or False

_____ 1. A microorganism is a tiny living plant or animal that cannot be seen with the naked eye.

_____ 2. A disease-producing microorganism is known as a nonpathogen.

_____ 3. Microorganisms grow best in an acidic environment.

_____ 4. Coughing and sneezing help to force pathogens from the body.

_____ 5. An alcohol-based hand rub should be used to sanitize hands that are visibly soiled.

_____ 6. OSHA stands for Occupational Safety and Health Administration.

_____ 7. A biohazard warning label must be fluorescent orange or an orange-red color.

_____ 8. Prescription eyeglasses are acceptable eye protection when handling blood.

_____ 9. Hepatitis B is an infection of the liver caused by a virus.

_____ 10. AIDS cannot be transmitted through casual contact.

?≣ **POSTTEST**

True or False

_____ 1. Bacteria and viruses are examples of microorganisms.

_____ 2. An anaerobe can exist only in the presence of oxygen.

_____ 3. The optimum growth temperature is the temperature at which a microorganism grows the best.

_____ 4. Medical asepsis is a practice that helps keep an area free from infection.

_____ 5. Resident flora are picked up in the course of daily activities and are usually pathogenic.

_____ 6. The purpose of the OSHA Standard is to prevent exposure of employees to bloodborne pathogens.

_____ 7. OSHA requires the Exposure Control Plan to be updated annually.

_____ 8. An engineering control is a physical or mechanical device used to remove health hazards from the workplace.

_____ 9. A reagent strip that has been used to test urine is an example of regulated medical waste.

_____ 10. Patients with chronic hepatitis B face an increased risk of developing pancreatitis.

A. Definitions

Directions: Match each medical term with its definition.

_____ 1. Aerobe

_____ 2. Anaerobe

_____ 3. Antiseptic

_____ 4. Asepsis

_____ 5. Bloodborne pathogens

_____ 6. Cilia

_____ 7. Contaminate

_____ 8. Exposure incident

_____ 9. Hand hygiene

_____ 10. Infection

_____ 11. Microorganism

_____ 12. Nonintact skin

_____ 13. Nonpathogen

_____ 14. Occupational exposure

_____ 15. Opportunistic infection

_____ 16. Optimal growth temperature

_____ 17. Pathogen

_____ 18. pH

_____ 19. Postexposure prophylaxis

_____ 20. Regulated medical waste

_____ 21. Reservoir host

_____ 22. Susceptible

_____ 23. Transient flora

A. A disease-producing microorganism

B. Microorganisms that reside on the superficial skin layers and are picked up in the course of daily activities

C. A microorganism that needs oxygen to live and grow

D. Reasonably anticipated skin, eye, mucous membrane, or parenteral contact with bloodborne pathogens or other potentially infectious materials that may result from the performance of an employee's duties

E. Free from infection or pathogens

F. Easily affected; lacking resistance

G. Skin that has a break in the surface

H. The temperature at which an organism grows best

I. The degree to which a solution is acidic or basic

J. A specific eye, mouth, other mucous membrane, nonintact skin, or parenteral contact with blood or other potentially infectious materials that results from an employee's duties

K. Pathogenic microorganisms capable of causing disease that are present in human blood

L. The condition in which the body, or part of it, is invaded by a pathogen

M. Any waste containing infectious material that may pose a threat to health and safety

N. Slender, hairlike processes that constantly beat toward the outside to remove microorganisms from the body

O. A microorganism that does not normally produce disease

P. A microscopic plant or animal

Q. A microorganism that grows best in the absence of oxygen

R. To soil or to make impure

S. The organism that becomes infected by a pathogen and also serves as a source of transfer of pathogens to others

T. An infection resulting from a defective immune system that cannot defend the body from pathogens normally found in the environment

U. An agent that inhibits the growth of or kills microorganisms

V. The process of cleaning or sanitizing the hands

W. Treatment administered to an individual after exposure to an infectious disease to prevent the disease

B. Word Parts

Directions: Indicate the meaning of each word part in the space provided. List as many medical terms as possible that incorporate the word part in the space provided.

Word Part	Meaning of Word Part	Medical Terms That Incorporate Word Part
1. aer/o		
2. an-		
3. anti-		
4. septic		
5. a-		
6. micro-		
7. non-		
8. path/o		
9. -gen		
10. para-		
11. enter/o		
12. -al		
13. peri-		
14. natal		
15. post-		

EVALUATION OF LEARNING

Directions: Fill in each blank with the correct answer.

1. List four examples of types of microorganisms.

2. Define medical asepsis.

3. What type of microorganisms may remain on an object that is considered medically aseptic?

4. What is the name given to the organism that uses organic or living substances for food?

5. Why do most microorganisms prefer a neutral pH?

6. List five examples of how microorganisms can enter the body.

_____

_____

_____

_____

_____

7. List three examples of how a microorganism can be transmitted from one person to another.

_____

_____

_____

8. List four examples of factors that would make a host more susceptible to the entrance of a pathogen.

_____

_____

_____

_____

9. List five protective devices of the body that prevent the entrance of microorganisms.

_____

_____

_____

10. What is the difference between resident flora and transient flora?

_____

_____

_____

11. List three examples of when handwashing should be performed in the medical office.

_____

_____

12. How does antiseptic handwashing sanitize the hands?

_____

_____

13. List five examples of when an alcohol-based hand rub may be used to sanitize the hands.

_____

_____

_____

14. What are the advantages and disadvantages of alcohol-based hand rubs?

_____

_____

15. List six medical aseptic practices the medical assistant should follow in the medical office.

_____

_____

_____

_____

_____

_____

_____

16. What are the advantages of latex gloves?

_____

_____

_____

17. What guidelines should be followed when working with gloves?

_____

_____

_____

_____

18. What does the acronym OSHA stand for, and what is the purpose of OSHA?

_____

_____

19. What is the purpose of the OSHA Occupational Exposure to Bloodborne Pathogens Standard?

_____

_____

20. Who must follow the OSHA Standard? List examples.

_____

_____

_____

21. What is the purpose of the Needlestick Safety and Prevention Act?

_____

_____

22. List five examples of other potentially infectious materials (OPIMs).

_____

_____

_____

_____

23. List examples of nonintact skin.

_____

_____

24. What is the purpose of the exposure control plan (ECP)?

_____

_____

25. List three examples of items to which a biohazard warning label must be attached.

_____

_____

26. What is the purpose of a sharps injury log? What types of offices must maintain this log?

_____

_____

27. Define an engineering control, and list three examples of engineering controls.

_____

_____

_____

28. What is a safer medical device?

_____

_____

29. What should be done before and after gloves are applied?

_____

30. List six guidelines that must be followed when using personal protective equipment (PPE).

_____

_____

_____

_____

_____

_____

31. List four guidelines that must be followed with respect to biohazard sharps containers.

_____

_____

_____

_____

32. What procedure should be followed when a sharps container located in an examining room becomes full? Explain the reason for your answer.

_____

_____

33. Explain how to prepare regulated medical waste for pickup by a medical waste service.

_____

_____

_____

34. How should regulated medical waste be stored while waiting for pickup by the medical waste service? Explain why.

_____

_____

_____

35. What information is included on a regulated medical waste tracking form?

_____

_____

_____

36. What is the most likely means of contracting hepatitis B in the health care setting?

_____

_____

37. What side effects may occur after the administration of a hepatitis B vaccine?

_____

_____

38. What postexposure prophylaxis (PEP) is recommended for an unvaccinated individual who has been exposed to hepatitis B?

_____

_____

_____

39. Why is chronic hepatitis C known as "an epidemic that occurred in the past?"

_____

_____

_____

40. How is HIV transmitted? How is it not transmitted?

_____

_____

_____

41. What is the CDC's definition of AIDS?

_____

_____

CRITICAL THINKING ACTIVITIES

A. Infection Process Cycle

Carefully review the infection process cycle and the requirements for growth needed by microorganisms. Create an environment in a medical office that would function to interrupt the infection process cycle and discourage the growth of pathogens.

_____

_____

_____

_____

B. Handwashing

Using the principles outlined in the handwashing procedure, explain what may happen under the following circumstances:

1. The medical assistant's uniform touches the sink during the handwashing procedure.

   _____

   _____

   _____

2. The hands are not held lower than the elbows during the handwashing procedure.

   _____

   _____

   _____

3. Friction is not used to wash the hands.

   _____

   _____

   _____

4. Water is splashed on the medical assistant's uniform during the handwashing procedure.

   _____

   _____

   _____

5. The medical assistant continually uses water that is too cold to wash hands.

   _____

   _____

   _____

6. The medical assistant turns off the running water with his or her bare hands.

   _____

   _____

   _____

7. The medical assistant does not clean his or her fingernails daily.

   _____

   _____

   _____

8. The medical assistant's skin becomes chapped.

   _____

   _____

   _____

C. Personal Protective Equipment: Gloves

In which of the following situations does OSHA require the use of clean disposable gloves? Indicate your answer by placing a checkmark in the space provided.

———— 1. Performing a urinalysis on a urine specimen that contains blood.

———— 2. Sanitizing operating scissors for sterilization.

———— 3. Performing a finger puncture.

———— 4. Performing a vision screening test on a school-aged child.

———— 5. Cleaning up a blood spill on a laboratory work table.

———— 6. Drawing blood from an elderly patient.

———— 7. Measuring the weight of a college student.

———— 8. Testing a blood specimen for glucose.

D. Personal Protective Equipment

Create a collage of items or articles that can and cannot be used as PPE following these guidelines:

1. Using items cut from a magazine, colored pencils, or markers, create a collage of items that are designated as PPE by OSHA.

2. On the reverse side of the sheet, create a collage of items or articles that are not permitted to be used as PPE.

3. In the classroom, choose a partner and trade sheets. For each PPE item, provide examples of the procedures or tasks which may require its use. For each item that is not PPE, explain why it should not be used as PPE.

Examples of PPE:

_____

_____

_____

_____

Not examples of PPE:

_____

_____

_____

_____

E. OSHA Standard

The following situations may occur in the medical office. For each situation, indicate an appropriate action to take that complies with the OSHA Bloodborne Pathogens Standard.

1. **Situation:** You just gave an injection to a patient, and after withdrawing the needle, you notice that there is no sharps container in the room.
   Action:

_____

_____

_____

2. **Situation:** You are getting ready to apply gloves and notice that you have a cut on your finger.
   Action:

   _____

   _____

   _____

3. **Situation:** You accidentally get some blood on your bare hands while removing your gloves.
   Action:

   _____

   _____

   _____

4. **Situation:** A part-time clinical medical assistant was just hired. She is not immunized against hepatitis B.
   Action:

   _____

   _____

   _____

5. **Situation:** A clinical medical assistant who has worked at the office for 5 years changes her mind and decides she wants the hepatitis B vaccine.
   Action:

   _____

   _____

   _____

6. **Situation:** You are wearing a protective laboratory coat over your scrubs. While performing a laboratory test, some blood splashes onto your lab coat, but it does not penetrate through to your scrubs.
   Action:

   _____

   _____

   _____

7. **Situation:** You go into an examining room and notice that the biohazard sharps container in that room is completely full.
   Action:

   _____

   _____

   _____

8. **Situation:** You have collected three tubes of blood from a patient using glass tubes. You accidentally drop one of the blood tubes, and it breaks.
   Action:

   _____

   _____

   _____

9. **Situation:** You are wearing a protective lab coat over your scrubs, and you are getting ready to leave for the day.
   Action:

   _____

   _____

   _____

10. **Situation:** You remove your gloves after giving an injection to a patient and accidentally discard them into the bio-hazard sharps container.
    Action:

    _____

    _____

    _____

F. Discarding Medical Waste

Indicate where each of the following (used) items should be discarded using these acronyms:

RWC: regular waste container
BSC: biohazard sharps container
BB: biohazard bag waste container

_____ 1. Urine testing strip

_____ 2. Lancet

_____ 3. Gloves with blood on them

_____ 4. Blood tube

_____ 5. Tongue depressor

_____ 6. Razor blade

_____ 7. Capillary pipet

_____ 8. Dressing saturated with blood

_____ 9. Patient drape

_____ 10. An empty urine container

_____ 11. Sutures caked with blood

_____ 12. Thermometer probe cover

_____ 13. Patient gown

_____ 14. Disposable diaper

_____ 15. Dressing saturated with a purulent discharge

_____ 16. Clean disposable gloves

_____ 17. Disposable vaginal speculum

_____ 18. An outdated vaccine

_____ 19. Syringe and needle

_____ 20. Examining table paper

G. Crossword Puzzle: Medical Asepsis and the OSHA Standard

Directions: Complete the crossword puzzle using the clues provided.

Across

1 Grows best without oxygen
5 Infection resulting from a defective immune system
6 HBV serious complication
8 Microorganism that causes disease
11 Normally live on the skin
12 Vaginal secretions (example)
16 Protector of public health
17 Can live dry for 1 week
19 Traps microorganisms
20 Lacking resistance
21 After exposure: may prevent disease
22 Health hazard eliminator
24 Eats "live stuff"

Down

2 Example of a microorganism
3 Body invasion by a pathogen
4 Found in antimicrobial soap
7 Way to prevent a needlestick injury
9 HIV screening test
10 Broken skin
13 #1 chronic viral disease in the United States
14 #1 aseptic practice
15 Scrubs are not this
17 Hepatitis B passive immunizing agent
18 Piercing of the skin barrier
23 Discard in a biohazard container

PRACTICE FOR COMPETENCY

Medical Asepsis

Procedure 17-1: Handwashing. Perform the handwashing procedure. List five medically aseptic steps that must be followed during this procedure.

1. _____

   _____

2. _____

   _____

3. _____

   _____

4. _____

   _____

5. _____

   _____

Procedure 17-2 : Alcohol-Based Hand Rub. Apply an alcohol-based hand rub. Practice applying a gel and a foam hand rub. List the brand names of the hand rubs you applied, and list the ingredients contained in them.

_____

_____

Procedure 17-3: Clean Disposable Gloves. Apply and remove clean disposable gloves. What size gloves fit you best?

_____

_____

Notes

Procedure 17-2: Applying an Alcohol-Based Hand Rub

Name: _____   Date: _____

Evaluated by: _____   Score: _____

Performance Objective

Outcome:	Apply an alcohol-based hand rub.
Conditions:	Given an alcohol-based hand rub.
Standards:	Time: 2 minutes. Student completed procedure in _____ minutes.
	Accuracy: Satisfactory score on the performance evaluation checklist.

Performance Evaluation Checklist

Trial 1	Trial 2	Point Value	Performance Standards
		●	Inspected the hands to make sure they are not visibly soiled.
		▷	Stated the procedure to follow if the hands are visibly soiled.
		●	Removed watch or pushed it up on the forearm.
		●	Removed rings.
			Applied the alcohol-based hand rub to the palm of one hand as follows:
		●	*Gel or lotion:* Applied an amount of gel or lotion approximately equal to the size of a dime.
		●	*Foam:* Applied an amount of foam approximately equal to the size of a walnut.
		▷	Explained why it is important not to use more than the recommended amount of hand rub.
		●	Thoroughly spread the hand rub over the surface of both hands up to ½ inch above the wrist.
		●	Spread the hand rub around and under the fingernails.
		▷	Explained why it is important to cover the entire surface of the hands.
		●	Rubbed the hands together until they were dry.
		●	Did not touch anything until the hands were dry.
		✱	Completed the procedure within 2 minutes.
			TOTALS

Evaluation of Student Performance

EVALUATION CRITERIA			COMMENTS
Symbol	**Category**	**Point Value**	
✴	Critical Step	16 points	
●	Essential Step	6 points	
▷	Theory Question	2 points	

Score calculation: 100 Points

− Points missed
_____
___ Score

Satisfactory score: 85 or above

CAAHEP Competencies Achieved

Psychomotor (Skills)

☑ III. 2. Practice Standard Precautions.
☑ IX. 8. Apply local, state, and federal health care legislation and regulation appropriate to the medical assisting practice setting.

Affective (Behavior)

☑ IX. 3. Recognize the importance of local, state, and federal legislation and regulations in the practice setting.

ABHES Competencies Achieved

☑ 4. f. Comply with federal, state, and local health laws and regulations.
☑ 9. b. Apply principles of aseptic techniques and infection control.
☑ 9. i. Use standard precautions.

18 Sterilization and Disinfection

CHAPTER ASSIGNMENTS

√ After Completing	Date Due	Textbook Pages	TEXTBOOK ASSIGNMENTS	Possible Points	Points You Earned
		267-296	Read Chapter 18: Sterilization and Disinfection		
		270 294	Read Case Study 1 Case Study 1 questions	5	
		280 294	Read Case Study 2 Case Study 2 questions	5	
		281 294-295	Read Case Study 3 Case Study 3 questions	5	
			TOTAL POINTS		
√ After Completing	**Date Due**	**Study Guide Pages**	**STUDY GUIDE ASSIGNMENTS (CTA = Critical Thinking Activity)**	**Possible Points**	**Points You Earned**
		241	Pretest	10	
		242	Term Key Term Assessment	17	
		243-245	Evaluation of Learning questions	28	
		246-247	CTA A: Material Safety Data Sheet	17	
		247-248	CTA B: Obtaining a Material Data Safety Sheet	10	
		249	CTA C: Sanitization	8	
		249-250	CTA D: Sterilization	10	
		252-254	CTA E: What Comes Next? Game (Record points earned)		
			e Evolve Site: Chapter 18 What Happens Now? (Record points earned)		
			e Evolve Site: Chapter 18 Quiz Show (Record points earned)		

√ After Completing	Date Due	Study Guide Page(s)	STUDY GUIDE ASSIGNMENTS	Possible Points	Points You Earned
			Evolve Site: Apply Your Knowledge questions (Record points earned)	10	
			Evolve Site: Video Evaluation	36	
		241	Posttest	10	
			ADDITIONAL ASSIGNMENTS		
			TOTAL POINTS		

√ When Assigned By Your Instructor	Study Guide Pages	Practices Required	LABORATORY ASSIGNMENTS (Procedure Number and Name)	Score*
	255	3	**Practice for Competency** 18-1: Sanitization of Instruments Textbook reference: pp. 275-279	
	257-259		**Evaluation of Competency** 18-1: Sanitization of Instruments	*
	255	Paper: 3 Muslin: 3	**Practice for Competency** 18-2: Wrapping Instruments Using Paper or Muslin Textbook reference: pp. 285-286	
	261-262		**Evaluation of Competency** 18-2: Wrapping Instruments Using Paper or Muslin	*
	255	3	**Practice for Competency** 18-3: Wrapping Instruments Using a Pouch Textbook reference: pp. 286-287	
	263-264		**Evaluation of Competency** 18-3: Wrapping Instruments Using a Pouch	*
	255	3	**Practice for Competency** 18-4: Sterilizing Articles in the Autoclave Textbook reference: pp. 291-293	
	265-267		**Evaluation of Competency** 18-4: Sterilizing Articles in the Autoclave	*
			ADDITIONAL ASSIGNMENTS	

Notes

Name _____   Date _____

True or False

_____ 1. A bacterial spore consists of a hard, thick-walled capsule that can resist adverse conditions.

_____ 2. The purpose of sanitization is to remove all microorganisms and spores from a contaminated article.

_____ 3. According to OSHA, gloves do not need to be worn during the sanitization process.

_____ 4. Glutaraldehyde (Cidex) is a high-level disinfectant.

_____ 5. High-level disinfection kills all microorganisms but not spores.

_____ 6. Sterilization is the process of destroying all forms of microbial life except for bacterial spores.

_____ 7. Autoclave tape indicates whether an autoclaved item is sterile.

_____ 8. The wrapper used to autoclave articles should prevent contaminants from getting in during handling and storage.

_____ 9. Tap water should be used in the autoclave.

_____ 10. The inside of the autoclave should be wiped every day with a damp cloth.

📄 **POSTTEST**

True or False

_____ 1. The agent used to destroy microorganisms on an article depends on the size of the article.

_____ 2. The purpose of the Hazard Communications Standard is to make sure that employees do not use hazardous chemicals in the workplace.

_____ 3. The Hazard Communications Standard requires that the label of a hazardous chemical include information on how to store and handle the chemical.

_____ 4. Stethoscopes must be decontaminated using a high-level disinfectant.

_____ 5. The most common temperature and pressure for autoclaving is 212°F at 15 lb of pressure per square inch.

_____ 6. A sterilization strip should be positioned in the center of a wrapped pack.

_____ 7. The best means of determining the effectives of the sterilization process are biologic indicators.

_____ 8. The proper time for sterilizing an article in the autoclave depends on what is being autoclaved.

_____ 9. A pack that has been in the storage cupboard for 4 weeks should be resterilized.

_____ 10. Ethylene oxide gas is used by medical manufacturers to sterilize disposable items.

Directions: Match each medical term with its definition.

_____ 1. Antiseptic

_____ 2. Autoclave

_____ 3. Contaminate

_____ 4. Critical item

_____ 5. Decontamination

_____ 6. Detergent

_____ 7. Disinfectant

_____ 8. Hazardous chemical

_____ 9. Incubate

_____ 10. Load

_____ 11. Material Safety Data Sheet

_____ 12. Noncritical item

_____ 13. Sanitization

_____ 14. Semicritical item

_____ 15. Spore

_____ 16. Sterilization

_____ 17. Thermolabile

A. To provide proper conditions for growth and development

B. To soil, stain, or pollute; to make impure

C. Easily affected or changed by heat

D. A substance that kills disease-producing microorganisms but not their spores (usually applied to living tissues)

E. An item that comes in contact with intact skin but not mucous membranes

F. A hard, thick-walled capsule formed by some bacteria that contains only the essential parts of the protoplasm of the bacterial cell

G. An item that comes in contact with sterile tissue or the vascular system

H. An apparatus for the sterilization of materials, using steam under pressure

I. An agent that cleanses by emulsifying dirt and oil

J. An item that comes in contact with nonintact skin or intact mucous membranes

K. The articles that are being sterilized

L. An agent used to destroy pathogenic microorganisms but not their spores (usually applied to inanimate objects)

M. A sheet that provides information regarding a chemical and its hazards, and measures to take to avoid injury and illness when handling the chemical

N. A process to remove organic matter from an article and to lower the number of microorganisms to a safe level as determined by public health requirements

O. The process of destroying all forms of microbial life, including bacterial spores

P. The use of physical or chemical means to remove or destroy pathogens on an item so that it is no longer capable of transmitting disease, making it safe to handle

Q. Any chemical that presents a threat to the health and safety of an individual coming into contact with it

Directions: Fill in each blank with the correct answer.

1. How does one determine what type of physical or chemical agent to use to destroy microorganisms on an article?

   _____

   _____

2. List two diseases that are caused by bacteria that produce spores.

   _____

   _____

3. What is the purpose of the Hazard Communication Standard?

   _____

   _____

4. List four examples of hazardous chemicals that may be used in the medical office.

   _____

   _____

5. What information must be included on a hazardous chemical label as required by the Hazard Communication Standard?

   _____

   _____

6. List and describe the information that must be included in a Material Safety Data Sheet.

   _____

   _____

   _____

   _____

   _____

   _____

   _____

   _____

7. What is the purpose of sanitizing an article?

   _____

   _____

8. What is the advantage of using the ultrasound method to clean instruments?

   _____

   _____

9. Why should gloves be worn during the sanitization procedure?

_____

_____

10. What is the definition of high-level disinfection?

_____

_____

11. List one example of an item that requires high-level disinfection. List one example of a high-level disinfectant.

_____

_____

12. List two examples of items that can be disinfected through intermediate-level disinfection. List one example of an intermediate-level disinfectant.

_____

_____

_____

13. List two examples of items that are disinfected by low-level disinfection.

_____

14. What is the purpose of the pressure used in the autoclaving process?

_____

_____

15. Why is it important that all air be removed from the autoclave during the sterilization process?

_____

_____

16. What temperature and pressure are the most commonly used to sterilize materials with the autoclave?

_____

_____

17. What information does the Centers for Disease Control and Prevention (CDC) recommend be recorded in an autoclave log regarding each cycle?

_____

_____

_____

18. What is the function of a sterilization indicator?

_____

_____

19. What is the purpose of wrapping articles to be autoclaved?

_____

_____

20. List two properties of a good wrapper for use in autoclaving.

_____

_____

21. List three examples of wrapping materials used for the autoclave and identify an advantage of each type.

_____

_____

_____

22. Why is more time needed to autoclave a large minor office surgery pack?

_____

_____

23. What is *event-related sterility*?

_____

_____

24. Describe the care an autoclave should receive on a daily basis.

_____

_____

_____

25. Why is a longer exposure period needed to ensure sterilization when using the dry-heat oven?

_____

_____

26. What effect does moist heat have on instruments with sharp cutting edges?

_____

27. How does the medical manufacturing industry use ethylene oxide gas sterilization?

_____

_____

_____

28. What guidelines must be followed when using cold sterilization?

_____

_____

_____

_____

CRITICAL THINKING ACTIVITIES

A. Material Safety Data Sheet

Refer to the Material Safety Data Sheet (MSDS) in the textbook (see Fig. 18-2), and answer the following questions.

1. When was this MSDS last revised?

_____

2. Is glutaraldehyde soluble in water?

_____

3. Describe the appearance and odor of glutaraldehyde.

_____

4. What is the pH of glutaraldehyde?

_____

5. Is glutaraldehyde flammable?

_____

6. Is glutaraldehyde stable?

_____

7. What conditions should be avoided with glutaraldehyde?

_____

8. How can glutaraldehyde enter the body?

_____

_____

9. What symptoms occur if glutaraldehyde does the following?

   a. Comes in contact with the skin _____

   b. Is splashed into the eyes _____

   c. Is inhaled _____

   d. Is ingested _____

10. What preexisting conditions can an individual possess that can be aggravated by glutaraldehyde?

_____

11. Does glutaraldehyde cause cancer?

_____

12. What are the emergency and first aid procedures for glutaraldehyde for the following?

   a. Skin _____

_____

b. Eyes _____

_____

_____

c. Inhalation _____

_____

_____

d. Ingestion _____

_____

_____

13. What should be done if glutaraldehyde is spilled?

_____

_____

_____

14. What is the disposal method for glutaraldehyde?

_____

_____

_____

15. How should glutaraldehyde be stored?

_____

_____

_____

16. What type of ventilation is needed when working with glutaraldehyde?

_____

17. What skin and eye protection should be taken with glutaraldehyde?

_____

_____

B. Obtaining a Material Safety Data Sheet

Obtain an MSDS for one of the following hazardous chemicals, and answer the questions.
To locate an MSDS on the Internet, enter the name of the chemical into a search engine with the abbreviation "MSDS." (Example: Cidex MSDS)

- Cidex
- MetriCide
- Cidex OPA
- CaviCide
- MadaCide
- Wavicide
- Biozide
- Sporox II
- Vesphene
- Envirocide
- Clorox bleach

1. What is the chemical name of this hazardous chemical?

   _____

2. What is the trade or brand name of this chemical?

   _____

3. Who manufactures this chemical?

   _____

4. What number would you call if an emergency occurred with this chemical?

   _____

5. What type of symptoms occur if this chemical does the following?

   a. Comes in contact with the skin _____

   b. Is splashed into the eyes _____

   c. Is inhaled _____

   d. Is ingested _____

6. What are the emergency and first aid procedures for this chemical?

   _____

   _____

7. What should be done if this chemical is spilled?

   _____

   _____

8. What is the disposal method for this chemical?

   _____

   _____

9. How should this chemical be stored?

   _____

   _____

10. What type of protection should be taken when working with this chemical?

    _____

    _____

C. Sanitization

For each of the following situations involving sanitization, write **C** if the technique is correct and **I** if the technique is incorrect. If the situation is correct, state the principle underlying the technique. If the situation is incorrect, explain what might happen if the technique was performed in the incorrect manner.

_____ 1. A contaminated surgical instrument is left in the examination room.

_____ 2. The medical assistant does not wear gloves when sanitizing surgical instruments.

_____ 3. The medical assistant piles instruments while preparing them for sanitization.

_____ 4. The medical assistant forgets to read the material safety data sheet before decontaminating some surgical instruments in Cidex.

_____ 5. The medical assistant uses laundry detergent to sanitize surgical instruments.

_____ 6. Dried blood is not completely cleansed from hemostatic forceps before they are sterilized in the autoclave.

_____ 7. The medical assistant checks all instruments for proper working condition before sterilizing them.

_____ 8. The medical assistant lubricates hemostatic forceps with a steam-penetrable lubricant before sterilizing them.

D. Sterilization

For each of the following situations involving sterilization of articles in the autoclave, write **C** if the technique is correct, and **I** if the technique is incorrect. If the situation is correct, state the principle underlying the technique. If the situation is incorrect, explain what might happen if the technique was performed in the incorrect manner.

_____ 1. The medical assistant opens a hemostat before placing it in a sterilization pouch.

_____ 2. Tap water is used to fill the water reservoir of the autoclave.

_____ 3. When loading the autoclave, the medical assistant places glass jars in an upright position.

_____

_____

_____ 4. The medical assistant places four sterilization pouches on top of each other in the autoclave.

_____

_____

_____ 5. The medical assistant places small packs to be sterilized approximately 1 to 3 inches apart in the autoclave.

_____

_____

_____ 6. Spore strips are placed in the autoclave where steam will penetrate them most easily.

_____

_____

_____ 7. The medical assistant begins timing the load in the autoclave after the proper temperature of 250°F has been reached.

_____

_____

_____ 8. The medical assistant removes the load from the autoclave while it is still wet.

_____

_____

_____ 9. The medical assistant notices a tear in one of the wrappers while removing articles from the autoclave. He or she rewraps and resterilizes the article.

_____

_____

_____ 10. The medical assistant notices that a sterilized wrapped article stored on the storage shelf has opened up. He or she retapes the pack and places it back on the storage shelf.

_____

_____

Notes

E. What Comes Next? Game

Object: The object of the game is to achieve sterilization of an article by determining the correct sequence of events in the sanitization and sterilization procedure.

Directions:
1. Cut out the game cards on the following page.
2. Make your cards unique by coloring and decorating them.
3. Review the sequence of steps in the sanitization and sterilization procedures.
4. Get into a group of three students.
5. Hold your game cards with the steps facing you.
6. Each player places the first step in the sanitization or sterilization procedure face down on the table.
7. When all players have placed a card on the table, turn the cards over.
8. Award yourself 5 points if you have correctly determined the proper step in the sequence. If you have a question regarding the correct answer, consult your instructor.
9. In turn, each player can earn an additional 5 points by stating a fact about that step in the procedure. For example, if the step is "Apply Gloves," a corresponding fact is that clean gloves and utility gloves must be worn during the sanitization procedure.
10. Keep track of your points on the Score Card provided.
11. Keep the cards in their proper sequence on the table, and continue the game until all of the game cards have been used.

WHAT COMES NEXT?
SCORE CARD

Name: _____

Recording Points:

Cross off a number each time you properly sequence a game card (starting with 5 and continuing in sequence). Cross off another number if you are able to state a fact about the step in the procedure. Your total points will be equal to the last number you crossed off. Record this number in the space provided, and check the level that you achieved.

Game Card Points:	
5	75
10	80
15	85
20	90
25	95
30	100
35	105
40	110
45	115
50	120
55	125
60	130
65	135
70	140

Total Points: _____

LEVEL:

≤ 100 to 120 points: **Sterile**—You got rid of all microorganisms and spores!
≤ 80 to 100 points: **Aseptic**—You got rid of the pathogenic microorganisms.
≤ 60 to 80 points: **Contaminated**—Your article is still contaminated.

Read MSDS	Apply gloves	Rinse contaminated instruments	Decontaminate instruments
Clean instruments manually	Thoroughly rinse instruments	Dry instruments	Check working order and lubricate instruments
Wrap instruments	Load the autoclave	Operate the autoclave	Store instruments

What comes next?

What comes next?

What comes next?

What comes next?

What comes next?

What comes next?

What comes next?

What comes next?

What comes next?

What comes next?

What comes next?

What comes next?

PRACTICE FOR COMPETENCY

Sterilization and Disinfection

Procedure 18-1: Sanitizing Instruments. Sanitize instruments. In the space provided, indicate the following:

A. Name of the disinfectant _____

B. Name of the instrument cleaner _____

C. Names of instruments sanitized _____

_____

_____

Procedures 18-2 and 18-3: Wrapping Articles for the Autoclave. Wrap articles for autoclaving. In the space provided, list the information you indicated on the label of each pack that includes the contents of the pack, the date, and your initials.

Information indicated on the label of the wrapped article:

_____

_____

_____

_____

_____

_____

Procedure 18-4: Sterilizing Articles in the Autoclave. Sterilize articles in the autoclave. In the space provided, indicate the articles you sterilized.

_____

_____

_____

_____

Notes

EVALUATION OF COMPETENCY

Procedure 18-1: Sanitization of Instruments

Name: _____   Date: _____

Evaluated by: _____   Score: _____

Performance Objective

Outcome:	Sanitize instruments.
Conditions:	Given the following: disposable gloves, utility gloves, contaminated instruments, chemical disinfectant and MSDS, disinfectant container, cleaning solution and MSDS, basin, nylon brush, wire brush, paper towels, cloth towel, and instrument lubricant.
Standards:	Time: 10 minutes. Student completed procedure in _____ minutes.
	Accuracy: Satisfactory score on the Performance Evaluation Checklist.

Performance Evaluation Checklist

Trial 1	Trial 2	Point Value	Performance Standards
		●	Reviewed the MSDS for hazardous chemicals being used.
		●	Applied gloves.
		●	Transported the contaminated instruments to the cleaning area.
		●	Applied heavy-duty utility gloves over the disposable gloves.
		▷	Stated the purpose of the utility gloves.
		●	Separated sharp instruments and delicate instruments from other instruments.
		▷	Explained why instruments should be separated.
		●	Immediately rinsed the instruments thoroughly under warm running water.
		▷	Stated why the instruments should be rinsed immediately.
			Decontaminated the instruments
		●	Checked the expiration date of the chemical disinfectant.
		▷	Explained why an expired disinfectant should not be used.
		●	Observed all personal safety precautions listed on the label.
		●	Followed label directions for proper mixing and use of the disinfectant.
		●	Labeled the disinfecting container with the name of the disinfectant and the reuse expiration date.
		●	Poured the disinfectant into the labeled container.
		●	Completely submerged the articles in the disinfectant.
		●	Covered the disinfectant container.

Trial 1	Trial 2	Point Value	Performance Standards
		▷	Stated the reason for covering the container.
		●	Disinfected the articles for 10 minutes.
		▷	Explained the reason for decontaminating the instruments.
			Cleaned the instruments: manual method
		●	Checked the expiration date of the cleaning agent.
		●	Observed all personal safety precautions.
		●	Followed label directions for proper use and mixing of the cleaning agent.
		●	Removed articles from disinfectant and placed them in the cleaning solution.
		●	Cleaned the surface of the instruments with a nylon brush.
		●	Cleaned grooves, crevices, or serrations with a wire brush.
		●	Removed stains using commercial stain remover.
		●	Scrubbed the instruments until they were visibly clean.
		▷	Explained why all organic matter must be removed.
			Cleaned the instruments: ultrasound method
		●	Prepared the cleaning solution in the ultrasonic cleaner.
		●	Observed all personal safety precautions listed on label.
		●	Removed the articles from the disinfectant.
		●	Separated instruments of dissimilar metals.
		●	Properly placed the instruments in the ultrasonic cleaner.
		●	Positioned hinged instruments in an open position.
		▷	Stated why hinged instruments must be in an open position.
		●	Ensured that sharp instruments did not touch other instruments.
		●	Checked to make sure all instruments were fully submerged.
		●	Placed the lid on the ultrasonic cleaner.
		●	Turned on the ultrasonic cleaner.
		●	Cleaned the instruments for the length of time recommended by the manufacturer.
		●	Removed the instruments from the machine.
		●	Rinsed each instrument thoroughly with warm water for 20 to 30 seconds.
		▷	Explained why instruments should be rinsed thoroughly.
		●	Dried each instrument with a paper towel.

Trial 1	Trial 2	Point Value	Performance Standards
			Completed the procedure:
		●	Placed instrument on a towel for additional drying.
		▷	Stated the reason for drying the instruments.
		●	Checked each instrument for defects and proper working condition.
		●	Lubricated hinged instruments in an open position.
		●	Opened and closed the instrument to distribute the lubricant.
		●	Placed the lubricated instrument on a towel to drain.
		▷	Stated the reason for lubricating instruments.
		●	Disposed of the cleaning solution according to the manufacturer's instructions.
		●	Removed both sets of gloves.
		●	Sanitized hands.
		●	Wrapped the instruments.
		●	Sterilized the instruments in the autoclave.
		✶	Completed the procedure within 10 minutes.
			TOTALS

Evaluation of Student Performance

EVALUATION CRITERIA			COMMENTS
Symbol	**Category**	**Point Value**	
✶	Critical Step	16 points	
●	Essential Step	6 points	
▷	Theory Question	2 points	

Score calculation: 100 Points

−   _____ Points missed

_____ Score

Satisfactory score: 85 or above

CAAHEP Competencies Achieved

Psychomotor (Skills)

☑ III. 5. Prepare items for autoclaving.

ABHES Competencies Achieved

☑ 9. b. Apply principles of aseptic techniques and infection control.

Notes

💿 **Procedure 18-2: Wrapping Instruments Using Paper or Muslin**

Name: _____   Date: _____

Evaluated by: _____   Score: _____

Performance Objective

Outcome:	Wrap an instrument for autoclaving.
Conditions:	Given the following: sanitized instrument, wrapping material, sterilization indicator strip, autoclave tape, and a permanent marker.
	Time: 5 minutes. Student completed procedure in _____ minutes.
Standards:	Accuracy: Satisfactory score on the performance evaluation checklist.

Performance Evaluation Checklist

Trial 1	Trial 2	Point Value	Performance Standards
		●	Sanitized hands.
		●	Assembled equipment.
		●	Selected the appropriate-sized wrapping material.
		●	Checked the expiration date on the sterilization indicator box.
		▷	Stated why outdated strips should not be used.
		●	Placed wrapping material on clean, flat surface.
		●	Turned the wrap in a diagonal position.
		●	Placed instrument in the center of wrapping material.
		●	Placed instruments with movable joints in an open position.
		▷	Stated why instruments with movable joints must be placed in an open position.
		●	Placed a sterilization indicator in the center of the pack.
		●	Folded wrapping material up from the bottom and doubled back a small corner.
		●	Folded over one edge of wrapping material and doubled back the corner.
		●	Folded over the other edge of wrapping material and doubled back the corner.
		●	Folded the pack up from the bottom and secured with autoclave tape.
		●	Ensured that the pack was firm enough for handling, but loose enough to permit proper circulation of steam.
		▷	Stated why instruments are wrapped for autoclaving.

Trial 1	Trial 2	Point Value	Performance Standards
		●	Labeled and dated the pack. Included your initials.
		▷	Stated the purpose of dating the pack.
		✳	Completed the procedure within 5 minutes.
			TOTALS

Evaluation of Student Performance

EVALUATION CRITERIA			COMMENTS
Symbol	**Category**	**Point Value**	
✳	Critical Step	16 points	
●	Essential Step	6 points	
▷	Theory Question	2 points	

Score calculation: 100 Points

−   _____ Points missed
_____
_____ Score

Satisfactory score: 85 or above

CAAHEP Competencies Achieved

Psychomotor (Skills)
☑ III. 5. Prepare items for autoclaving.

ABHES Competencies Achieved

☑ 9. h. Wrap items for autoclaving.

Procedure 18-3: Wrapping Instruments Using a Pouch

Name: _____   Date: _____

Evaluated by: _____   Score: _____

Performance Objective

Outcome:	Wrap an instrument for autoclaving.
Conditions:	Given the following: sanitized instrument, sterilization pouch, and a permanent marker.
Standards:	Time: 5 minutes. Student completed procedure in _____ minutes.
	Accuracy: Satisfactory score on the performance evaluation checklist.

Performance Evaluation Checklist

Trial 1	Trial 2	Point Value	Performance Standards
		●	Sanitized hands.
		●	Assembled equipment.
		●	Selected the appropriate-sized pouch.
		●	Placed the pouch on a clean, flat surface.
		●	Labeled and dated the pack. Included your initials.
		●	Inserted the instrument into the open end of the pouch.
		●	Sealed the pouch.
		●	Sterilized the pack in the autoclave.
		▷	Stated how long the pack is sterile once it has been autoclaved.
		★	Completed the procedure within 5 minutes.
			TOTALS

Evaluation of Student Performance

EVALUATION CRITERIA			COMMENTS
Symbol	Category	Point Value	
✶	Critical Step	16 points	
●	Essential Step	6 points	
▷	Theory Question	2 points	

Score calculation: 100 Points

－ _____ Points missed

_____ Score

Satisfactory score: 85 or above

CAAHEP Competencies Achieved

Psychomotor (Skills)
☑ III. 5. Prepare items for autoclaving.

ABHES Competencies Achieved

☑ 9. h. Wrap items for autoclaving.

Procedure 18-4: Sterilizing Articles in the Autoclave

Name: _____   Date: _____

Evaluated by: _____   Score: _____

Performance Objective

Outcome:	Sterilize articles in the autoclave.
Conditions:	Using an autoclave.
	Time: 10 minutes. Student completed procedure in _____ minutes.
Standards:	Accuracy: Satisfactory score on the performance evaluation checklist.

Performance Evaluation Checklist

Trial 1	Trial 2	Point Value	Performance Standards
		●	Assembled equipment.
		●	Checked the water level in the autoclave.
		●	Properly loaded the autoclave.
		▷	Stated how far apart to place small packs and large packs.
		▷	Explained two ways for positioning pouches in the autoclave.
			Manually operated the autoclave:
		●	Determined the sterilizing time for the type of articles being autoclaved.
		●	Turned on the autoclave.
		●	Filled the chamber with water.
		●	Closed and latched the door.
		●	Set the timing control.
		▷	Stated when the timer should be set.
		●	Vented the chamber of steam.
		●	Dried the load.
		▷	Stated the reason for drying the load.
			Automatically operated the autoclave:
		●	Closed and latched the door.
		●	Turned on the autoclave.

265

Trial 1	Trial 2	Point Value	Performance Standards
		●	Determined the sterilization program.
		●	Pressed the appropriate program button.
		●	Pressed the start button.
		▷	Stated the purpose of each control or indicator on the autoclave.
			Completed the procedure:
		●	Turned off the autoclave.
		●	Removed the load with heat-resistant gloves.
		▷	Stated the reason for using heat-resistant gloves.
		●	Inspected the packs as they were removed for damage.
		▷	Explained what should be done if a pack is torn.
		●	Checked the sterilization indicators on the outside of the packs.
		●	Recorded information in the autoclave log.
		●	Stored the articles in a clean dust-proof area.
		●	Placed the most recently sterilized packs behind previously sterilized packs.
		●	Maintained appropriate daily care of the autoclave.
		▷	Described the care the autoclave should receive each day.
		✱	Completed the procedure within 10 minutes.
			TOTALS

Evaluation of Student Performance

EVALUATION CRITERIA			COMMENTS
Symbol	Category	Point Value	
✱	Critical Step	16 points	
●	Essential Step	6 points	
▷	Theory Question	2 points	

Score calculation: 100 Points

−   _____ Points missed

_____ Score

Satisfactory score: 85 or above

CAAHEP Competencies Achieved

Psychomotor (Skills)
☑ III. 6. Perform sterilization procedures.
Affective (Behavior)

☑ IX. 3. Recognize the importance of local, state, and federal legislation and regulations in the practice setting.

ABHES Competencies Achieved

☑ 9. o. (4) Perform sterilization techniques.

Notes

19 Vital Signs

√ After Completing	Date Due	Textbook Pages	TEXTBOOK ASSIGNMENTS	Possible Points	Points You Earned
		297-347	Read Chapter 19: Vital Signs		
		316 344	Read Case Study 1 Case Study 1 questions	5	
		320 344	Read Case Study 2 Case Study 2 questions	5	
		332 344	Read Case Study 3 Case Study 3 questions	5	
			TOTAL POINTS		

√ After Completing	Date Due	Study Guide Pages	STUDY GUIDE ASSIGNMENTS (CTA = Critical Thinking Activity)	Possible Points	Points You Earned
		273	Pretest	10	
		274-275 275-276	Key Term Assessment A. Definitions B. Word Parts (Add 1 point for each medical term)	55 30	
		277-286	Evaluation of Learning questions	90	
		286-287	CTA A: Measurement of Body Temperature	18	
		288	CTA B: Alterations in Body Temperature	5	
		288	CTA C: Pulse Sites	6	
		289	CTA D: Pulse and Respiratory Rates	3	
		289-290	CTA E: Pulse Oximetry	18	
		291	CTA F: Blood Pressure Measurement	6	
		291-292	CTA G: Proper BP Cuff Selection	12	
		292	CTA H: Reading Blood Pressure Values	24	
			Evolve Site: Under Pressure (Record points earned)		

√ After Completing	Date Due	Study Guide Pages	STUDY GUIDE ASSIGNMENTS (CTA = Critical Thinking Activity)	Possible Points	Points You Earned
		292-293	CTA I: Interpreting Blood Pressure Readings	10	
		293	CTA J: Hypertension	20	
		294	CTA K: Crossword Puzzle	30	
			Evolve Site: Road to Recovery Game Vital Signs Terminology (Record points earned)		
			Evolve Site: Animations	20	
			Evolve Site: Apply Your Knowledge questions (Record points earned)	11	
			Evolve Site: Video Evaluation	86	
		273	Posttest	10	
			ADDITIONAL ASSIGNMENTS		
			TOTAL POINTS		

√ When Assigned By Your Instructor	Study Guide Pages	Practices Required	LABORATORY ASSIGNMENTS	Score*
	295-296	5	**Practice for Competency** 19-1: Measuring Oral Body Temperature—Electronic Thermometer Textbook reference: pp. 305-307	
	297-299		**Evaluation of Competency** 19-1: Measuring Oral Body Temperature—Electronic Thermometer	*
	295-296	3	**Practice for Competency** 19-2: Measuring Axillary Body Temperature—Electronic Thermometer Textbook reference: pp. 307-308	
	301-302		**Evaluation of Competency** 19-2: Measuring Axillary Body Temperature—Electronic Thermometer	*
	295-296	3	**Practice for Competency** 19-3: Measuring Rectal Body Temperature—Electronic Thermometer Textbook reference: pp. 308-309	
	303-305		**Evaluation of Competency** 19-3: Measuring Rectal Body Temperature—Electronic Thermometer	*
	295-296	5	**Practice for Competency** 19-4: Measuring Aural Body Temperature—Tympanic Membrane Thermometer Textbook reference: pp. 310-312	
	307-308		**Evaluation of Competency** 19-4: Measuring Aural Body Temperature—Tympanic Membrane Thermometer	*
	295-296	5	**Practice for Competency** 19-5: Measuring Temporal Body Temperature Textbook reference: pp. 312-314	
	309-310		**Evaluation of Competency** 19-5: Measuring Temporal Body Temperature	*
	295-296	10	**Practice for Competency** 19-6: Measuring Pulse and Respiration Textbook reference: pp. 326-327	
	311-312		**Evaluation of Competency** 19-6: Measuring Pulse and Respiration	*
	295-296	5	**Practice for Competency** 19-7: Measuring Apical Pulse Textbook reference: p. 328	

√ When Assigned By Your Instructor	Study Guide Pages	Practices Required	LABORATORY ASSIGNMENTS	Score*
	313-314		**Evaluation of Competency** 19-7: Measuring Apical Pulse	*
	295-296	5	**Practice for Competency** 19-8: Performing Pulse Oximetry Textbook reference: pp. 329-330	
	315-317		**Evaluation of Competency** 19-8: Performing Pulse Oximetry	*
	295-296	10	**Practice for Competency** 19-9: Measuring Blood Pressure Textbook reference: pp. 339-342	
	319-321		**Evaluation of Competency** 19-9: Measuring Blood Pressure	*
			ADDITIONAL ASSIGNMENTS	

Measuring Body Temperature

Measure body temperature with each of the following types of thermometers, and record results in the chart provided.

Procedures 19-1, 19-2, and 19-3: Electronic Thermometer (Oral, Axillary, and Rectal)

Procedure 19-4: Tympanic Membrane Thermometer (Aural)

Procedure 19-5: Temporal Artery Thermometer

Measuring Pulse, Respiration, and Oxygen Saturation

Procedure 19-6: Pulse and Respiration. Measure the radial pulse and respiration. Describe the rhythm and volume of the pulse. Describe the rhythm and depth of the respirations. Record the results in the chart provided.

Procedure 19-7: Apical Pulse. Measure apical pulse. Describe the rhythm and volume of the pulse. Record the results in the chart provided.

Procedure 19-8: Pulse Oximetry. Measure the oxygen saturation level and record the results in the chart provided.

Measuring Blood Pressure

Procedure 19-9: Blood Pressure. Measure blood pressure. Record results in the chart provided.

CHART	
Date	

CHART	
Date	

296

Procedure 19-1: Measuring Oral Body Temperature—Electronic Thermometer

Name: _____ Date: _____

Evaluated by: _____ Score: _____

Performance Objective

Outcome:	Measure oral body temperature.
Conditions:	Given the following: electronic thermometer and oral probe, probe cover, and a waste container.
Standards:	Time: 5 minutes. Student completed procedure in _____ minutes.
	Accuracy: Satisfactory score on the Performance Evaluation Checklist.

Performance Evaluation Checklist

Trial 1	Trial 2	Point Value	Performance Standards
		●	Sanitized hands.
		●	Assembled equipment.
		●	Removed thermometer from its storage base.
		●	Attached oral probe to thermometer unit.
		●	Inserted probe into the thermometer.
		●	Greeted the patient and introduced yourself.
		●	Identified the patient and explained the procedure.
		●	Asked the patient if he/she has ingested hot or cold beverages.
		▷	Explained what to do if the patient has recently ingested a hot or cold beverage.
		●	Removed probe from the thermometer.
		▷	Explained what occurs when probe is removed from the thermometer.
		●	Attached probe cover to probe.
		▷	Stated the purpose of the probe cover.
		●	Correctly inserted the probe in patient's mouth.
		●	Instructed the patient to keep the mouth closed.
		▷	Explained why the mouth should be kept closed.
		●	Held probe in place until an audible tone was heard.
		●	Noted patient's temperature reading on display screen.
		●	Removed probe from patient's mouth.

Trial 1	Trial 2	Point Value	Performance Standards
		●	Discarded probe cover in a regular waste container.
		●	Did not allow fingers to come in contact with cover.
		●	Returned probe to the thermometer unit.
		▷	Stated what occurs when probe is returned to the thermometer.
		●	Returned the thermometer unit to its storage base.
		●	Sanitized hands.
		●	Charted the results correctly.
		★	The temperature recording was identical to the reading on the display screen.
		▷	Stated the normal body temperature range for an adult (97°F to 99°F).
		★	Completed the procedure within 5 minutes.
			TOTALS

	CHART	
Date		

Evaluation of Student Performance

EVALUATION CRITERIA			COMMENTS
Symbol	Category	Point Value	
★	Critical Step	16 points	
●	Essential Step	6 points	
▷	Theory Question	2 points	

Score calculation: 100 points

−   _____ points missed

_____ Score

Satisfactory score: 85 or above

CAAHEP Competencies Achieved

Psychomotor (Skills)
☑ I. 1. Obtain vital signs.

Affective (Behavior)

☑ I. 1. Apply critical thinking skills in performing patient assessment and care.

ABHES Competencies Achieved

☑ 9. c. Take vital signs.

Notes

Procedure 19-2: Measuring Axillary Body Temperature—Electronic Thermometer

Name: _____

Date: _____

Evaluated by: _____

Score: _____

Performance Objective

Outcome:	Measure axillary body temperature.
Conditions:	Given the following: electronic thermometer and oral probe, probe cover, and a waste container
Standards:	Time: 5 minutes. Student completed procedure in _____ minutes.
	Accuracy: Satisfactory score on the Performance Evaluation Checklist.

Performance Evaluation Checklist

Trial 1	Trial 2	Point Value	Performance Standards
		●	Sanitized hands.
		●	Assembled equipment.
		●	Removed thermometer from its storage base.
		●	Attached oral probe to thermometer unit.
		●	Inserted probe into the thermometer.
		●	Greeted the patient and introduced yourself.
		●	Identified the patient and explained the procedure.
		●	Removed clothing from patient's shoulder and arm.
		●	Made sure that the axilla was dry.
		●	Removed probe from the thermometer.
		●	Attached probe cover to probe.
		●	Placed probe in the center of the patient's axilla.
		●	Ensured that the arm was held close to the body.
		▷	Explained why the arm must be held close to the body.
		●	Held probe in place until an audible tone was heard.
		●	Removed probe from patient's axilla.
		●	Noted patient's temperature reading on display screen.
		●	Discarded probe cover in a regular waste container.
		●	Did not allow fingers to come in contact with cover.

Trial 1	Trial 2	Point Value	Performance Standards
		●	Returned probe to the thermometer unit.
		●	Returned the thermometer unit to its storage base.
		●	Sanitized hands.
		●	Charted the results correctly.
		✶	Temperature recording was identical to the reading on the display screen.
		✶	Completed the procedure within 5 minutes.
			TOTALS

CHART

Date	

Evaluation of Student Performance

EVALUATION CRITERIA			COMMENTS
Symbol	**Category**	**Point Value**	
✶	Critical Step	16 points	
●	Essential Step	6 points	
▷	Theory Question	2 points	

Score calculation: 100 points

− _____ points missed

_____ Score

Satisfactory score: 85 or above

CAAHEP Competencies Achieved

Psychomotor (Skills)
☑ I. 1. Obtain vital signs.

Affective (Behavior)
☑ I. 1. Apply critical thinking skills in performing patient assessment and care.

ABHES Competencies Achieved

☑ 9. c. Take vital signs.

Procedure 19-3: Measuring Rectal Body Temperature—Electronic Thermometer

Name: _____   Date: _____

Evaluated by: _____   Score: _____

Performance Objective

Outcome:	Measure rectal body temperature.
Conditions:	Given the following: electronic thermometer, rectal probe, probe cover, lubricant, disposable gloves, tissues, and a waste container.
Standards:	Time: 5 minutes. Student completed procedure in _____ minutes.
	Accuracy: Satisfactory score on the Performance Evaluation Checklist.

Performance Evaluation Checklist

Trial 1	Trial 2	Point Value	Performance Standards
		●	Sanitized hands.
		●	Assembled equipment.
		●	Removed thermometer from its storage base.
		●	Attached rectal probe to thermometer unit.
		●	Inserted probe into the thermometer.
		●	Greeted the patient and introduced yourself.
		●	Identified the patient and explained the procedure.
		●	Applied gloves.
		▷	Stated the reason for applying gloves.
		●	Positioned and draped the patient.
		▷	Explained how to position an adult and an infant.
		●	Removed probe from the thermometer.
		●	Attached probe cover to probe.
		●	Applied lubricant up to a level of 1 inch.
		▷	Stated the purpose of the lubricant.
		●	Instructed patient to lie still.
		●	Separated the buttocks and properly inserted the thermometer.

Trial 1	Trial 2	Point Value	Performance Standards
		▷	Stated how far the thermometer should be inserted for adults, children, and infants.
		●	Held probe in place until an audible tone was heard.
		●	Removed the probe in the same direction as it was inserted.
		●	Noted patient's temperature reading on display screen.
		●	Discarded probe cover in a regular waste container.
		▷	Explained why the cover can be discarded in a regular waste container.
		●	Returned probe to the thermometer unit.
		●	Returned the thermometer unit to its storage base.
		●	Wiped the anal area with tissues.
		●	Removed gloves and sanitized hands.
		●	Charted the results correctly.
		★	The temperature recording was identical to the reading on the display screen.
		★	Completed the procedure within 5 minutes.
			TOTALS

CHART	
Date	

Evaluation of Student Performance

EVALUATION CRITERIA			COMMENTS
Symbol	Category	Point Value	
★	Critical Step	16 points	
●	Essential Step	6 points	
▷	Theory Question	2 points	

Score calculation: 100 points

— _____ points missed

_____ Score

Satisfactory score: 85 or above

CAAHEP Competencies Achieved

Psychomotor (Skills)
☑ I. 1. Obtain vital signs.

Affective (Behavior)
☑ I. 1. Apply critical thinking skills in performing patient assessment and care.

ABHES Competencies Achieved

☑ 9. c. Take vital signs.

Notes

Procedure 19-4: Measuring Aural Body Temperature—Tympanic Membrane Thermometer

Name: _____ Date: _____

Evaluated by: _____ Score: _____

Performance Objective

Outcome:	Measure aural body temperature.
Conditions:	Given the following: tympanic membrane thermometer, probe cover, and a waste container.
Standards:	Time: 5 minutes. Student completed procedure in _____ minutes.
	Accuracy: Satisfactory score on the Performance Evaluation Checklist.

Performance Evaluation Checklist

Trial 1	Trial 2	Point Value	Performance Standards
		●	Sanitized hands.
		●	Assembled equipment.
		●	Greeted the patient and introduced yourself.
		●	Identified the patient and explained the procedure.
		●	Removed thermometer from its storage base.
		●	Checked to make sure the probe lens was clean and intact.
		▷	Stated what might occur if the lens was dirty.
		●	Placed a cover on the probe.
		▷	Explained the purpose of the probe cover.
		●	Observed the screen to determine if the thermometer is ready to use.
		●	Held the thermometer in the dominant hand.
		●	Straightened the patient's ear canal with the nondominant hand.
		▷	Explained the purpose of straightening the ear canal.
		●	Inserted the probe into the patient's ear canal and sealed the opening without causing the patient discomfort.
		●	Pointed the tip of the probe toward the opposite temple.
		▷	Stated the reason for pointing the probe toward the opposite temple.
		●	Asked the patient to remain still.
		●	Depressed the activation button for 1 full second or until an audible tone is heard.
		●	Removed the thermometer from the ear canal and noted the patient's temperature on the display screen.

Trial 1	Trial 2	Point Value	Performance Standards
		▷	Stated what should be done if the temperature seems too low.
		●	Disposed of the probe cover in a waste container.
		●	Replaced the thermometer in its storage base.
		▷	Explained the reason for storing the thermometer in its base.
		●	Sanitized hands.
		●	Charted the results correctly.
		✶	The temperature recording was identical to the reading on the display screen.
		✶	Completed the procedure within 5 minutes.
			TOTALS

CHART	
Date	

Evaluation of Student Performance

EVALUATION CRITERIA			COMMENTS
Symbol	Category	Point Value	
✶	Critical Step	16 points	
●	Essential Step	6 points	
▷	Theory Question	2 points	

Score calculation: 100 points

−   _____ points missed

_____ Score

Satisfactory score: 85 or above

CAAHEP Competencies Achieved

Psychomotor (Skills)
☑ I. 1. Obtain vital signs.

Affective (Behavior)
☑ I. 1. Apply critical thinking skills in performing patient assessment and care.

ABHES Competencies Achieved

☑ 9. c. Take vital signs.

EVALUATION OF COMPETENCY

Procedure 19-5: Measuring Temporal Body Temperature

Name: _____   Date: _____

Evaluated by: _____   Score: _____

Performance Objective

Outcome:	Measure temporal body temperature.
Conditions:	Given the following: temporal artery thermometer, disposable probe cover, antiseptic wipe, waste container.
Standards:	Time: 5 minutes. Student completed procedure in _____ minutes.
	Accuracy: Satisfactory score on the Performance Evaluation Checklist.

Performance Evaluation Checklist

Trial 1	Trial 2	Point Value	Performance Standards
		●	Sanitized the hands and assembled equipment.
		●	Greeted the patient and introduced yourself.
		●	Identified the patient and explained the procedure.
		●	Checked to make sure the probe lens is clean and intact.
		▷	Stated why the lens should be clean.
		●	Placed a disposable cover onto the probe or cleaned the probe with an antiseptic wipe and allowed it to dry.
		●	Selected an appropriate site.
		●	Brushed away any hair that is covering the scanning sites.
		▷	Explained why hair must be brushed away.
		●	Held the thermometer in the dominant hand with the thumb on the scan button.
		●	Gently positioned the probe of the thermometer on the center of the patient's forehead.
		●	Depressed the scan button and kept it depressed for the entire measurement.
		▷	Stated why the scan button must be continually depressed.
		●	Slowly and gently slid the probe straight across the forehead midway between the eyebrow and the upper hairline.
		●	Continued until the hairline was reached making sure to keep the probe flush against the forehead.
		●	Keeping the button depressed, lifted the probe from the forehead and placed it behind the earlobe for 1 to 2 seconds.
		▷	Stated why the probe is placed behind the earlobe.

309

Trial 1	Trial 2	Point Value	Performance Standards
		●	Released the scan button and noted the temperature on the display screen.
		●	Disposed of the probe cover in a regular waste container.
		●	Wiped the probe with an antiseptic wipe and allowed it to dry.
		●	Sanitized hands.
		●	Charted the results correctly.
		✶	The temperature recording was identical to the reading on the display screen.
		●	Stored the thermometer in a clean, dry area.
		✶	Completed the procedure within 5 minutes.
			TOTALS

CHART	
Date	

Evaluation of Student Performance

EVALUATION CRITERIA			COMMENTS
Symbol	**Category**	**Point Value**	
✶	Critical Step	16 points	
●	Essential Step	6 points	
▷	Theory Question	2 points	

Score calculation: 100 points

− _____ points missed

_____ Score

Satisfactory score: 85 or above

CAAHEP Competencies Achieved

Psychomotor (Skills)
☑ I. 1. Obtain vital signs.

Affective (Behavior)
☑ I. 1. Apply critical thinking skills in performing patient assessment and care.

ABHES Competencies Achieved

☑ 9. c. Take vital signs.

Procedure 19-6: Measuring Pulse and Respiration

Name: _____   Date: _____

Evaluated by: _____   Score: _____

Performance Objective

Outcome:	Measure radial pulse and respiration.
Conditions:	Using a watch with a second hand.
Standards:	Time: 5 minutes. Student completed procedure in _____ minutes.
	Accuracy: Satisfactory score on the performance evaluation checklist.

Performance Evaluation Checklist

Trial 1	Trial 2	Point Value	Performance Standards
		●	Sanitized hands.
		●	Greeted the patient and introduced yourself.
		●	Identified the patient and explained the procedure.
		●	Observed patient for any signs that might affect the pulse rate or respiratory rate.
		▷	Stated two factors that would increase the pulse rate.
		●	Positioned the patient in a comfortable position.
		●	Placed three middle fingertips over the radial pulse site.
		▷	Explained why the pulse should not be taken with the thumb.
		●	Applied moderate, gentle pressure until the pulse was felt.
		▷	Stated what will occur if too much pressure is applied over the radial artery.
		●	Counted the pulse for 30 seconds and made a mental note of the number.
		●	Determined the rhythm and volume of the pulse.
		▷	Stated when the pulse should be measured for a full minute.
		●	Continued to hold the fingers on the patient's wrist.
		▷	Explained why respirations should be taken without the patient's awareness.
		●	Observed the rise and fall of patient's chest.
		●	Counted the number of respirations for 30 seconds and made a mental note of the number.
		▷	Stated what makes up one respiration.
		●	Determined the rhythm and depth of the respirations.
		●	Observed the patient's color.

Trial 1	Trial 2	Point Value	Performance Standards
		●	Sanitized hands.
		●	Multiplied the pulse and respiration values by 2.
		●	Charted the results correctly.
		✴	The pulse rate was within ± 2 beats of the evaluator's reading.
		✴	The respiratory rate was within 1 respiration of the evaluator's measurement.
		▷	Stated the normal adult range for the pulse rate (60 to 100 beats/min).
		▷	Stated the normal adult range for the respiratory rate (12 to 20 respirations/minute).
		✴	Completed the procedure within 5 minutes.
			TOTALS

CHART

Date	

Evaluation of Student Performance

EVALUATION CRITERIA			COMMENTS
Symbol	Category	Point Value	
✴	Critical Step	16 points	
●	Essential Step	6 points	
▷	Theory Question	2 points	

Score calculation: 100 points

− _____ points missed

_____ Score

Satisfactory score: 85 or above

CAAHEP Competencies Achieved

Psychomotor (Skills)
☑ I. 1. Obtain vital signs.

Affective (Behavior)
☑ I. 1. Apply critical thinking skills in performing patient assessment and care.

ABHES Competencies Achieved

☑ 9. c. Take vital signs.

Procedure 19-7: Measuring Apical Pulse

Name: _____   Date: _____

Evaluated by: _____   Score: _____

Performance Objective

Outcome:	Measure apical pulse.
Conditions:	Given the following: stethoscope and antiseptic wipe.
Standards:	Using a watch with a second hand.
	Time: 5 minutes. Student completed procedure in _____ minutes.
	Accuracy: Satisfactory score on the Performance Evaluation Checklist.

Performance Evaluation Checklist

Trial 1	Trial 2	Point Value	Performance Standards
		●	Sanitized hands.
		●	Greeted the patient and introduced yourself.
		●	Identified the patient and explained the procedure.
		●	Observed the patient for any signs that might affect the pulse rate.
		●	Assembled equipment.
		●	Rotated the chest piece to the bell position.
		●	Cleaned earpieces and chest piece with antiseptic wipe.
		▷	Stated the reason for cleaning stethoscope with an antiseptic.
		●	Positioned patient.
		●	Asked the patient to unbutton or remove his or her shirt.
		●	Warmed chest piece of the stethoscope.
		▷	Explained the reason for warming chest piece.
		●	Inserted earpieces of stethoscope in a forward position in the ears.
		▷	Explained why the earpieces must be directed forward.
		●	Placed the chest piece over the apex of the heart.
		▷	Described the location of the apex of the heart.
		●	Counted the number of heartbeats for 30 seconds and multiplied by 2.
		✳	The reading was within ±2 beats of the evaluator's reading.
		●	Sanitized hands.

313

Trial 1	Trial 2	Point Value	Performance Standards
		●	Charted the results correctly.
		●	Cleaned earpieces and chest piece with an antiseptic wipe.
		★	Completed the procedure within 5 minutes.
			TOTALS

	CHART	
Date	

Evaluation of Student Performance

EVALUATION CRITERIA			COMMENTS
Symbol	**Category**	**Point Value**	
★	Critical Step	16 points	
●	Essential Step	6 points	
▷	Theory Question	2 points	

Score calculation: 100 points

−   _____ points missed

    ___ Score

Satisfactory score: 85 or above

CAAHEP Competencies Achieved

Psychomotor (Skills)
☑ I. 1. Obtain vital signs.

Affective (Behavior)
☑ I. 1. Apply critical thinking skills in performing patient assessment and care.

ABHES Competencies Achieved

☑ 9. c. Take vital signs.

Procedure 19-8: Performing Pulse Oximetry

Name: _____   Date: _____

Evaluated by: _____   Score: _____

Performance Objective

Outcome:	Perform pulse oximetry.
Conditions:	Given the following: handheld pulse oximeter, reusable finger probe, and an antiseptic wipe.
Standards:	Time: 5 minutes. Student completed procedure in _____ minutes.
	Accuracy: Satisfactory score on the Performance Evaluation Checklist.

Performance Evaluation Checklist

Trial 1	Trial 2	Point Value	Performance Standards
		●	Sanitized hands and assembled equipment.
		●	Ensured the probe opened and closed smoothly and that the windows were clean.
		●	Disinfected the probe windows and platforms and allowed them to dry.
		▷	Stated the purpose of disinfecting the probe windows.
		●	If necessary, connected the probe to the cable.
		●	Connected the cable to the monitor.
		●	Did not lift or carry the monitor by the cable.
		●	Greeted the patient and introduced yourself.
		●	Identified the patient and explained the procedure.
		●	Seated the patient in a chair with the lower arm supported and the palm facing down.
		▷	Explained why the arm should be supported.
		●	Selected an appropriate finger to apply the probe.
		●	Observed the patient's finger to make sure it is free of dark fingernail polish or an artificial nail.
		●	Checked to make sure the patient's fingertip is clean.
		●	Checked to make sure the patient's finger is not cold.
		▷	Explained what to do if the patient's finger is cold
		●	Made sure that ambient light will not interfere with the measurement.
		▷	Explained why ambient light should be avoided.
		●	Positioned the probe securely on the fingertip.

Trial 1	Trial 2	Point Value	Performance Standards
		●	Allowed the cable to lay across the back of the hand and parallel to the arm of the patient.
		●	Instructed the patient to remain still and to breathe normally.
		▷	Stated why the patient must remain still.
		●	Turned on the pulse oximeter.
		●	Waited while the oximeter went through its power-on self-test (POST).
		▷	Explained what to do if the oximeter fails the POST.
		●	Allowed several seconds for the oximeter to detect the pulse and calculate the oxygen saturation.
		●	Ensured that the pulse strength indicator fluctuates with each pulsation and that the pulse signal is strong.
		▷	Stated what should be done if the oximeter is unable to locate a pulse.
		●	Left the probe in place until the oximeter displayed a reading.
		●	Noted the oxygen saturation value and pulse rate.
		✶	The reading was identical to the evaluator's reading.
		▷	Stated the normal oxygen saturation level of a healthy adult (95% to 99%).
		●	Removed the probe from the patient's finger and turned off the oximeter.
		●	Sanitized hands.
		●	Charted the results correctly.
		●	Disconnected the cable from the monitor.
		●	Disinfected the probe with an antiseptic wipe.
		●	Properly stored the monitor in a clean dry area.
		✶	Completed the procedure within 5 minutes.
			TOTALS

	Chart	
Date		

Evaluation of Student Performance

<table>
<tr><td colspan="3" align="center">**EVALUATION CRITERIA**</td><td rowspan="2" align="center">**COMMENTS**</td></tr>
<tr><td align="center">**Symbol**</td><td align="center">**Category**</td><td align="center">**Point Value**</td></tr>
<tr><td align="center">✱</td><td align="center">Critical Step</td><td align="center">16 points</td><td></td></tr>
<tr><td align="center">●</td><td align="center">Essential Step</td><td align="center">6 points</td><td></td></tr>
<tr><td align="center">▷</td><td align="center">Theory Question</td><td align="center">2 points</td><td></td></tr>
</table>

Score calculation: 100 points

         –   _____ points missed

             ___ Score

Satisfactory score: 85 or above

CAAHEP Competencies Achieved

Psychomotor (Skills)
☑ I. 1. Obtain vital signs.

Affective (Behavior)
☑ I. 1. Apply critical thinking skills in performing patient assessment and care.

ABHES Competencies Achieved

☑ 9. c. Take vital signs.

Notes

Procedure 19-9: Measuring Blood Pressure

Name: _____ Date: _____

Evaluated by: _____ Score: _____

Performance Objective

Outcome:	Measure blood pressure.
Conditions:	Given the following: stethoscope, sphygmomanometer, and an antiseptic wipe.
Standards:	Time: 5 minutes. Student completed procedure in _____ minutes.
	Accuracy: Satisfactory score on the Performance Evaluation Checklist.

Performance Evaluation Checklist

Trial 1	Trial 2	Point Value	Performance Standards
		●	Sanitized hands.
		●	Assembled equipment.
		●	Rotated the chest piece to the diaphragm position.
		●	Cleaned earpieces and chest piece of stethoscope with an antiseptic wipe.
		●	Greeted the patient and introduced yourself.
		●	Identified the patient and explained the procedure.
		●	Observed patient for any signs that might influence the blood pressure reading.
		▷	Listed signs that would influence the blood pressure reading.
		●	Determined how high to pump the cuff (palpated systolic pressure or checking the patient's chart).
		●	Positioned patient in a sitting position with the legs uncrossed.
		●	Made sure that the patient's arm was uncovered.
		▷	Explained why blood pressure should not be taken over clothing.
		●	Positioned patient's arm at heart level with the palm facing up.
		●	Selected the proper cuff size.
		▷	Explained how to determine the proper cuff size.
		●	Located the brachial pulse with the fingertips.
		▷	Stated the location of the brachial pulse.
		●	Centered bladder over the brachial pulse site.

Trial 1	Trial 2	Point Value	Performance Standards
		▷	Explained why the bladder should be centered over the brachial pulse site.
		●	Placed cuff on patient's arm 1 to 2 inches above bend in elbow.
		●	Wrapped cuff smoothly and snugly around patient's arm and secured it.
		●	Positioned self and/or manometer for direct viewing and at a distance of no more than 3 feet.
		●	Instructed the patient not to talk.
		●	Inserted earpieces of stethoscope in a forward position in the ears.
		●	Located the brachial pulse again.
		▷	Stated the purpose of locating the brachial pulse again.
		●	Placed diaphragm of the stethoscope over the brachial pulse site to make a tight seal.
		▷	Explained why there should be good contact of the chest piece with the skin.
		●	Made sure chest piece was not touching cuff.
		▷	Explained why the chest piece should not touch the cuff.
		●	Closed valve on bulb by turning thumbscrew to the right.
		●	Rapidly pumped air into cuff up to a level of 20 to 30 mm Hg above the palpated or previously measured systolic pressure.
		●	Released pressure at a moderate, steady rate by turning thumbscrew to the left.
		●	Heard and noted the first clear tapping sound (systolic pressure).
		●	Continued to deflate the cuff for another 10 mm Hg.
		●	Heard and noted the point on the scale at which the sounds ceased (diastolic pressure).
		●	Quickly and completely deflated cuff to zero and removed earpieces from ears.
		▷	Stated how long to wait before taking the blood pressure again on the same arm.
		●	Carefully removed cuff from patient's arm.
		●	Sanitized hands.
		●	Charted the results correctly.
		✱	The reading was within ± 2 mm Hg of the evaluator's reading.
		▷	Stated the normal blood pressure for an adult (less than 120/80 mm Hg).
		●	Cleaned earpieces and chest piece with an antiseptic wipe.
		✱	Completed the procedure within 5 minutes.
			TOTALS

CHART	
Date	

Evaluation of Student Performance

EVALUATION CRITERIA			COMMENTS
Symbol	Category	Point Value	
✱	Critical Step	16 points	
●	Essential Step	6 points	
▷	Theory Question	2 points	

Score calculation: 100 points

− _____ points missed

_____ Score

Satisfactory score: 85 or above

CAAHEP Competencies Achieved

Psychomotor (Skills)
☑ I. 1. Obtain vital signs.

Affective (Behavior)
☑ I. 1. Apply critical thinking skills in performing patient assessment and care.

ABHES Competencies Achieved

☑ 9. c. Take vital signs.

Notes

20 The Physical Examination

CHAPTER ASSIGNMENTS

√ After Completing	Date Due	Textbook Pages	TEXTBOOK ASSIGNMENTS	Possible Points	Points You Earned
		348-383	Read Chapter 20: The Physical Examination		
		353 381	Read Case Study 1 Case Study 1 questions	5	
		353 381	Read Case Study 2 Case Study 2 questions	5	
		378 381-382	Read Case Study 3 Case Study 3 questions	5	
			TOTAL POINTS		

√ After Completing	Date Due	Study Guide Pages	STUDY GUIDE ASSIGNMENTS (CTA = Critical Thinking Activity)	Possible Points	Points You Earned
		327	Pretest	10	
		328 328	Key Term Assessment A. Definitions B. Word Parts (Add 1 point for each medical term)	17 9	
		329-332	Evaluation of Learning questions	31	
		332	CTA A: Preparation of the Examining Room	10	
		333	CTA B: Reading Weight Measurements	15	
			Evolve Site: By the Pound (Record points earned)		
		334	CTA C: Reading Height Measurements	11	
			Evolve Site: Feet and Inches (Record points earned)		
		335	CTA D: Calculating BMI	12	
		335	CTA E: Dear Gabby	10	
		336	CTA F: Patient Positions	10	
			Evolve Site: Let's Get Physical (Record points earned)		
		336	CTA G: Examination Techniques	10	
		337	CTA H: Otoscope	4	

√ After Completing	Date Due	Study Guide Pages	STUDY GUIDE ASSIGNMENTS (CTA = Critical Thinking Activity)	Possible Points	Points You Earned
		337	CTA I: Crossword Puzzle	25	
			Evolve Site: Apply Your Knowledge questions	10	
			Evolve Site: Video Evaluation	54	
		327	Posttest	10	
			ADDITIONAL ASSIGNMENTS		
			TOTAL POINTS		

√ When Assigned By Your Instructor	Study Guide Pages	Practices Required	LABORATORY ASSIGNMENTS (Procedure Number and Name)	Score*
	339-340	5	**Practice for Competency** 20-1: Measuring Weight and Height Textbook reference: pp. 359-340	
	341-343		**Evaluation of Competency** 20-1: Measuring Weight and Height	*
	339-340		**Practice for Competency** 20-A: Body Mechanics Textbook reference: pp. 361-363	
	345-347		**Evaluation of Competency** 20-A: Body Mechanics	*
	339-340	3	**Practice for Competency** 20-2: Sitting Position Textbook reference: p. 364	
	349-350		**Evaluation of Competency** 20-2: Sitting Position	*
	339-340	3	**Practice for Competency** 20-3: Supine Position Textbook reference: pp. 364-365	
	351-352		**Evaluation of Competency** 20-3: Supine Position	*
	339-340	3	**Practice for Competency** 20-4: Prone Position Textbook reference: pp. 365-366	
	353-354		**Evaluation of Competency** 20-4: Prone Position	*
	339-340	3	**Practice for Competency** 20-5: Dorsal Recumbent Position Textbook reference: pp. 366-367	
	355-356		**Evaluation of Competency** 20-5: Dorsal Recumbent Position	*
	339-340	3	**Practice for Competency** 20-6: Lithotomy Position Textbook reference: pp. 367-368	
	357-358		**Evaluation of Competency** 20-6: Lithotomy Position	*
	339-340	3	**Practice for Competency** 20-7: Sims Position Textbook reference: p. 369	
	359-360		**Evaluation of Competency** 20-7: Sims Position	*
	339-340	3	**Practice for Competency** 20-8: Knee-Chest Position Textbook reference: p. 370	
	361-362		**Evaluation of Competency** 20-8: Knee-Chest Position	*

√ When Assigned By Your Instructor	Study Guide Pages	Practices Required	LABORATORY ASSIGNMENTS (Procedure Number and Name)	Score*
	339-340	3	**Practice for Competency** 20-9: Fowler's Position Textbook reference: p. 371	
	363-364		**Evaluation of Competency** 20-9: Fowler's Position	*
	339-340	3	**Practice for Competency** 20-10: Wheelchair Transfer Textbook reference: pp. 372-376	
	365-367		**Evaluation of Competency** 20-10: Wheelchair Transfer	*
	339-340	3	**Practice for Competency** 20-11: Assisting with the Physical Examination Textbook reference: pp. 378-380	
	369-372		**Evaluation of Competency** 20-11: Assisting with the Physical Examination	*
			ADDITIONAL ASSIGNMENTS	

Procedure 20-1: Measuring Weight and Height

Name: _____   Date: _____

Evaluated by: _____   Score: _____

Performance Objective

Outcome:	Measure weight and height.
Conditions:	Given a paper towel.
	Using an upright balance scale.
Standards:	Time: 5 minutes. Student completed procedure in _____ minutes.
	Accuracy: Satisfactory score on the performance evaluation checklist.

Performance Evaluation Checklist

Trial 1	Trial 2	Point Value	Performance Standards
			Weight
		●	Sanitized hands.
			Checked the balance scale for accuracy
		●	Verified that the upper and lower weights were on zero.
		●	Looked at the indicator point to make sure the scale is balanced.
		▷	Stated what will be observed if the scale is balanced.
		▷	Explained what to do if the indicator point rests below the center.
		▷	Explained what to do if the indicator point rests above the center.
		▷	Stated what occurs if the scale is not balanced.
		●	Greeted the patient and introduced yourself.
		●	Identified the patient and explained the procedure.
		●	Instructed patient to remove shoes and heavy outer clothing.
		●	Placed paper towel on the scale.
		●	Assisted patient onto the scale.
		●	Instructed patient not to move.
			Balanced the scale
		●	Moved the lower weight to the groove that did not cause the indicator point to drop to the bottom of the balance area.
		▷	Stated why the lower weight should be seated firmly in its groove.

Trial 1	Trial 2	Point Value	Performance Standards
		●	Slid the upper weight slowly until the indicator point came to a rest at the center of the balance area.
		●	Read the results to the nearest quarter pound. Jotted down this value or made a mental note of it.
		★	The reading was identical to the evaluator's reading.
		●	Asked the patient to step off the scale.
			Height
		●	Slid the calibration rod until it was above the patient's height.
		●	Opened the measuring bar to its horizontal position.
		●	Instructed the patient to step onto the scale platform with his or her back to the scale.
		●	Instructed patient to stand erect and to look straight ahead.
		●	Carefully lowered the measuring bar until it rested gently on top of the patient's head.
		●	Verified that the bar was in a horizontal position.
		●	Instructed the patient to step down and put on his or her shoes.
		●	Read the marking to the nearest quarter inch. Jotted down this value or made a mental note of it.
		★	The reading was identical to the evaluator's reading.
		●	Returned the measuring bar to its vertical position.
		●	Slid the calibration rod to its lowest position.
		●	Returned the weights to zero.
		●	Sanitized hands.
		●	Charted the results correctly.
		★	Completed the procedure within 5 minutes.
			TOTALS
			CHART
	Date		

Evaluation of Student Performance

EVALUATION CRITERIA			COMMENTS
Symbol	Category	Point Value	
★	Critical Step	16 points	
●	Essential Step	6 points	
▷	Theory Question	2 points	

Score calculation: 100 points

        −   points missed

                  Score

Satisfactory score: 85 or above

CAAHEP Competencies Achieved

Psychomotor (Skills)

☑ IV. 6. Prepare a patient for procedures and/or treatments.

Affective (Behavior)

☑ IV. 1. Demonstrate empathy in communicating with patients, family, and staff.
☑ IV. 9. Recognize and protect personal boundaries in communicating with others.

ABHES Competencies Achieved

☑ 8. bb. Are impartial and show empathy when dealing with patients.
☑ 9. l. Prepare patient for examinations and treatments.

Notes

Procedure 20-A: Body Mechanics

Name: _____   Date: _____

Evaluated by: _____   Score: _____

Performance Objective

Outcome:	Demonstrate proper body mechanics while standing, sitting, and lifting an object.
Conditions:	Given the following: object for lifting.
	Using a chair.
Standards:	Time: 10 minutes. Student completed procedure in _____ minutes.
	Accuracy: Satisfactory score on the performance evaluation checklist.

Performance Evaluation Checklist

Trial 1	Trial 2	Point Value	Performance Standards
			Standing
		●	Wore comfortable low-heeled shoes that provide good support.
		●	Held the head erect at the midline of the body.
		●	Maintained the back as straight as possible with the pelvis tucked inward.
		●	The chest is forward with the shoulders back and the abdomen drawn in and kept flat.
		▷	Stated the purpose of standing correctly.
		●	Knees are slightly flexed.
		●	Feet are pointing forward and parallel to each other about 3 inches apart.
		▷	Explained the reason for proper positioning of the feet.
		●	Arms are positioned comfortably at the side.
		●	Weight of the body is evenly distributed over both feet.
			Sitting
		●	Sat in a chair with a firm back.
		●	Back and buttocks are supported against the back of the chair.
		●	Body weight is evenly distributed over the buttocks and thighs.
		●	A small pillow or rolled towel is used.
		▷	Stated the use of the pillow or rolled towel.

Trial 1	Trial 1	Point Value	Performance Standards
		●	Feet are flat on the floor.
		●	Knees are level with the hips.
		▷	Explained what to do if prolonged sitting is required.
			Lifting
		●	Determined the weight of the object.
		▷	Stated the purpose of determining the weight of an object before lifting it.
		●	Stood in front of the object with the feet 6 to 8 inches apart.
		●	The toes are pointed outward and one foot is slightly forward.
		●	Tightened the stomach and gluteal muscles in preparation for the lift.
		●	Bent the body at the knees and hips.
		▷	Stated the purpose of bending the body at the knees and hips.
		●	Grasped the object firmly with both hands.
		●	Lifted the object smoothly with the leg muscles while keeping the back straight.
		▷	Stated why the leg muscles and not the back muscles should be used to lift the object.
		●	Held the object as close to the body as possible at waist level.
		▷	Stated why the object should not be lifted higher than the chest.
		●	Turned by pivoting the whole body.
		●	Made sure the area of transport of the object is dry and free of clutter.
		●	Lowered the object slowly while bending from the knees.
		★	Completed the procedures within 10 minutes.
			TOTALS

Evaluation of Student Performance

EVALUATION CRITERIA			COMMENTS
Symbol	Category	Point Value	
✱	Critical Step	16 points	
●	Essential Step	6 points	
▷	Theory Question	2 points	

Score calculation: 100 points

        −   points missed

           Score

Satisfactory score: 85 or above

CAAHEP Competencies Achieved

Psychomotor (Skills)
☑ XI. 3. Develop a personal (patient and employee) safety plan.
☑ XI. 11. Use proper body mechanics.

ABHES Competencies Achieved

☑ 4. e. Perform risk management procedures.

Notes

Chapter **20**   **The Physical Examination**

Procedure 20-2: Sitting Position

Name: _____   Date: _____

Evaluated by: _____   Score: _____

Performance Objective

Outcome:	Position and drape an individual in the sitting position.
Conditions:	Given the following: a patient gown and a drape.
	Using an examining table.
Standards:	Time: 5 minutes. Student completed procedure in _____ minutes.
	Accuracy: Satisfactory score on the performance evaluation checklist.

Performance Evaluation Checklist

Trial 1	Trial 2	Point Value	Performance Standards
		●	Sanitized hands.
		●	Greeted the patient and introduced yourself.
		●	Identified the patient.
		●	Explained what type of examination or procedure will be performed.
		●	Provided patient with a patient gown.
		●	Instructed patient to remove clothing and to put on a patient gown with the opening in front.
		▷	Stated what qualities the disrobing facility should have.
		●	Pulled out the footrest and assisted the patient into a sitting position.
		●	The patient's buttocks and thighs were firmly supported on the edge of the table.
		●	Placed a drape over the patient's thighs and legs.
		●	Assisted the patient off the table after the examination.
		●	Returned the footrest to its normal position.
		●	Instructed the patient to get dressed.
		●	Discarded the gown and drape in a waste container.
		▷	Stated one use of the sitting position.
		★	Completed the procedure within 5 minutes.
			TOTALS

Evaluation of Student Performance

EVALUATION CRITERIA			COMMENTS
Symbol	Category	Point Value	
✱	Critical Step	16 points	
●	Essential Step	6 points	
▷	Theory Question	2 points	

Score calculation: 100 points

      −   points missed

           _____

           ___ Score

Satisfactory score: 85 or above

CAAHEP Competencies Achieved

Psychomotor (Skills)
☑ IV. 6. Prepare a patient for procedures and/or treatments.
☑ XI. 11. Use proper body mechanics.

Affective (Behavior)
☑; IV. 4. Demonstrate awareness of the territorial boundaries of the person with whom communicating.

ABHES Competencies Achieved

☑ 9. 1. Prepare patient for examinations and treatments.

Procedure 20-3: Supine Position

Name: _____   Date: _____

Evaluated by: _____   Score: _____

Performance Objective

Outcome:	Position and drape an individual in the supine position.
Conditions:	Given the following: a patient gown and a drape.
	Using an examining table.
Standards:	Time: 5 minutes. Student completed procedure in _____ minutes.
	Accuracy: Satisfactory score on the performance evaluation checklist.

Performance Evaluation Checklist

Trial 1	Trial 2	Point Value	Performance Standards
		●	Sanitized hands.
		●	Greeted the patient and introduced yourself.
		●	Identified the patient.
		●	Explained what type of examination or procedure will be performed.
		●	Provided patient with a patient gown.
		●	Instructed patient to remove clothing and to put on a patient gown with the opening in front.
		●	Pulled out the footrest and assisted the patient into a sitting position.
		●	Placed a drape over the patient's thighs and legs.
		●	Asked the patient to move back on the table.
		●	Pulled out the table extension while supporting the patient's lower legs.
		●	Asked the patient to lie down on his or her back with the legs together.
		●	Placed the patient's arms above the head or alongside the body.
		●	Positioned the drape lengthwise over the patient.
		▷	Stated the purpose of the drape.
		●	Moved the drape according to the body parts being examined.
		●	Assisted the patient back into a sitting position after the examination.
		●	Slid the table extension back into place while supporting the patient's lower legs.
		●	Assisted the patient from the examining table.

Trial 1	Trial 2	Point Value	Performance Standards
		●	Returned the footrest to its normal position.
		●	Instructed the patient to get dressed.
		●	Discarded the gown and drape in a waste container.
		▷	Stated one use of the supine position.
		✱	Completed the procedure within 5 minutes.
			TOTALS

Evaluation of Student Performance

EVALUATION CRITERIA			COMMENTS
Symbol	**Category**	**Point Value**	
✱	Critical Step	16 points	
●	Essential Step	6 points	
▷	Theory Question	2 points	

Score calculation: 100 points

        −   _____ points missed

                _____ Score

Satisfactory score: 85 or above

CAAHEP Competencies Achieved

Psychomotor (Skills)
☑ IV. 6. Prepare a patient for procedures and/or treatments.
☑ XI. 11. Use proper body mechanics.

Affective (Behavior)
☑ IV. 4. Demonstrate awareness of the territorial boundaries of the person with whom communicating.

ABHES Competencies Achieved

☑ 9. 1. Prepare patient for examinations and treatments.

Procedure 20-4: Prone Position

Name: _____

Date: _____

Evaluated by: _____

Score: _____

Performance Objective

Outcome:	Position and drape an individual in the prone position.
Conditions:	Given the following: a patient gown and a drape.
	Using an examining table.
Standards:	Time: 5 minutes. Student completed procedure in _____ minutes.
	Accuracy: Satisfactory score on the performance evaluation checklist.

Performance Evaluation Checklist

Trial 1	Trial 2	Point Value	Performance Standards
		●	Sanitized hands.
		●	Greeted the patient and introduced yourself.
		●	Identified the patient.
		●	Explained what type of examination or procedure will be performed.
		●	Provided patient with a patient gown.
		●	Instructed patient to remove clothing and to put on a patient gown with the opening in back.
		●	Pulled out the footrest and assisted the patient into a sitting position.
		●	Placed a drape over the patient's thighs and legs.
		●	Asked the patient to move back on the table.
		●	Pulled out the table extension while supporting the patient's lower legs.
		●	Asked the patient to lie down on his or her back.
		●	Positioned the drape lengthwise over the patient.
		●	Asked the patient to turn onto his or her stomach by rolling toward you.
		●	Provided assistance.
		▷	Stated the reason for providing assistance.
		●	Positioned the patient with his or her legs together and the head turned to one side.
		●	Placed the patient's arms above the head or alongside the body.

Trial 1	Trial 2	Point Value	Performance Standards
		●	Adjusted the drape as needed.
		●	Moved the drape according to the body parts being examined.
		●	Assisted the patient into the supine position after the examination.
		●	Assisted the patient into a sitting position.
		●	Slid the table extension back into place while supporting the patient's lower legs.
		●	Assisted the patient from the examining table.
		●	Returned the footrest to its normal position.
		●	Instructed the patient to get dressed.
		●	Discarded the gown and drape in a waste container.
		▷	Stated one use of the prone position.
		✳	Completed the procedure within 5 minutes.
			TOTALS

Evaluation of Student Performance

EVALUATION CRITERIA			COMMENTS
Symbol	**Category**	**Point Value**	
✳	Critical Step	16 points	
●	Essential Step	6 points	
▷	Theory Question	2 points	

Score calculation: 100 points

− _____ points missed

_____ Score

Satisfactory score: 85 or above

CAAHEP Competencies Achieved

Psychomotor (Skills)
☑ IV. 6. Prepare a patient for procedures and/or treatments.
☑ XI. 11. Use proper body mechanics.

Affective (Behavior)
☑ IV. 4. Demonstrate awareness of the territorial boundaries of the person with whom communicating.

ABHES Competencies Achieved

☑ 9. 1. Prepare patient for examinations and treatments.

Procedure 20-5: Dorsal Recumbent Position

Name: _____ Date: _____

Evaluated by: _____ Score: _____

Performance Objective

Outcome:	Position and drape an individual in the dorsal recumbent position.
Conditions:	Given the following: a patient gown and a drape.
	Using an examining table.
Standards:	Time: 5 minutes. Student completed procedure in _____ minutes.
	Accuracy: Satisfactory score on the performance evaluation checklist.

Performance Evaluation Checklist

Trial 1	Trial 2	Point Value	Performance Standards
		●	Sanitized hands.
		●	Greeted the patient and introduced yourself.
		●	Identified the patient.
		●	Explained what type of examination or procedure will be performed.
		●	Provided patient with a patient gown.
		●	Instructed patient to remove clothing and to put on a patient gown with the opening in front.
		●	Pulled out the footrest and assisted the patient into a sitting position.
		●	Placed a drape over the patient's thighs and legs.
		●	Asked the patient to move back on the table.
		●	Pulled out the table extension while supporting the patient's lower legs.
		●	Asked the patient to lie down on his or her back.
		●	Placed the patient's arms above their head or alongside the body.
		●	Positioned the drape diagonally over the patient.
		●	Asked the patient to bend the knees and place each foot at the edge of the table with the soles of the feet flat on the table.
		●	Provided assistance.
		●	Pushed in the table extension and the footrest.

Trial 1	Trial 2	Point Value	Performance Standards
		●	Adjusted the drape as needed.
		●	Folded back the center corner of the drape when the physician was ready to examine the patient.
		●	Pulled out the footrest and the table extension after the examination.
		●	Assisted the patient back into a supine position and then into a sitting position.
		●	Slid the table extension back into place while supporting the patient's lower legs.
		●	Assisted the patient from the examining table.
		●	Returned the footrest to its normal position.
		●	Instructed the patient to get dressed.
		●	Discarded the gown and drape in a waste container.
		▷	Stated one use of the dorsal recumbent position.
		✱	Completed the procedure within 5 minutes.
			TOTALS

Evaluation of Student Performance

EVALUATION CRITERIA			COMMENTS
Symbol	**Category**	**Point Value**	
✱	Critical Step	16 points	
●	Essential Step	6 points	
▷	Theory Question	2 points	

Score calculation: 100 points

     −   _____ points missed

         ____ Score

Satisfactory score: 85 or above

CAAHEP Competencies Achieved

Psychomotor (Skills)
☑ IV. 6. Prepare a patient for procedures and/or treatments.
☑ XI. 11. Use proper body mechanics.

Affective (Behavior)
☑ IV. 4. Demonstrate awareness of the territorial boundaries of the person with whom communicating.

ABHES Competencies Achieved

☑ 9. l. Prepare patient for examinations and treatments.

Procedure 20-6: Lithotomy Position

Name: _____   Date: _____

Evaluated by: _____   Score: _____

Performance Objective

Outcome:	Position and drape an individual in the lithotomy position.
Conditions:	Given the following: a patient gown and a drape.
	Using an examining table.
Standards:	Time: 5 minutes. Student completed procedure in _____ minutes.
	Accuracy: Satisfactory score on the performance evaluation checklist.

Performance Evaluation Checklist

Trial 1	Trial 2	Point Value	Performance Standards
		●	Sanitized hands.
		●	Greeted the patient and introduced yourself.
		●	Identified the patient.
		●	Explained what type of examination or procedure will be performed.
		●	Provided patient with a patient gown.
		●	Instructed patient to remove clothing and to put on a patient gown with the opening in front.
		●	Pulled out the footrest and assisted the patient into a sitting position.
		●	Placed a drape over the patient's thighs and legs.
		●	Asked the patient to move back on the table.
		●	Pulled out the table extension while supporting the patient's lower legs.
		●	Asked the patient to lie down on his or her back.
		●	Placed the patient's arms above head or alongside body.
		●	Positioned the drape diagonally over the patient.
		●	Pulled out the stirrups and positioned them at an angle.
		●	Positioned the stirrups so that they were level with the examining table and pulled out approximately 1 foot from the edge of the table.
		●	Asked the patient to bend the knees and place each foot into a stirrup.
		●	Provided assistance.
		●	Pushed in the table extension and the footrest.
		●	Instructed the patient to slide buttocks to the edge of the table and to rotate thighs outward as far as is comfortable.

357

Trial 1	Trial 2	Point Value	Performance Standards
		●	Repositioned the drape as needed.
		●	Folded back the center corner of the drape when the physician was ready to examine the genital area.
		●	After completion of the examination, pulled out the footrest and the table extension.
		●	Asked the patient to slide the buttocks back from the end of the table.
		●	Lifted the patient's legs out of the stirrups at the same time and placed them on the table extension.
		▷	Stated why both legs should be lifted at the same time.
		●	Returned stirrups to the normal position.
		●	Assisted the patient back into a sitting position.
		●	Slid the table extension back into place while supporting the patient's lower legs.
		●	Assisted the patient from the examining table.
		●	Returned the footrest to its normal position.
		●	Instructed the patient to get dressed.
		●	Discarded the gown and drape in a waste container.
		▷	Stated one use of the lithotomy position.
		✱	Completed the procedure within 5 minutes.
			TOTALS

Evaluation of Student Performance

EVALUATION CRITERIA			COMMENTS
Symbol	**Category**	**Point Value**	
✱	Critical Step	16 points	
●	Essential Step	6 points	
▷	Theory Question	2 points	

Score calculation: 100 points

− _____ points missed

_____ Score

Satisfactory score: 85 or above

CAAHEP Competencies Achieved

Psychomotor (Skills)
☑ IV. 6. Prepare a patient for procedures and/or treatments.
☑ XI. 11. Use proper body mechanics.

Affective (Behavior)
☑ IV. 4. Demonstrate awareness of the territorial boundaries of the person with whom communicating.

ABHES Competencies Achieved

☑ 9. l. Prepare patient for examinations and treatments.

Procedure 20-7: Sims Position

Name: _____   Date: _____

Evaluated by: _____   Score: _____

Performance Objective

Outcome:	Position and drape an individual in the Sims position.
Conditions:	Given the following: a patient gown and a drape.
	Using an examining table.
Standards:	Time: 5 minutes. Student completed procedure in _____ minutes.
	Accuracy: Satisfactory score on the performance evaluation checklist.

Performance Evaluation Checklist

Trial 1	Trial 2	Point Value	Performance Standards
		●	Sanitized hands.
		●	Greeted the patient and introduced yourself.
		●	Identified the patient.
		●	Explained what type of examination or procedure will be performed.
		●	Provided patient with a patient gown.
		●	Instructed patient to remove clothing and to put on a patient gown with the opening in back.
		●	Pulled out the footrest and assisted the patient into a sitting position.
		●	Placed a drape over the patient's thighs and legs.
		●	Asked the patient to move back on the table.
		●	Pulled out the table extension while supporting the patient's lower legs.
		●	Asked the patient to lie down on his or her back.
		●	Positioned the drape lengthwise over the patient.
		●	Asked the patient to turn onto the left side.
		●	Provided assistance.
		●	Positioned the left arm behind the body and the right arm forward with the elbow bent.
		●	Assisted the patient in flexing the legs with the right leg flexed sharply and the left leg flexed slightly.
		●	Adjusted the drape by folding back the drape to expose the anal area when the physician was ready to examine the patient.

Trial 1	Trial 2	Point Value	Performance Standards
		●	Assisted the patient into a supine position and then into a sitting position following the examination.
		●	Slid the table extension back into place while supporting the patient's lower legs.
		●	Assisted the patient from the examining table.
		●	Returned the footrest to its normal position.
		●	Instructed the patient to get dressed.
		●	Discarded the gown and drape in a waste container.
		▷	Stated one use of the Sims position.
		✶	Completed the procedure within 5 minutes.
			TOTALS

Evaluation of Student Performance

EVALUATION CRITERIA			COMMENTS
Symbol	**Category**	**Point Value**	
✶	Critical Step	16 points	
●	Essential Step	6 points	
▷	Theory Question	2 points	

Score calculation: 100 points

    −   _____ points missed

    _____ Score

Satisfactory score: 85 or above

CAAHEP Competencies Achieved

Psychomotor (Skills)

☑ IV. 6. Prepare a patient for procedures and/or treatments.
☑ XI. 11. Use proper body mechanics.

Affective (Behavior)
☑ IV. 4. Demonstrate awareness of the territorial boundaries of the person with whom communicating.

ABHES Competencies Achieved

☑ 9. 1. Prepare patient for examinations and treatments.

Procedure 20-8: Knee-Chest Position

Name: _____   Date: _____

Evaluated by: _____   Score: _____

Performance Objective

Outcome:	Position and drape an individual in the knee-chest position.
Conditions:	Given the following: a patient gown and a drape.
	Using an examining table.
Standards:	Time: 5 minutes. Student completed procedure in _____ minutes.
	Accuracy: Satisfactory score on the performance evaluation checklist.

Performance Evaluation Checklist

Trial 1	Trial 2	Point Value	Performance Standards
		●	Sanitized hands.
		●	Greeted the patient and introduced yourself.
		●	Identified the patient.
		●	Explained what type of examination or procedure will be performed.
		●	Provided patient with a patient gown.
		●	Instructed patient to remove clothing and to put on a patient gown with the opening in back.
		●	Pulled out the footrest and assisted the patient into a sitting position.
		●	Placed a drape over the patient's thighs and legs.
		●	Asked the patient to move back on the table.
		●	Pulled out the table extension while supporting the patient's lower legs.
		●	Assisted the patient into the supine position and then into the prone position.
		●	Positioned the drape diagonally over the patient.
		●	Asked the patient to bend the arms at the elbows and rest them alongside the head.
		●	Asked the patient to elevate the buttocks while keeping the back straight.
		●	Turned the patient's head to one side, with the weight of the body supported by the chest.
		●	Used a pillow for additional support, if needed.
		●	Separated the knees and lower legs approximately 12 inches.

361

Trial 1	Trial 2	Point Value	Performance Standards
		●	Adjusted the drape diagonally as needed.
		●	Folded back a small portion of the drape to expose the anal area when the physician was ready to examine the patient.
		●	Assisted the patient into a prone position and then into a supine position after the examination.
		●	Allowed the patient to rest in a supine position before sitting up.
		▷	Stated why the patient should be allowed to rest.
		●	Assisted the patient into a sitting position.
		●	Slid the table extension back into place while supporting the patient's lower legs.
		●	Assisted the patient from the examining table.
		●	Returned the footrest to its normal position.
		●	Instructed the patient to get dressed.
		●	Discarded the gown and drape in a waste container.
		▷	Stated one use of the knee-chest position.
		★	Completed the procedure within 5 minutes.
			TOTALS

Evaluation of Student Performance

EVALUATION CRITERIA			COMMENTS
Symbol	**Category**	**Point Value**	
★	Critical Step	16 points	
●	Essential Step	6 points	
▷	Theory Question	2 points	

Score calculation: 100 points

－   _____ points missed

_____ Score

Satisfactory score: 85 or above

CAAHEP Competencies Achieved

Psychomotor (Skills)
☑ IV. 6. Prepare a patient for procedures and/or treatments.
☑ XI. 11. Use proper body mechanics.

Affective (Behavior)
☑ IV. 4. Demonstrate awareness of the territorial boundaries of the person with whom communicating.

ABHES Competencies Achieved

☑ 9. 1. Prepare patient for examinations and treatments.

Procedure 20-9: Fowler's Position

Name: _____   Date: _____

Evaluated by: _____   Score: _____

Performance Objective

Outcome:	Position and drape an individual in the Fowler's position.
Conditions:	Given the following: a patient gown and a drape.
	Using an examining table.
Standards:	Time: 5 minutes. Student completed procedure in _____ minutes.
	Accuracy: Satisfactory score on the performance evaluation checklist.

Performance Evaluation Checklist

Trial 1	Trial 2	Point Value	Performance Standards
		●	Sanitized hands.
		●	Greeted the patient and introduced yourself.
		●	Identified the patient.
		●	Explained what type of examination or procedure will be performed.
		●	Provided patient with a patient gown.
		●	Instructed patient to remove clothing and to put on a patient gown with the opening in front.
		●	Positioned the head of the table at a 45-degree angle for a semi-Fowler's position or at a 90-degree angle for a full Fowler's position.
		●	Pulled out the footrest and assisted the patient into a sitting position.
		●	Placed a drape over the patient's thighs and legs.
		●	Pulled out the table extension while supporting the patient's lower legs.
		●	Asked the patient to lean back against the table head.
		●	Provided assistance.
		●	Positioned the drape lengthwise over the patient.
		●	Moved the drape according to the body parts being examined.
		●	Assisted the patient into a sitting position after the examination.
		●	Slid the table extension back into place while supporting the patient's lower legs.

Trial 1	Trial 2	Point Value	Performance Standards
		●	Assisted the patient from the examining table.
		●	Instructed the patient to get dressed.
		●	Returned the head of the table and the footrest to their normal positions.
		●	Discarded the gown and drape in a waste container.
		▷	Stated one use of the Fowler's position.
		✶	Completed the procedure within 5 minutes.
			TOTALS

Evaluation of Student Performance

EVALUATION CRITERIA			COMMENTS
Symbol	**Category**	**Point Value**	
✶	Critical Step	16 points	
●	Essential Step	6 points	
▷	Theory Question	2 points	

Score calculation: 100 points

− _____ points missed

_____ Score

Satisfactory score: 85 or above

CAAHEP Competencies Achieved

Psychomotor (Skills)

☑ IV. 6. Prepare a patient for procedures and/or treatments.
☑ XI. 11. Use proper body mechanics.

Affective (Behavior)
☑ IV. 4. Demonstrate awareness of the territorial boundaries of the person with whom communicating.

ABHES Competencies Achieved

☑ 9. 1. Prepare patient for examinations and treatments.

Procedure 20-10: Wheelchair Transfer

Name: _____ Date: _____

Evaluated by: _____ Score: _____

Performance Objective

Outcome:	Transfer a patient from a wheelchair to the examining table and from the examining table to a wheelchair.
Conditions:	Given the following: transfer belt.
	Using an examining table and a wheelchair.
Standards:	Time: 10 minutes. Student completed procedure in _____ minutes.
	Accuracy: Satisfactory score on the performance evaluation checklist.

Performance Evaluation Checklist

Trial 1	Trial 2	Point Value	Performance Standards
			Transferring to the examining table:
		●	Sanitized hands.
		●	Greeted the patient and introduced yourself.
		●	Identified the patient and explained the procedure.
		●	Determined whether the patient has the mental and physical capability to perform the transfer.
		●	Estimated the weight of the patient and whether he or she can assist in the transfer.
		●	Assessed your ability to safely make the transfer.
		▷	Stated factors that would prevent you from making the transfer.
		●	Wrapped the transfer belt around the patient's waist and fastened it.
		●	The belt was snug with just enough space to allow the fingers to be inserted comfortably.
		▷	Stated why the belt should be snug.
		●	With the patient's stronger side next to the table, positioned the wheelchair at a 45-degree angle to the end of the examining table.
		●	If the table is height-adjustable, adjusted it to the same height as the wheelchair or slightly lower.
		●	If the table is not height-adjustable, pulled out the footrest.
		●	Locked the brakes of the wheelchair.
		▷	Stated why the brakes should be locked.
		●	Folded back the wheelchair footrests.
		●	Informed the patient what to do during the transfer.

Trial 1	Trial 2	Point Value	Performance Standards
		●	Made sure the patient's feet were flat on the floor.
		●	Stood in front of the patient with the feet 6 to 8 inches apart, with one foot slightly forward and the knees bent.
		●	Asked the patient to place his or her arms on the armrests of the wheelchair and to lean forward.
		●	Grasped the transfer belt on either side of the patient's waist using an underhand grasp.
		▷	Stated the purpose of the transfer belt.
		●	Instructed the patient to push off the armrests and into a standing position on the count of 3.
		●	Straightened the knees and assisted the patient to a standing position by pulling upward on the transfer belt.
		●	Kept the back straight lifted with the knees, arms, and legs, and not the back.
		●	Pivoted and positioned the patient's buttocks and back of the legs toward the examining table.
		●	Instructed the patient to step backward onto the footrest, one foot at a time.
		●	Gradually lowered the patient into a sitting position on the examining table.
		●	Removed the transfer belt.
		●	Unlocked the wheelchair and moved it out of the way.
		●	Pushed in the footrest of the examining table.
		●	Stayed with the patient to prevent falls.
			Transferring to the wheelchair:
		●	Wrapped the transfer belt snugly around the patient's waist and fastened it.
		●	Positioned the wheelchair at a 45-degree angle to the end of the examining table.
		●	If the table is height-adjustable, adjusted it to the same height as the wheelchair or slightly lower.
		●	If the table is not height-adjustable, pulled out the footrest.
		●	Locked the wheelchair in place and folded back the footrests, if needed.
		●	Informed the patient what to do during the transfer.
		●	Stood in front of the patient with the feet 6 to 8 inches apart, with one foot slightly forward and the knees bent.
		●	Asked the patient to place his or her arms on your shoulders.
		●	Did not allow the patient to place his or her arms around your neck.
		●	Grasped the transfer belt on either side of the patient's waist using an underhand grasp.
		●	Instructed the patient to stand on the count of 3.

Trial 1	Trial 2	Point Value	Performance Standards
		●	Straightened your knees and assisted the patient to a standing position by pulling upward on the transfer belt.
		●	Instructed the patient to step down from the footrest, one foot at a time.
		●	Pivoted the patient until the back of the legs are against the seat of the wheelchair.
		●	Asked the patient to grasp the armrests of the wheelchair.
		●	Gradually lowered the patient into the wheelchair by bending at the knees.
		●	Removed the transfer belt and made sure the patient was comfortable.
		●	Repositioned the wheelchair footrests and assisted the patient in placing his or her feet in them.
		●	Unlocked the wheelchair.
		●	Pushed in the footrest of the examining table.
		✱	Completed the procedure within 10 minutes.
			TOTALS

Evaluation of Student Performance

EVALUATION CRITERIA			COMMENTS
Symbol	Category	Point Value	
✱	Critical Step	16 points	
●	Essential Step	6 points	
▷	Theory Question	2 points	

Score calculation: 100 points

−   points missed

_____

____ Score

Satisfactory score: 85 or above

CAAHEP Competencies Achieved

Psychomotor (Skills)
☑ IV. 6. Prepare a patient for procedures and/or treatments.
☑ XI. 11. Use proper body mechanics.

Affective (Behavior)
☑ IV. 4. Demonstrate awareness of the territorial boundaries of the person with whom communicating.

ABHES Competencies Achieved

☑ 5. b. Identify and respond appropriately when working/caring for patients with special needs.
☑ 9. l. Prepare patient for examinations and treatments.
☑ 9. q. Instruct patients with special needs.

Notes

Chapter **20** **The Physical Examination**

Procedure 20-11: Assisting with the Physical Examination

Name: _____ Date: _____

Evaluated by: _____ Score: _____

Performance Objective

Outcome:	Prepare the patient and assist with a physical examination.
Conditions:	Given the following: equipment for the type of examination to be performed, patient examination gown, and drapes.
	Using an examining table.
Standards:	Time: 20 minutes. Student completed procedure in _____ minutes.
	Accuracy: Satisfactory score on the performance evaluation checklist.

Performance Evaluation Checklist

Trial 1	Trial 2	Point Value	Performance Standards
		●	Prepared examination room.
		●	Sanitized hands.
		●	Assembled all necessary equipment.
		●	Arranged instruments in a neat and orderly manner.
		●	Obtained the patient's medical record.
		●	Went to the waiting room, and asked the patient to come back.
		●	Escorted the patient to the examination room.
		●	Asked the patient to be seated.
		●	Greeted the patient and introduced yourself.
		●	Identified the patient by full name and date of birth.
		▷	Stated why a calm and friendly manner should be used.
		●	Seated yourself facing the patient at a distance of 3 to 4 feet.
		●	Obtained and recorded patient symptoms.
		●	Measured vital signs and charted results.
		▷	Stated the adult normal range for temperature (97°F to 99°F), pulse (60 to 100 beats/min), respiration (12 to 20 breaths/min), and blood pressure (<120/80 mm Hg).
		●	Measured weight and height, and charted results.
		●	Asked patient if he or she needs to void.

Trial 1	Trial 2	Point Value	Performance Standards
		▷	Stated why the patient should be asked to void.
		●	Instructed patient to remove all clothing and put on an examining gown.
		●	Informed the patient that the physician will be in soon.
		●	Left the room to provide patient with privacy.
		●	Made patient's medical record available to the physician.
		●	Checked to make sure patient is ready to be seen.
		●	Informed physician that the patient is ready.
			Assisted the physician:
		●	Ensured the patient was in a sitting position on examination table.
		●	Handed the ophthalmoscope to the physician when requested.
		●	Dimmed the lights when the physician was ready to use the ophthalmoscope.
		▷	Stated why the lights are dimmed.
		▷	Stated the proper use of the ophthalmoscope.
		●	Handed the otoscope to the examiner when requested.
		▷	Stated the proper use of the otoscope.
		●	Is able to change the speculum and bulb in the otoscope.
		●	Handed the tongue depressor to the examiner when requested.
		●	Offered reassurance to patient as needed.
		●	Positioned patient as required for examination of the remaining body systems.
			Assisted and instructed patient:
		●	Allowed patient to rest in a sitting position before getting off the examining table.
		▷	Stated why the patient should be allowed to rest before getting off the table.
		●	Assisted patient off the examining table.
		●	Instructed patient to get dressed.
		●	Provided patient with any necessary instructions.
		▷	Stated what type of instructions may need to be relayed to the patient.
		●	Sanitized hands and charted any instructions given to the patient.
		●	Escorted the patient to the reception area.

Trial 1	Trial 2	Point Value	Performance Standards
			Cleaned the examination room:
		●	Discarded paper on the examining table and unrolled a fresh length.
		●	Discarded all disposable supplies into an appropriate waste container.
		●	Checked to make sure ample supplies are available.
		●	Removed reusable equipment for sanitization, sterilization, or disinfection.
		✱	Completed the procedure within 20 minutes.
			TOTALS

	CHART
Date	

Evaluation of Student Performance

EVALUATION CRITERIA			COMMENTS
Symbol	Category	Point Value	
✱	Critical Step	16 points	
●	Essential Step	6 points	
▷	Theory Question	2 points	

Score calculation: 100 points

− _____ points missed

_____ Score

Satisfactory score: 85 or above

CAAHEP Competencies Achieved

Psychomotor (Skills)
☑ I. 10. Assist physician with patient care.
☑ IV. 5. Instruct patients according to their needs to promote health maintenance and disease prevention.
☑ IV. 6. Prepare a patient for procedures and/or treatments.
☑ IV. 12. Develop and maintain a current list of community resources related to patients' health care needs.
☑ V. 9. Perform routine maintenance of office equipment with documentation.
☑ XI. 11. Use proper body mechanics.

Affective (Behavior)
☑ I. 3. Demonstrate respect for diversity in approaching patients and families.
☑ IV. 2. Apply active listening skills.
☑ IV. 3. Use appropriate body language and other nonverbal skills in communicating with patients, family, and staff.
☑ IV. 8. Analyze communications in providing appropriate responses or feedback.
☑ IV. 10. Demonstrate respect for individual diversity, incorporating awareness of one's own biases in areas including gender, race, religion, age, and economic status.
☑ X. 3. Demonstrate awareness of diversity in providing patient care.

ABHES Competencies Achieved

☑ 6. g. Analyze the effect of hereditary, cultural, and environmental influences.
☑ 8. x. Maintain medical facility.
☑ 8. y. Perform routine maintenance of administrative and clinical equipment.
☑ 8. z. Maintain inventory equipment and supplies.
☑ 8. aa. Are attentive, listen, and learn.
☑ 8. cc. Communicate on the recipient's level of comprehension.
☑ 8. ii. Recognize and respond to verbal and nonverbal communication.
☑ 8. kk. Adapt to individualized needs.
☑ 9. k. Prepare and maintain examination and treatment area.
☑ 9. l. Prepare patient for examinations and treatments.
☑ 9. m. Assist physician with routine and specialty examinations and treatments.
☑ 9. p. Advise patients of office policies and procedures.
☑ 9. r. Teach patients methods of health promotion and disease prevention.

21 Eye and Ear Assessment and Procedures

CHAPTER ASSIGNMENTS

√ After Completing	Date Due	Textbook Pages	TEXTBOOK ASSIGNMENTS	Possible Points	Points You Earned
		384-408	Read Chapter 21: Eye and Ear Assessment and Procedures		
		389 406	📝 Read Case Study 1 Case Study 1 questions	5	
		393 406	📝 Read Case Study 2 Case Study 2 questions	5	
		397 406-407	📝 Read Case Study 3 Case Study 3 questions	5	
			TOTAL POINTS		

√ After Completing	Date Due	Study Guide Pages	STUDY GUIDE ASSIGNMENTS (CTA = Critical Thinking Activity)	Possible Points	Points You Earned
		377	📄 Pretest	10	
		378	🔑 Key Term Assessment A. Definitions B. Word Parts (Add 1 point for each medical term)	13 11	
		379-381	📝 Evaluation of Learning questions	22	
		381	CTA A: Measuring Distance Visual Acuity	6	
		381-382	CTA B: Interpreting Visual Acuity Results	4	
		382	CTA C: Charting Visual Acuity Results	4	
		382-383	CTA D: Ear Procedures	8	
		383	CTA E: Dear Gabby	10	
		384	CTA F: Crossword Puzzle	20	
		385-388	CTA G: Eye and Ear Conditions	40	
			e Evolve Site: Animations	20	
			e Evolve Site: Apply Your Knowledge questions	10	

√ After Completing	Date Due	Study Guide Pages	STUDY GUIDE ASSIGNMENTS (CTA = Critical Thinking Activity)	Possible Points	Points You Earned
			Evolve Site: Video Evaluation	70	
		377	Posttest	10	
			ADDITIONAL ASSIGNMENTS		
			TOTAL POINTS		

√ When Assigned By Your Instructor	Study Guide Pages	Practices Required	LABORATORY ASSIGNMENTS (Procedure Number and Name)	Score*
	389-390	5	**Practice for Competency** 21-1: Assessing Distance Visual Acuity—Snellen Chart Textbook reference: pp. 390-391	
	391-393		**Evaluation of Competency** 21-1: Assessing Distance Visual Acuity—Snellen Chart	*
	389-390	3	**Practice for Competency** 21-2: Assessing Color Vision: Ishihara Test Textbook reference: pp. 391-392	
	395-397		**Evaluation of Competency** 21-2: Assessing Color Vision: Ishihara Test	*
	389-390	3	**Practice for Competency** 21-3: Performing an Eye Irrigation Textbook reference: pp. 394-395	
	399-401		**Evaluation of Competency** 21-3: Performing an Eye Irrigation	*
	389-390	3	**Practice for Competency** 21-4: Performing an Eye Instillation Textbook reference: pp. 396-397	
	403-404		**Evaluation of Competency** 21-4: Performing an Eye Instillation	*
	389-390	3	**Practice for Competency** 21-5: Performing an Ear Irrigation Textbook reference: pp. 402-403	
	405-407		**Evaluation of Competency** 21-5: Performing an Ear Irrigation	*
	389-390	3	**Practice for Competency** 21-6: Performing an Ear Instillation Textbook reference: pp. 404-405	
	409-410		**Evaluation of Competency** 21-6: Performing an Ear Instillation	*
			ADDITIONAL ASSIGNMENTS	

Notes

Name _____   Date _____

True or False

_____ 1. Refraction refers to the bending of light rays so that they can be focused on the retina.

_____ 2. A person who is farsighted has a condition known as *myopia*.

_____ 3. An optometrist can perform eye surgery.

_____ 4. The Snellen eye test is conducted at a distance of 20 feet.

_____ 5. The Snellen eye chart should be positioned at the medical assistant's eye level.

_____ 6. An eye instillation may be performed to treat an eye infection.

_____ 7. Conjunctivitis caused by a bacterium is not contagious.

_____ 8. The most specific type of hearing test is the tuning fork test.

_____ 9. Serous otitis media can result in a conductive hearing loss.

_____ 10. An ear instillation may be performed to treat an ear infection.

? POSTTEST

True or False

_____ 1. A person who cannot see objects close up has a condition known as amblyopia.

_____ 2. Visual acuity refers to sharpness of vision.

_____ 3. Presbyopia is a decrease in the elasticity of the lens due to the aging process.

_____ 4. An optician fills prescriptions for eyeglasses.

_____ 5. The Snellen Big E chart is used with school-aged children.

_____ 6. The most common color vision defects are congenital in nature.

_____ 7. The external auditory canal of an adult is straightened by pulling the ear downward and backward.

_____ 8. The range of frequencies for normal speech is 300 to 4000 Hz.

_____ 9. Intense noise can result in a sensorineural hearing loss.

_____ 10. Tympanometry is used to diagnose patients with auditory nerve damage.

A. Definitions

Directions: Match each medical term with its definition.

_____ 1. Astigmatism

_____ 2. Audiometer

_____ 3. Canthus

_____ 4. Cerumen

_____ 5. Hyperopia

_____ 6. Impacted

_____ 7. Instillation

_____ 8. Irrigation

_____ 9. Myopia

_____ 10. Otoscope

_____ 11. Presbyopia

_____ 12. Refraction

_____ 13. Tympanic membrane

A. The washing of a body canal with a flowing solution

B. A decrease in the elasticity of the lens that occurs with aging, resulting in a decreased ability to focus on close objects

C. Farsightedness

D. The deflection or bending of light rays by a lens

E. The junction of the eyelids at either corner of the eye

F. Nearsightedness

G. The dropping of a liquid into a body cavity

H. An instrument for examining the external ear canal and tympanic membrane

I. Earwax

J. An instrument used to quantitatively measure hearing acuity for the various frequencies of sound waves

K. A thin, semitransparent membrane located between the external ear canal and the middle ear that receives and transmits sound waves

L. A refractive error that causes distorted and blurred vision for both near and far objects due to a cornea that is oval shaped

M. Wedged firmly together so as to be immovable

B. Word Parts

Directions: Indicate the meaning of each word part in the space provided. List as many medical terms as possible that incorporate the word part in the space provided.

Word Part	Meaning of Word Part	Medical Terms That Incorporate Word Part
1. a-		
2. stigma/a		
3. -ism		
4. audi/o		
5. -meter		
6. hyper-		
7. -opia		
8. ot/o		
9. -scope		
10. tympan/o		
11. -ic		

Directions: Fill in each blank with the correct answer.

1. What is visual acuity?

   _____

   _____

2. What type of symptoms might be experienced with myopia?

   _____

   _____

3. What methods can be used to correct myopia?

   _____

   _____

4. What causes an individual with astigmatism to have distorted and blurred vision?

   _____

   _____

5. What are each of the following eye professionals qualified to perform?

   a. Ophthalmologist

   _____

   _____

   b. Optometrist

   _____

   _____

   c. Optician

   _____

   _____

6. What condition can be detected by measuring distance visual acuity?

   _____

7. What type of patient would warrant use of the Snellen Big E eye chart? (Give two examples.)

   _____

   _____

8. Explain the significance of the top number and bottom number next to each line of letters on the Snellen eye chart.

   _____

   _____

9. List two conditions that can be detected by measuring near visual acuity.

_____

_____

10. Explain the difference between congenital and acquired color vision defects.

_____

_____

_____

11. What is a polychromatic plate?

_____

_____

_____

12. List three reasons for performing eye irrigation.

_____

_____

_____

13. List three reasons for performing eye instillation.

_____

_____

_____

14. What is the range of frequencies for normal speech?

_____

_____

15. List five conditions that may cause conductive hearing loss.

_____

_____

_____

16. List four conditions that may result in sensorineural hearing loss.

_____

_____

17. What information is obtained through audiometry?

_____

_____

_____

18. What information is obtained through tympanometry?

_____

_____

_____

19. List three reasons for performing ear irrigation.

_____

_____

20. List three reasons for performing ear instillation.

_____

21. Explain how impacted cerumen is removed from the ear.

_____

_____

_____

22. Explain how to straighten the external auditory canal in an adult and in children 3 years old or younger.

_____

_____

_____

CRITICAL THINKING ACTIVITIES

A. Measuring Distance Visual Acuity

For each of the following situations, write **C** if the technique is correct and **I** if the technique is incorrect.

_____ 1. The patient is not given an opportunity to study the Snellen chart before beginning the test.

_____ 2. The Snellen chart is positioned at the medical assistant's eye level.

_____ 3. The patient is instructed to use his or her hand to cover the eye that is not being tested.

_____ 4. The medical assistant instructs the patient to close the eye that is not being tested.

_____ 5. The first line that the medical assistant asks the patient to identify is the 20/20 line.

_____ 6. The medical assistant observes the patient for signs of squinting or leaning forward during the test.

B. Interpreting Visual Acuity Results

1. A patient has a distance visual acuity reading of 20/30 in the right eye. Using this information, answer the following questions:

   a. How far was the patient from the eye chart?

   _____

   b. At what distance would a person with normal acuity be able to read this line?

   _____

2. A patient has a distance visual acuity reading of 20/10 in the left eye. Using this information, answer the following questions:

a. How far was the patient from the eye chart?

_____

b. At what distance would a person with normal acuity be able to read this line?

_____

C. Charting Visual Acuity Results

Properly chart the distance visual acuity results in the spaces provided. In all cases, the line indicated is the smallest line the patient could read at a distance of 20 feet.

1. The patient read the line marked 20/30 with the right eye with two errors; with the left eye, the patient read the line marked 20/30 with one error. The patient was wearing corrective lenses.

_____

_____

2. The patient read the line marked 20/20 with the right eye with one error; with the left eye, the patient read the line marked 20/20 with no errors. The patient was wearing corrective lenses.

_____

_____

3. The patient read the line marked 20/40 with the right eye with two errors; with the left eye, the patient read the line marked 20/30 with one error. The patient exhibited squinting and frowning during the test. The patient was not wearing corrective lenses.

_____

_____

4. The patient read the line marked 20/15 with the right eye with no errors; with the left eye, the patient read the line marked 20/20 with one error. The patient was not wearing corrective lenses.

_____

_____

D. Ear Procedures

Explain the principle for each of the following procedures.

Ear Irrigation

1. Positioning the patient's head so that it is tilted toward the affected ear

_____

_____

2. Cleansing the outer ear before irrigating

_____

_____

3. Straightening the external auditory canal

_____

_____

4. Injecting the irrigating solution toward the roof of the ear canal

_____

_____

_____

5. Making sure not to obstruct the canal opening

_____

_____

_____

Ear Instillation

6. Positioning the patient's head so that it is tilted toward the unaffected ear

_____

_____

_____

7. Instructing the patient to lie on the unaffected side after the instillation

_____

_____

_____

8. Placing a cotton wick in the patient's ear

_____

_____

_____

E. Dear Gabby

Gabby has a middle ear infection and is not feeling well. She wants you to fill in for her. In the space provided, respond to the following letter.

Dear Gabby:

I am dating the sweetest and dearest man. "Mike" has only one flaw. He likes loud music. He had those big boom boxes installed in his car. When we drive somewhere in his car, he blasts the music. Sometimes, when we are driving down a street, people even turn around to see where the loud music is coming from. The music hurts my ears, and I cannot think straight. My ears even start ringing when we go on a trip. When I am talking to Mike, he says I mumble, and I have to speak extra loud around him. I keep telling Mike that the loud music is going to damage our hearing, but he says that we are way too young for that and that only old people have trouble hearing. Please help me Gabby, because I love going on trips with Mike, but not if my ears hurt afterward.

Signed, Ears Are Ringing

_____

_____

_____

_____

_____

_____

_____

_____

_____

_____

F. Crossword Puzzle: Eye and Ear

Directions: Complete the crossword puzzle using the clues provided.

Across

1 Decreased lens elasticity
3 Fills eyeglasses prescriptions
8 Color blind test
10 Impacted cerumen may cause this
13 Fixed stapes
15 Assesses mobility of eardrum
16 Drum in your ear
17 Earwax
18 Music that is too loud may cause this
19 Normal DVA
20 Has an S shape

Down

2 Physician who diagnoses and treats eye disorders
4 Instrument that measures hearing
5 A cause of pink eye
6 Caught it!
7 Fluid in middle ear
9 Middle ear infection
11 Cannot see far away
12 Sharpness of vision
14 Measurement for sound

G. Eye and Ear Conditions

1. You and your classmates work at a large clinic. It is National Eye and Ear Week. The physicians at your clinic ask you to develop for their patients informative, creative, and colorful brochures about eye and ear conditions. Choose a condition, and design a brochure using the blank Frequently Asked Questions (FAQ) brochure provided on the following page. Each student in the class should select a different topic. On a separate sheet of paper, write three true or false questions related to the information in your brochure.

2. Present your brochure to the class. After all the brochures have been presented, each student should ask three questions to the entire class to see how well the class understands eye and ear conditions. (*Note:* You can take notes during the presentations and refer to them when answering the questions.)

Eye

1. Amblyopia (lazy eye)
2. Age-related macular degeneration
3. Astigmatism
4. Blepharitis
5. Cataracts
6. CMV retinitis
7. Corneal ulcer
8. Corneal abrasion
9. Strabismus (crossed-eyed)
10. Diabetic retinopathy
11. Drooping eyelids (ptosis)
12. Dry eyes
13. Floaters and spots
14. Glaucoma
15. Keratoconus
16. Ocular hypertension
17. Presbycusis
18. Retinal detachment
19. Retinitis pigmentosa
20. Stye

Ear

1. Acute mastoiditis
2. External otitis
3. Meniere's disease
4. Noise-induced hearing loss
5. Serous otitis media

Notes

FAQ on:

Q: **A:**

Q: **A:**

Q: **A:**

Q: **A:**

Q:

A:

Q:

A:

Illustration

Q:

A:

Q:

A:

Chapter **21** **Eye and Ear Assessment and Procedures**

Eye Assessment and Procedures

Procedure 21-1: Distance Visual Acuity. Assess distance visual acuity using a Snellen eye chart, and record results in the chart provided. Circle any readings that indicate distance visual acuity above or below average.

Procedure 21-2: Color Vision. Assess color vision, and record results in the chart provided. Circle any abnormal results.

Procedure 21-3: Eye Irrigation. Perform an eye irrigation, and record the procedure in the chart provided.

Procedure 21-4: Eye Instillation. Perform an eye instillation, and record the procedure in the chart provided.

Ear Procedures

Procedure 21-5: Ear Irrigation. Perform an ear irrigation, and record the procedure in the chart provided.

Procedure 21-6: Ear Instillation. Perform an ear instillation, and record the procedure in the chart provided.

CHART	
Date	

	CHART
Date	

Procedure 21-1: Assessing Distance Visual Acuity—Snellen Chart

Name: _____   Date: _____

Evaluated by: _____   Score: _____

Performance Objective

Outcome:	Assess distance visual acuity.
Conditions:	Given the following: Snellen eye chart, eye occluder, and an antiseptic wipe.
	Time: 5 minutes. Student completed procedure in _____ minutes.
Standards:	Accuracy: Satisfactory score on the performance evaluation checklist.

Performance Evaluation Checklist

Trial 1	Trial 2	Point Value	Performance Standards
		●	Sanitized hands.
		●	Assembled equipment.
		●	Disinfected the eye occluder with an antiseptic wipe.
		●	Greeted the patient and introduced yourself.
		●	Identified the patient and explained the procedure.
		●	Determined if patient wears corrective lenses and instructed patient to leave them on during the test.
		●	Positioned patient 20 feet from the eye chart.
		●	Positioned the center of the eye chart at patient's eye level.
		●	Instructed patient to cover the left eye with the occluder and to keep the left eye open.
		▷	Stated how the occluder should be positioned if the patient wears glasses.
		▷	Explained why the patient's left eye should remain open.
		●	Instructed patient not to squint during the test.
		▷	Explained why the patient should not squint during the test.
		●	Asked patient to identify the 20/70 line, using the right eye.
		▷	Stated why the test should begin with a line that is above the 20/20 line.
		●	Proceeded down the chart if the patient identified the 20/70 line or proceeded up the chart if the patient was unable to identify the 20/70 line.

Trial 1	Trial 2	Point Value	Performance Standards
		●	Continued until the smallest line of letters that the patient could read was reached.
		●	Observed patient for any unusual symptoms.
		●	Jotted down the numbers next to the smallest line read by the patient.
		●	Asked patient to cover the right eye and to keep the right eye open.
		●	Measured visual acuity in the left eye.
		●	Jotted down the numbers next to the smallest line read by the patient.
		✶	The visual acuity measurements were identical to the evaluator's measurements.
		●	Charted the results correctly.
		●	Disinfected the occluder with an antiseptic wipe.
		●	Sanitized hands.
		✶	Completed the procedure within 5 minutes.
			TOTALS

CHART	
Date	

Evaluation of Student Performance

EVALUATION CRITERIA			COMMENTS
Symbol	**Category**	**Point Value**	
✶	Critical Step	16 points	
●	Essential Step	6 points	
▷	Theory Question	2 points	

Score calculation: 100 points

− _____ points missed

_____ Score

Satisfactory score: 85 or above

CAAHEP Competencies Achieved

Psychomotor (Skills)
☑ IV. 6. Prepare a patient for procedures and/or treatments.

Affective (Behavior)
☑ I. 2. Use language/verbal skills that enable patient's understanding.
☑ IV. 7. Demonstrate recognition of the patient's level of understanding in communications.

ABHES Competencies Achieved

☑ 8. cc. Communicate on the recipient's level of comprehension.
☑ 9. l. Prepare patient for examinations and treatments.

Notes

Procedure 21-2: Assessing Color Vision—Ishihara Test

Name: _____   Date: _____

Evaluated by: _____   Score: _____

Performance Objective

Outcome:	Assess color vision.
Conditions:	Given an Ishihara book of color plates and a cotton swab.
Standards:	Time: 10 minutes. Student completed procedure in _____ minutes.
	Accuracy: Satisfactory score on the performance evaluation checklist.

Performance Evaluation Checklist

Trial 1	Trial 2	Point Value	Performance Standards
		●	Sanitized hands.
		●	Assembled equipment.
		●	Conducted the test in a quiet room illuminated by natural daylight.
		▷	Stated why natural daylight should be used.
		●	Greeted the patient and introduced yourself.
		●	Identified the patient.
		●	Explained the procedure using the practice plate.
		▷	Stated the purpose of the practice plate.
		●	Held the first plate 30 inches from the patient at a right angle to the patient's line of vision.
		●	Instructed patient to keep both eyes open.
		●	Told patient that he or she would have 3 seconds to identify each plate.
		●	Asked the patient to identify the number on the plate.
		●	Asked the patient to trace plates that have a winding line with a cotton swab.
		▷	Stated why a cotton swab should be used to make the tracing.
		●	Recorded the results after identification of each plate.

Trial 1	Trial 2	Point Value	Performance Standards
		●	Continued until the patient viewed all plates.
		●	Charted the results correctly.
		✳	The results were identical to the evaluator's results.
		●	Returned the Ishihara book to its proper place, storing it in a closed position.
		▷	Explained why the book should be stored in a closed position.
		✳	Completed the procedure within 10 minutes.
			TOTALS
CHART				
Date		

CHART		
Plate No.	Normal Person	Results
1	12	
2	8	
3	5	
4	29	
5	74	
6	7	
7	45	
8	2	
9	X	
10	16	
11	Traceable	
Date :		
Evaluated by :		

(From Bonewit-West K: *Study guide for clinical medical assistants*, ed 8, St. Louis, 2011, Saunders.)

Evaluation of Student Performance

<table>
<tr><th colspan="3">EVALUATION CRITERIA</th><th rowspan="2">COMMENTS</th></tr>
<tr><th>Symbol</th><th>Category</th><th>Point Value</th></tr>
<tr><td>✱</td><td>Critical Step</td><td>16 points</td><td></td></tr>
<tr><td>●</td><td>Essential Step</td><td>6 points</td><td></td></tr>
<tr><td>▷</td><td>Theory Question</td><td>2 points</td><td></td></tr>
</table>

Score calculation: 100 points

         −   points missed
                _____ Score

Satisfactory score: 85 or above

CAAHEP Competencies Achieved

Psychomotor (Skills)
☑ IV. 6. Prepare a patient for procedures and/or treatments.

Affective (Behavior)
☑ I. 2. Use language/verbal skills that enable patients' understanding.
☑ IV. 7. Demonstrate recognition of the patient's level of understanding in communications.

ABHES Competencies Achieved

☑ 8. cc. Communicate on the recipient's level of comprehension.
☑ 9. 1. Prepare patient for examinations and treatments.

Notes

Procedure 21-3: Performing an Eye Irrigation

Name: _____   Date: _____

Evaluated by: _____   Score: _____

Performance Objective

Outcome:	Perform an eye irrigation.
Conditions:	Given the following: disposable (nonpowdered) gloves, irrigating solution, solution container, disposable rubber bulb syringe, basin, moisture-resistant towel, and sterile gauze pads.
Standards:	Time: 5 minutes. Student completed procedure in _____ minutes.
	Accuracy: Satisfactory score on the Performance Evaluation Checklist.

Performance Evaluation Checklist

Trial 1	Trial 2	Point Value	Performance Standards
		●	Sanitized hands.
		●	Assembled equipment.
		●	Checked the solution label with the physician's instructions.
		●	Checked expiration date of the solution.
		▷	Stated the reason for checking the expiration date.
		●	Warmed the irrigating solution to body temperature.
		▷	Explained why the solution should be at body temperature.
		●	Checked the label a second time and poured the solution into a basin.
		●	Checked the label a third time before returning the container to storage.
		●	Greeted the patient and introduced yourself.
		●	Identified the patient and explained the procedure.
		●	Asked patient to remove glasses or contact lenses.
		●	Positioned patient in a lying or sitting position.
		●	Placed a moisture-resistant towel on the patient's shoulder.
		●	Positioned a basin tightly against the patient's cheek under the affected eye.
		●	Asked patient to tilt head in the direction of the affected eye and hold the basin in place.
		▷	Explained why patient's head is turned in the direction of the affected eye.
		●	Applied nonpowdered gloves.

Trial 1	Trial 2	Point Value	Performance Standards
		▷	Stated why nonpowdered gloves should be used.
		●	Cleansed the eyelids from inner to outer canthus.
		▷	Stated why eyelids are cleansed.
		●	Filled irrigating syringe.
		●	Instructed patient to keep both eyes open and to look at a focal point.
		▷	Stated the reason for looking at a focal point.
		●	Separated eyelids.
		●	Held tip of syringe 1 inch above the eye at the inner canthus.
		●	Allowed solution to flow over the eye at a moderate rate from the inner canthus to the outer canthus and directed solution to the lower conjunctiva.
		▷	Explained why the syringe should be directed toward the lower conjunctiva.
		●	Did not allow syringe to touch the eye.
		●	Refilled the syringe and continued irrigating until the desired results were obtained or all the solution was used.
		●	Dried eyelids with gauze pad from inner to outer canthus.
		●	Removed gloves and sanitized hands.
		●	Charted the procedure correctly.
		▷	Stated the abbreviation for both eyes (OU), the right eye (OD), and the left eye (OS).
		●	Returned equipment.
		★	Completed the procedure within 5 minutes.
			TOTALS

CHART

Date	

Evaluation of Student Performance

EVALUATION CRITERIA			COMMENTS
Symbol	**Category**	**Point Value**	
✶	Critical Step	16 points	
●	Essential Step	6 points	
▷	Theory Question	2 points	

Score calculation: 100 points

          −   points missed

             _____ Score

Satisfactory score: 85 or above

CAAHEP Competencies Achieved

Psychomotor (Skills)
☑ II. 1. Prepare proper dosages of medication for administration.
☑ IV. 6. Prepare a patient for procedures and/or treatments.

Affective (Behavior)
☑ II. 1. Verify ordered doses/dosages prior to administration.
☑ IV. 5. Demonstrate sensitivity appropriate to the message being delivered.

ABHES Competencies Achieved

☑ 8. bb. Are impartial and show empathy when dealing with patients.
☑ 9. d. Recognize and understand various treatment protocols.
☑ 9. l. Prepare patient for examinations and treatments.

Notes

Procedure 21-4: Performing an Eye Instillation

Name: _____   Date: _____

Evaluated by: _____   Score: _____

Performance Objective

Outcome:	Perform an eye instillation.
Conditions:	Given the following: disposable (nonpowdered) gloves, ophthalmic medication, tissues, and gauze pads.
Standards:	Time: 5 minutes. Student completed procedure in _____ minutes.
	Accuracy: Satisfactory score on the Performance Evaluation Checklist.

Performance Evaluation Checklist

Trial 1	Trial 2	Point Value	Performance Standards
		●	Sanitized hands.
		●	Assembled equipment.
		●	Checked the drug label when removing it from storage.
		▷	Stated what word must appear on the medication label.
		●	Checked drug label and dosage against the physician's instructions.
		●	Checked the expiration date of the medication.
		●	Greeted the patient and introduced yourself.
		●	Identified the patient and explained the procedure.
		●	Positioned patient in a sitting or supine position.
		●	Applied nonpowdered gloves.
		●	Prepared the medication.
		●	Checked the drug label and removed the cap.
		●	Asked patient to look up and exposed the lower conjunctival sac.
		▷	Explained the reason for asking patient to look up.
		●	Drew the skin of the cheek downward and exposed the conjunctival sac.
		●	Inserted the medication correctly.
		▷	Explained how to instill eyedrops and ointment.
		●	Instructed patient to close eyes gently and move eyeballs.
		▷	Stated the reason for closing the eyes and moving the eyeballs.

Trial 1	Trial 2	Point Value	Performance Standards
		●	Told patient that the instillation may temporarily blur vision.
		●	Dried eyelids with a gauze pad from inner to outer canthus.
		●	Removed gloves and sanitized hands.
		●	Charted the procedure correctly.
		●	Returned equipment.
		✱	Completed the procedure within 5 minutes.
			TOTALS

	CHART
Date	

Evaluation of Student Performance

EVALUATION CRITERIA			COMMENTS
Symbol	**Category**	**Point Value**	
✱	Critical Step	16 points	
●	Essential Step	6 points	
▷	Theory Question	2 points	

Score calculation: 100 points

– _____ points missed

_____ Score

Satisfactory score: 85 or above

CAAHEP Competencies Achieved

Psychomotor (Skills)
☑ II. 1. Prepare proper dosages of medication for administration.
☑ IV. 6. Prepare a patient for procedures and/or treatments.

Affective (Behavior)
☑ II. 1. Verify ordered doses/dosages prior to administration.
☑ IV. 5. Demonstrate sensitivity appropriate to the message being delivered.

ABHES Competencies Achieved

☑ 8. bb. Are impartial and show empathy when dealing with patients.
☑ 9. d. Recognize and understand various treatment protocols.
☑ 9. l. Prepare patient for examinations and treatments.

Procedure 21-5: Performing an Ear Irrigation

Name: _____   Date: _____

Evaluated by: _____   Score: _____

Performance Objective

Outcome:	Perform an ear irrigation.
Conditions:	Given the following: disposable gloves, irrigating solution, solution container, irrigating syringe, ear basin, moisture-resistant towel, gauze pads, and ear wick.
Standards:	Time: 10 minutes. Student completed procedure in _____ minutes.
	Accuracy: Satisfactory score on the performance evaluation checklist.

Performance Evaluation Checklist

Trial 1	Trial 2	Point Value	Performance Standards
		●	Sanitized hands.
		●	Assembled equipment.
		●	Checked the label of the irrigating solution with the physician's instructions.
		●	Checked expiration date of the solution.
		●	Warmed the irrigating solution to body temperature.
		▷	Stated the reason for warming the irrigating solution.
		●	Checked the label a second time and poured the solution into a basin.
		●	Checked the label a third time before returning the container to storage.
		●	Greeted the patient and introduced yourself.
		●	Identified the patient and explained the procedure.
		●	Positioned patient in a sitting position.
		●	Placed a towel on patient's shoulder under ear to be irrigated.
		●	Positioned basin under affected ear and asked patient to hold it in place.
		●	Asked patient to tilt head toward the affected ear.
		▷	Explained why the head should be tilted toward the affected ear.
		●	Applied gloves.
		●	Cleansed the outer ear.
		▷	Explained why the outer ear should be cleansed.
		●	Filled the irrigating syringe.

Trial 1	Trial 2	Trial 2	Performance Standards
		●	Expelled air from syringe.
		▷	Explained why air should be expelled from syringe.
		●	Properly straightened the ear canal.
		▷	Stated why the canal must be straightened.
		●	Inserted syringe tip into the ear.
		●	Did not insert the syringe too deeply.
		●	Made sure that tip of syringe did not obstruct the canal opening.
		▷	Stated why the canal should not be obstructed.
		●	Injected the irrigating solution toward the roof of the ear canal.
		▷	Stated why solution should be injected toward roof of the canal.
		●	Refilled the syringe and continued irrigating until the desired results were obtained or all the solution was used.
		●	Observed the returning solution to note the material present and the amount.
		●	Dried outside of the ear with a gauze pad.
		●	Informed patient that the ear will feel sensitive.
		●	Instructed patient to lie on the affected side on treatment table.
		▷	Explained why patient should lie on the affected side.
		●	Inserted a cotton wick loosely in the ear canal for 15 minutes.
		▷	Stated the purpose of the cotton wick.
		●	Removed gloves and sanitized hands.
		●	Charted the procedure correctly.
		▷	Stated the abbreviation for both ears (AU), the right ear (AD), and the left ear (AS).
		●	Returned equipment.
		✶	Completed the procedure within 10 minutes.
			TOTALS

		CHART	
	Date		

Evaluation of Student Performance

EVALUATION CRITERIA			COMMENTS
Symbol	**Category**	**Point Value**	
✳	Critical Step	16 points	
●	Essential Step	6 points	
▷	Theory Question	2 points	

Score calculation: 100 points

      −   _____ points missed

             _____ Score

Satisfactory score: 85 or above

CAAHEP Competencies Achieved

Psychomotor (Skills)
☑ II. 1. Prepare proper dosages of medication for administration.
☑ IV. 6. Prepare a patient for procedures and/or treatments.

Affective (Behavior)
☑ II. 1. Verify ordered doses/dosages prior to administration.
☑ IV. 5. Demonstrate sensitivity appropriate to the message being delivered.

ABHES Competencies Achieved

☑ 8. bb. Are impartial and show empathy when dealing with patients.
☑ 9. d. Recognize and understand various treatment protocols.
☑ 9. l. Prepare patient for examinations and treatments.

Notes

Procedure 21-6: Performing an Ear Instillation

Name: _____   Date: _____

Evaluated by: _____   Score: _____

Performance Objective

Outcome:	Perform an ear instillation.
Conditions:	Given the following: disposable gloves, otic medication, and gauze pad.
Standards:	Time: 5 minutes. Student completed procedure in _____ minutes.
	Accuracy: Satisfactory score on the Performance Evaluation Checklist.

Performance Evaluation Checklist

Trial 1	Trial 2	Point Value	Performance Standards
		●	Sanitized hands.
		●	Assembled equipment.
		●	Checked the drug label when removing the medication from storage.
		▷	Stated what word must appear on the medication label.
		●	Checked the drug label and dosage against the physician's instructions.
		●	Checked the expiration date of the medication.
		▷	Explained what might occur if the medication is outdated.
		●	Greeted the patient and introduced yourself.
		●	Identified the patient and explained the procedure.
		●	Positioned patient in a sitting position.
		●	Warmed the eardrops with your hands.
		●	Applied gloves.
		●	Mixed medication if required, by shaking the container.
		●	Checked the drug label and removed the cap.
		●	Asked the patient to tilt the head in the direction of the unaffected ear.
		●	Properly straightened the ear canal.
		▷	Stated the reason for straightening the canal.
		●	Placed tip of dropper at the opening of the ear canal and inserted the proper amount of medication.
		●	Instructed patient to lie on the unaffected side for 2 to 3 minutes.

409

Trial 1	Trial 2	Point Value	Performance Standards
		▷	Explained why patient should lie on the unaffected side.
		●	Placed a moistened cotton wick loosely in the ear canal for 15 minutes.
		▷	Stated the reason for moistening the wick.
		●	Removed gloves and sanitized hands.
		●	Charted the procedure correctly.
		●	Returned equipment.
		★	Completed the procedure within 5 minutes.
			TOTALS

CHART	
Date	

Evaluation of Student Performance

EVALUATION CRITERIA			COMMENTS
Symbol	**Category**	**Point Value**	
★	Critical Step	16 points	
●	Essential Step	6 points	
▷	Theory Question	2 points	

Score calculation: 100 points

     −   points missed

         _____ Score

Satisfactory score: 85 or above

CAAHEP Competencies Achieved

Psychomotor (Skills)
☑ II. 1. Prepare proper dosages of medication for administration.
☑ IV. 6. Prepare a patient for procedures and/or treatments.

Affective (Behavior)
☑ II. 1. Verify ordered doses/dosages prior to administration.
☑ IV. 5. Demonstrate sensitivity appropriate to the message being delivered.

ABHES Competencies Achieved

☑ 8. bb. Are impartial and show empathy when dealing with patients.
☑ 9. d. Recognize and understand various treatment protocols.
☑ 9. l. Prepare patient for examinations and treatments.

Physical Agents to Promote Tissue Healing

CHAPTER ASSIGNMENTS

√ After Completing	Date Due	Textbook Pages	TEXTBOOK ASSIGNMENTS	Possible Points	Points You Earned
		409-426	Read Chapter 22: Physical Agents to Promote Tissue Healing		
		412 425	Read Case Study 1 Case Study 1 questions	5	
		420 425-426	Read Case Study 2 Case Study 2 questions	5	
			TOTAL POINTS		

√ After Completing	Date Due	Study Guide Pages	STUDY GUIDE ASSIGNMENTS (CTA = Critical Thinking Activity)	Possible Points	Points You Earned
		415	Pretest	10	
		416	Term Key Term Assessment	9	
		416-418	Evaluation of Learning questions	15	
		418	CTA A: Dear Gabby	10	
		419	CTA B: Crutch Guidelines	8	
		419-420	CTA C: Accessibility for Physical Disabilities	7	
		421	CTA D: Crossword Puzzle	25	
		422-424	CTA E: Bone and Joint Conditions	40	
			Evolve Site: Animations	20	
			Evolve Site: Quiz Show (Record points earned)		
			Evolve Site: Apply Your Knowledge questions	10	
			Evolve Site: Video Evaluation	63	
		415	Posttest	10	

√ After Completing	Date Due	Study Guide Pages	STUDY GUIDE ASSIGNMENTS (CTA = Critical Thinking Activity)	Possible Points	Points You Earned
			ADDITIONAL ASSIGNMENTS		
			TOTAL POINTS		

√ When Assigned By Your Instructor	Study Guide Page(s)	Practices Required	LABORATORY ASSIGNMENTS (Procedure Number and Name)	Score*
	425-426	3	**Practice for Competency** 22-1: Applying a Heating Pad Textbook reference: p. 413	
	427-428		**Evaluation of Competency** 22-1: Applying a Heating Pad	*
	425-426	3	**Practice for Competency** 22-2: Applying a Hot Soak Textbook reference: pp. 413-414	
	429-430		**Evaluation of Competency** 22-2: Applying a Hot Soak	*
	425-426	3	**Practice for Competency** 22-3: Applying a Hot Compress Textbook reference: pp. 414-415	
	431-432		**Evaluation of Competency** 22-3: Applying a Hot Compress	*
	425-426	3	**Practice for Competency** 22-4: Applying an Ice Bag Textbook reference: pp. 415-416	
	433-434		**Evaluation of Competency** 22-4: Applying an Ice Bag	*
	425-426	3	**Practice for Competency** 22-5: Applying a Cold Compress Textbook reference: pp. 416-417	
	435-436		**Evaluation of Competency** 22-5: Applying a Cold Compress	*
	425-426	3	**Practice for Competency** 22-6: Applying a Chemical Pack Textbook reference: p. 417	
	437-438		**Evaluation of Competency** 22-6: Applying a Chemical Pack	*
	425-426	3	**Practice for Competency** 22-7: Measuring for Axillary Crutches Textbook reference: p. 421	
	439-440		**Evaluation of Competency** 22-7: Measuring for Axillary Crutches	*
	425-426	3 × for each gait	**Practice for Competency** 22-8: Instructing a Patient in Crutch Gaits Textbook reference: pp. 422-424	
	441-443		**Evaluation of Competency** 22-8: Instructing a Patient in Crutch Gaits	*
	425-426	Cane: 3 Walker: 3	**Practice for Competency** 22-9 and 22-10: Instructing a Patient in the Use of a Cane and Walker Textbook reference: p. 425	

√ When Assigned By Your Instructor	Study Guide Page(s)	Practices Required	LABORATORY ASSIGNMENTS (Procedure Number and Name)	Score*
	445-446		**Evaluation of Competency** 22-9 and 22-10: Instructing a Patient in the Use of a Cane and Walker	*
			ADDITIONAL ASSIGNMENTS	

Name _____ Date _____

True or False

_____ 1. A hot compress is an example of moist heat.

_____ 2. Erythema is redness of the skin caused by dilation of superficial blood vessels.

_____ 3. The local application of cold may be used to relieve muscle spasms.

_____ 4. Heat is often prescribed by the physician for black eyes.

_____ 5. The medical assistant should instruct the patient to adjust the heating pad to a higher setting if it no longer feels warm.

_____ 6. Chemical cold packs should be stored in the refrigerator.

_____ 7. Forearm crutches are often used by patients with cerebral palsy.

_____ 8. The three-point gait is the most stable and slowest crutch gait.

_____ 9. Ambulation refers to the inability to walk.

_____ 10. A patient using crutches should be instructed to support his or her weight against the axilla.

📋 POSTTEST

True or False

_____ 1. The recommended time for the application of heat is 15 to 30 minutes.

_____ 2. The local application of heat results in constriction of blood vessels in the area where it is applied.

_____ 3. An exudate is a discharge produced by the body's tissues.

_____ 4. After immersing a patient's foot in a hot soak, the medical assistant should add crushed ice to the soak.

_____ 5. A patient with diabetes mellitus may have more than usual sensitivity to the local application of heat.

_____ 6. An ice bag should be filled with large pieces of ice.

_____ 7. If axillary crutches have been fitted properly, the elbow will be flexed at an angle of 30 degrees.

_____ 8. Walkers are primarily used by pediatric patients.

_____ 9. Incorrectly fitted crutches may cause crutch palsy.

_____ 10. A cane should be held on the strong side of the body.

Chapter **22** **Physical Agents to Promote Tissue Healing**

Directions: Match each medical term with its definition.

_____ 1. Ambulation

_____ 2. Compress

_____ 3. Edema

_____ 4. Erythema

_____ 5. Exudate

_____ 6. Soak

_____ 7. Sprain

_____ 8. Strain

_____ 9. Suppuration

A. A discharge produced by the body's tissues
B. An overstretching of a muscle caused by trauma
C. A soft, moist, absorbent cloth that is folded in several layers and applied to a part of the body in the local application of heat or cold
D. Walking or moving from one place to another
E. The direct immersion of a body part in water or a medicated solution
F. The retention of fluid in the tissues, resulting in swelling
G. Reddening of the skin caused by dilation of superficial blood vessels in the skin
H. Trauma to a joint that causes injury to the ligaments
I. The process of pus formation

EVALUATION OF LEARNING

Directions: Fill in each blank with the correct answer.

1. State whether the following is an example of dry heat, moist heat, dry cold, or moist cold.

   a. Hot compress

   _____

   b. Ice bag

   _____

   c. Heating pad

   _____

   d. Chemical hot pack

   _____

   e. Cold compress

   _____

2. List three factors that must be taken into consideration when applying heat or cold.

   _____

   _____

3. How does the local application of heat to an affected area for a short period of time influence the following?

   a. The diameter of the blood vessels in the affected area

   _____

   b. The blood supply to the affected area

   _____

   c. Tissue metabolism in the affected area

   _____

4. What happens to the diameter of blood vessels if heat is applied for a prolonged period (more than 1 hour)?

_____

_____

5. List three reasons for applying heat locally.

_____

_____

_____

6. How does the local application of cold for a short period of time to an affected area influence the following?

   a. The diameter of the blood vessels in the affected area

   _____

   _____

   b. The blood supply to the affected area

   _____

   _____

   c. Tissue metabolism in the affected area

   _____

   _____

7. List two reasons for applying cold locally.

_____

_____

8. What factors does the physician take into consideration when prescribing an ambulatory assistive device?

_____

_____

9. Describe one advantage of the forearm crutch.

_____

10. What may occur if axillary crutches are not fitted properly?

_____

_____

11. List eight guidelines that must be followed during crutch use to ensure safety.

_____

_____

_____

_____

_____

_____

_____

_____

Chapter **22** **Physical Agents to Promote Tissue Healing**

12. List one use for each of the following crutch gaits:

    a. Four-point gait _____

    b. Three-point gait _____

    c. Swing-to gait _____

13. List and describe the three types of canes.

_____

_____

14. List two reasons for prescribing a cane.

_____

15. List two reasons for prescribing a walker.

_____

_____

CRITICAL THINKING ACTIVITIES

A. Dear Gabby

Gabby was called out of town unexpectedly and wants you to fill in for her. In the space provided, respond to the following letter.

Dear Gabby:

I am 15 years old and in the 10th grade. I need your help. I have a backpack; my dad weighed it and said it was 40 pounds. I only weigh 105 pounds. My back and neck hurt from lugging it around. I have to walk almost one-half mile to the bus stop. I do not have time to use my locker between classes because it is down a flight of stairs and at the end of the hall. Once, when I started using my locker, my science teacher got mad at me because I was late getting to class. Gabby, what should I do?

Signed,

Pain in the Neck

_____

_____

_____

_____

_____

_____

_____

_____

_____

_____

B. Crutch Guidelines

Each of the following patients is wearing a long leg cast because of a broken tibia and is using wooden axillary crutches to ambulate. Evaluate the crutch technique being practiced by each patient. Write **C** if the technique is correct and **I** if the technique is incorrect. If the technique is correct, explain why it should be performed this way. If incorrect, indicate what may happen from performing the technique in this manner.

1. Andy Morris wears Nike sports shoes when ambulating with his crutches.

   _____

   _____

2. Juliet Wright does not stand up straight when using her crutches.

   _____

   _____

3. Miguel Saldivia puts his weight on the axilla when getting around on his crutches.

   _____

   _____

4. Lindy Campbell has a lot of decorative throw rugs in her house, and she does not want to remove them.

   _____

   _____

5. Andrew Spence likes to move quickly on his crutches so he advances them forward about 20 inches with each step when using the swing-through gait.

   _____

   _____

6. Hanna Romes has tingling in her hands but thinks it is just part of what happens when one uses crutches.

   _____

   _____

7. Tamra Hetrick pads both the shoulder rests and the handgrips of her crutches.

   _____

   _____

8. Erica Anderson's crutch tips get wet but she does not take the time to dry them before going into a shopping mall.

   _____

   _____

C. Accessibility for Physical Disabilities

Next to each of the following facilities, list the features you have observed that facilitate accessibility of individuals with a physical disability.

1. Schools

   _____

   _____

2. Grocery stores

_____

_____

3. Shopping malls

_____

_____

4. Movie theaters

_____

_____

5. Restaurants

_____

_____

6. Doctors' offices

_____

_____

7. Community parks

_____

_____

D. Crossword Puzzle: Physical Agents to Promote Tissue Healing

Directions: Complete the crossword puzzle using the clues provided.

Across

1 Cold prescribed for this condition
6 Red skin
7 Overstretching of a muscle
9 "Too long" crutches may cause this
11 Cold blood vessels do this
14 Retention of fluid
15 Slow crutch gait
18 Do not use heat for this condition
19 Are more sensitive to cold
22 Walking
23 Prevents low back pain
24 Examples: standard, tripod, or quad
25 Elbow flexion for crutches

Down

2 Example of dry cold
3 Condition that causes impaired circulation
4 Transfers weight from legs to arms
5 Discharge
8 Cane handle should be level with this
10 Broken leg crutch gait
12 Pus formation
13 Heat often prescribed for this condition
16 Application of heat promotes this
17 Needed after knee replacement
20 Warm blood vessels do this
21 Maximum minutes for heat application

E. Bone and Joint Conditions

1. It is National Bone and Joint Week. The mayor has asked you and your classmates to develop informative, creative, and colorful brochures for the community about bone and joint conditions. Choose a condition below and design a brochure using the blank Frequently Asked Questions (FAQs) brochure provided on the following page. Each student in the class should select a different topic. On a separate sheet of paper, write three true or false questions relating to the information in your brochure.

2. Present your brochure to the class. After all the brochures have been presented, each student should ask the three questions to the entire class to see how well the class understands bone and joint conditions. (*Note:* You can take notes during the presentations and refer to them when answering the questions.)

1. Bursitis
2. Congenital hip dysplasia
3. Epicondylitis
4. Fibromyalgia
5. Gout
6. Hammer toe
7. Herniated disk
8. Juvenile rheumatoid arthritis
9. Knee replacement surgery
10. Kyphosis
11. Osteoarthritis
12. Osteomyelitis
13. Osteoporosis
14. Paget's disease
15. Rheumatoid arthritis
16. Scoliosis
17. Sprain
18. Strain
19. Tendonitis

FAQ on:

Q: 　　　　　　　　A:

Q: 　　　　　　　　A:

Q: 　　　　　　　　A:

Q: 　　　　　　　　A:

Q:

A:

Q:

A:

Illustration

Q:

A:

Q:

A:

Local Application of Heat and Cold

Procedures 22-1, 22-2, and 22-3: Application of Heat. Apply the following heat treatments, and record the procedure in the chart provided: heating pad, hot soak, hot compress, and chemical hot pack.

Procedures 22-4, 22-5, and 22-6: Application of Cold. Apply the following cold treatments, and record the results in the chart provided: ice bag, cold compress, and chemical cold pack.

Ambulatory Aids

Procedure 22-7: Axillary Crutch Measurement. Measure an individual for axillary crutches, and record the procedure in the chart provided.

Procedure 22-8: Crutch Gaits. Instruct an individual in mastering the following crutch gaits: four-point, two-point, three-point, swing-to, and swing-through. Record the procedure in the chart provided.

Procedure 22-9: Cane. Instruct an individual in the use of a cane, and record the procedure in the chart provided.

Procedure 22-10: Walker. Instruct an individual in the use of a walker, and record the procedure in the chart provided.

	Chart
Date	

Chart	
Date	

Procedure 22-1: Applying a Heating Pad

Name: _____   Date: _____

Evaluated by: _____   Score: _____

Performance Objective

Outcome:	Apply a heating pad.
Conditions:	Given a heating pad with a protective covering.
Standards:	Time: 5 minutes. Student completed procedure in _____ minutes.
	Accuracy: Satisfactory score on the performance evaluation checklist.

Performance Evaluation Checklist

Trial 1	Trial 2	Point Value	Performance Standards
		●	Sanitized hands.
		●	Assembled equipment.
		●	Greeted the patient and introduced yourself.
		●	Identified the patient and explained the procedure.
		●	Placed the heating pad in protective covering.
		●	Connected the plug to electrical outlet and set selector switch to the proper setting.
		●	Placed heating pad on patient's affected body area and asked how the temperature felt.
		●	Instructed patient not to lie on the pad or turn the temperature setting higher.
		▷	Stated why patient should be instructed not to lie on heating pad.
		▷	Explained why patient may want to increase the temperature.
		●	Checked patient's skin periodically.
		●	Administered treatment for the proper length of time as designated by physician.
		●	Sanitized hands.
		●	Charted the procedure correctly.
		●	Properly cared for and returned equipment to its storage place.
		✱	Completed the procedure within 5 minutes.
			TOTALS

EVALUATION CRITERIA			COMMENTS
Symbol	**Category**	**Point Value**	
✶	Critical Step	16 points	
●	Essential Step	6 points	
▷	Theory Question	2 points	

Score calculation: 100 points

−   _____ points missed

_____ Score

Satisfactory score: 85 or above

CAAHEP Competencies Achieved

Psychomotor (Skills)
☑ IV. 2. Report relevant information to others succinctly and accurately.
☑ IV. 6. Prepare a patient for procedures and/or treatments.

Affective (Behavior)
☑ I. 1. Apply critical thinking skills in performing patient assessment and care.

ABHES Competencies Achieved

☑ 8. cc. Communicate on the recipient's level of comprehension.
☑ 9. d. Recognize and understand various treatment protocols.
☑ 9. l. Prepare patient for examinations and treatments.

Procedure 22-2: Applying a Hot Soak

Name: _____ Date: _____

Evaluated by: _____ Score: _____

Performance Objective

Outcome:	Apply a hot soak.
Conditions:	Given the following: soaking solution, bath thermometer, basin, and bath towels.
Standards:	Time: 10 minutes. Student completed procedure in _____ minutes.
	Accuracy: Satisfactory score on the performance evaluation checklist.

Performance Evaluation Checklist

Trial 1	Trial 2	Point Value	Performance Standards
		●	Sanitized hands.
		●	Assembled equipment.
		●	Checked the label on the solution container.
		●	Warmed the soaking solution.
		●	Greeted the patient and introduced yourself.
		●	Identified the patient and explained the procedure.
		●	Filled basin one-half to two-thirds full with the warmed soaking solution.
		●	Checked temperature of the solution with a bath thermometer.
		▷	Stated the safe temperature range that should be used for an adult patient (105°F to 110°F).
		●	Assisted patient in a comfortable position and padded side of the basin with towel.
		●	Slowly and gradually immersed affected body part into the solution and asked patient how the temperature felt.
		●	Kept the solution at a constant temperature by removing cooler solution and adding hot solution.
		●	Placed a hand between patient and solution when adding more solution.
		●	Stirred the solution with your hand while pouring it.
		●	Checked patient's skin periodically.
		●	Applied hot soak for the proper length of time as designated by physician.
		●	Completely dried affected part.

429

Trial 1	Trial 2	Point Value	Performance Standards
		●	Sanitized hands.
		●	Charted the procedure correctly.
		●	Properly cared for and returned equipment to its storage place.
		✱	Completed the procedure within 10 minutes.
			TOTALS

	CHART
Date	

Evaluation of Student Performance

EVALUATION CRITERIA			COMMENTS
Symbol	**Category**	**Point Value**	
✱	Critical Step	16 points	
●	Essential Step	6 points	
▷	Theory Question	2 points	

Score calculation: 100 points

−   points missed

_____ Score

Satisfactory score: 85 or above

CAAHEP Competencies Achieved

Psychomotor (Skills)
☑ IV. 2. Report relevant information to others succinctly and accurately.
☑ IV. 6. Prepare a patient for procedures and/or treatments.

Affective (Behavior)
☑ I. 1. Apply critical thinking skills in performing patient assessment and care.

ABHES Competencies Achieved

☑ 8. cc. Communicate on the recipient's level of comprehension.
☑ 9. d. Recognize and understand various treatment protocols.
☑ 9. l. Prepare patient for examinations and treatments.

Procedure 22-3: Applying a Hot Compress

Name: _____ Date: _____

Evaluated by: _____ Score: _____

Performance Objective

Outcome:	Apply a hot compress.
Conditions:	Given the following: solution for the compresses, bath thermometer, basin, washcloths, and a towel.
Standards:	Time: 10 minutes. Student completed procedure in _____ minutes.
	Accuracy: Satisfactory score on the Performance Evaluation Checklist.

Performance Evaluation Checklist

Trial 1	Trial 2	Point Value	Performance Standards
		●	Sanitized hands.
		●	Assembled equipment.
		●	Checked the label on the solution container.
		●	Warmed the soaking solution.
		●	Greeted the patient and introduced yourself.
		●	Identified the patient and explained the procedure.
		●	Filled basin half full with the warmed solution.
		●	Checked temperature of the solution with a bath thermometer.
		▷	Stated the safe temperature range that should be used for an adult patient (105°F to 110°F).
		●	Completely immersed the compress in the solution.
		●	Squeezed excess solution from compress.
		●	Applied compress to affected body part and asked patient how the temperature felt.
		●	Placed additional compresses in the solution.
		●	Repeated the application every 2 to 3 minutes for the duration of time specified by physician.
		●	Checked patient's skin periodically.
		●	Checked temperature of the solution periodically, removed cooler fluid, and added hot fluid if needed.
		●	Administered treatment for proper length of time as designated by a physician.

Trial 1	Trial 2	Point Value	Performance Standards
		●	Thoroughly dried affected part.
		●	Sanitized hands.
		●	Charted the procedure correctly.
		●	Properly cared for and returned equipment to its storage place.
		✳	Completed the procedure within 10 minutes.
			TOTALS

CHART	
Date	

Evaluation of Student Performance

EVALUATION CRITERIA			COMMENTS
Symbol	**Category**	**Point Value**	
✳	Critical Step	16 points	
●	Essential Step	6 points	
▷	Theory Question	2 points	

Score calculation: 100 points

–   points missed
_____
___ Score

Satisfactory score: 85 or above

CAAHEP Competencies Achieved

Psychomotor (Skills)
☑ IV. 2. Report relevant information to others succinctly and accurately.
☑ IV. 6. Prepare a patient for procedures and/or treatments.

Affective (Behavior)
☑ I. 1. Apply critical thinking skills in performing patient assessment and care.

ABHES Competencies Achieved

☑ 8. cc. Communicate on the recipient's level of comprehension.
☑ 9. d. Recognize and understand various treatment protocols.
☑ 9. l. Prepare patient for examinations and treatments.

Name: _____   Date: _____

Evaluated by: _____   Score: _____

Performance Objective

Outcome:	Apply an ice bag.
Conditions:	Given the following: ice bag and protective covering, and small pieces of ice.
Standards:	Time: 10 minutes. Student completed procedure in _____ minutes.
	Accuracy: Satisfactory score on the Performance Evaluation Checklist.

Performance Evaluation Checking

Trial 1	Trial 2	Point Value	Performance Standards
		●	Sanitized hands.
		●	Assembled equipment.
		●	Greeted the patient and introduced yourself.
		●	Identified the patient and explained the procedure.
		●	Checked ice bag for leakage.
		●	Filled bag one-half to two-thirds full with small pieces of ice.
		▷	Explained why small pieces of ice are used.
		●	Expelled air from bag.
		▷	Explained the reason for expelling air from bag.
		●	Placed the bag in protective covering.
		▷	Stated the purpose of placing bag in protective covering.
		●	Placed bag on affected body area and asked patient how the temperature felt.
		●	Checked patient's skin periodically.
		▷	Listed skin changes that would warrant removal of bag.
		●	Refilled bag with ice and changed protective covering when needed.
		●	Administered treatment for the proper length of time as designated by physician.
		●	Sanitized hands.
		●	Charted the procedure correctly.

Chapter **22** **Physical Agents to Promote Tissue Healing**

Trial 1	Trial 2	Point Value	Performance Standards
		●	Properly cared for and returned equipment to its storage place.
		★	Completed the procedure within 10 minutes.
			TOTALS

CHART

Date	

Evaluation of Student Performance

EVALUATION CRITERIA			COMMENTS
Symbol	**Category**	**Point Value**	
★	Critical Step	16 points	
●	Essential Step	6 points	
▷	Theory Question	2 points	

Score calculation: 100 points

−   _____ points missed

_____ Score

Satisfactory score: 85 or above

CAAHEP Competencies Achieved

Psychomotor (Skills)
☑ IV. 2. Report relevant information to others succinctly and accurately.
☑ IV. 6. Prepare a patient for procedures and/or treatments.

Affective (Behavior)
☑ I. 1. Apply critical thinking skills in performing patient assessment and care.

ABHES Competencies Achieved

☑ 8. cc. Communicate on the recipient's level of comprehension.
☑ 9. d. Recognize and understand various treatment protocols.
☑ 9. l. Prepare patient for examinations and treatments.

Name: _____ Date: _____

Evaluated by: _____ Score: _____

Performance Objective

Outcome:	Apply a cold compress.
Conditions:	Given the following: ice cubes, a basin, and washcloths.
Standards:	Time: 10 minutes. Student completed procedure in _____ minutes.
	Accuracy: Satisfactory score on the Performance Evaluation Checklist.

Performance Evaluation Checklist

Trial 1	Trial 2	Point Value	Performance Standards
		●	Sanitized hands.
		●	Assembled equipment.
		●	Checked the label on the solution.
		●	Greeted the patient and introduced yourself.
		●	Identified the patient and explained the procedure.
		●	Placed large ice cubes in basin and added the solution until the basin is half full.
		▷	Explained why larger pieces of ice are used.
		●	Completely immersed the compress in the solution.
		●	Squeezed excess solution from compress.
		●	Applied compress to affected body part and asked patient how the temperature felt.
		●	Placed additional compresses in the solution.
		●	Repeated the application every 2 to 3 minutes for the duration of time specified by physician.
		●	Checked patient's skin periodically.
		●	Added ice if needed to keep the solution cold.
		●	Administered treatment for proper length of time as designated by physician.
		●	Thoroughly dried affected part.
		●	Sanitized hands.

Trial 1	Trial 2	Point Value	Performance Standards
		●	Charted the procedure correctly.
		●	Properly cared for and returned equipment to its storage place.
		✳	Completed the procedure within 10 minutes.
			TOTALS

	CHART
Date	

Evaluation of Student Performance

EVALUATION CRITERIA			COMMENTS
Symbol	**Category**	**Point Value**	
✳	Critical Step	16 points	
●	Essential Step	6 points	
▷	Theory Question	2 points	

Score calculation: 100 points

    −   _____ points missed

       _____ Score

Satisfactory score: 85 or above

CAAHEP Competencies Achieved

Psychomotor (Skills)
☑ IV. 2. Report relevant information to others succinctly and accurately.
☑ IV. 6. Prepare a patient for procedures and/or treatments.

Affective (Behavior)
☑ I. 1. Apply critical thinking skills in performing patient assessment and care.

ABHES Competencies Achieved

☑ 8. cc. Communicate on the recipient's level of comprehension.
☑ 9. d. Recognize and understand various treatment protocols.
☑ 9. l. Prepare patient for examinations and treatments.

Procedure 22-6: Applying a Chemical Pack

Name: _____ Date: _____

Evaluated by: _____ Score: _____

Performance Objective

Outcome:	Apply a chemical cold and hot pack.
Conditions:	Given a chemical cold and hot pack.
Standards:	Time: 5 minutes. Student completed procedure in _____ minutes.
	Accuracy: Satisfactory score on the Performance Evaluation Checklist.

Performance Evaluation Checklist

Trial 1	Trial 2	Point Value	Performance Standards
		●	Sanitized hands.
		●	Assembled equipment.
		●	Greeted the patient and introduced yourself.
		●	Identified the patient and explained the procedure.
		●	Shook the crystals to the bottom of bag.
		●	Squeezed bag firmly to break inner water bag.
		●	Shook bag vigorously to mix the contents.
		●	Covered bag with a protective covering.
		●	Applied bag to affected area.
		●	Checked the patient's skin periodically.
		●	Administered treatment for the proper length of time.
		●	Discarded bag in an appropriate receptacle.
		●	Sanitized hands.
		●	Charted the procedure correctly.
		✱	Completed the procedure within 5 minutes.
			TOTALS

Evaluation of Student Performance

EVALUATION CRITERIA			COMMENTS
Symbol	**Category**	**Point Value**	
✱	Critical Step	16 points	
●	Essential Step	6 points	
▷	Theory Question	2 points	

Score calculation: 100 points

− _____ points missed

_____ Score

Satisfactory score: 85 or above

CAAHEP Competencies Achieved

Psychomotor (Skills)
☑ IV. 2. Report relevant information to others succinctly and accurately.
☑ IV. 6. Prepare a patient for procedures and/or treatments.

Affective (Behavior)
☑ I. 1. Apply critical thinking skills in performing patient assessment and care.

ABHES Competencies Achieved

☑ 8. cc. Communicate on the recipient's level of comprehension.
☑ 9. d. Recognize and understand various treatment protocols.
☑ 9. l. Prepare patient for examinations and treatments.

Procedure 22-7: Measuring for Axillary Crutches

Name: _____ Date: _____

Evaluated by: _____ Score: _____

Performance Objective

Outcome:	Measure an individual for axillary crutches.
Conditions:	Given the following: axillary crutches and a tape measure.
Standards:	Time: 10 minutes. Student completed procedure in _____ minutes.
	Accuracy: Satisfactory score on the Performance Evaluation Checklist.

Performance Evaluation Checklist

Trial 1	Trial 2	Point Value	Performance Standards
		●	Asked patient to stand erect.
		●	Positioned crutches with the tips at a distance of 2 inches in front of, and 4 to 6 inches to the side of, each foot.
		●	Adjusted crutch length so that the shoulder rests were approximately 1½ to 2 inches below the axilla.
		●	Asked the patient to support his or her weight by the handgrips.
		●	Adjusted the handgrips so that patient's elbow was flexed approximately 30 degrees.
		●	Checked the fit of the crutches by placing two fingers between the top of the crutch and patient's axilla.
		●	Charted the procedure correctly.
		✱	Completed the procedure within 10 minutes.
			TOTALS

	CHART	
Date		

Evaluation of Student Performance

EVALUATION CRITERIA			COMMENTS
Symbol	Category	Point Value	
✴	Critical Step	16 points	
●	Essential Step	6 points	
▷	Theory Question	2 points	

Score calculation: 100 points

−   points missed
_____
___ Score

Satisfactory score: 85 or above

CAAHEP Competencies Achieved

Psychomotor (Skills)
☑ IV. 6. Prepare a patient for procedures and/or treatments.

Affective (Behavior)
☑ I. 1. Apply critical thinking skills in performing patient assessment and care.

ABHES Competencies Achieved

☑ 5. b. Identify and respond appropriately when working/caring for patients with special needs.

Procedure 22-8: Instructing a Patient in Crutch Gaits

Name: _____ Date: _____

Evaluated by: _____ Score: _____

Performance Objective

Outcome:	Instruct an individual in the following crutch gaits: four-point, two-point, three-point, swing-to, and swing-through.
Conditions:	Given axillary crutches.
Standards:	Time: 15 minutes. Student completed procedure in _____ minutes.
	Accuracy: Satisfactory score on the Performance Evaluation Checklist.

Performance Evaluation Checklist

Trial 1	Trial 2	Point Value	Performance Standards
			Tripod Position
			Instructed patient:
		●	Stand erect and face straight ahead.
		●	Place the tips of crutches 4 to 6 inches in front of, and 4 to 6 inches to side of, each foot.
		▷	Stated one use of the tripod position.
			Four-Point Gait
			Instructed patient:
		●	Begin in the tripod position.
		●	Move the right crutch forward.
		●	Move the left foot forward to the level of the left crutch.
		●	Move the left crutch forward.
		●	Move the right foot forward to the level of the right crutch.
		●	Repeat the above sequence.
		▷	Stated one use of the four-point gait.
			Two-Point Gait
			Instructed patient:
		●	Begin in the tripod position.
		●	Move the left crutch and the right foot forward at the same time.
		●	Move the right crutch and left foot forward at the same time.

Trial 1	Trial 2	Point Value	Performance Standards
		●	Repeat the above sequence.
		▷	Stated one use of the two-point gait.
			Three-Point Gait
			Instructed patient:
		●	Begin in the tripod position.
		●	Move both crutches and the affected leg forward.
		●	Move the unaffected leg forward while balancing weight on both crutches.
		●	Repeat the above sequence.
		▷	Stated two uses of the three-point gait.
			Swing-To Gait
			Instructed patient:
		●	Begin in the tripod position.
		●	Move both crutches forward together.
		●	Lift and swing body to the crutches.
		●	Repeat the above sequence.
		▷	Stated one use of the swing-to gait.
			Swing-Through Gait
			Instructed patient:
		●	Begin in the tripod position.
		●	Move both crutches forward together.
		●	Lift and swing body past the crutches.
		●	Repeat the above sequence.
		▷	Stated one use of the swing-through gait.
		★	Completed the procedure within 15 minutes.
			TOTALS

		CHART	
	Date		

Evaluation of Student Performance

EVALUATION CRITERIA			COMMENTS
Symbol	**Category**	**Point Value**	
✱	Critical Step	16 points	
●	Essential Step	6 points	
▷	Theory Question	2 points	

Score calculation: 100 points

        −   points missed
                ─────────────
            ___ Score

Satisfactory score: 85 or above

CAAHEP Competencies Achieved

Psychomotor (Skills)
☑ IV. 5. Instruct patients according to their needs to promote health maintenance and disease prevention.
☑ IV. 6. Prepare a patient for procedures and/or treatments.

Affective (Behavior)
☑ I. 2. Use language/verbal skills that enable patients' understanding.
☑ IV. 6. Demonstrate awareness of how an individual's personal appearance affects anticipated responses.

ABHES Competencies Achieved

☑ 9. q. Instruct patients with special needs.

Notes

Procedures 22-9 and 22-10: Instructing a Patient in Use of a Cane and Walker

Name: _____ Date: _____

Evaluated by: _____ Score: _____

Performance Objective

Outcome:	Instruct an individual in the use of a cane and walker.
Conditions:	Given the following: a cane and a walker.
Standards:	Time: 10 minutes. Student completed procedure in _____ minutes.
	Accuracy: Satisfactory score on the Performance Evaluation Checklist.

Performance Evaluation Checklist

Trial 1	Trial 2	Point Value	Performance Standards
			Cane
			Instructed patient:
		●	Hold the cane on the strong side of body.
		●	Place tip of the cane 4 to 6 inches to the side of foot.
		●	Move the cane forward approximately 12 inches.
		●	Move the affected leg forward to the level of the cane.
		●	Move strong leg forward and ahead of the cane and weak leg.
		●	Repeat the above sequence.
		▷	Stated one condition for which a cane is used.
			Walker
			Instructed patient:
		●	Pick up the walker and move it forward approximately 6 inches.
		●	Move the right foot and then the left foot up to the walker.
		●	Repeat the above sequence.
		▷	Stated one condition for which a walker is used.
		★	Completed the procedure within 10 minutes.
			TOTALS

Date	

Evaluation of Student Performance

EVALUATION CRITERIA			COMMENTS
Symbol	**Category**	**Point Value**	
✶	Critical Step	16 points	
●	Essential Step	6 points	
▷	Theory Question	2 points	

Score calculation: 100 points

       −   points missed
               _____ Score

Satisfactory score: 85 or above

CAAHEP Competencies Achieved

Psychomotor (Skills)
☑ IV. 5. Instruct patients according to their needs to promote health maintenance and disease prevention.
☑ IV. 6. Prepare a patient for procedures and/or treatments.

Affective (Behavior)
☑ I. 2. Use language/verbal skills that enable patients' understanding.
☑ IV. 6. Demonstrate awareness of how an individual's personal appearance affects anticipated responses.

ABHES Competencies Achieved

☑ 9. q. Instruct patients with special needs.

---

23 The Gynecologic Examination and Prenatal Care

√ After Completing	Date Due	Textbook Pages	TEXTBOOK ASSIGNMENTS	Possible Points	Points You Earned
		427-469	Read Chapter 23: The Gynecologic Examination and Prenatal Care		
		430 465	Read Case Study 1 Case Study 1 questions	5	
		447 465	Read Case Study 2 Case Study 2 questions	5	
		455 465-466	Read Case Study 3 Case Study 3 questions	5	
		459 466	Read Case Study 4 Case Study 4 questions	5	
			TOTAL POINTS		

√ After Completing	Date Due	Study Guide Pages	STUDY GUIDE ASSIGNMENTS (CTA = Critical Thinking Activity)	Possible Points	Points You Earned
		451	Pretest	10	
		452-453 453	Key Term Assessment A. Definitions B. Word Parts (Add 1 point for each medical term)	47 22	
		454-460	Evaluation of Learning questions	48	
		460-461	CTA A: Breast Cancer (5 points per question)	15	
			Evolve Site: What's on Your Tray? (Record points earned)		
		462-464	CTA B: Methods of Contraception (3 points per each method)	42	
		464-468	CTA C: Herpesvirus and Human Papillomavirus (40 points per brochure)	80	
		469	CTA D: Signs and Symptoms of Pregnancy	16	

√ After Completing	Date Due	Study Guide Pages	STUDY GUIDE ASSIGNMENTS (CTA = Critical Thinking Activity)	Possible Points	Points You Earned
		469	CTA E: Calculation of the Expected Date of Delivery	5	
		470	CTA F: Nutrition During Pregnancy	8	
		470-471	CTA G: Minor Discomforts of Pregnancy	10	
		471-472	CTA H: Health Promotion During Pregnancy	7	
		473	CTA I: Breast feeding	8	
		473	CTA J: Prenatal Ultrasound	5	
		474	CTA K: Crossword Puzzle	19	
			e Evolve Site: Road to Recovery Game OB/GYN Terminology (Record points earned)		
			e Evolve Site: Animations	20	
			e Evolve Site: Apply Your Knowledge questions	12	
			e Evolve Site: Video Evaluation	48	
		451	Posttest	10	
			ADDITIONAL ASSIGNMENTS		
			TOTAL POINTS		

√ When Assigned By Your Instructor	Study Guide Pages	Practices Required	LABORATORY ASSIGNMENTS (Procedure Number and Name)	Score*
	475	5	**Practice for Competency** 23-1: Breast Self-Examination Instructions Textbook reference: pp. 438-440	
	483-486		**Evaluation of Competency** 23-1: Breast Self-Examination Instructions	*
	475-476	5	**Practice for Competency** 23-2: Assisting with a Gynecologic Examination Textbook reference: pp. 440-444	
	487-491		**Evaluation of Competency** 23-2: Assisting with a Gynecologic Examination	*
	477-482	5	**Practice for Competency** 23-3: Assisting with a Return Prenatal Examination Textbook reference: pp. 462-464	
	493-495		**Evaluation of Competency** 23-3: Assisting with a Return Prenatal Examination	*
			ADDITIONAL ASSIGNMENTS	

Notes

Procedure 23-1: Breast Self-Examination Instructions

Name: _____   Date: _____

Evaluated by: _____   Score: _____

Performance Objective

Outcome:	Instruct a patient in the procedure for performing a breast self-examination.
Conditions:	Small pillow.
Standards:	Time: 10 minutes. Student completed procedure in _____ minutes.
	Accuracy: Satisfactory score on the performance evaluation checklist.

Performance Evaluation Checklist

Trial 1	Trial 2	Point Value	Performance Standards
		●	Greeted the patient and introduced yourself.
		●	Identified patient and explained that you will be instructing the patient in a BSE.
		●	Explained the purpose of the exam, when to perform it, and the three methods of examination.
		▷	Explained why three methods are used to examine the breasts.
			Instructed patient:
			1. Before a mirror
		●	Remove clothing from the waist up.
		●	Place arms at sides and inspect the breasts.
		●	Inspect for a change in size or shape; swelling, puckering, or dimpling; change in skin texture; nipple retraction; change in nipple size or position compared with other breast.
		▷	Described what may cause puckering or dimpling of the skin.
		●	Slowly raise arms over head and inspect the breasts.
		▷	Stated what should normally occur when the arms are moved at the same time.
		●	Rest palms on hips, press down firmly, and inspect the breasts.
		▷	Stated the purpose of flexing the chest muscles.
		●	Gently squeeze each nipple and look for a discharge.
			2. Lying down
		●	Place a pillow (or folded towel) under right shoulder.
		●	Place right hand behind head.

Trial 1	Trial 2	Point Value	Performance Standards
		▷	Stated the purpose of the pillow and hand placement.
		●	Use the finger pads of the middle three fingers of the left hand.
		▷	Explained why the finger pads should be used.
		●	Use small rotating motions and continuous firm pressure.
		●	Use one of the following patterns to move around the breast: circular, vertical strip, or wedge.
		▷	Stated why a pattern is used.
			Circular pattern:
		●	Visualize breast as a clock face.
		●	Start at outside edge of breast.
		●	Proceed clockwise until you return to starting point.
		●	Move in 1 inch, and repeat the circle.
		●	Continue until nipple is reached.
			Vertical strip:
		●	Divide breast into strips.
		●	Start at underarm.
		●	Slowly move fingers down until they are below the breast.
		●	Move fingers 1 inch toward middle and move back up.
		●	Repeat until entire breast has been examined.
			Wedge:
		●	Divide breasts into wedges.
		●	Start at outer edge of breast.
		●	Move fingers toward the nipple and back to edge of breast.
		●	Repeat until entire breast has been examined.
			Use the following techniques during the examination:
		●	Press firmly enough to feel the different breast tissues.
		●	Palpate for lumps, hard knots, or thickening.
		▷	Explained how normal breast tissue feels.
		●	Examine the entire chest area from your collarbone to the base of a properly fitted bra and from the breastbone to the underarm.
		●	Pay special attention to the area between the breast and underarm including the underarm itself.
		▷	Explained why the underarm should be examined.

Trial 1	Trial 2	Point Value	Performance Standards
		●	Continue the examination until every part of the right breast has been examined, including the nipple.
		●	Repeat the procedure on the left breast, with a pillow or rolled towel under the left shoulder, the left hand behind the head, and using the right hand to palpate.
			3. In the shower
		●	Gently lather each breast.
		▷	Explained why the breasts should be examined in the shower.
		●	Place right hand behind head.
		●	Use the finger pads of the middle three fingers of the left hand.
		●	Use small, rotating motions and continuous, firm pressure.
		●	Use your preferred pattern to thoroughly examine the right breast and underarm for lumps, hard knots, or thickening.
		●	Repeat the procedure on the left breast using the pads of your right fingers.
		●	Instructed the patient to report any lumps or changes to the physician immediately.
		▷	Explained why it is important to report changes immediately.
		●	Charted the procedure correctly.
		✱	Completed the procedure within 10 minutes.
			TOTALS

CHART

Date	

Evaluation of Student Performance

<table>
<tr><th colspan="3">EVALUATION CRITERIA</th><th>COMMENTS</th></tr>
<tr><th>Symbol</th><th>Category</th><th>Point Value</th><td rowspan="8"></td></tr>
<tr><td>✱</td><td>Critical Step</td><td>16 points</td></tr>
<tr><td>●</td><td>Essential Step</td><td>6 points</td></tr>
<tr><td>▷</td><td>Theory Question</td><td>2 points</td></tr>
<tr><td>Score calculation:</td><td colspan="2">100 points</td></tr>
<tr><td></td><td colspan="2">−   points missed</td></tr>
<tr><td></td><td colspan="2">_____ Score</td></tr>
<tr><td colspan="3">Satisfactory score: 85 or above</td></tr>
</table>

CAAHEP Competencies Achieved

Psychomotor (Skills)
☑ IV. 5. Instruct patients according to their needs to promote health maintenance and disease prevention.
☑ IV. 9. Document patient education.

Affective (Behavior)
☑ I. 2. Use language/verbal skills that enable patients' understanding.
☑ IV. 3. Use appropriate body language and other nonverbal skills in communicating with patients, family, and staff.

ABHES Competencies Achieved

☑ 8. e. Locate resources and information for patients and employers.
☑ 8. cc. Communicate on the recipient's level of comprehension.
☑ 8. ii. Recognize and respond to verbal and nonverbal communication.
☑ 9. r. Teach patients methods of health promotion and disease prevention.

Procedure 23-2: Assisting with a Gynecologic Examination

Name: _____   Date: _____

Evaluated by: _____   Score: _____

Performance Objective

Outcome:	Assist with a gynecologic examination.
Conditions:	Using an examining table. Given the following: disposable gloves, examining gown and drape, disposable vaginal speculum, lubricant, gauze pads, Hemoccult slide and developing solution, tissues, biohazard waste container, cytology request form, biohazard specimen transport bag. *Direct-Smear Method:* ThinPrep vial, plastic spatula, and endocervical brush or cytology broom. *Liquid-Prep Method:* ThinPrep vial, plastic spatula, and endocervical brush or cytology broom.
Standards:	Time: 15 minutes. Student completed procedure in _____ minutes. Accuracy: Satisfactory score on the Performance Evaluation Checklist.

Performance Evaluation Checklist

Trial 1	Trial 2	Point Value	Performance Standards
		●	Sanitized hands.
		●	Assembled equipment.
		●	Completed as much of the cytology request form as possible.
			Prepared collection materials:
		●	*Pap smear method:* Identified the slides on the frosted edge.
		●	*Liquid-prep method:* Checked the expiration date and labeled the vial.
		●	Greeted the patient and introduced yourself.
		●	Escorted the patient to the examining room.
		●	Identified the patient.
		●	Asked patient if she has any problems or concerns and charted the information.
		●	Completed the cytology request by asking necessary questions.
		●	Measured vital signs and height and weight and charted the results correctly.
			Prepared patient for the examination:
		●	Asked patient if she needs to empty bladder.
		▷	Explained why the bladder should be empty for the examination.

Trial 1	Trial 2	Point Value	Performance Standards
		●	Instructed the patient to undress and put on the examining gown with opening in front.
		●	Informed patient that physician would be in soon.
		●	Left the room to provide patient privacy.
		●	Made medical record available for review by the physician.
		●	Checked to make sure patient is ready.
		●	Informed physician that the patient was ready.
			Assisted the physician:
		●	Positioned and draped patient in a supine position for the breast examination.
		●	Positioned and draped patient in the lithotomy position for the pelvic examination.
		●	Prepared the vaginal speculum and handed it to the physician.
		●	Prepared the light for physician.
		●	Handed vaginal speculum to physician.
		●	Reassured patient and helped her to relax during the examination.
		▷	Explained why patient should be relaxed during the examination.
			Assisted with Pap specimen collection:
		●	Applied gloves.
			1. Direct smear method
		●	Held each slide for the physician to smear the specimen on it.
		●	Immediately fixed the slides.
		●	Allowed slides to dry and placed them in a slide container.
			2a. ThinPrep spatula and brush method
		●	Held the vial to receive the collection device from the physician.
		●	Correctly rinsed each collection device in the liquid preservative.
		▷	Explained why the collection device should be swirled vigorously.
		●	Discarded each collection device in a biohazard waste container.
		●	Tightened the cap on the vial.
			2b. ThinPrep broom method
		●	Held the vial to receive the broom from the physician.
		●	Correctly rinsed the broom in the liquid preservative.
		●	Discarded the broom in a biohazard waste container.
		●	Tightened the cap on the vial.

Trial 1	Trial 2	Point Value	Performance Standards
			3. SurePath spatula and brush method
		•	Held the vial to receive each collection device from the physician.
		•	Broke off or disconnected tip of each collection device.
		•	Discarded each handle in a regular waste container.
		•	Tightened cap on the vial.
			Assisted with the remainder of the examination:
		•	Removed light source.
		•	Discarded vaginal speculum in a biohazard waste container.
		•	Provided the physician with lubricant for the bimanual and rectal-vaginal examinations.
		•	Assisted as required with the collection of the fecal occult blood specimen.
		•	Assisted the patient into a sitting position and allowed her to rest.
		▷	Explained why the patient should be allowed to rest.
		•	Offered the patient tissues to remove lubricant from the perineum.
		•	Assisted patient from the examining table.
		•	Instructed patient to get dressed.
		•	Informed patient of the method used by the medical office to relay test results.
		•	Tested the fecal occult blood specimen and charted the results.
		•	Prepared Pap specimen for transport to the laboratory.
		•	Placed specimen in a biohazard specimen bag and sealed the bag.
		•	Inserted the cytology requisition into the outside pocket of bag.
		•	Placed bag in appropriate location for pickup by the laboratory.
		•	Charted the transport of the Pap specimen to an outside laboratory.
		•	Cleaned the examining room.
		✶	Completed the procedure within 15 minutes.
			TOTALS
CHART			
Date			

EVALUATION CRITERIA			COMMENTS
Symbol	**Category**	**Point Value**	
★	Critical Step	16 points	
●	Essential Step	6 points	
▷	Theory Question	2 points	

Score calculation: 100 points

             –   points missed

                  ___ Score

Satisfactory score: 85 or above

CAAHEP Competencies Achieved

Psychomotor (Skills)

☑ I. 10. Assist physician with patient care.
☑ IV. 5. Instruct patients according to their needs to promote health maintenance and disease prevention.
☑ IV. 6. Prepare a patient for procedures and/or treatments.

Affective (Behavior)

☑ III. 3. Show awareness of patients' concerns.
☑ IV. 1. Demonstrate empathy in communicating with patients, family, and staff.

ABHES Competencies Achieved

☑ 8. bb. Are impartial and show empathy when dealing with patients.
☑ 9. f. Screen and follow up patient test results.
☑ 9. k. Prepare and maintain examination and treatment area.
☑ 9. l. Prepare patient for examinations and treatments.
☑ 9. m. Assist physician with routine and specialty examinations and treatments.

GYN CYTOLOGY REQUISITION

THOMAS WOODSIDE, MD
501 MAIN ST
ST. LOUIS, MO 63146
(314) 883–0093

PATIENT INFO

Patient's Name (Last)	(First)	(MI)	Date of Birth MO	DAY	YR	Collection Time : AM PM	Collection Date MO	DAY	YR	Patient's ID #

Patient's Address   Phone

City   State   ZIP

RESP. PARTY

Name of Responsible Party (if different from patient)

Address of Responsible Party   APT #

City   State   ZIP

INSURANCE

Patient's Relationship to Responsible Party   ☐ 1. Self   ☐ 2. Spouse   ☐ 3. Child   ☐ 4. Other

Insurance Comany Name   Plan   Carrier Code

Subscriber/Member #   Location   Group #

Insurance Address   Physician's Provider #

City   State   ZIP

Employer's Name or Number   Insured SSN

Diagnosis/Signs/Symptoms in ICD-9 Format (Highest Specificity)

REQUIRED

ICD-9 codes are the internationally accepted method of describing the clinical picture of the patient. All diagnoses should be provided by the ordering physician or his or her authorized designee. The following is a partial list of of common diagnoses in ICD-9 format. Most third party payers require an ICD-9 code to indicate the medical necessity of the test(s) and or profile(s) ordered. For a complete list of all ICD-9 codes, please refer to a current ICD-9 manual.

V76.2	Routine Cervical Pap Smear	616.0	Cervicitis	626.8	Abnormal Bleeding
V15.89	High Risk Cervical Screening	616.10	Vaginitis	627.1	Postmenopausal Bleeding
V22.2	Pregnancy	617.0	Endometriosis, Uterus	627.3	Atrophic Vaginitis
079.4	Human Papillomavirus	622.1	Dysplasia, Cervix	795.0	Abnormal Cervical Pap Smear
180.0	Malignant Neoplasm, Cervix	623.0	Dysplasia, Vagina		

COLLECTION METHOD

Liquid Based Prep
192055 ☐ Thin Prep Pap Test

192039 ☐ Thin Prep Pap Test w/reflex to HPV Hybrid Capture when ASC-US or SIL

192047 ☐ Thin Prep Pap Test w/reflex to high-risk only HPV Hybrid Capture when ASC-US

Pap Smear
009100 ☐ 1 Slide   009191 ☐ 2 Slides

Pap Smear and Maturation Index
009209 ☐ 1 Slide   190074 ☐ 2 Slides

SOURCE OF SPECIMEN

☐ Cervical
☐ Endocervical
☐ Vaginal

Date LMP
____ / ____ / ____
Mo   Day   Year

COLLECTION TECHNIQUE

☐ Spatula
☐ Brush
☐ Broom
☐ Other
_____

PATIENT HISTORY

☐ Pregnant
☐ Lactating
☐ Oral Contraceptives
☐ Postmenopausal
☐ Hormone Replacement Therapy

☐ PMP Bleeding
☐ Postpartum
☐ IUD
☐ Postcoital Bleeding
☐ DES Exposure
☐ Previous Abnormal Pap Test

☐ Other _____

PREVIOUS TREATMENT   Date/Results

☐ None
☐ Colposcopy and Bx _____
☐ Cryosurgery _____
☐ LEEP _____
☐ Laser Vaporization _____
☐ Conization _____
☐ Hysterectomy _____
☐ Radiation _____
☐ Chemotherapy _____

(From Bonewit-West K: *Study guide for clinical medical assistants,* ed 8, St. Louis, 2011, Saunders.)

Chapter **23**   **The Gynecologic Examination and Prenatal Care**

Notes

Procedure 23-3: Assisting with a Return Prenatal Examination

Name: _____ Date: _____

Evaluated by: _____ Score: _____

Performance Objective

Outcome:	Prepare the patient and assist with a return prenatal examination.
Conditions:	Using an examining table. Given the following: centimeter tape measure, Doppler fetal pulse detector, ultrasound coupling agent, paper towel, disposable vaginal speculum, disposable gloves, lubricant, gauze pads, examining gown and drape, and a biohazard waste container.
Standards:	Time: 15 minutes. Student completed procedure in _____ minutes. Accuracy: Satisfactory score on the Performance Evaluation Checklist.

Performance Evaluation Checklist

Trial 1	Trial 2	Point Value	Performance Standards
		●	Sanitized hands.
		●	Set up the tray for the prenatal examination.
		●	Greeted the patient and introduced yourself.
		●	Identified patient and explained the procedure.
		●	Asked the patient to obtain a urine specimen.
		●	Escorted the patient to the examining room and asked her to be seated.
		●	Asked the patient if she has experienced any problems since her last visit and recorded information in the prenatal record.
		●	Measured patient's blood pressure and charted the results correctly.
		●	Weighed the patient and charted the results correctly.
		▷	Stated the importance of weighing the patient.
		●	Instructed and prepared patient for the examination.
		●	Left room to provide patient with privacy.
		●	Made medical record available for review by the physician.
		●	Tested the urine specimen for glucose and protein, and charted the results correctly.
		●	Checked to make sure the patient is ready to be seen by physician.
		●	Informed physician that patient is ready.
		▷	Stated how the physician can be informed that the patient is ready.
		●	Assisted patient into a supine position and properly draped her.

493

Trial 1	Trial 2	Point Value	Performance Standards
			Assisted physician during the examination:
		•	Handed physician the tape measure for determination of fundal height.
		•	Applied coupling gel to the patient's abdomen and handedphysician Doppler device.
		•	Removed gel from patient's abdomen.
		•	Cleaned the probe head of the Doppler device.
		•	Assisted patient into the lithotomy position if a vaginal specimen is to be obtained or if vaginal examination is to be performed.
			After completion of the examination:
		•	Assisted patient into a sitting position and allowed her to rest.
		•	Assisted patient from examining table.
		•	Provided patient teaching and explanation of physician's instructions as required.
		•	Escorted patient to the reception area.
		•	Cleaned the examining room in preparation for the next patient.
		•	Prepared any specimens collected for transport to an outside laboratory.
		✱	Completed the procedure within 15 minutes.
			TOTALS
			CHART
Date			

Evaluation of Student Performance

EVALUATION CRITERIA			COMMENTS
Symbol	**Category**	**Point Value**	
✱	Critical Step	16 points	
•	Essential Step	6 points	
▷	Theory Question	2 points	
Score calculation:	100 points		
	− points missed		
	___ Score		
Satisfactory score: 85 or above			

494

CAAHEP Competencies Achieved

Psychomotor (Skills)

☑ I. 10. Assist physician with patient care.
☑ II. 2. Maintain laboratory test results using flow sheets.
☑ IV. 1. Use reflection, restatement, and clarification techniques to obtain a patient history.
☑ IV. 5. Instruct patients according to their needs to promote health maintenance and disease prevention.
☑ IV. 6. Prepare a patient for procedures and/or treatments.
☑ IX. 7. Document accurately in the patient record.

Affective (Behavior)

☑ IV. 2. Apply active listening skills.
☑ IV. 8. Analyze communications in providing appropriate responses or feedback.

ABHES Competencies Achieved

☑ 4. a. Document accurately.
☑ 8. e. Locate resources and information for patients and employers.
☑ 8. ff. Interview effectively.
☑ 9. f. Screen and follow up patient test results.
☑ 9. k. Prepare and maintain examination and treatment area.
☑ 9. l. Prepare patient for examinations and treatments.
☑ 9. m. Assist physician with routine and specialty examinations and treatments.
☑ 9. r. Teach patients methods of health promotion and disease prevention.

PATIENT'S NAME _____

INTERVAL PRENATAL HISTORY

Date 20___	Weeks Gestation	Height of Fundus (cm)	Weight	B/P	Urine Glucose	Urine Protein	FHT	Vaginal Examination	Presentation	Edema	Discharge	Bleeding	Contractions	Fetal Activity	NST	Next Appt.	Initials

(From Bonewit-West K: *Study guide for clinical medical assistants,* ed 8, St. Louis, 2011, Saunders.)

Chapter **23** **The Gynecologic Examination and Prenatal Care**

Notes

24 The Pediatric Examination

CHAPTER ASSIGNMENTS

√ After Completing	Date Due	Textbook Pages	TEXTBOOK ASSIGNMENTS	Possible Points	Points You Earned
		470-497	Read Chapter 24: The Pediatric Examination		
		472 495	Read Case Study 1 Case Study 1 questions	5	
		482 495	Read Case Study 2 Case Study 2 questions	5	
		488 495	Read Case Study 3 Case Study 3 questions	5	
			TOTAL POINTS		

√ After Completing	Date Due	Study Guide Pages	STUDY GUIDE ASSIGNMENTS (CTA = Critical Thinking Activity)	Possible Points	Points You Earned
		501	Pretest	10	
		502	Term Key Term Assessment	12	
		502-505	Evaluation of Learning questions	30	
		505	CTA A: Pediatric Weight	7	
			Evolve Site: Pounds and Ounces (Record points earned)		
		505	CTA B: Pediatric Length	8	
			Evolve Site: Inch by Inch (Record points earned)		
		506	CTA C: Growth Charts	18	
		506-507	CTA D: Motor and Social Development (5 points per each category)	65	
		507	CTA E: Intramuscular Injection	15	
		507-508	CTA F: Vaccine Information Statement	10	
		508-509	CTA G: Locating and Interpreting a Vaccine Information Statement	20	

√ After Completing	Date Due	Study Guide Pages	STUDY GUIDE ASSIGNMENTS (CTA = Critical Thinking Activity)	Possible Points	Points You Earned
		509-510	CTA H: Immunization Administration Record	40	
		511	CTA I: Crossword Puzzle	28	
			Evolve Site: Apply Your Knowledge questions (Record points earned)	10	
			Evolve Site: Video Evaluation	31	
		501	Posttest	10	
			ADDITIONAL ASSIGNMENTS		
			TOTAL POINTS		

√ When Assigned By Your Instructor	Study Guide Pages	Practices Required	LABORATORY ASSIGNMENTS (Procedure Number and Name)	Score*
	513	3	**Practice for Competency** 24-A: Carrying an Infant Textbook reference: p. 473	
	517-518		**Evaluation of Competency** 24-A: Carrying an Infant	*
	514	5	**Practice for Competency** 24-1: Measuring the Weight and Length of an Infant Textbook reference: pp. 476-477	
	519-521		**Evaluation of Competency** 24-1: Measuring the Weight and Length of an Infant	*
	515-516	5	**Practice for Competency** 24-2: Measuring Head and Chest Circumference of an Infant Textbook reference: pp. 477-478	
	523-524		**Evaluation of Competency** 24-2: Measuring Head and Chest Circumference of an Infant	*
	514	5	**Practice for Competency** 24-3: Calculating Growth Percentiles Textbook reference: pp. 478-480	
	525-526		**Evaluation of Competency** 24-3: Calculating Growth Percentiles	*
	515-516	5	**Practice for Competency** 24-4: Applying a Pediatric Urine Collector Textbook reference: pp. 483-484	
	527-529		**Evaluation of Competency** 24–4: Applying a Pediatric Urine Collector	*
			ADDITIONAL ASSIGNMENTS	

Notes

Name _____   Date _____

True or False

_____ 1. A pediatrician is a medical doctor who specializes in the diagnosis and treatment of disease in children.

_____ 2. The first well-child visit is usually scheduled 1 week after birth.

_____ 3. Length is measured with the child standing with his or her back to the measuring device.

_____ 4. Blood pressure should be taken for a child starting at 8 years of age.

_____ 5. It is best not to tell a child that an immunization will hurt.

_____ 6. The vastus lateralis muscle site is recommended for administering an injection to an infant.

_____ 7. An MMR injection includes the following immunizations: measles, meningitis, and rubella.

_____ 8. A Vaccine Information Statement explains the benefits and risks of a vaccine in lay terminology.

_____ 9. The hepatitis B vaccine can be given to a newborn.

_____ 10. The blood specimen for a newborn screening test is obtained from the infant's earlobe.

POSTTEST

True or False

_____ 1. A well-child visit is also referred to as a health maintenance visit.

_____ 2. A reason for weighing a child is to determine proper medication dosage.

_____ 3. Growth charts can be used to identify children with growth abnormalities.

_____ 4. Measuring pediatric blood pressure helps to identify children at risk for type 1 diabetes.

_____ 5. Using a blood pressure cuff that is too large for the child can result in a falsely low reading.

_____ 6. The length of the needle used for a pediatric IM injection depends on the amount of medication being administered.

_____ 7. The resistance of the body to pathogenic microorganisms or their toxins is known as *inflammation*.

_____ 8. The recommended route of administration for an MMR vaccine is subcutaneous.

_____ 9. Before administering a pediatric immunization, the National Childhood Vaccine Injury Act (NCVIA) requires that the parent sign a consent form.

_____ 10. If phenylketonuria (PKU) is left untreated, it can lead to malnutrition.

Directions: Match each medical term with its definition.

_____ 1. Immunity

_____ 2. Immunization

_____ 3. Infant

_____ 4. Length

_____ 5. Pediatrician

_____ 6. Pediatrics

_____ 7. Preschooler

_____ 8. School-age child

_____ 9. Toddler

_____ 10. Toxoid

_____ 11. Vaccine

_____ 12. Vertex

A. A physician who specializes in the care and development of children and the diagnosis and treatment of children's diseases

B. A child between 1 and 3 years old

C. The top of the head

D. The resistance of the body to the effects of a harmful agent such as a pathogenic microorganism or its toxins

E. The branch of medicine that deals with the care and development of children and the diagnosis and treatment of children's diseases

F. A suspension of attenuated or killed microorganisms administered to an individual to prevent an infectious disease

G. The process of becoming immune or of rendering an individual immune through the use of a vaccine or toxoid

H. The measurement from the vertex of the head to the heel of the foot in a supine position

I. A toxin that has been treated by heat or chemicals to destroy its harmful properties administered to an individual to prevent an infectious disease

J. A child from birth to 12 months old

K. A child from 3 to 6 years old

L. A child from 6 to 12 years old

EVALUATION OF LEARNING

Directions: Fill in each blank with the correct answer.

1. What are the components of the well-child visit?

_____

_____

2. What is the usual schedule for well-child visits?

_____

_____

_____

3. What is the purpose of the sick-child visit?

_____

_____

4. What procedures are often performed by the medical assistant during pediatric office visits?

_____

_____

_____

5. Why is it important for the medical assistant to develop a rapport with the pediatric patient?

_____

_____

_____

6. List the two positions that can be used to safely carry an infant.

_____

7. Why is it important to measure the growth (weight and height or length) of the child during each office visit?

_____

8. What is the difference between height and length?

_____

_____

9. What is the purpose of measuring head circumference?

_____

_____

10. What is the primary use of growth charts?

_____

_____

11. What is the primary cause of childhood obesity?

_____

12. What problems are associated with childhood obesity?

_____

_____

13. List five guidelines for preventing childhood obesity.

_____

_____

_____

14. According to the American Academy of Pediatrics, at what age and how often should blood pressure be measured in children?

_____

_____

15. What is the importance of measuring blood pressure in children?

_____

_____

16. What criteria must be followed to determine the correct cuff size for a child?

_____

_____

17. What occurs if the blood pressure cuff is too small or too large?

_____

_____

18. What three factors must be taken into consideration when determining if a child has hypertension?

_____

_____

_____

19. List three reasons for collecting a urine specimen from a child.

_____

_____

_____

20. Why should the child's genitalia be cleansed before applying a pediatric urine collector?

_____

_____

21. What gauge and length (range) of needle are recommended for giving an intramuscular injection to a child?

_____

22. Why is the dorsogluteal site not recommended for use as an intramuscular injection site in infants and young children?

_____

_____

_____

23. Why is the vastus lateralis muscle recommended as a good site for giving an intramuscular injection to an infant or young child?

_____

_____

_____

24. What is the difference between a vaccine and a toxoid?

_____

_____

_____

25. According to the American Academy of Pediatrics, what immunizations are recommended for each of the following pediatric patients?

a. 2-month-old infant: _____

b. 6-month-old infant: _____

c. 12-month-old infant: _____

d. 5-year-old child: _____

504

26. What information must be provided to parents as required by the NCVIA?

_____

_____

27. According to the NCVIA, what information must be recorded in the patient's medical record after a pediatric immunization has been administered?

_____

_____

_____

28. The newborn screening test screens for which metabolic diseases?

_____

_____

29. What are the symptoms of PKU if left untreated?

_____

30. Why can the PKU screening test be performed earlier on infants on formula compared with breast-fed babies?

_____

_____

CRITICAL THINKING ACTIVITIES

A. Pediatric Weight

Locate the following weight values on your pediatric scale. Place a check mark next to each one after it has been correctly located.

1. 7 lb, 9 oz   _____

2. 8 lb, 5 oz   _____

3. 12 lb, 10 oz   _____

4. 15 lb, 11 oz   _____

5. 19 lb, 7 oz   _____

6. 23 lb, 6 oz   _____

7. 25 lb, 3 oz   _____

B. Pediatric Length

Locate the following length values on your pediatric measuring device. Place a check mark next to each after it has been correctly located.

1. 20½ inches   _____

2. 22½ inches   _____

3. 24 inches   _____

4. 25¾ inches   _____

5. 28½ inches   _____

6. 31 inches   _____

7. 33¼ inches   _____

8. 36½ inches   _____

C. Growth Charts

Matthew Williams, age 2 years (24 months), has had health maintenance visits at the intervals listed below. His length and weight measurements were taken during each visit and are recorded here. Plot these on the growth chart on page 480 of your textbook. You can also print out a growth chart from your computer by going to the following website: www.cdc.gov/growthcharts. Calculate the percentile for each and record it in the space provided. (*Note:* His birth weight was 7 lb, 8 oz and his length was 20 inches.)

Well-Child Visit

Age	Weight	Percentile	Length	Percentile
1 month	9 lb, 10 oz		22 in	
2 months	12 lb, 4 oz		23½ in	
4 months	16 lb, 5 oz		25¼ in	
6 months	18 lb, 8 oz		27 in	
9 months	22 lb, 4 oz		29¼ in	
12 months	24 lb, 4 oz		30½ in	
15 months	26 lb, 8 oz		31½ in	
18 months	27 lb		32½ in	
24 months	28 lb		35¾ in	

D. Motor and Social Development

Using a reference source, describe the motor and social development of the age groups listed here. The first one is done for you.

Age	Motor and Social Development
Birth to 3 months	Raises head but not stable, can turn head from side to side, activities are limited to reflexes, cries when hungry, responsive social smile, coos, eyes can focus on an object and follow a moving object 180 degrees.
4 to 6 months	
7 to 9 months	
10 to 12 months	
1 year	
2 years	
3 years	
4 years	
5 years	

Age	Motor and Social Development
6 years	
7 years	
8 to 10 years	
Preadolescent	
Adolescent	

E. Intramuscular Injection

How would you prepare the following children for an intramuscular injection of penicillin to reduce apprehension and fear? Table 24-2, Techniques for Interacting with Children, on page 473 of your textbook can be used as a reference for this activity.

a. Katie Waugh, age 5

_____

_____

_____

b. Patrick Williams, age 8

_____

_____

_____

c. Julie Anderson, age 15

_____

_____

_____

F. Vaccine Information Statement

Refer to the Diphtheria, Tetanus, and Pertussis Vaccine Information Statement (VIS) in your textbook (pages 490 and 491), and answer the following questions:

1. How does an individual contract tetanus?

_____

_____

2. What are the symptoms of the following diseases?

a. Diphtheria _____

b. Tetanus _____

c. Pertussis _____

3. Why is DTaP now used instead of DTP?

_____

_____

4. What is the immunization schedule for DTaP?

_____

_____

5. Who should not get a DTaP immunization?

_____

_____

6. What does Td protect against, and what is the recommended immunization schedule for Td?

_____

_____

7. What mild problems may occur from a DTaP vaccine?

_____

_____

8. What moderate problems may occur from a DTaP vaccine?

_____

_____

9. What should be done if the patient develops fever and pain after receiving a DTaP?

_____

_____

10. What should be done if a moderate or severe reaction occurs after a DTaP immunization?

_____

_____

G. Locating and Interpreting a Vaccine Information Statement

Obtain a VIS for a vaccine that you would like to know more about (other than the DTaP vaccine already included in your textbook). List the information that would be important for a parent to know before this immunization is administered to his or her child. The following Internet sites can be used to obtain a VIS:

www.cdc.gov/vaccines/pubs/vis
www.immunize.org/vis

Name of Immunization: _____

Publication Date: _____

Information to Relay to a Parent:

_____

_____

_____

_____

_____

_____

_____

_____

_____

_____

H. Immunization Administration Record

Complete the following immunization record form for an infant at his or her 2-month, 4-month, and 6-month visits using Figure 24-11 (immunization schedule) in the textbook to determine which immunizations are administered during these well-child visits. The website (www.immunize.org/catg.d/p2022.pdf) provides an example of a completed immunization admistration form to assist you in completing this form.

IMMUNIZATION ADMINISTRATION RECORD

Name _____
(first)   (MI)   (last)

DOB _____

Physician _____

Address _____

_____

SITE ABBREVIATIONS:

RVL: Right vastus lateralis

LVL: Left vastus lateralis

RD: Right deltoid

LD: Left deltoid

PO: By mouth

IN: Intranasal

Vaccine	Type of Vaccine[1] (generic abbreviation)	Date Given (mo/day/yr)	Dose	Site	Vaccine		Vaccine Information Statement		Signature and Title of Vaccinator
					Lot #	Mfr.	Date on VIS	Date Given	
Hepatitis B[2] (e.g., HepB, Hib-HepB, DTaP-HepB-IPV) Give IM.									
Diphtheria, Tetanus, Pertussis[2] (e.g., DTaP, DTaP-Hib, DTaP-HepB-IPV, DT, DTaP-HiB-IPV, Tdap, DTaP-IPV, Td) Give IM.									
Haemophilus influenzae type b[2] (e.g., Hib, Hib-HepB, DTaP-HiB-IPV, DTaP-Hib) Give IM.									
Polio[2] (e.g., IPV, DTaP-HepB-IPV, DTaP-HiB-IPV, DTaP-IPV) Give IPV SC or IM. Give all others IM.									
Pneumococcal (e.g., PCV, conjugate; PPV, polysaccharide) Give PCV IM. Give PPV SC or IM.									
Rotavirus Give oral.									
Measles, Mumps, Rubella (e.g., MMR, MMRV) Give SC.									
Varicella (e.g., Var, MMRV) Give SC.									
Hepatitis A (HepA) Give IM									
Meningococcal (e.g., MCV4, MPSV4) Give MCV4 IM and MPSV4 SC.									
Human papillomavirus (e.g., HPV) Give IM									
Influenza (e.g., TIV, inactivated; LAIV, live attenuated) Give TIV IM. Give LAIV IN.									
Other									

1. Record the generic abbreviation for the type of vaccine given (e.g., DTaP-Hib, PCV), not the trade name.
2. For combination vaccines, fill in a row for each separate antigen in the combination.

(Modified from Bonewit-West K: *Study Guide for clinical procedures for medical assistants,* ed 8, St. Louis, 2011, Saunders.)

I. Crossword Puzzle: The Pediatric Examination

Directions: Complete the crossword puzzle using the clues provided.

ACROSS

1 Right size for child's BP?
3 Title expires at 1 year
6 Child's vaccine act
9 German measles
10 Not for pregnant women
13 Whooping cough
16 PKU puncture site
17 3-in-1 vaccine
20 Do not weigh infant in this
21 Stand up straight
22 Begin at 3
23 First breast milk
24 Baby doctor
25 MMR administration route
26 Can give at birth vaccine
27 Injection site for infants

DOWN

1 Hold-me position
2 Not a kid reward
4 Common immunization side effect
5 From 1 to 3
7 Resistance to microorganisms
8 No phenylalanine enzyme
11 Vertex to heel
12 Child's work
14 Childhood obesity can cause this
15 Not caused by chickens
18 Fights with a microorganism
19 Immunization explainer

Notes

Procedure 24-A: Carrying an Infant

Practice the procedure for carrying an infant, using a pediatric training mannequin in the following positions: cradle and upright.

Carrying Position	Number Of Practices

Procedures 24-1 and 24-3: Weight, Length, and Growth Charts

1. **Weight and Length.** Measure the weight of an infant using a pediatric training mannequin. Record the results in the chart provided.
2. **Growth Charts.** Calculate growth percentiles on a growth chart using the values presented below. Assume these values were taken from the same (female) child over the course of her first year of life.

Age	Weight	Length
2 months	9 pounds	21 inches
4 months	11 pounds, 8 ounces	23½ inches
6 months	14 pounds, 8 ounces	25¼ inches
9 months	18 pounds, 8 ounces	27¼ inches
12 months	21 pounds, 6 ounces	28¾ inches

CHART	
Date	

Procedure 24-2: Head and Chest Circumference. Measure the head and chest circumference of an infant using a pediatric training mannequin. Record the results in the chart provided.

Procedure 24-4: Pediatric Urine Collector. Practice the procedure for applying a pediatric urine collector, using a pediatric training mannequin. Record the procedure in the chart provided.

	CHART
Date	

CHART	
Date	

Procedure 24-A: Carrying an Infant

Name: _____   Date: _____

Evaluated by: _____   Score: _____

Performance Objective

Outcome:	Carry an infant in the following positions: cradle and upright.
Conditions:	Given a pediatric training mannequin.
Standards:	Time: 5 minutes. Student completed procedure in _____ minutes.
	Accuracy: Satisfactory score on the performance evaluation checklist.

Performance Evaluation Checklist

Trial 1	Trial 2	Point Value	Performance Standards
			Cradle position:
		●	Slid the left hand and arm under infant's back.
		●	Grasped infant's upper arm from behind.
		●	Encircled infant's upper arm with the thumb and fingers.
		●	Supported infant's head, shoulders, and back on your arm.
		●	Slipped the right arm up and under the infant's buttocks.
		●	Cradled infant in your arms with the infant's body resting against your chest.
			Upright position:
		●	Slipped the right hand under infant's head and shoulders.
		●	Spread the fingers apart to support infant's head and neck.
		●	Slipped the left forearm under infant's buttocks.
		●	Allowed infant to rest against your chest.
		✱	Completed the procedure within 5 minutes.
			TOTALS
		CHART	
Date			

Evaluation of Student Performance

EVALUATION CRITERIA			COMMENTS
Symbol	**Category**	**Point Value**	
★	Critical Step	16 points	
●	Essential Step	6 points	
▷	Theory Question	2 points	

Score calculation: 100 points

– _____ points missed

_____ Score

Satisfactory score: 85 or above

CAAHEP Competencies Achieved

Psychomotor (Skills)
☑ IV. 6. Prepare a patient for procedures and/or treatments.

Affective (Behavior)
☑ IV. 1. Demonstrate empathy in communicating with patients, family, and staff.

ABHES Competencies Achieved

☑ 9. 1. Prepare patient for examinations and treatments.

Procedure 24-1: Measuring the Weight and Length of an Infant

Name: _____ Date: _____

Evaluated by: _____ Score: _____

Performance Objective

Outcome:	Measure the weight and length of an infant.
Conditions:	Using a pediatric training mannequin and a pediatric balance scale (table model).
	Given a paper protector.
Standards:	Time: 5 minutes. Student completed procedure in _____ minutes.
	Accuracy: Satisfactory score on the performance evaluation checklist.

Performance Evaluation Checklist

Trial 1	Trial 2	Point Value	Performance Standards
			Weight:
		●	Sanitized hands.
		●	Greeted the infant's parent and introduced yourself.
		●	Identified the infant.
		●	Explained the procedure to the child's parent.
		●	Based on the medical office policy asked parent to: a. Remove infant's clothing and put on a dry diaper. b. Remove infant's clothing including the diaper.
		▷	Stated why the infant should not be weighed with a wet diaper.
		●	Unlocked pediatric scale and placed a clean paper protector on it.
		▷	Stated the purpose of the paper protector.
		●	Checked the balance scale for accuracy.
		▷	Stated the purpose for balancing the scale.
		●	Gently placed infant on his or her back on the scale.
		●	Placed one hand slightly above infant.
		●	Balanced scale.
		●	Read results while infant was lying still.
		●	Jotted down value or made a mental note of it.
		✱	The reading was identical to the evaluator's reading.

Trial 1	Trial 2	Point Value	Performance Standards
		●	Returned balance to its resting position and locked the scale.
			Length:
		●	Placed the vertex of infant's head against the headboard at the zero mark.
		●	Asked parent to hold infant's head in position.
		●	Straightened infant's knees and placed soles of infant's feet firmly against the upright footboard.
		●	Read infant's length in inches from the measure.
		●	Jotted down value or made a mental note of it.
		✶	The reading was identical to the evaluator's reading.
		●	Removed infant from the scale and handed him or her to the parent.
		●	Returned headboard and footboard to their resting positions.
		●	Sanitized hands.
		●	Charted the results correctly.
		✶	Completed the procedure within 5 minutes.
			TOTALS
			CHART
Date	

Evaluation of Student Performance

EVALUATION CRITERIA			COMMENTS
Symbol	**Category**	**Point Value**	
✶	Critical Step	16 points	
●	Essential Step	6 points	
▷	Theory Question	2 points	

Score calculation: 100 points

     −   _____ points missed

        _____ Score

Satisfactory score: 85 or above

CAAHEP Competencies Achieved

Psychomotor (Skills)
☑ IV. 6. Prepare a patient for procedures and/or treatments.

Affective (Behavior)
☑ I. 2. Use language/verbal skills that enable patients' understanding.
☑ IV. 7. Demonstrate recognition of the patient's level of understanding in communications.

ABHES Competencies Achieved

☑ 5. f. Identify and discuss developmental stages of life.
☑ 8. cc. Communicate on the recipient's level of comprehension.
☑ 9. l. Prepare patient for examinations and treatments.

Notes

Procedure 24-2: Measuring Head and Chest Circumference of an Infant

Name: _____   Date: _____

Evaluated by: _____   Score: _____

Performance Objective

Outcome:	Measure the head and chest circumference of an infant.
Conditions:	Given a flexible, nonstretch tape measure (in centimeters).
Standards:	Time: 5 minutes. Student completed procedure in _____ minutes.
	Accuracy: Satisfactory score on the performance evaluation checklist.

Performance Evaluation Checklist

Trial 1	Trial 2	Point Value	Performance Standards
			Measurement of head circumference:
		●	Sanitized hands.
		●	Assembled equipment.
		●	Positioned the infant.
		▷	Stated what positions can be used to measure head circumference.
		●	Positioned the measuring device around the infant's head.
		●	The tape measure was placed slightly above the eyebrows and pinna of the ears, and around the occipital prominence at the back of the skull.
		●	Read the results in centimeters (or inches).
		●	Jotted down value or made a mental note of it.
		✱	The reading was identical to the evaluator's reading.
		●	Sanitized hands.
		●	Charted the results correctly.
			Measurement of chest circumference:
		●	Positioned the infant on his or her back on the examining table.
		●	Encircled the measuring device around the infant's chest at the nipple line.
		●	Ensured that the measuring device was snug but not too tight.

Trial 1	Trial 2	Point Value	Performance Standards
		●	Read the results in centimeters (or inches).
		●	Jotted down this value or made a mental note of it.
		✱	The reading was identical to the evaluator's reading.
		●	Charted the results correctly.
		✱	Completed the procedure within 5 minutes.
			TOTALS

CHART

Date	

Evaluation of Student Performance

EVALUATION CRITERIA			COMMENTS
Symbol	**Category**	**Point Value**	
✱	Critical Step	16 points	
●	Essential Step	6 points	
▷	Theory Question	2 points	

Score calculation: 100 points

     −   _____ points missed

        _____ Score

Satisfactory score: 85 or above

CAAHEP Competencies Achieved

Psychomotor (Skills)
☑ IV. 6. Prepare a patient for procedures and/or treatments.

Affective (Behavior)
☑ I. 1. Apply critical thinking skills in performing patient assessment and care.

ABHES Competencies Achieved

☑ 9. 1. Prepare patient for examinations and treatments.

Procedure 24-3: Calculating Growth Percentiles

Name: _____   Date: _____

Evaluated by: _____   Score: _____

Performance Objective

Outcome:	Plot a pediatric growth value on a growth chart.
Conditions:	Given a pediatric growth chart.
Standards:	Time: 5 minutes. Student completed procedure in _____ minutes.
	Accuracy: Satisfactory score on the performance evaluation checklist.

Performance Evaluation Checklist

Trial 1	Trial 2	Point Value	Performance Standards
		●	Selected the proper growth chart.
		●	Located the child's age in the horizontal column at the bottom of the chart.
		●	Located the growth value in the vertical column under the appropriate category.
		●	Drew a (imaginary) vertical line from the child's age mark and an imaginary horizontal line from the growth mark.
		●	Found the site at which the two lines intersected on the graph.
		●	Placed a dot on this site.
		●	Determined the percentile by following the curved percentile line upward.
		●	Read the value located on the right side of the chart.
		●	Estimated the results if the value did not fall exactly on a percentile line.
		●	Charted the results correctly.
		✴	The value was within ±2 percentage points of the evaluator's determination.
		✴	Completed the procedure within 5 minutes.
			TOTALS

Evaluation of Student Performance

EVALUATION CRITERIA			COMMENTS
Symbol	**Category**	**Point Value**	
✳	Critical Step	16 points	
●	Essential Step	6 points	
▷	Theory Question	2 points	

Score calculation: 100 points

      −   _____ points missed

        ___ Score

Satisfactory score: 85 or above

CAAHEP Competencies Achieved

Psychomotor (Skills)
☑ II. 3. Maintain growth charts.

Affective (Behavior)
☑ II. 2. Distinguish between normal and abnormal test results.

ABHES Competencies Achieved

☑ 5. f. Identify and discuss developmental stages of life.
☑ 8. hh. Receive, organize, prioritize, and transmit information expediently.

Procedure 24-4: Applying a Pediatric Urine Collector

Name: _____ Date: _____

Evaluated by: _____ Score: _____

Performance Objective

Outcome:	Apply a pediatric urine collector.
Conditions:	Using a pediatric training mannequin.
	Given the following: disposable gloves, personal antiseptic wipes, pediatric urine collector bag, urine specimen container and label, and a waste container.
Standards:	Time: 10 minutes. Student completed procedure in _____ minutes.
	Accuracy: Satisfactory score on the performance evaluation checklist.

Performance Evaluation Checklist

Trial 1	Trial 2	Point Value	Performance Standards
		●	Sanitized hands.
		●	Assembled equipment.
		●	Greeted the child's parent and introduced yourself.
		●	Identified the child and explained the procedure to the parent.
		●	Applied gloves.
		●	Positioned child on his or her back with legs spread apart.
			Cleanse the area and apply the bag:
			Females
		●	Cleansed each side of the meatus with a separate wipe using a front-to-back motion.
		●	Cleansed directly down the middle with a third wipe.
		●	Discarded each wipe after cleansing.
		▷	Stated the reason for cleansing the urinary meatus.
		●	Allowed the area to dry completely.
		▷	Explained why the area should be allowed to dry.
		●	Removed paper backing from urine collector bag.
		●	Placed the bottom of the adhesive ring on the perinuem and work upward.
		●	Firmly pressed the adhesive surface firmly to the skin surrounding the external genitalia.

527

Trial 1	Trial 2	Point Value	Performance Standards
		●	Made sure there was no puckering.
		●	Opening of the bag was placed directly over the urinary meatus.
		●	Excess length of the bag was positioned toward the feet.
			Males
		●	Retracted the foreskin of the penis if the child is not circumcised.
		●	Cleansed each side of the urethral orifice with a separate wipe.
		●	Cleansed directly over the urethral orifice.
		●	Cleansed the scrotum.
		●	Discarded each wipe after cleansing.
		●	Allowed the area to dry completely.
		●	Removed the paper backing from urine collector bag.
		●	Positioned the bag so that child's penis and scrotum are projected through the opening of the bag.
		●	Firmly pressed the adhesive surface firmly to the skin.
		●	Excess length of the bag was positioned toward the feet.
			Completed the procedure:
		●	Loosely diapered child.
		●	Checked bag every 15 minutes until urine specimen was obtained.
		●	Gently removed collector bag from top to bottom.
		●	Cleansed genital area with a personal antiseptic wipe and rediapered child.
		●	Transferred urine specimen into specimen container and tightly applied the lid.
		●	Applied label to the container.
		●	Disposed of collector bag in a regular waste container.
		●	Tested the specimen or prepared it for transfer to an outside laboratory.
		▷	Explained why the urine specimen should not be allowed to stand at room temperature.
		●	Removed gloves and sanitized hands.
		●	Charted the procedure correctly.
		✱	Completed the procedure within 5 minutes.
			TOTALS

528

Chapter **24** **The Pediatric Examination**

Copyright © 2013, 2009 by Saunders, an imprint of Elsevier Inc. All rights reserved.

CHART	
Date	

Evaluation of Student Performance

EVALUATION CRITERIA			COMMENTS
Symbol	**Category**	**Point Value**	
✳	Critical Step	16 points	
●	Essential Step	6 points	
▷	Theory Question	2 points	
Score calculation: 100 points − ____ points missed ____ Score			
Satisfactory score: 85 or above			

CAAHEP Competencies Achieved

Psychomotor (Skills)
☑ IV. 6. Prepare a patient for procedures and/or treatments.

Affective (Behavior)
☑ III. 2. Explain the rationale for performance of a procedure to the patient.

ABHES Competencies Achieved

☑ 10. d. Collect, label, and process specimens.

Notes

25 Minor Office Surgery

CHAPTER ASSIGNMENTS

√ After Completing	Date Due	Textbook Pages	TEXTBOOK ASSIGNMENTS	Possible Points	Points You Earned
		498-548	Read Chapter 25: Minor Office Surgery		
		519 546	Read Case Study 1 Case Study 1 questions	5	
		528 546	Read Case Study 2 Case Study 2 questions	5	
		541 547	Read Case Study 3 Case Study 3 questions	5	
			TOTAL POINTS		

√ After Completing	Date Due	Study Guide Pages	STUDY GUIDE ASSIGNMENTS (CTA = Critical Thinking Activity)	Possible Points	Points You Earned
		535	Pretest	10	
		536	Term Key Term Assessment A. Definitions B. Word Parts (Add 1 point for each medical term)	26 9	
		537-541	Evaluation of Learning questions	47	
		542-543	CTA A: Medical and Surgical Asepsis	10	
		543	CTA B: Violation of Surgical Asepsis	10	
		544-545	CTA C: Surgical Instruments (2 points each)	22	
			Evolve Site: It's Instrumental (Record points earned)		
			Evolve Site: Keep it Sterile (Record points earned)		
		546	CTA D: Pioneers in Surgical Asepsis (5 points each)	15	
		546-547	CTA E: Patient Instruction Sheet	20	

√ After Completing	Date Due	Study Guide Pages	STUDY GUIDE ASSIGNMENTS (CTA = Critical Thinking Activity)	Possible Points	Points You Earned
		548	CTA F: Crossword Puzzle	24	
			e Evolve Site: Apply Your Knowledge questions	10	
			e Evolve Site: Video Evaluation	69	
		535	📰 Posttest	10	
			ADDITIONAL ASSIGNMENTS		
			TOTAL POINTS		

√ When Assigned By Your Instructor	Study Guide Pages	Practices Required	LABORATORY ASSIGNMENTS (Procedure Number and Name)	Score*
	549-550	5	**Practice for Competency** 25-1: Applying and Removing Sterile Gloves Textbook reference: pp. 506-507	
	551-552		**Evaluation of Competency** 25-1: Applying and Removing Sterile Gloves	*
	549-550	5	**Practice for Competency** 25-2: Opening a Sterile Package Textbook reference: pp. 508-509	
	553-554		**Evaluation of Competency** 25-2: Opening a Sterile Package	*
	549-550	5	**Practice for Competency** Using Commercially Prepared Sterile Packages Textbook reference: p. 505	
	555-556		**Evaluation of Competency** Using Commercially Prepared Sterile Packages	*
	549-550	3	**Practice for Competency** 25-3: Pouring a Sterile Solution Textbook reference: p. 510	
	557-558		**Evaluation of Competency** 25-3: Pouring a Sterile Solution	*
	549-550	5	**Practice for Competency** 25-4: Changing a Sterile Dressing Textbook reference: pp. 513-515	
	559-561		**Evaluation of Competency** 25-4: Changing a Sterile Dressing	*
	549-550	Sutures: 3 Staples: 3	**Practice for Competency** 25-5: Removing Sutures and Staples Textbook reference: pp. 519-521	
	563-565		**Evaluation of Competency** 25-5: Removing Sutures and Staples	*
	549-550	3	**Practice for Competency** 25-6: Applying and Removing Adhesive Skin Closures Textbook reference: pp. 522-525	
	567-570		**Evaluation of Competency** 25-6: Applying and Removing Adhesive Skin Closures	*

√ When Assigned By Your Instructor	Study Guide Pages	Practices Required	LABORATORY ASSIGNMENTS (Procedure Number and Name)	Score*
	549-550	5	**Practice for Competency** 25-7: Assisting with Minor Office Surgery Textbook reference: pp. 530-533	
	571-574		**Evaluation of Competency** 25-7: Assisting with Minor Office Surgery	*
	549-550	Each bandage turn: 3	**Practice for Competency** 25-A: Bandage Turns Textbook reference: pp. 543-545	
	575-577		**Evaluation of Competency** 25-A: Bandage Turns	*
			ADDITIONAL ASSIGNMENTS	

Name _____ Date _____

True or False

_____ 1. Surgical asepsis refers to practices that keep objects and areas free from all microorganisms.

_____ 2. Something that is sterile is contaminated if it comes in contact with a pathogen.

_____ 3. Reaching over a sterile field is a violation of sterile technique.

_____ 4. An incision is a jagged tearing of the tissues.

_____ 5. The skin is the first line of defense of the body.

_____ 6. One of the local signs of inflammation is fever.

_____ 7. Sutures approximate the edges of a wound until proper healing occurs.

_____ 8. A biopsy is usually performed to determine if an infection is present.

_____ 9. An ingrown toenail can be caused by shoes that are too tight.

_____ 10. One of the functions of a bandage is to hold a dressing in place.

?≡ POSTTEST

True or False

_____ 1. Measuring a patient's temperature requires the use of surgical asepsis.

_____ 2. Hemostatic forceps are used to clamp off blood vessels.

_____ 3. An instrument with a ratchet should be kept in a closed position when not in use.

_____ 4. The physician would most likely order a tetanus booster for an abrasion.

_____ 5. Inflammation is the protective response of the body to trauma and the entrance of foreign substances.

_____ 6. A serous exudate is red in color.

_____ 7. Size 4-0 sutures have a smaller diameter than size 3 sutures.

_____ 8. Sebaceous cysts are commonly found on the palm of the hand.

_____ 9. Colposcopy is frequently used to evaluate lesions of the cervix.

_____ 10. Cryosurgery is used in the treatment of cervical cancer.

A. Definitions

Directions: Match each medical term with its definition.

_____	1. Abrasion	A.	A protective response of the body to trauma and the entrance of foreign matter
_____	2. Abscess	B.	To cause a sterile object or surface to become unsterile
_____	3. Absorbable suture	C.	A wound made by a sharp pointed object piercing the skin
_____	4. Approximation	D.	The condition in which the body is invaded by a pathogen
_____	5. Bandage	E.	A collection of pus in a cavity surrounded by inflamed tissue
_____	6. Biopsy	F.	The arrest of bleeding by natural or artificial means
_____	7. Capillary action	G.	Free of all living microorganisms and bacterial spores
_____	8. Colposcope	H.	A wound in which the tissues are torn apart, leaving ragged and irregular edges
_____	9. Colposcopy	I.	A lighted instrument with a binocular magnifying lens used to examine the vagina and cervix
_____	10. Contaminate	J.	A localized staphylococcal infection that originates deep within a hair follicle; also known as a boil
_____	11. Contusion	K.	An injury to the tissues under the skin that causes blood vessels to rupture, allowing blood to seep into the tissues
_____	12. Cryosurgery	L.	The surgical removal and examination of tissue from the living body
_____	13. Fibroblast	M.	A wound in which the outer layers of the skin are damaged
_____	14. Forceps	N.	The action that causes liquid to rise along a wick, a tube, or a gauze dressing
_____	15. Furuncle	O.	A two-pronged instrument for grasping and squeezing
_____	16. Hemostasis	P.	Practices that keep objects and areas sterile or free from microorganisms
_____	17. Incision	Q.	A break in the continuity of an external or internal surface caused by physical means
_____	18. Infection	R.	The therapeutic use of freezing temperatures to destroy abnormal tissue
_____	19. Inflammation	S.	The visual examination of the vagina and cervix using a lighted instrument with a magnifying lens
_____	20. Laceration	T.	Suture material that is gradually digested and absorbed by the body
_____	21. Nonabsorbable suture	U.	The process of bringing two parts, such as tissue, together through the use of sutures or other means
_____	22. Puncture	V.	A strip of woven material used to wrap or cover a part of the body
_____	23. Sterile	W.	A clean cut caused by a cutting instrument
_____	24. Surgery	X.	Suture material that is not absorbed by the body
_____	25. Surgical asepsis	Y.	An immature cell from which connective tissue can develop
_____	26. Wound	Z.	The branch of medicine that deals with operative and manual procedures for correction of deformities and defects, repair of injuries, and diagnosis and treatment of certain diseases

B. Word Parts

Directions: Indicate the meaning of each word part in the space provided. List as many medical terms as possible that incorporate the word part in the space provided.

Word Part	Meaning of Word Part	Medical Terms That Incorporate Word Part
1. bi/o		
2. -opsy		
3. colp/o		
4. -scope		
5. -scopy		
6. cry/o		
7. fibr/o		
8. hem/o		
9. stasis		

Directions: Fill in each blank with the correct answer.

1. List the characteristics of a minor surgical procedure.

_____

_____

_____

_____

2. List the responsibilities of the medical assistant during a minor surgical operation.

_____

_____

_____

_____

3. What is the purpose of serrations found on some instruments?

_____

_____

4. What is the difference in function between mosquito hemostatic forceps and standard hemostatic forceps?

_____

_____

_____

5. List five guidelines that should be followed in caring for instruments.

_____

_____

_____

_____

6. What is the difference between a closed and an open wound?

_____

_____

7. Why does a puncture wound encourage the growth of tetanus bacteria?

_____

_____

8. What is the purpose of inflammation?

_____

_____

9. List the four local signs that occur during inflammation.

_____

10. What occurs during the inflammatory phase of wound healing?

_____

_____

11. What occurs during the granulation phase of wound healing?

_____

_____

12. What occurs during the maturation phase of wound healing?

_____

13. What is an exudate?

_____

_____

14. Describe the appearance of the following types of exudates:

    a. Serous _____

    b. Sanguineous _____

    c. Purulent _____

    d. Serosanguineous _____

    e. Purosanguineous _____

15. List two functions of a sterile dressing.

_____

_____

16. The names and sizes of sutures are listed. In each set, circle the suture that has the smaller diameter:

    a. 4-0 silk

       2-0 silk

    b. 0 chromic surgical gut

       3-0 chromic surgical gut

    c. 2-0 polypropylene

       2 polypropylene

17. List five examples of materials used for nonabsorbable sutures.

_____

_____

18. What is a swaged needle? List advantages of using a swaged needle.

_____

_____

19. Why are sutures inserted in the head and neck generally removed sooner than other sutures?

_____

_____

20. List two advantages of using surgical skin staples to approximate a wound.

_____

_____

21. List three advantages of adhesive skin closures.

_____

_____

_____

22. What is the purpose of preparing the patient's skin before minor office surgery?

_____

23. What is the purpose of a fenestrated drape?

_____

_____

24. What is the name of the local anesthetic most frequently used in the medical office during minor office surgery.

_____

25. Explain how an instrument should be handed to the physician during minor office surgery.

_____

26. What is a sebaceous cyst, and what causes it to form?

_____

_____

27. What is the purpose of using gauze packing or a rubber Penrose drain after incising a localized infection?

_____

_____

28. What is the difference between congenital nevi and acquired nevi?

_____

_____

29. What are skin tags? Where are they most frequently found on the body?

_____

_____

_____

30. Describe the appearance of dysplastic nevi. What concern exists with dysplastic nevi?

_____

_____

_____

31. List the characteristics of melanoma.

_____

_____

_____

32. What are the most common methods used to remove moles?

_____

_____

33. What is the purpose of a biopsy?

_____

_____

34. What is an ingrown toenail?

_____

_____

35. List three causes of an ingrown toenail.

_____

_____

_____

36. List two reasons for performing a colposcopy.

_____

_____

37. What is the purpose of performing a cervical punch biopsy?

_____

_____

38. List the postoperative instructions that must be relayed to the patient after a cervical punch biopsy.

_____

_____

_____

39. List two uses of cryosurgery.

_____

_____

40. List the postoperative instructions that must be relayed to the patient after cervical cryosurgery.

_____

_____

_____

41. List three functions of a bandage.

_____

_____

_____

42. List four guidelines to follow when applying a bandage.

_____

_____

_____

_____

43. List four signs that may indicate a bandage is too tight.

_____

_____

_____

_____

44. Why should the medical assistant be careful when applying an elastic bandage?

_____

_____

45. What is the purpose of reversing the spiral during a spiral-reverse turn?

_____

_____

46. List two uses of the figure-eight bandage turn.

_____

_____

47. What type of bandage turn is used to anchor a bandage?

_____

CRITICAL THINKING ACTIVITIES

A. Medical and Surgical Asepsis

Refer to Chapter 17, and describe the difference between medical asepsis and surgical asepsis.

_____

_____

_____

Which technique (medical asepsis or surgical asepsis) would be employed during the following procedures? For procedures requiring surgical asepsis, indicate which of the following reasons necessitate the use of surgical asepsis: caring for broken skin, penetrating a skin surface, or entering a body cavity that is normally sterile.

1. Administering oral medication

_____

_____

2. Inserting sutures

_____

_____

3. Measuring oral temperature

_____

_____

4. Applying a bandage to the forearm

_____

_____

5. Performing a needle biopsy

_____

_____

6. Removing a sebaceous cyst

_____

_____

7. Obtaining a Pap specimen

_____

_____

8. Inserting a urinary catheter

_____

_____

9. Incision and drainage of an abscess

_____

_____

10. Applying a dressing to an open wound

_____

_____

B. Violation of Surgical Asepsis

In the situations that follow, the principles of surgical asepsis have been violated. In the space provided, explain why the techniques should not be performed in this manner.

1. Placing a sterile 4 × 4 gauze pad within the 1-inch border around the sterile field

_____

_____

2. Wearing rings during the application of sterile gloves

_____

_____

3. Talking over a sterile field

_____

_____

4. Reaching over a sterile field

_____

_____

5. Holding sterile gauze below waist level

_____

_____

6. Not palming the label when pouring an antiseptic solution

_____

_____

7. Spilling an antiseptic solution on the sterile field

_____

_____

8. Passing a soiled dressing over the sterile field

_____

_____

9. Placing a vial of Xylocaine on the sterile field

_____

_____

10. Using bare hands to arrange articles on the sterile field

_____

_____

543

C. Surgical Instruments

In the space provided, state the name and use of each of the following types of surgical instruments. Identify any of the following parts present on each instrument by labeling the instrument: box lock, spring handle, ratchets, serrations, cutting edge, and teeth.

1. Name: _____

   Use: _____

   _____

2. Name: _____

   Use: _____

   _____

3. Name: _____

   Use: _____

   _____

4. Name: _____

   Use: _____

   _____

5. Name: _____

   Use: _____

   _____

6. Name: _____

   Use: _____

   _____

7. Name: _____

   Use: _____

   _____

8. Name: _____

   Use: _____

   _____

9. Name: _____

   Use: _____

   _____

10. Name: _____

   Use: _____

   _____

11. Name: _____

   Use: _____

   _____

D. Pioneers In Surgical Asepsis

Using a reference source, describe the contributions the following men made to medicine, especially regarding surgical asepsis:

1. Ignaz Semmelweis

_____

_____

_____

2. Louis Pasteur

_____

_____

_____

3. Joseph Lister

_____

_____

_____

E. Patient Instruction Sheet

1. You are working for a surgeon who would like you to develop a patient instruction sheet for minor surgery. Select one of the minor operations provided. Using the following instruction sheet, develop a sheet that would be informative and visually appealing to a patient. Be as creative as possible in designing your sheet.

2. Select a partner. Have your partner play the role of a patient who is going to have the minor surgery performed, and explain the information on the sheet. Ask the patient to sign the sheet, and witness the patient's signature.

   Minor office operations

   a. Sebaceous cyst removal
   b. Mole removal
   c. Needle biopsy
   d. Ingrown toenail removal
   e. Colposcopy and biopsy
   f. Cervical cryosurgery

PATIENT INSTRUCTION SHEET

NAME OF THE PROCEDURE:

DESCRIPTION OF PROCEDURE:

PURPOSE OF THE PROCEDURE:

HOW TO PREPARE FOR THE PROCEDURE:

WHAT TO DO FOLLOWING THE PROCEDURE:

I have received and understand the above instructions:

Patient's Signature _____

Witness: _____ Date: _____

547

F. Crossword Puzzle: Minor Office Surgery

Directions: Complete the crossword puzzle using the clues presented below.

(From Bonewit West K: *Study guide for clinical procedures for medical assistants*, ed 8, St. Louis, 2011, Saunders.)

Across

1 Drape with a hole
4 Produces collagen
6 Clean, smooth cut
8 Boil
9 Sac containing oil secretions
14 Pus formation
15 Clamps off blood vessels
17 Local anesthetic brand name
20 Pus in a cavity
22 Tetanus may grow here
23 A local sign of inflammation
24 Bring together

Down

2 Free of all MOs and spores
3 Bruise
5 Scrape
7 Exudate containing blood
10 Suture/needle combination
11 Tx for chronic cervicitis
12 Father of modern surgery
13 Ragged and irregular wound
16 Discovered penicillin
18 Position for colposcopy
19 Antiseptic brand name
21 Nonabsorbable suture material

Sterile Technique

Procedure 25-1: Applying and Removing Sterile Gloves. Apply and remove sterile gloves.

Procedure 25-2: Sterile Package. Open a sterile package. Add a sterile article to a sterile field using a commercially prepared peel-apart package. Practice each of the methods used to transfer articles to a sterile field as shown in Figure 25-4 of your textbook.

Procedure 25-3: Sterile Solution. Pour a sterile solution into a container on a sterile field.

Minor Surgical Procedures

Procedure 25-4: Sterile Dressing. Change a sterile dressing and record the procedure in the chart provided.

Procedure 25-5: Suture and Staple Removal. Practice the procedure for removing sutures and staples, and record the procedure in the chart provided.

Procedure 25-6: Adhesive Skin Closures. Practice the procedure for applying and removing adhesive skin closures, and record the procedure in the chart provided.

Procedure 25-7: Assisting with Minor Office Surgery. Obtain eight index cards. For each of the following minor office surgeries, indicate (on one side of the card) the equipment and supplies required for the side table. On the other side of the card, indicate the equipment and supplies required for the sterile tray setup. Set up a surgical tray for the procedures listed using your index cards. In the chart provided, record the instructions relayed to the patient following the surgery.

a. Suture insertion

b. Sebaceous cyst removal

c. Incision and drainage of a localized infection

d. Mole removal

e. Needle biopsy

f. Ingrown toenail removal

g. Colposcopy

h. Cervical punch biopsy

i. Cervical cryosurgery

Procedure 25-A: Bandage Turns. Practice the following bandage turns:

a. Circular turn

b. Spiral turn

c. Spiral-reverse turn

d. Figure-eight turn

e. Recurrent turn

CHART	
Date	

549

CHART	
Date	

Procedure 25-1: Applying and Removing Sterile Gloves

Name: _____ Date: _____

Evaluated by: _____ Score: _____

Performance Objective

Outcome:	Apply and remove sterile gloves.
Conditions:	Given the appropriate-sized sterile gloves.
	Using a clean flat surface.
Standards:	Time: 5 minutes. Student completed procedure in _____ minutes.
	Accuracy: Satisfactory score on the Performance Evaluation Checklist.

Performance Evaluation Checklist

Trial 1	Trial 2	Point Value	Performance Standards
			Application of gloves:
		●	Removed rings and washed hands with an antimicrobial soap.
		▷	Explained why the hands should be washed.
		●	Selected the appropriate-sized gloves.
		▷	Explained what may occur if the gloves are too small or too large.
		●	Placed the glove package on a clean flat surface.
		●	Opened the sterile glove package without touching the inside of the wrapper.
		●	Picked up the first glove on the inside of the cuff without contaminating.
		▷	Explained why the inside of the cuff can be touched with the bare hand.
		●	Did not touch the outside of the glove with the bare hand.
		●	Stepped back and pulled on glove and allowed the cuff to remain turned back on itself.
		●	Picked up the second glove by slipping sterile gloved fingers under its cuff and grasping the opposite side with the thumb.
		▷	Stated how the previous step prevents contamination.
		●	Pulled the glove on and turned back the cuff.
		●	Turned back the cuff of the first glove without contaminating it.
		●	Adjusted the gloves to a comfortable position.
		●	Inspected the gloves for tears.
		▷	Explained what should be done if a glove is torn.
			Removal of gloves:

551

Trial 1	Trial 2	Point Value	Performance Standards
		●	Grasped the outside of the right glove 1 to 2 inches from the top with the gloved left hand.
		●	Slowly pulled right glove off the hand.
		●	Pulled the right glove free and scrunched it into a ball with the gloved left hand.
		●	Placed index and middle fingers of the right hand on the inside of left glove.
		●	Did not allow the clean hand to touch the outside of the glove.
		●	Pulled the glove off the left hand, enclosing the balled-up right glove.
		●	Discarded both gloves in an appropriate waste container.
		▷	Stated how to discard gloves if they are visibly contaminated with blood.
		●	Sanitized hands.
		✳	Completed the procedure within 5 minutes.
			TOTALS

Evaluation of Student Performance

EVALUATION CRITERIA			COMMENTS
Symbol	**Category**	**Point Value**	
✳	Critical Step	16 points	
●	Essential Step	6 points	
▷	Theory Question	2 points	

Score calculation: 100 points

−   _____ points missed

_____ Score

Satisfactory score: 85 or above

CAAHEP Competencies Achieved

Psychomotor (Skills)

☑ III. 3. Select appropriate barrier/personal protective equipment (PPE) for potentially infectious situations.

ABHES Competencies Achieved

☑ 9. b. Apply principles of aseptic techniques and infection control.
☑ 9. i. Use standard precautions.

EVALUATION OF COMPETENCY

Procedure 25-2: Opening a Sterile Package

Name: _____   Date: _____

Evaluated by: _____   Score: _____

Performance Objective

Outcome:	Open a sterile package.
Conditions:	Given a sterile package.
	Using a clean flat surface.
Standards:	Time: 5 minutes. Student completed procedure in _____ minutes.
	Accuracy: Satisfactory score on the Performance Evaluation Checklist.

Performance Evaluation Checklist

Trial 1	Trial 2	Point Value	Performance Standards
		●	Sanitized hands.
		●	Assembled equipment.
		●	Checked pack to make sure it is not wet, torn, or opened.
		●	Checked the autoclave tape on the pack.
		▷	Stated the purpose of autoclave tape.
		●	Positioned the pack on the table so that the top flap of wrapper will open away from the body.
		●	Removed the fastener on wrapped package and discarded it.
		●	Opened the first flap away from the body.
		●	Opened the left and right flaps without contaminating contents.
		●	Opened the flap closest to the body.
		●	In all cases, touched only the outside of the wrapper.
		●	In all cases, did not reach over the sterile contents of the package.
		▷	Stated why the medical assistant should not reach over the contents of the package.
		●	Adjusted the sterile wrapper by the corners as needed.

		●	Checked the sterilization indicator on the inside of the pack.	
		▷	Stated the reason for checking the sterilization indicator.	
		✱	Completed the procedure within 5 minutes.	
			TOTALS	

Evaluation of Student Performance

EVALUATION CRITERIA			COMMENTS
Symbol	**Category**	**Point Value**	
✱	Critical Step	16 points	
●	Essential Step	6 points	
▷	Theory Question	2 points	

Score calculation: 100 points

− _____ points missed

_____ Score

Satisfactory score: 85 or above

CAAHEP Competencies Achieved

Psychomotor (Skills)

☑ I. 10. Assist physician with patient care.

ABHES Competencies Achieved

☑ 9. n. Assist physician with minor office surgical procedures.

Using Commercially Prepared Sterile Packages

Name: _____   Date: _____

Evaluated by: _____   Score: _____

Performance Objective

Outcome:	Add a sterile article to a sterile field from a peel-apart package by ejecting its contents onto the field.
Conditions:	Given the following: peel-apart package and a sterile field.
Standards:	Time: 3 minutes. Student completed procedure in _____ minutes.
	Accuracy: Satisfactory score on the Performance Evaluation Checklist.

Performance Evaluation Checklist

Trial 1	Trial 2	Point Value	Performance Standards
		●	Sanitized hands.
		●	Grasped the two unsterile flaps of the peel-pack between thumbs.
		●	Pulled the package apart using a rolling-outward motion.
		▷	Stated what parts of the peel-pack must remain sterile.
		●	Stepped back slightly from the sterile field.
		▷	Explained the reason for stepping back.
		●	Gently ejected contents of the peel-pack onto the center of the sterile field.
		✱	Completed the procedure within 3 minutes.
			TOTALS

EVALUATION CRITERIA			COMMENTS
Symbol	**Category**	**Point Value**	
✱	Critical Step	16 points	
●	Essential Step	6 points	
▷	Theory Question	2 points	

Score calculation: 100 points

– _____ points missed

_____ Score

Satisfactory score: 85 or above

CAAHEP Competencies Achieved

Psychomotor (Skills)

☑ I. 10. Assist physician with patient care.

ABHES Competencies Achieved

☑ 9. n. Assist physician with minor office surgical procedures.

Procedure 25-3: Pouring a Sterile Solution

Name: _____   Date: _____

Evaluated by: _____   Score: _____

Performance Objective

Outcome:	Pour a sterile solution.
Conditions:	Given the following: sterile solution, sterile container, and a sterile towel.
Standards:	Time: 5 minutes. Student completed procedure in _____ minutes.
	Accuracy: Satisfactory score on the Performance Evaluation Checklist.

Performance Evaluation Checklist

Trial 1	Trial 2	Point Value	Performance Standards
		●	Checked the label of the solution.
		●	Checked expiration date on the solution.
		▷	Explained why an outdated solution should not be used.
		●	Checked solution label a second time.
		●	Palmed the label of the bottle.
		▷	Explained why the label should be palmed.
		●	Removed cap and placed it on a flat surface with the open end up.
		▷	Stated why cap should be placed with the open end up.
		●	Rinsed the lip of the bottle.
		▷	Explained why the lip of the bottle should be rinsed.
		●	Poured the proper amount of solution into a sterile container at a height of 6 inches.
		●	Did not allow the neck of the bottle to come in contact with container.
		●	Did not allow any of the solution to splash onto the sterile field.
		▷	Explained why the sterile solution should not be allowed to splash onto the sterile field.
		●	Replaced cap on container without contaminating.
		●	Checked the label a third time.
		★	Completed the procedure within 5 minutes.
			TOTALS

Evaluation of Student Performance

EVALUATION CRITERIA			COMMENTS
Symbol	Category	Point Value	
✶	Critical Step	16 points	
●	Essential Step	6 points	
▷	Theory Question	2 points	

Score calculation: 100 points

‒ _____ points missed

_____ Score

Satisfactory score: 85 or above

CAAHEP Competencies Achieved

Psychomotor (Skills)

☑ I. 10. Assist physician with patient care.

ABHES Competencies Achieved

☑ 9. n. Assist physician with minor office surgical procedures.

Procedure 25-4: Changing a Sterile Dressing

Name: _____   Date: _____

Evaluated by: _____   Score: _____

Performance Objective

Outcome:	Change a sterile dressing.
Conditions:	Given the following: Mayo stand, biohazard waste container, clean and disposable gloves, antiseptic swabs, sterile gloves, plastic waste bag, adhesive tape and scissors, sterile dressing, and thumb forceps.
Standards:	Time: 10 minutes. Student completed procedure in _____ minutes.
	Accuracy: Satisfactory score on the Performance Evaluation Checklist.

Performance Evaluation Checklist

Trial 1	Trial 2	Point Value	Performance Standards
		●	Washed hands with an antimicrobial soap.
		●	Assembled equipment.
		●	Set up nonsterile items on a side table or counter.
		●	Positioned the plastic waste bag in a convenient location.
		●	Greeted the patient and introduced yourself.
		●	Identified patient and explained the procedure.
		●	Instructed patient not to move during procedure.
		●	Adjusted the light.
		●	Applied clean gloves.
		●	Loosened the tape and carefully removed soiled dressing by pulling it upward.
		●	Did not touch inside of dressing next to the wound.
		▷	Explained why the inside of the dressing should not be touched.
		▷	Described what should be done if the dressing is stuck to the wound.
		●	Placed soiled dressing in the waste bag without touching outside of bag.
		●	Inspected the wound.
		▷	Stated what type of inspection should be performed.
		●	Opened the antiseptic swabs and placed the pouch in a convenient location or held the pouch in your hand.

		•	Applied the antiseptic to the wound.
		•	Used a new swab for each motion.
		•	Discarded each contaminated swab in the waste bag after use.
		•	Removed gloves and discarded them without contaminating.
		•	Sanitized hands and prepared the sterile field.
		•	Instructed patient not to talk, laugh, sneeze, or cough over the sterile field.
		•	Opened sterile glove package and applied sterile gloves.
		•	Picked up sterile dressing from the tray using sterile gloves or sterile forceps.
		•	Placed sterile dressing over the wound by lightly dropping it in place.
		•	Did not move dressing after dropping it in place.
		▷	Explained why the dressing should be dropped onto the wound and then not moved.
		•	Discarded gloves (and forceps) in the waste bag.
		•	Applied hypoallergenic tape to hold sterile dressing in place.
		•	Provided the patient with written wound care instructions.
		•	Instructed patient in wound care.
		▷	Described the wound care that should be relayed to the patient.
		•	Asked patient to sign instruction sheet.
		•	Witnessed the patient's signature.
		•	Gave a signed copy to the patient.
		•	Filed original in the patient's medical record.
		▷	Stated the purpose of filing original in patient's chart.
		•	Returned equipment.
		•	Disposed of plastic bag in a biohazard waste container.
		•	Sanitized hands.
		•	Charted the procedure correctly.
		★	Completed the procedure within 10 minutes.
			TOTALS

CHART	
Date	

Evaluation of Student Performance

EVALUATION CRITERIA			COMMENTS
Symbol	**Category**	**Point Value**	
✱	Critical Step	16 points	
●	Essential Step	6 points	
▷	Theory Question	2 points	

Score calculation: 100 points

      −   _____ points missed

           ____ Score

Satisfactory score: 85 or above

CAAHEP Competencies Achieved

Psychomotor (Skills)

☑ IV. 5. Instruct patients according to their needs to promote health maintenance and disease prevention.
☑ IV. 6. Prepare a patient for procedures and/or treatments.
☑ IV. 8. Document patient care.
☑ IV. 9. Document patient education.

Affective (Behavior)

☑ III. 2. Explain the rationale for performance of a procedure to the patient.
☑ III. 3. Show awareness of patients' concerns regarding their perceptions related to the procedure being performed.

ABHES Competencies Achieved

☑ 4. a. Document accurately.
☑ 8. cc. Communicate on the recipient's level of comprehension.
☑ 9. l. Prepare patient for examinations and treatments.
☑ 9. r. Teach patients methods of health promotion and disease prevention.

Notes

EVALUATION OF COMPETENCY

Procedure 25-5: Removing Sutures and Staples

Name: _____   Date: _____

Evaluated by: _____   Score: _____

Performance Objective

Outcome:	Remove sutures and staples.
Conditions:	Given the following: Mayo stand, antiseptic swabs, clean and disposable gloves, sterile 4 × 4 gauze, surgical tape, biohazard waste container, suture removal kid, and staple removal kit.
Standards:	Time: 10 minutes. Student completed procedure in _____ minutes.
	Accuracy: Satisfactory score on the Performance Evaluation Checklist.

Performance Evaluation Checklist

Trial 1	Trial 2	Point Value	Performance Standards
		●	Washed hands with an antimicrobial soap.
		●	Assembled equipment.
		●	Greeted the patient and introduced yourself.
		●	Identified patient and explained the procedure.
		●	Positioned the patient as required.
		●	Adjusted the light.
		●	Checked to make sure the sutures (or staples) were intact.
		●	Checked to make sure the incision line was approximated and free from infection.
		▷	Explained what to do if the incision line is not approximated.
		●	Opened the suture or staple removal kit.
		●	Applied clean gloves.
		●	Cleaned the incision line with antiseptic swabs using a new swab for each motion.
		●	Allowed the skin to dry.
		●	Informed the patient that he or she would feel a pulling sensation as each suture (or staple) is removed.
			Removed sutures as follows:
		●	Picked up the knot of suture with thumb forceps.
		●	Placed curved tip of suture scissors under the suture.

563

		●	Cut suture below the knot on the side of suture closest to the skin.	
		●	Gently pulled suture out of the skin, using a smooth, continuous motion.	
		●	Did not allow any portion of suture previously on the outside to be pulled through the tissue lying beneath the incision line.	
		●	Placed the suture on the gauze.	
		●	Repeated above sequence until all sutures were removed.	
			Removed staples as follows:	
		●	Gently placed the jaws of the staple remover under the staple.	
		●	Squeezed the staple handles until they were fully closed.	
		●	Lifted the staple remover upward to remove the staple.	
		●	Placed staple on gauze.	
		●	Continued until all the staples were removed.	
		●	Counted number of sutures or staples and checked number with chart.	
		●	Cleansed the site with an antiseptic swab.	
		●	Applied adhesive skin closures if directed by physician.	
		●	Applied DSD, directed to do so by physician.	
		●	Disposed of sutures or staples and gauze in biohazard waste container.	
		●	Removed gloves and sanitized hands.	
		●	Charted the procedure correctly.	
		✶	Completed the procedure within 10 minutes.	
			TOTALS	

CHART	
Date	

Evaluation of Student Performance

EVALUATION CRITERIA			COMMENTS
Symbol	Category	Point Value	
✱	Critical Step	16 points	
●	Essential Step	6 points	
▷	Theory Question	2 points	

Score calculation: 100 points

−   points missed
_____
___ Score

Satisfactory score: 85 or above

CAAHEP Competencies Achieved

Psychomotor (Skills)

☑ IV. 5. Instruct patients according to their needs to promote health maintenance and disease prevention.
☑ IV. 6. Prepare a patient for procedures and/or treatments.
☑ IV. 8. Document patient care.

Affective (Behavior)

☑ III. 3. Show awareness of patients' concerns regarding their perceptions related to the procedure being performed.
☑ IV. 1. Demonstrate empathy in communicating with patients, family, and staff.

ABHES Competencies Achieved

☑ 4. a. Document accurately.
☑ 8. bb. Are impartial and show empathy when dealing with patients.
☑ 8. cc. Communicate on the recipient's level of comprehension.
☑ 9. l. Prepare patient for examinations and treatments.
☑ 9. r. Teach patients methods of health promotion and disease prevention.

Notes

Procedure 25-6: Applying and Removing Adhesive Skin Closures

Name: _____   Date: _____

Evaluated by: _____   Score: _____

Performance Objective

Outcome:	Apply and remove adhesive skin closures.
Conditions:	Given the following: clean and disposable gloves, sterile gloves, antiseptic solution, surgical scrub brush, antiseptic swabs, tincture of benzoin, sterile cotton-tipped applicator, adhesive skin closure strips, sterile 4 × 4 gauze pads, surgical tape, and a biohazard waste container.
Standards:	Time: 10 minutes. Student completed procedure in _____ minutes.
	Accuracy: Satisfactory score on the Performance Evaluation Checklist.

Performance Evaluation Checklist

Trial 1	Trial 2	Point Value	Performance Standards
			Application of adhesive skin closures:
		●	Washed hands with an antimicrobial soap.
		●	Assembled equipment.
		●	Checked expiration date on the adhesive skin closures.
		●	Greeted patient and introduced yourself.
		●	Identified patient and explained the procedure.
		●	Positioned the patient as required.
		●	Adjusted the light.
		●	Applied clean gloves.
		●	Inspected the wound for redness, swelling, and drainage.
		●	Scrubbed the wound with an antiseptic solution.
		●	Allowed the skin to dry or patted dry with gauze pads.
		●	Applied antiseptic using a new swab for each motion.
		●	Allowed the skin to dry.
		▷	Explained why the skin must be completely dry.
		●	Applied tincture of benzoin without letting it touch the wound.
		▷	Stated the purpose of tincture of benzoin.
		●	Allowed the skin to dry.

		•	Removed gloves and washed hands.	
		•	Opened the package of adhesive strips and laid them on a flat surface.	
		•	Applied sterile gloves and teared tab off card of strips.	
		•	Peeled a strip of tape off the card.	
		•	Checked to make sure the skin surface was dry.	
		•	Positioned the first strip over the center of the wound.	
		•	Secured one end of the strip to the skin by pressing down firmly on the tape.	
		•	Stretched the strip across the incision until the edges of the wound were approximated.	
		•	Secured the strip to the skin on the other side of the wound.	
		•	Applied the second strip on one side of center strip at an 18-inch interval.	
		•	Applied a third strip at a 18-inch interval on the other side of the center strip.	
		•	Continued applying the strips at 18-inch intervals until the edges of the wound were approximated.	
		▷	Explained why the strips should be spaced at 18-inch intervals.	
		•	Applied two closures approximately ½-inch from the ends of the strips.	
		▷	Stated the purpose of applying a strip along each edge.	
		•	Applied a sterile dressing over the strips if indicated by the physician.	
		•	Removed gloves and sanitized hands.	
		•	Provided patient with written wound care instructions.	
		•	Explained the wound care instructions.	
		•	Asked patient to sign instruction sheet and witnessed patient's signature.	
		•	Gave a signed copy to the patient and filed original in the patient's medical record.	
		•	Charted the procedure correctly.	
			Removal of adhesive skin closures:	
		•	Sanitized hands.	
		•	Greeted patient and introduced yourself.	
		•	Identified patient and explained the procedure.	

			●	Positioned the patient as required.
			●	Adjusted the light.
			●	Checked to make sure the incision line was approximated and free from infection.
			●	Positioned a 4 × 4 gauze pad in a convenient location.
			●	Applied clean gloves.
			●	Peeled off each half of the strip from the outside toward the wound margin.
			●	Stabilized the skin with one finger.
			●	Gently lifted the strip up and away from the wound and placed it on the gauze.
			●	Continued until all closures were removed.
			●	Cleansed the site with an antiseptic swab.
			●	Applied a sterile dressing if indicated by the physician.
			●	Disposed of strips and gauze in a biohazard waste container.
			●	Removed gloves and sanitized hands.
			●	Charted the procedure correctly.
			✱	Completed the procedure within 10 minutes.
				TOTALS

CHART	
Date	

EVALUATION CRITERIA			COMMENTS
Symbol	**Category**	**Point Value**	
✳	Critical Step	16 points	
●	Essential Step	6 points	
▷	Theory Question	2 points	

Score calculation: 100 points

−   points missed

_____

          Score

Satisfactory score: 85 or above

CAAHEP Competencies Achieved

Psychomotor (Skills)

☑ IV. 5. Instruct patients according to their needs to promote health maintenance and disease prevention.
☑ IV. 6. Prepare a patient for procedures and/or treatments.
☑ IV. 8. Document patient care

Affective (Behavior)

☑ III. 2. Explain the rationale for performance of a procedure to the patient.
☑ III. 3. Show awareness of patients' concerns regarding their perceptions about the procedure being performed.

ABHES Competencies Achieved

☑ 4. a. Document accurately.
☑ 8. bb. Are impartial and show empathy when dealing with patients.
☑ 8. cc. Communicate on the recipient's level of comprehension.
☑ 9. l. Prepare patient for examinations and treatments.
☑ 9. r. Teach patients methods of health promotion and disease prevention.

Procedure 25-7: Assisting with Minor Office Surgery

Name: _____ Date: _____

Evaluated by: _____ Score: _____

Performance Objective

Outcome:	Set up the surgical tray and assist with minor office surgery.
Conditions:	Given a Mayo stand, biohazard waste container, and the instruments and supplies required for a specific minor office surgery as designed by the instructor.
Standards:	Time: 15 minutes. Student completed procedure in _____ minutes.
	Accuracy: Satisfactory score on the Performance Evaluation Checklist.

Performance Evaluation Checklist

Trial 1	Trial 2	Point Value	Performance Standards
		●	Determined the type of minor office surgery to be performed.
		●	Prepared examining room.
		●	Sanitized hands.
		●	Set up articles required that are not sterile on a side table or counter.
		●	Labeled the specimen container (if included in the setup).
		●	Washed hands with an antimicrobial soap.
		●	Set up the minor office surgery tray on a clean, dry, flat surface, using the principles of surgical asepsis.
		Prepackaged sterile setup	
		●	Selected the appropriate package from supply shelf and placed it on a flat surface.
		●	Opened the setup using the inside of wrapper as the sterile field.
		●	Checked the sterilization indicator on inside of pack.
		●	Added any additional articles required for the surgery and covered tray setup with a sterile towel.
		Transferring articles to a sterile field:	
		●	Placed sterile towel on a flat surface by two corner ends, making sure not to contaminate it.
		●	Transferred sterile articles to the field, using peel-apart packages.
		●	Applied sterile glove.
		●	Arranged articles neatly on the sterile field with sterile glove.

			•	Checked to make sure all articles were available on the sterile field.
			•	Covered the tray setup with a sterile towel without allowing arms to pass over the sterile field.
				Prepared the patient:
			•	Greeted the patient and introduced yourself.
			•	Identified patient, explained the procedure, and reassured the patient.
			•	Asked patient if he or she needs to void before the surgery.
			•	Instructed patient on clothing removal.
			•	Instructed patient not to move during procedure or to talk, laugh, sneeze, or cough over the sterile field.
			•	Positioned patient as required for the type of surgery to be performed.
			•	Adjusted the light so that it was focused on the operative site.
				Prepared the patient's skin:
			•	Applied clean disposable gloves.
			•	Shaved skin (if required).
			•	Cleansed skin with an antiseptic solution.
			•	Rinsed and dried the area.
			•	Applied antiseptic using antiseptic swabs.
			•	Allowed the skin to dry.
			•	Removed gloves and sanitized hands.
			•	Checked to make sure that everything was ready and informed physician.
				Assisted the physician:
			•	Uncovered the tray setup.
			•	Opened the outer glove wrapper for physician.
			•	Held the vial while physician withdrew the local anesthetic.
			•	Adjusted the light as required.
			•	Restrained patient (e.g., child).
			•	Relaxed and reassured patient.
			•	Handed instruments and supplies to physician. Sterile gloves required.

			●	Kept the sterile field neat and orderly. Sterile gloves required.
			●	Held basin for physician to deposit soiled instruments and supplies. Clean gloves required.
			●	Retracted tissue. Sterile gloves required.
			●	Sponged blood from operative site. Sterile gloves required.
			●	Added instruments and supplies as necessary to the sterile field.
			●	Held specimen container to accept specimen. Clean gloves required.
			●	Cut ends of suture material after insertion by physician. Sterile gloves required.
				After surgery:
			●	Applied sterile dressing to the surgical wound if ordered by physician.
			●	Stayed with patient as a safety precaution.
			●	Assisted and instructed patient as required.
			●	Verified that patient understood postoperative instructions.
			●	Provided patient with verbal and written wound care instructions.
			▷	Stated the patient instructions that should be relayed for wound and suture care.
			●	Asked patient to sign instruction sheet and witnessed the patient's signature.
			●	Gave a signed copy to the patient and filed original in patient's medical record.
			●	Relayed information regarding the return visit
			●	Assisted patient off table.
			●	Instructed patient to get dressed.
			●	Prepared any specimens collected for transfer to the laboratory with a completed biopsy request.
			●	Charted correctly.
			●	Cleaned examining room.
			●	Discarded disposable contaminated articles in a biohazard waste container.
			●	Sanitized and sterilized instruments.
			★	Completed the procedure within 15 minutes.
				TOTALS

CHART

CHART	
Date	

Evaluation of Student Performance

EVALUATION CRITERIA			COMMENTS
Symbol	**Category**	**Point Value**	
✱	Critical Step	16 points	
●	Essential Step	6 points	
▷	Theory Question	2 points	

Score calculation: 100 points

− _____ points missed

_____ Score

Satisfactory score: 85 or above

CAAHEP Competencies Achieved

Psychomotor (Skills)

☑ I. 10. Assist physician with patient care.
☑ IV. 5. Instruct patients according to their needs to promote health maintenance and disease prevention.
☑ IV. 6. Prepare a patient for procedures and/or treatments.
☑ IV. 8. Document patient care.
☑ IX. 1. Respond to issues of confidentiality.

Affective (Behavior)

☑ III. 2. Explain the rationale for performance of a procedure to the patient.
☑ III. 3. Show awareness of patients' concerns regarding their perceptions related to the procedure being performed.
☑ IV. 6. Demonstrate awareness of how an individual's personal appearance affects anticipated responses.
☑ IX. 3. Recognize the importance of local, state, and federal legislation and regulations in the practice setting.

ABHES Competencies Achieved

☑ 4. a. Document accurately.
☑ 4. f. Comply with federal, state, and local health laws and regulations.
☑ 8. bb. Are impartial and show empathy when dealing with patients.
☑ 8. cc. Communicate on the recipient's level of comprehension.
☑ 9. e. Recognize emergencies and treatments and minor office surgical procedures.
☑ l. Prepare patient for examinations and treatments.
☑ 9. n. Assist physician with minor office surgical procedures.
☑ 9. r. Teach patients methods of health promotion and disease prevention.

Procedure 25-A: Bandage Turns

Name: _____   Date: _____

Evaluated by: _____   Score: _____

Performance Objective

Outcome:	Apply the following bandage turns: circular, spiral, spiral-reverse, figure-eight, and recurrent.
Conditions:	Given the following: a roller bandage and an elastic bandage.
Standards:	Time: 15 minutes. Student completed procedure in _____ minutes.
	Accuracy: Satisfactory score on the Performance Evaluation Checklist.

Performance Evaluation Checklist

Trial 1	Trial 2	Point Value	Performance Standards
			Circular turn:
		●	Placed the end of a bandage on a slant.
		●	Encircled the body part while allowing the corner of the bandage to extend.
		●	Turned down corner of bandage.
		●	Made another circular turn around the body part.
		▷	Stated a use of the circular turn.
			Spiral turn:
		●	Anchored bandage using a circular turn.
		●	Encircled the body part while keeping bandage at a slant.
		●	Carried each spiral turn upward at a slight angle.
		●	Overlapped each previous turn by one half to two thirds of the width of the bandage.
		▷	Stated a use of the spiral turn.
			Spiral-reverse turn:
		●	Anchored bandage using a circular turn.
		●	Encircled the body part while keeping bandage at a slant.
		●	Reversed the spiral turn using the thumb or index finger.
		●	Directed bandage downward and folded it on itself.
		●	Kept bandage parallel to the lower edge of the previous turn.

		●	Overlapped each previous turn by two thirds the width of the bandage.	
		▷	Stated a use of the spiral-reverse turn.	
			Figure-eight turn:	
		●	Anchored bandage using a circular turn.	
		●	Slanted bandage turns to alternately ascend and descend around the body part.	
		●	Crossed the turns over one another in the middle to resemble a figure eight	
		●	Overlapped each previous turn by two thirds of the width of the bandage.	
		▷	Stated a use of the figure-eight turn.	
			Recurrent turn:	
		●	Anchored bandage using two circular turns.	
		●	Passed bandage back and forth over the tip of the body part being bandaged.	
		●	Overlapped each previous turn by two thirds of the width of the bandage.	
		▷	Stated a use of the recurrent turn.	
		✱	Completed the procedure within 15 minutes.	
			TOTALS	

CHART	
Date	

Evaluation of Student Performance

EVALUATION CRITERIA			COMMENTS
Symbol	**Category**	**Point Value**	
✱	Critical Step	16 points	
●	Essential Step	6 points	
▷	Theory Question	2 points	

Score calculation: 100 points

−   _____ points missed

_____ Score

Satisfactory score: 85 or above

CAAHEP Competencies Achieved

Psychomotor (Skills)

☑ IV. 5. Instruct patients according to their needs to promote health maintenance and disease prevention.
☑ IV. 6. Prepare a patient for procedures and/or treatments.

Affective (Behavior)

☑ I. 1. Apply critical thinking skills in performing patient assessment and care.

ABHES Competencies Achieved

☑ 9. l. Prepare patient for examinations and treatments.
☑ 9. r. Teach patients methods of health promotion and disease prevention.

Notes

26 Administration of Medication and Intravenous Therapy

CHAPTER ASSIGNMENTS

√ After Completing	Date Due	Textbook Pages	TEXTBOOK ASSIGNMENTS	Possible Points	Points You Earned
		549-618	Read Chapter 26: Administration of Medication and Intravenous Therapy		
		555 616	🖼 Read Case Study 1 Case Study 1 questions	5	
		577 616	🖼 Read Case Study 2 Case Study 2 questions	5	
		590 617	🖼 Read Case Study 3 Case Study 3 questions	5	
			TOTAL POINTS		

√ After Completing	Date Due	Study Guide Pages	STUDY GUIDE ASSIGNMENTS (CTA = Critical Thinking Activity)	Possible Points	Points You Earned
		585	📰 Pretest	10	
		586 587	🔑 Term Key Term Assessment A. Definitions B. Word Parts 　(Add 1 point for each medical term)	30 18	
		587-593	📋 Evaluation of Learning questions	65	
		593-596	CTA A: Using the PDR	34	
		597-598	CTA B: Locating Information in a Drug Insert	12	
		598	CTA C: Drug Classifications (3 points each)	30	
			𝑒 Evolve Site: Road to Recovery: Drug Categories		
		598	CTA D: Medication Record	20	
		599	CTA E: Seven Rights of Medication Administration	35	
			𝑒 Evolve Site: Script It! (Record points earned)		
		600	CTA F: Liquid Measurement	11	

√ After Completing	Date Due	Study Guide Pages	STUDY GUIDE ASSIGNMENTS (CTA = Critical Thinking Activity)	Possible Points	Points You Earned
		600	CTA G: Parts of a Needle and Syringe	11	
			e Evolve Site: Take the Plunge (Record points earned)		
		600-601	CTA H: Hypodermic Syringe Calibrations	10	
			e Evolve Site: Which Needle? (Record points earned)		
		601	CTA I: Insulin Syringe Calibrations	20	
		601-602	CTA J: Tuberculin Syringe Calibrations	30	
			e Evolve Site: Draw It Up! (Record points earned)		
		602	CTA K: Syringe and Needle Labels (3 points each)	12	
		602	CTA L: Angle of Insertion for Injections	3	
		602-603	CTA M: Preparing and Administering Parenteral Medication	18	
		603-604	CTA N: Measuring Mantoux Test Reactions	5	
		605	CTA O: Interpreting Mantoux Test Reactions	11	
		605	CTA P: Anaphylactic Reaction	20	
		606-621	CTA Q: Researching Drugs (5 points per drug researched)	200	
		622	CTA R: Crossword Puzzle	34	
			e Evolve Site: Animations	20	
			e Evolve Site: Apply Your Knowledge questions	10	
			e Evolve Site: Video Evaluation	60	
		585	Posttest	10	
			ADDITIONAL ASSIGNMENTS		
			TOTAL POINTS		

580

√ After Completing	Date Due	Study Guide Pages	**STUDY GUIDE ASSIGNMENTS** **Drug Dose Calculation:** **Supplemental Education for** **Chapter 26**	Possible Points	Points You Earned
		653	Unit 1: The Metric System A. Units of Measurement	10	
		654	Unit 1: The Metric System B. Metric Abbreviations	10	
		654	Unit 1: The Metric System C. Metric Notation	20	
		655	Unit 2: The Apothecary System A. Units of Measurement	14	
		655	Unit 2: The Apothecary System B. Apothecary Abbreviations	10	
		656	Unit 2: The Apothecary System C. Apothecary Notation	20	
		656	Unit 3: The Household System A. Units of Measurements	4	
		657	Unit 4: Medication Orders A. Medical Abbreviations	30	
		658-659	Unit 4: Medication Orders B. Interpreting Medication Orders (3 points each)	30	
		659-660	Unit 5: Converting Units of Measurement A. Using Conversion Tables (2 points each)	50	
		660-662	Unit 5: Converting Units of Measurement B. Converting Units within the Metric System (2 points each)	40	
		662-664	Unit 5: Converting Units of Measurement C. Converting Units Within the Apothecary System (2 points each)	50	
		664-666	Unit 5: Converting Units of Measurement D. Converting Units Within the Household System (2 points each)	20	
		666-668	Unit 6: Ratio and Proportion A. Ratio and Proportion Guidelines (6 points each)	48	

Chapter **26** **Administration of Medication and Intravenous Therapy**

√ After Completing	Date Due	Study Guide Pages	STUDY GUIDE ASSIGNMENTS Drug Dose Calculation: Supplemental Education for Chapter 26	Possible Points	Points You Earned
		669-670	Unit 6: Ratio and Proportion B. Converting Units Using Ratio and Proportion (2 points each)	40	
		670-676	Unit 7: Determining Drug Dose A. Oral Administration (2 points each)	30	
		676-679	Unit 7: Determining Drug Dose B. Parenteral Administration (2 points each)	20	
			ADDITIONAL ASSIGNMENTS		
			TOTAL POINTS		

√ When Assigned By Your Instructor	Study Guide Pages	Practices Required	LABORATORY ASSIGNMENTS (Procedure Number and Name)	Score*
	623-626	5	**Practice for Competency** 26-1: Administering Oral Medication Textbook reference: pp. 581-582	
	627-629		**Evaluation of Competency** 26-1: Administering Oral Medication	*
	623-626	Vial: 5 Ampule: 5	**Practice for Competency** 26-2: Preparing an Injection Textbook reference: pp. 591-594	
	631-633		**Evaluation of Competency** 26-2: Preparing an Injection	*
	623-626	3	**Practice for Competency** 26-3: Reconstituting Powdered Drugs Textbook reference: p. 595	
	635-636		**Evaluation of Competency** 26-3: Reconstituting Powdered Drugs	*
	623-626	5	**Practice for Competency** 26-4: Administering a Subcutaneous Injection Textbook reference: pp. 596-597	
	637-639		**Evaluation of Competency** 26-4: Administering a Subcutaneous Injection	*
	623-626	5	**Practice for Competency** 26-5: Administering an Intramuscular Injection Textbook reference: pp. 598-599	
	641-643		**Evaluation of Competency** 26-5: Administering an Intramuscular Injection	*
	623-626	5	**Practice for Competency** 26-6: Z-Tract Intramuscular Injection Technique Textbook reference: p. 600	
	645-647		**Evaluation of Competency** 26-6: Z-Tract Intramuscular Injection Technique	*
	623-626	5	**Practice for Competency** 26-7: Administering an Intradermal Injection Textbook reference: pp. 611-614	

Chapter **26** **Administration of Medication and Intravenous Therapy**

√ When Assigned By Your Instructor	Study Guide Pages	Practices Required	LABORATORY ASSIGNMENTS (Procedure Number and Name)	Score*
	649-652		Evaluation of Competency 26-7: Administering an Intradermal Injection	*
			ADDITIONAL ASSIGNMENTS	

Procedure 26-1: Administering Oral Medication

Name: _____   Date: _____

Evaluated By: _____   Score: _____

Performance Objective

Outcome:	Administer oral solid and liquid medication.
Conditions:	Given the following: appropriate medication, medicine cup, and a medication tray.
Standards:	Time: 5 minutes. Student completed procedure in _____ minutes.
	Accuracy: Satisfactory score on the Performance Evaluation Checklist.

Performance Evaluation Checklist

Trial 1	Trial 2	Point Value	Performance Standards
		●	Sanitized hands.
		●	Assembled equipment.
		●	Worked in a quiet, well-lit atmosphere.
		●	Selected the correct medication from the shelf.
		●	Compared the medication with the physician's instructions.
		●	Checked the drug label.
		●	Checked the expiration date.
		●	Calculated the correct dose to be given, if needed.
		●	Removed the bottle cap.
		●	Checked the drug label and poured the medication.
			Solid medication
		✳	Poured the correct number of capsules or tablets into the bottle cap.
		▷	Explained why the medication is poured into the bottle cap.
		●	Transferred the medication to a medicine cup.
			Liquid medication
		●	Placed lid of bottle on a flat surface with the open end facing up.
		●	Palmed the surface of the drug label.
		▷	Explained why the surface of the drug label should be palmed.
		●	Placed thumbnail at the proper calibration on medicine cup.

Trial 1	Trial 2	Point Value	Performance Standards
		●	Held medicine cup at eye level.
		✱	Poured the correct amount of medication and read the dose at the lowest level of the meniscus.
		●	Replaced the bottle cap.
		●	Checked the drug label and returned the medication to its storage location.
		●	Greeted the patient and introduced yourself.
		●	Identified the patient and explained the procedure.
		●	Handed the medicine cup to the patient.
		●	Offered water to patient.
		▷	Stated one instance when water should not be offered.
		●	Remained with patient until the medication was swallowed.
		●	Sanitized hands.
		●	Charted the procedure correctly.
		✱	Completed the procedure within 10 minutes.
			TOTALS

CHART

Date	

Evaluation of Student Performance

EVALUATION CRITERIA			COMMENTS
Symbol	**Category**	**Point Value**	
✱	Critical Step	16 points	
●	Essential Step	6 points	
▷	Theory Question	2 points	

Score calculation: 100 points

−   points missed
_____
___Score

Satisfactory score: 85 or above

CAAHEP Competencies Achieved

Psychomotor (Skills)
☑ I. 8. Administer oral medications.
☑ II. 1. Prepare proper dosages of medication for administration.
☑ IX. 7. Document accurately in the patient record.

Affective (Behavior)
☑ II. 1. Verify ordered doses or dosages before administration.
☑ IX. 2. Demonstrate awareness of the consequences of not working within the legal scope of practice.

ABHES Competencies Achieved

☑ 4. a. Document accurately.
☑ 9. j. Prepare and administer oral and parenteral medications as directed by physician.

Notes

Procedure 26-2: Preparing an Injection

Name: _____   Date: _____

Evaluated By: _____   Score: _____

Performance Objective

Outcome:	Prepare an injection from an ampule and a vial.
Conditions:	Given the following: medication ordered by the physician, needle and syringe, antiseptic wipe, and medication tray.
Standards:	Time: 10 minutes. Student completed procedure in _____ minutes.
	Accuracy: Satisfactory score on the Performance Evaluation Checklist.

Performance Evaluation Checklist

Trial 1	Trial 2	Point Value	Performance Standards
		●	Sanitized hands.
		●	Assembled equipment.
		●	Worked in a quiet, well-lit atmosphere.
		★	Selected the proper medication from its storage location.
		●	Checked the drug label.
		●	Compared the medication with the physician's instructions.
		●	Checked the expiration date.
		★	Calculated the correct dose to be given, if needed.
		●	Opened syringe and needle packages.
		●	Assembled needle and syringe if necessary.
		●	Made sure that needle is attached firmly to syringe and moved the plunger back and forth.
		●	Checked the drug label a second time.
		●	If required, mixed the medication.
			Withdrew medication from a vial
		●	Removed metal or plastic cap if vial is new.
		●	Cleansed the rubber stopper of the vial with an antiseptic wipe and allowed it to dry.
		●	Placed vial in an upright position on a flat surface.

Trial 1	Trial 2	Point Value	Performance Standards
		●	Removed the needle guard.
		●	Drew air into syringe equal to the amount of medication to be withdrawn.
		●	Inserted needle through rubber stopper until it reached the empty space between stopper and the fluid level.
		●	Pushed down on plunger to inject air into the vial.
		●	Kept needle above the fluid level.
		▷	Explained why air must be injected into the vial.
		●	Inverted the vial while holding onto syringe and plunger.
		✶	Held syringe at eye level and withdrew the proper amount of medication.
		●	Kept the needle opening below the fluid level.
		▷	Explained why the needle opening must be kept below the fluid level.
		●	Removed any air bubbles in syringe by tapping barrel with the fingertips.
		▷	Explained why air bubbles should be removed from the syringe.
		●	Removed any air remaining at the top of syringe by pushing the plunger forward.
		●	Removed the needle from rubber stopper and replaced the needle guard.
		●	If required, removed the needle and replaced it with a new needle.
		●	Checked the drug label for a third time and returned the medication to its storage location.
			Withdrew medication from an ampule
		●	Removed regular needle from syringe and attached a filter needle.
		▷	Stated the purpose of a filter needle.
		●	Cleansed the neck of the vial with an antiseptic wipe.
		●	Tapped the stem of the ampule lightly to remove any medication in the neck of ampule.
		●	Checked the medication label a second time.
		●	Placed piece of gauze around the neck of ampule.
		●	Broke off the stem by snapping it quickly and firmly away from the body.
		●	Discarded the stem and gauze in a biohazard sharps container.
		●	Placed the ampule on a flat surface.
		●	Removed the needle guard.
		●	Inserted needle opening below the fluid level.
		✶	Withdrew the proper amount of medication.
		●	Kept needle opening below the fluid level.

Trial 1	Trial 2	Point Value	Performance Standards
		▷	Explained why needle opening must be kept below the fluid level.
		●	Removed needle from ampule and replaced needle guard.
		●	Checked drug label for a third time.
		●	Discarded the ampule in a biohazard sharps container.
		●	Removed the filter needle and reapplied the regular needle (and guard) to the syringe.
		●	Tapped the syringe to remove air bubbles.
		●	Removed needle guard and expelled air remaining at the top of syringe.
		●	Replaced the needle guard.
		✴	Completed the procedure within 10 minutes.
			TOTALS

Evaluation of Student Performance

EVALUATION CRITERIA			COMMENTS
Symbol	**Category**	**Point Value**	
✴	Critical Step	16 points	
●	Essential Step	6 points	
▷	Theory Question	2 points	

Score calculation: 100 points

— _____ points missed

_____ Score

Satisfactory score: 85 or above

CAAHEP Competencies Achieved

Psychomotor (Skills)
☑ II. 1. Prepare proper dosages of medication for administration.

Affective (Behavior)
☑ II. 1. Verify ordered doses or dosages before administration.

ABHES Competencies Achieved

☑ 9. j. Prepare and administer oral and parenteral medications as directed by physician.

Chapter **26** **Administration of Medication and Intravenous Therapy**

Notes

Procedure 26-3: Reconstituting Powdered Drugs

Name: _____   Date: _____

Evaluated By: _____   Score: _____

Performance Objective

Outcome:	Reconstitute a powdered drug for parenteral administration.
Conditions:	Given the following: vial containing the powdered drug, reconstituting liquid, and a needle and syringe.
Standards:	Time: 5 minutes. Student completed procedure in _____ minutes.
	Accuracy: Satisfactory score on the Performance Evaluation Checklist.

Performance Evaluation Checklist

Trial 1	Trial 2	Point Value	Performance Standards
		●	Sanitized hands.
		●	Assembled equipment.
		✳	Selected the proper medication from its storage location.
		●	Checked the drug label.
		●	Compared the medication with the physician's instructions.
		●	Checked the expiration date.
		✳	Calculated the correct dose to be given, if needed.
		●	Opened syringe and needle packages.
		●	Assembled needle and syringe, if necessary.
		●	Made sure that the needle is attached firmly to syringe and moved the plunger back and forth.
		●	Checked the drug label a second time.
		●	Withdrew an amount of air equal to the amount of liquid to be injected into the vial from the vial containing the powdered drug.
		●	Injected the air into the vial of diluent.
		✳	Inverted the diluent vial and withdrew the proper amount of liquid into the syringe.
		●	Removed air bubbles from the syringe and removed the needle from the vial.
		●	Inserted the needle into the powdered drug vial.
		●	Injected the diluent into the vial.
		●	Removed the needle from the vial and discarded the syringe and needle in a biohazard sharps container.

635

Trial 1	Trial 2	Point Value	Performance Standards
		●	Rolled the vial between hands to mix it.
		●	Labeled multiple-dose vials with the date of preparation and your initials.
		●	Administered the medication.
		●	Stored multiple-dose vials as indicated in the manufacturer's instructions.
		▷	Explained the importance of checking the date of preparation of a reconstituted multiple-dose vial before administering it.
		✹	Completed the procedure within 5 minutes.
			TOTALS

Evaluation of Student Performance

EVALUATION CRITERIA			COMMENTS
Symbol	**Category**	**Point Value**	
✹	Critical Step	16 points	
●	Essential Step	6 points	
▷	Theory Question	2 points	

Score calculation: 100 points

−   _____ points missed

___ Score

Satisfactory score: 85 or above

CAAHEP Competencies Achieved

Psychomotor (Skills)
☑ II. 1. Prepare proper dosages of medication for administration.

Affective (Behavior)
☑ II. 1. Verify ordered doses/dosages prior to administration.

ABHES Competencies Achieved

☑ 9. j. Prepare and administer oral and parenteral medications as directed by physician.

Procedure 26-4: Administering a Subcutaneous Injection

Name: _____   Date: _____

Evaluated By: _____   Score: _____

Performance Objective

Outcome:	Administer a subcutaneous injection.
Conditions:	Given the following: appropriate medication, appropriate needle and syringe, antiseptic wipe, 2 × 2 gauze pad, disposable gloves, and a biohazard sharps container.
Standards:	Time: 5 minutes. Student completed procedure in _____ minutes.
	Accuracy: Satisfactory score on the Performance Evaluation Checklist.

Performance Evaluation Checklist

Trial 1	Trial 2	Point Value	Performance Standards
		●	Sanitized hands.
		●	Prepared the injection.
		●	Greeted the patient and introduced yourself.
		●	Identified the patient and explained the procedure and purpose of the injection.
		●	Selected an appropriate subcutaneous injection site.
		▷	Stated the sites that can be used to administer a subcutaneous injection.
		●	Cleansed area with an antiseptic wipe and allowed it to dry completely.
		▷	Explained why the site should be allowed to dry.
		●	Applied gloves.
		●	Removed needle guard.
		●	Properly positioned the hand on area surrounding the injection site.
		▷	Explained when the area should be grasped and when it should be held taut.
		●	Inserted needle to the hub at a 45-degree or 90-degree angle (depending on the length of the needle) with a quick, smooth motion.
		▷	Explained how needle length determines the angle of insertion for a subcutaneous injection.
		●	Removed the hand from the skin.
		▷	Explained why the hand should be removed from the skin.
		✱	Aspirated to make sure that the needle was not in a blood vessel.

637

Trial 1	Trial 2	Point Value	Performance Standards
		▷	Explained what should be done if needle is in a blood vessel.
		●	Injected the medication slowly and steadily.
		▷	Described what would happen if the medication were injected rapidly.
		●	Placed an antiseptic wipe or gauze pad gently over the injection site and removed needle quickly at the same angle as insertion.
		▷	Explained why the needle should be removed at the angle of insertion.
		●	Applied gentle pressure to the injection site.
		▷	Stated why the site should not be vigorously massaged.
		●	Activated the safety shield on the needle.
		●	Properly disposed of needle and syringe.
		●	Removed gloves and sanitized hands.
		●	Charted the procedure correctly.
		●	Remained with patient to make sure there were no unusual reactions.
		▷	Stated the steps to follow if the patient has been given an allergy injection.
		✶	Completed the procedure within 5 minutes.
			TOTALS

	CHART
Date	

Evaluation of Student Performance

EVALUATION CRITERIA			COMMENTS
Symbol	Category	Point Value	
✶	Critical Step	16 points	
●	Essential Step	6 points	
▷	Theory Question	2 points	

Score calculation: 100 points

− _____ points missed

_____ Score

Satisfactory score: 85 or above

Chapter **26** **Administration of Medication and Intravenous Therapy**

CAAHEP Competencies Achieved

Psychomotor (Skills)

☑ I. 7. Select proper sites for administering parenteral medication.
☑ I. 9. Administer parenteral (excluding IV) medications.
☑ IX. 7. Document accurately in the patient record.
☑ XI. 5. Demonstrate proper use of the following equipment: c. Sharps disposal containers.

Affective (Behavior)

☑ III. 3. Show awareness of patients' concerns regarding their perceptions related to the procedure being performed.

ABHES Competencies Achieved

☑ 4. a. Document accurately.
☑ 9. j. Prepare and administer oral and parenteral medications as directed by physician.

Notes

Procedure 26-5: Administering an Intramuscular Injection

Name: _____   Date: _____

Evaluated By: _____   Score: _____

Performance Objective

Outcome:	Administer an intramuscular injection.
Conditions:	Given the following: appropriate medication, appropriate needle and syringe, antiseptic wipe, 2 × 2 gauze pad, disposable gloves, and a biohazard sharps container.
Standards:	Time: 5 minutes. Student completed procedure in _____ minutes.
	Accuracy: Satisfactory score on the Performance Evaluation Checklist.

Performance Evaluation Checklist

Trial 1	Trial 2	Point Value	Performance Standards
		●	Sanitized hands.
		●	Prepared the injection.
		●	Greeted the patient and introduced yourself.
		●	Identified the patient and explained the procedure and purpose of the injection.
			Located the intramuscular injection sites
		✶	Dorsogluteal
		✶	Deltoid
		✶	Vastus lateralis
		✶	Ventrogluteal
		▷	Stated what tissue layer of the body the medication will be injected into.
		●	Cleansed area with an antiseptic wipe and allowed it to dry completely.
		●	Applied gloves.
		●	Removed needle guard.
		●	Stretched the skin taut over the injection site.
		▷	Explained why the skin should be stretched taut.
		●	Held the barrel of syringe like a dart and inserted needle quickly at a 90-degree angle to the patient's skin with a firm motion.
		●	Inserted the needle to the hub.
		▷	Explained why the needle should be inserted at a 90-degree angle and to the hub.
		✶	Aspirated to make sure that the needle was not in a blood vessel.

641

Trial 1	Trial 2	Point Value	Performance Standards
		▷	Described what would happen if the medication was injected into a blood vessel.
		●	Injected the medication slowly and steadily.
		●	Placed an antiseptic wipe or gauze pad gently over the injection site and removed needle quickly at the same angle as insertion.
		●	Applied gentle pressure to the injection site.
		▷	Stated the reason for applying pressure to the injection site.
		●	Activated the safety shield on the needle.
		●	Properly disposed of needle and syringe.
		●	Removed gloves and sanitized hands.
		●	Charted the procedure correctly.
		▷	Stated the purpose of the lot number on the medication vial.
		●	Remained with patient to make sure there were no unusual reactions.
		✱	Completed the procedure within 5 minutes.
			TOTALS

CHART

Date	

Evaluation of Student Performance

EVALUATION CRITERIA			COMMENTS
Symbol	Category	Point Value	
✱	Critical Step	16 points	
●	Essential Step	6 points	
▷	Theory Question	2 points	

Score calculation: 100 points

− _____ points missed

_____ Score

Satisfactory score: 85 or above

Chapter **26** **Administration of Medication and Intravenous Therapy**

Notes

Procedure 26-6: Z-Track Intramuscular Injection Technique

Name: _____   Date: _____

Evaluated By: _____   Score: _____

Performance Objective

Outcome:	Administer an intramuscular injection using the Z-track method.
Conditions:	Given the following: appropriate medication, appropriate needle and syringe, antiseptic wipe, disposable gloves, and a biohazard sharps container.
Standards:	Time: 5 minutes. Student completed procedure in _____ minutes.
	Accuracy: Satisfactory score on the Performance Evaluation Checklist.

Performance Evaluation Checklist

Trial 1	Trial 2	Point Value	Performance Standards
		●	Sanitized hands.
		●	Prepared the injection.
		●	Greeted the patient and introduced yourself.
		●	Identified the patient and explained the procedure and purpose of the injection.
		●	Selected and properly located the intramuscular injection site.
		●	Cleansed area with an antiseptic wipe and allowed it to dry completely.
		●	Applied gloves.
		●	Removed needle guard.
		●	Pulled the skin away laterally from the injection site with the nondominant hand approximately 1 to 1½ inches.
		●	Inserted needle quickly and smoothly at a 90-degree angle.
		★	Aspirated to make sure that the needle was not in a blood vessel.
		●	Injected the medication slowly and steadily.
		●	Waited 10 seconds before withdrawing the needle.
		▷	Explained why there should be a 10-second waiting period.
		●	Withdrew needle quickly at the same angle as that of insertion.
		●	Released the traction on the skin.
		▷	Described what occurs when the skin traction is released.
		●	Did not apply pressure to the injection site.

Trial 1	Trial 2	Point Value	Performance Standards
		▷	Stated why pressure should not be applied to the injection site.
		●	Activated the safety shield on the needle.
		●	Properly disposed of needle and syringe.
		●	Removed gloves and sanitized hands.
		●	Charted the procedure correctly.
		●	Remained with patient to make sure there were no unusual reactions.
		★	Completed the procedure within 5 minutes.
			TOTALS

CHART	
Date	

Evaluation of Student Performance

EVALUATION CRITERIA			COMMENTS
Symbol	**Category**	**Point Value**	
★	Critical Step	16 points	
●	Essential Step	6 points	
▷	Theory Question	2 points	

Score calculation: 100 points

− _____ points missed

_____ Score

Satisfactory score: 85 or above

CAAHEP Competencies Achieved

Psychomotor (Skills)
- ☑ I. 7. Select proper sites for administering parenteral medication.
- ☑ I. 9. Administer parenteral (excluding IV) medications.
- ☑ IX. 7. Document accurately in the patient record.
- ☑ XI. 5. Demonstrate proper use of the following equipment: c. Sharps disposal containers.

Affective (Behavior)
- ☑ III. 3. Show awareness of patients' concerns regarding their perceptions related to the procedure being performed.

ABHES Competencies Achieved

- ☑ 4. a. Document accurately.
- ☑ 9. j. Prepare and administer oral and parenteral medications as directed by physician.

Notes

Procedure 26-7: Administering an Intradermal Injection

Name: _____   Date: _____

Evaluated By: _____   Score: _____

Performance Objective

Outcome:	Administer an intradermal injection and read the test results.
Conditions:	Given the following: skin testing solution, appropriate needle and syringe, antiseptic wipe, 2 × 2 gauze pad, disposable gloves, millimeter ruler, TB skin test record card, and a biohazard sharps container.
Standards:	Time: 5 minutes. Student completed procedure in _____ minutes.
	Accuracy: Satisfactory score on the Performance Evaluation Checklist.

Performance Evaluation Checklist

Trial 1	Trial 2	Point Value	Performance Standards
		●	Sanitized hands.
		●	Prepared the injection.
		●	Greeted the patient and introduced yourself.
		●	Identified the patient and explained the procedure and purpose of the injection.
		●	Selected an appropriate intradermal injection site.
		▷	Stated the recommended sites for an intradermal injection.
		●	Cleansed area with an antiseptic wipe and allowed it to dry completely.
		●	Applied gloves.
		●	Removed needle guard.
		●	Stretched the skin taut at the site of administration.
		▷	Explained why the skin is held taut.
		●	Inserted needle at an angle of 10 to 15 degrees and with the bevel upward.
		●	The bevel of the needle just penetrated the skin.
		▷	Stated why the bevel should face upward.
		●	Injected the medication slowly and steadily, ensuring that a wheal formed (approximately 6 to 10 mm in diameter).
		▷	Explained what to do if a wheal does not form.
		●	Placed an antiseptic wipe or gauze pad gently over the injection site and removed the needle quickly at the same angle as that of insertion.

649

Trial 1	Trial 2	Point Value	Performance Standards
		●	Did not apply pressure to the injection site.
		▷	Explained why pressure should not be applied to the site.
		●	Activated the safety shield on the needle.
		●	Properly disposed of needle and syringe.
		●	Removed gloves and sanitized hands.
		●	Remained with patient to make sure that there were no unusual reactions.
			Allergy skin tests
		●	Read the test results within 20 to 30 minutes.
		●	Inspected and palpated the site of the skin tests.
		●	Interpreted the skin test results.
		●	Charted the procedure correctly.
			Mantoux tuberculin test
		●	Informed the patient to return in 48 to 72 hours to have the results read.
		▷	Stated what must be done if the patient does not return to have the results read.
		●	Instructed the patient in the care of the test site.
		▷	Stated the instructions that must be relayed to the patient.
		●	Charted the procedure correctly.
			Reading Mantoux test results
		●	Greeted the patient and introduced yourself.
		●	Identified the patient and explained the procedure.
		●	Worked in a quiet, well-lit atmosphere.
		●	Checked the patient's chart to determine the site of administration of the test.
		●	Sanitized hands and applied gloves.
		●	Positioned patient's arm on a firm surface with the arm flexed at the elbow.
		●	Located the application site.
		●	Gently rubbed the fingertip over the test site.
		●	If induration is present, rubbed the area lightly, going from the area of normal skin to the indurated area to assess the size of the indurated area.
		●	Measured the diameter of the induration with a millimeter ruler.
		✱	The measurement was recorded in millimeters and was identical to the evaluator's measurement.

Trial 1	Trial 2	Point Value	Performance Standards
		●	Removed gloves and sanitized hands.
		●	Charted the results correctly.
		●	Completed a TB test record card and gave it to the patient.
		✱	Completed the procedure within 10 minutes.
			TOTALS
			CHART
Date			

TUBERCULOSIS TEST RECORD

Name

Date Admin:

Date Read:

MANTOUX TEST   RESULT

_____ mm

Logan Family Practice
401 St. George St.
St. Augustine, FL 32084
(555) 824-3933

Performed by _____

(From Bonewit-West K: *Study guide for clinical procedures for medical assistants*, ed 8, St. Louis, 2011, Saunders.)

Evaluation of Student Performance

EVALUATION CRITERIA			COMMENTS
Symbol	**Category**	**Point Value**	
✱	Critical Step	16 points	
●	Essential Step	6 points	
▷	Theory Question	2 points	
Score calculation: 100 points			
− _____ points missed			
_____ Score			
Satisfactory score: 85 or above			

CAAHEP Competencies Achieved
Psychomotor (Skills)
☑ I. 7. Select proper sites for administering parenteral medication.
☑ I. 9. Administer parenteral (excluding IV) medications.
☑ IX. 7. Document accurately in the patient record.
☑ XI. 5. Demonstrate proper use of the following equipment: c. Sharps disposal containers.
Affective (Behavior)
☑ III. 3. Show awareness of patients' concerns regarding their perceptions related to the procedure being performed.

ABHES Competencies Achieved
☑ 4. a. Document accurately.
☑ 9. j. Prepare and administer oral and parenteral medications as directed by physician.

DRUG DOSE CALCULATION: SUPPLEMENTAL EDUCATION FOR CHAPTER 26

This section is designed as supplemental education for Chapter 26 (Administration of Medication) in your textbook. Completion of these exercises will enable you to calculate drug dose effectively and accurately, which is essential for administering the proper amount of medication to patients and preventing medication errors. Because each unit builds on the next one; therefore, you should become completely familiar with each step before proceeding to the next.

Learning Objectives

After completing this chapter, you should be able to:

1. Identify metric abbreviations

2. Indicate dose quantity using metric notation guidelines

3. Identify apothecary abbreviations

4. Indicate dose quantity using apothecary notations

5. Identify common medical abbreviations used in writing medication orders

6. Interpret medication orders

7. Convert units of measurement within the following systems: metric, apothecary, and household

8. Convert units of measurement using ratio and proportion

9. Convert units of measurement between the metric, apothecary, and household systems

10. Determine oral drug dose

11. Determine parenteral drug dose

UNIT 1: THE METRIC SYSTEM

A. Units of Measurement: Practice Problems

The basic units of measurement in the metric system are the gram, liter, and meter. The gram is a unit of weight used to measure solids, the liter is a unit volume used to measure liquids, and the meter is a unit of length used to measure distance. In the space provided, indicate whether each of the following metric units of measurement is a unit of weight (W), volume (V), or length (L).

_____ 1. milligram

_____ 2. cubic centimeter

_____ 3. meter

_____ 4. kilogram

_____ 5. liter

_____ 6. milliliter

_____ 7. kiloliter

_____ 8. millimeter

_____ 9. microgram

_____ 10. gram

B. Metric Abbreviations: Practice Problems

Review the metric abbreviations in your textbook before completing these problems. In the space provided, indicate the correct abbreviation for each of the metric units of measurement.

_____ 1. milligram

_____ 2. gram

_____ 3. kilogram

_____ 4. liter

_____ 5. cubic centimeter

_____ 6. microgram

_____ 7. milliliter

C. Metric Notation: Practice Problems

To read prescriptions and medication orders, to record medication administration, and to avoid medication errors, the MA must be able to use metric notation guidelines. Review the Metric Notation Guidelines on page 567 of your textbook before completing the following practice problems. In the space provided, use metric notation guidelines to indicate the dose quantities.

_____ 1. 25 milligrams

_____ 2. 5 grams

_____ 3. 1½ liters

_____ 4. 1 cubic centimeter

_____ 5. 10 milliliters

_____ 6. ½ gram

_____ 7. 50 milligrams

_____ 8. ½ cubic centimeter

_____ 9. 4 milliliters

_____ 10. 2 kilograms

_____ 11. 120 milliliters

_____ 12. 3 cubic centimeters

_____ 13. ½ gram

_____ 14. 250 milligrams

_____ 15. ½ liter

_____ 16. 500 milliliters

_____ 17. 1 cubic centimeter

_____ 18. 5 kilograms

_____ 19. 2½ grams

_____ 20. 10 milligrams

UNIT 2: THE APOTHECARY SYSTEMS

A. Units of Measurement: Practice Problems

The basic units of measurement in the apothecary system are the grain, minim, and inch. The grain is a unit of weight used to measure solids, the minim is a unit of volume used to measure liquids, and the inch is a unit of length used to measure distance. In the space provided, indicate whether each of the following units of measurement is a unit of weight (W), volume (V), or length (L).

_____ 1. grain

_____ 2. inch

_____ 3. minim

_____ 4. fluid dram

_____ 5. foot

_____ 6. quart

_____ 7. ounce

_____ 8. gallon

_____ 9. yard

_____ 10. fluid ounce

_____ 11. pound

_____ 12. pint

_____ 13. dram

_____ 14. mile

B. Apothecary Abbreviations: Practice Problems

Review the apothecary abbreviations in your textbook before completing these problems. In the space provided, indicate the correct abbreviation or symbol for each of the apothecary units of measurement listed below.

_____ 1. grain

_____ 2. dram

_____ 3. ounce

_____ 4. minim

_____ 5. fluid dram

_____ 6. fluid ounce

_____ 7. pint

_____ 8. quart

_____ 9. gallon

_____ 10. inch

C. Apothecary Notation: Practice Problems

Although the apothecary system is used less frequently than the metric system, the MA must still be able to use apothecary notation guidelines. Review the Apothecary Notation Guidelines on p. 568 of your textbook before completing the practice problems. In the space provided, use apothecary notations to indicate the following dose quantities.

_____ 1. 4 ounces

_____ 2. 10 grains

_____ 3. 5 drams

_____ 4. ½ ounce

_____ 5. 6 fluid drams

_____ 6. 7½ grains

_____ 7. 3½ ounces

_____ 8. 10 minims

_____ 9. 3 fluid ounces

_____ 10. 2 drams

_____ 11. ¼ grain

_____ 12. 16 ounces

_____ 13. 12 minims

_____ 14. 1 dram

_____ 15. 9 fluid drams

_____ 16. 4 grains

_____ 17. 8 drams

_____ 18. 32 fluid ounces

_____ 19. 30 minims

_____ 20. 8 ounces

UNIT 3: THE HOUSEHOLD SYSTEM

The household system is more complicated and less accurate for administering medication than the metric and apothecary systems. However, most individuals are familiar with this system because of its frequent use in the United States. This system of measurement may be the only one the patient can fully relate to and therefore may safely use to administer liquid medication at home.

A. Units of Measurement: Practice Problems

Volume is the only household unit of measurement used to administer medication. The basic unit of liquid volume is the drop. The remaining units, in order of increasing volume, are the teaspoon, tablespoon, ounce, cup, and glass. In the space provided, indicate the correct abbreviation for each of the household units of measurement listed.

_____ 1. drop

_____ 2. teaspoon

_____ 3. tablespoon

_____ 4. ounce

A. Medical Abbreviations: Practice Problems

To safely administer medication, the MA must be completely familiar with common medical abbreviations. Review Table 26-5 in your textbook before completing the following practice problems. In the space provided, write the meaning of the following medical abbreviations.

_____ 1. NPO

_____ 2. prn

_____ 3. AS

_____ 4. hs

_____ 5. tab

_____ 6. OD

_____ 7. ac

_____ 8. pc

_____ 9. qid

_____ 10. c̄

_____ 11. OU

_____ 12. s̄

_____ 13. bid

_____ 14. tid

_____ 15. qh

_____ 16. gtts

_____ 17. qd

_____ 18. q4h

_____ 19. AU

_____ 20. qs

_____ 21. IM

_____ 22. caps

_____ 23. qod

_____ 24. po

_____ 25. OS

_____ 26. ad lib

_____ 27. a̅a̅

_____ 28. DAW

_____ 29. INH

_____ 30. OTC

B. Interpreting Medication Orders: Practice Problems

To safely administer medication and instruct patients on administering medication at home, the MA must be able to interpret medication orders. Interpret the following medication orders, and using a drug reference, indicate the drug category based on action and a brand name for each medication.

1. Tetracycline 250 mg po qid × 10 days

   _____

   Drug category: _____

   Brand name: _____

2. Lansoprazole 30 mg po qd ac

   _____

   Drug category: _____

   Brand name: _____

3. Alprazolam 0.25 mg po tid

   _____

   Drug category: _____

   Brand name: _____

4. Diltiazem 50 mg po q4h

   _____

   Drug category: _____

   Brand name: _____

5. Ciprofloxacin 500 mg q12h

   _____

   Drug category: _____

   Brand name: _____

6. Hydrocodone/acetaminophen 5 mg q4h prn

   _____

   Drug category: _____

   Brand name: _____

7. Furosemide 40 mg po q AM

   _____

   Drug category: _____

   Brand name: _____

8. Paroxetine 20 mg po qd in AM

   _____

   Drug category: _____

   Brand name: _____

9. Cetirizine 5 mg po qd

_____

Drug category: _____

Brand name: _____

10. Cyclobenzaprine 10 mg po tid × 1 wk

_____

Drug category: _____

Brand name: _____

UNIT 5: CONVERTING UNITS OF MEASUREMENT

A. Using Conversion Tables

Changing from one unit of measurement to another is known as *conversion*. Conversion is required when medication is ordered in one unit of measurement and the medication label expresses the drug strength in a different unit. The dose quantity must be mathematically translated or converted to the unit of measurement of the medication on hand. For example, if the physician orders 5 grams of an oral solid medication and the medication label expresses the drug strength in milligrams, the MA must convert the grams into milligrams to know how much medication to administer. Converting units of measurement can be classified as follows:

1. Conversion of units within a measurement system

2. Conversion of units from one measurement system to another

Converting units within a measurement system allows a quantity to be expressed in a different but equal unit of measurement within the same system. An example of converting between units of weight within the metric system is as follows: 1 gram is equal to 1000 milligrams.

Converting from one measurement system to another allows a quantity to be expressed in a unit of measurement of another system. An example of a conversion between the apothecary and metric systems is as follows: 1 grain (apothecary system) is equivalent to 60 milligrams (metric system). Methods used to convert units of measurement are presented in this unit and in Unit 6.

Conversion requires the use of a conversion table to indicate the equivalent values between units of measurement. The practice problems that follow can assist you in attaining competency in using conversion tables.

Conversion Tables: Practice Problems

Refer to the conversion tables at the end of this chapter. Locate and record the equivalent value for each of the units of measurement listed. In the space provided, indicate the conversion table you used to locate the equivalent value (e.g., metric, apothecary, metric to apothecary).

		ANSWER	CONVERSION TABLE
1. 1 g	=	_____ mg	_____
2. 1 ounce	=	_____ drams	_____
3. 1 tablespoon	=	_____ teaspoons	_____
4. 1 grain	=	_____ mg	_____
5. 1 liter	=	_____ mL	_____
6. 1 dram	=	_____ grains	_____
7. 1 pint	=	_____ fluid ounces	_____
8. 1 teaspoon	=	_____ drops	_____
9. 1 mL	=	_____ cc	_____
10. 1 mL	=	_____ minims	_____
11. 1 fluid ounce	=	_____ mL	_____

Chapter **26** **Administration of Medication and Intravenous Therapy**

12. 1 kg   =   _____ g   _____

13. 1 fluid dram =   _____ minims   _____

14. 1 gallon   =   _____ quarts   _____

15. 1 ounce   =   _____ tablespoons _____

16. 1 quart   =   _____ pints   _____

17. 1 fluid dram =   _____ mL   _____

18. 1 g   =   _____ grains   _____

19. 1 quart   =   _____ mL   _____

20. 1 drop   =   _____ minims   _____

21. 1 fluid ounce =   _____ tablespoons _____

22. 1 fluid dram =   _____ teaspoons _____

23. 1 tablespoon =   _____ fluid drams _____

24. 1 kg   =   _____ pounds   _____

25. 1 glass   =   _____ mL   _____

B. Converting Units Within the Metric System

Drug administration often requires conversion within the metric system to prepare the correct dose. Metric conversion involves converting a larger unit to a smaller unit (e.g., grams to milligrams) or converting a smaller unit to a larger unit (e.g., milliliters to liters). Methods used to convert one metric unit to another are described in the next sections.

Converting a Larger Unit to a Smaller Unit

Converting a larger unit to a smaller unit within the metric system can be accomplished using one of three methods. The method chosen is based on personal preference and the level of difficulty of the conversion problem. For example, more difficult problems require the use of ratio and proportion as the method of conversion. Examples of converting a larger unit to a smaller unit are as follows:

1. grams to milligrams
2. liters to milliliters
3. kilograms to grams

METHODS OF CONVERSION: To convert a larger unit to a smaller unit within the metric system, use one of the following:

Method 1: Multiply the unit to be changed by 1000.
Method 2: Move the decimal point of the unit to be changed three places to the right.
Method 3: Ratio and proportion (see Unit 6).

GUIDELINE: When converting a larger unit to a smaller unit, expect the quantity to become larger. Use this guideline to assist in making accurate conversions. The problems illustrate this guideline.

EXAMPLES

PROBLEM   2 L = _____ mL
Method 1:   Multiply the unit to be changed by 1000.
               $2 \times 1000 = 2000$ mL
Method 2:   Move the decimal point of the unit to be changed three places to the right.
               2.0 0 0. = 2000 mL

Answer   2 L = 2000 mL

PROBLEM   4 g = _____ mg
Method 1:   Multiply the unit to be changed by 1000.
                 $4 \times 1000 = 4000$ mg
Method 2:   Move the decimal point of the unit to be changed three places to the right.
                 4.0 0 0. = 4000 mg

> ***Answer***   4 g = 4000 mg

Converting a Smaller Unit to a Larger Unit

Converting a smaller unit to a larger unit within the metric system can be accomplished using one of three methods of conversion as outlined below. Examples of converting a smaller unit to a larger unit are as follows:

1. milligrams to grams
2. milliliters to liters
3. grams to kilograms

> METHOD OF CONVERSION: To convert a smaller unit to a larger unit within the metric system, use one of the following:
>
> *Method 1*: Divide the unit to be changed by 1000.
> *Method 2*: Move the decimal point of the unit to be changed three places to the left.
> *Method 3*: Ratio and proportion (see Unit 6).
>
> GUIDELINE: When converting a smaller unit to a larger unit, expect the quantity to become smaller. The problems illustrate this guideline.

EXAMPLES

PROBLEM   250 mg = _____ g
Method 1:   Divide the unit to be changed by 1000.
                 $250 \div 1000 = 0.25$ g
Method 2:   Move the decimal point of the unit to be changed three places to the left.
                 .2 5 0. = 0.25 g

> ***Answer***   250 mg = 0.25 g

PROBLEM   1500 mL = _____ L
Method 1:   Divide the unit to be changed by 1000.
                 $1500 \div 1000 = 1.5$ L
Method 2:   Move the decimal point of the unit to be changed three places to the left.
                 1.5 0 0. = 1.5 L

> ***Answer***   1500 mL = 1.5 L

Converting Units Within the Metric System: Practice Problems

Directions: Convert the following metric units of measurement using Method 1 or Method 2. In the space provided, indicate if the conversion is going from a larger to smaller unit (L→S) or smaller to larger unit (S→L), and indicate the conversion table you used.

		ANSWER	**CONVERSION TABLE**
1. 1 g	=	_____ mg	_____
2. 750 mg	=	_____ g	_____
3. 2 kg	=	_____ g	_____
4. 1000 g	=	_____ kg	_____

661

5. 1.5 L = _____ mL _____

6. 250 mL = _____ L _____

7. 5 g = _____ mg _____

8. 0.25 kg = _____ g _____

9. 1000 mg = _____ g _____

10. 2.5 g = _____ mg _____

11. 475 mL = _____ L _____

12. 0.05 g = _____ mg _____

13. 0.5 L = _____ mL _____

14. 1000 mL = _____ L _____

15. 500 g = _____ kg _____

16. 50 mg = _____ g _____

17. 1 L = _____ mL _____

18. 40 g = _____ mg _____

19. 50 mL = _____ L _____

20. 1 kg = _____ g _____

C. Converting Units Within the Apothecary System

Drug administration may sometimes require conversion within the apothecary system to prepare the correct dose. Apothecary conversion involves converting a larger unit to a smaller unit (e.g., drams to grains) or converting a smaller unit to a larger unit (e.g., ounces to pounds). Methods used to convert one apothecary unit to another are described below.

Converting a Larger Unit to a Smaller Unit

Converting a larger unit to a smaller unit within the apothecary system is accomplished through either the equivalent value method or the ratio and proportion method. Examples of converting a larger unit to a smaller unit follow:

Weight	*Volume*
drams to grains	fluid drams to minims
ounces to drams	fluid ounces to fluid drams
pounds to ounces	pints to fluid ounces
	quarts to pints
	gallons to quarts

> METHOD OF CONVERSION: To convert a larger unit to a smaller unit within the apothecary system, use one of the following:
>
> *Method 1:*
> a. Look at Table 26-2 (Apothecary Conversion) at the end of this chapter to determine the equivalent value between the two units of measurement.
> b. Multiply the equivalent value by the number next to the larger unit of measurement.
> *Method 2:* Ratio and proportion (see Unit 6).

EXAMPLES

PROBLEM   4 drams = _____ grains

Method 1:

a. Look at the conversion table to determine the equivalent value:

  1 dram = 60 grains

  60 = the equivalent value

b. Multiply the equivalent value by the number next to the larger unit of measurement:

  4 × 60 = 240 grains

> **Answer**   4 drams = 240 grams

PROBLEM   1½ pints = _____ fluid ounces
Method 1:
   a. Look at the conversion table to determine the equivalent value:
      1 pint = 16 fluid ounces
      16 = the equivalent value
   b. Multiply the equivalent value by the number next to the larger unit of measurement:
      1.5 × 16 = 24 fluid ounces

> *Answer*   1½ pints = 24 fluid ounces

Converting a Smaller Unit to a Larger Unit

Converting a smaller unit to a larger unit within the apothecary system also can be accomplished using the equivalent value method or the ratio and proportion method. Examples of converting from a smaller unit to a larger unit follow:

Weight	*Volume*
grains to drams	minims to fluid drams
drams to ounces	fluid drams to fluid ounces
ounces to pounds	fluid ounces to pints
	pints to quarts
	quarts to gallons

> METHOD OF CONVERSION: To convert a smaller unit to a larger unit within the apothecary system, use one of the following:
>
> *Method 1*:
> a. Look at Table 26-2 (Apothecary Conversion) at the end of this chapter to determine the equivalent value between the two units of measurement.
> b. Divide the equivalent value into the number next to the smaller unit of measurement.
> *Method 2*: Ratio and proportion (see Unit 6).

EXAMPLES

PROBLEM   30 grains = _____ drams
Method 1:
   a. Look at the conversion table to determine the equivalent value:
      60 grains = 1 dram
      60 = the equivalent value
   b. Divide the equivalent value into the number next to the smaller unit of measurement:
      30 ÷ 60 = ½ dram

> *Answer*   30 grains = ½ dram

PROBLEM   16 fluid drams = _____ fluid ounces
Method 1:
   a. Look at the conversion table to determine the equivalent value:
      8 fluid drams = 1 fluid ounce
      8 = the equivalent value
   b. Divide the equivalent value into the number next to the smaller unit of measurement:
      16 ÷ 8 = 2 fluid ounces

> *Answer* 16 fluid drams = 2 fluid ounces

Converting Units Within the Apothecary: Practice Problems

Convert the apothecary units of measurement using the equivalent value method of conversion. In the space provided, indicate the equivalent value for each problem.

		ANSWER	EQUIVALENT VALUE
1. 2 quarts	=	_____ pints	_____
2. 4 drams	=	_____ grains	_____
3. ½ ounce	=	_____ drams	_____
4. 300 grains	=	_____ drams	_____
5. 2 fluid drams	=	_____ minims	_____
6. 8 pints	=	_____ quarts	_____
7. 16 drams	=	_____ ounces	_____
8. 24 fluid drams	=	_____ fluid ounces	_____
9. 18 ounces	=	_____ pounds	_____
10. 32 fluid ounces	=	_____ pints	_____
11. ½ quart	=	_____ pints	_____
12. ½ dram	=	_____ grains	_____
13. 3 ounces	=	_____ drams	_____
14. 210 grains	=	_____ drams	_____
15. 4 ½ fluid drams	=	_____ minims	_____
16. 3 pints	=	_____ quarts	_____
17. 4 drams	=	_____ ounces	_____
18. 24 ounces	=	_____ pounds	_____
19. 8 fluid ounces	=	_____ pints	_____
20. 2 quarts	=	_____ gallons	_____
21. 120 minims	=	_____ fluid drams	_____
22. 2 fluid ounces	=	_____ fluid drams	_____
23. ½ pound	=	_____ ounces	_____
24. 4 pints	=	_____ fluid ounces	_____
25. 2 gallons	=	_____ quarts	_____

D. Converting Units Within the Household System

Household system conversion involves converting a larger unit to a smaller unit (e.g., tablespoons to teaspoons) or converting a smaller unit to a larger unit (e.g., tablespoons to ounces). Methods used to convert one unit to another are described.

Converting a Larger Unit to a Smaller Unit

Converting a larger unit to a smaller unit within the household system is accomplished using the equivalent value method or the ratio and proportion method. The method chosen is based on personal preference and on the level of difficulty of the conversion problem. Examples of converting a larger unit to a smaller unit follow:

Volume:
teaspoons to drops
tablespoons to teaspoons
ounces to teaspoons
ounces to tablespoons
teacup to ounces
glass to ounces

METHOD OF CONVERSION: To convert a larger unit to a smaller unit within the household system, use one of the following:

Method 1:

a. Look at Table 26-3 (Household Conversion) at the end of this chapter to determine the equivalent value between the two units of measurement.

b. Multiply the equivalent value by the number next to the larger unit of measurement.

Method 2: Ratio and proportion (see Unit 6)

EXAMPLES

PROBLEM   2 tablespoons = _____ teaspoons

Method 1:

    a. Look at the conversion table to determine the equivalent value:

      1 tablespoon = 3 teaspoons

      3 = the equivalent value

    b. Multiply the equivalent value by the number next to the larger unit of measurement:

      $2 \times 3 = 6$ teaspoons

> ***Answer*** 2 tablespoons = 6 teaspoons

PROBLEM   ½ teaspoon = _____ drops

Method 1:

    a. Look at the conversion table to determine the equivalent value:

      1 teaspoon = 60 drops

      60 = the equivalent value

    b. Multiply the equivalent value by the number next to the larger unit of measurement:

      $½ \times 60 = 30$ drops

> ***Answer***   ½ tablespoon = 30 drops

Converting a Smaller Unit to a Larger Unit

Converting a smaller unit to a larger unit within the household system is accomplished using the equivalent value method or the ratio and proportion method. Examples of converting from a smaller unit to a larger unit follow:

Volume

drops to teaspoons
teaspoons to tablespoons
teaspoons to ounces
tablespoons to ounces
ounces to teacups
ounces to glasses

METHOD OF CONVERSION: To convert a smaller unit to a larger unit within the household system, use one of the following:

Method 1:

a. Look at Table 26-3 (Household Conversion) at the end of this chapter to determine the equivalent value between the two units of measurement.

b. Divide the equivalent value into the number next to the smaller unit of measurement.

Method 2: Ratio and proportion (see Unit 6).

EXAMPLES

PROBLEM   4 tablespoons = _____ ounces

Method 1:
   a. Look at the conversion table to determine the equivalent value:
      1 ounce = 2 tablespoons
      2 = the equivalent value
   b. Divide the equivalent value into the number next to the smaller unit of measurement:
      4 ÷ 2 = 2 ounces

Answer	4 tablespoon = 2 ounces

PROBLEM   24 ounces = _____ glasses

Method 1:
   a. Look at the conversion table to determine the equivalent value:
      1 glass = 8 ounces
      8 = the equivalent value
   b. Divide the equivalent value into the number next to the smaller unit of measurement:
      24 ÷ 8 = 3 glasses

Answer	24 ounces = 3 glasses

Converting Units Within the Household System: Practice Problems

Directions: Convert the following household units of measurement using the equivalent value method of conversion. In the space provided, indicate the equivalent value for each problem.

			ANSWER	EQUIVALENT VALUE
1. 12 teaspoons	=		_____ ounces	_____
2. 4 ounces	=		_____ glasses	_____
3. 90 drops	=		_____ teaspoons	_____
4. ½ ounce	=		_____ tablespoons	_____
5. 6 teaspoons	=		_____ tablespoons	_____
6. 3 tablespoons	=		_____ ounces	_____
7. 18 ounces	=		_____ teacups	_____
8. ½ ounce	=		_____ teaspoons	_____
9. 3 tablespoons	=		_____ teaspoons	_____
10. ½ teaspoon	=		_____ drops	_____

UNIT 6: RATIO AND PROPORTION

Ratio and proportion are used to convert units of measurement. This method of conversion has the advantage of clarifying the mathematical rationale for the methods of conversion previously presented. It is also useful in converting units of measurement that are more difficult to calculate, such as converting between systems, such as when converting an apothecary unit of measurement to a metric unit of measurement.

A. Ratio and Proportion Guidelines

Some guidelines must be followed when using ratio and proportion:

1. A **ratio** is composed of two related numbers separated by a colon. It indicates the relationship between two quantities or numbers. The ratio example shows a relationship between milligrams and grams (i.e., 1000 mg = 1 g).

   EXAMPLE   1000 mg : 1 g

666

2. A **proportion** shows the relationship between two equal ratios. The proportion consists of two ratios separated by an equal sign (=), which indicates that the two ratios are equal. This proportion example shows the relationship between two equal ratios of milligrams and grams.

EXAMPLE   1000 mg : 1 g = 2000 mg : 2 g

3. The units of measurement in the two ratios of a proportion must be expressed in the same sequence. The correct sequencing in the proportion example is mg : g = mg : g, *not* mg : g = g : mg.

EXAMPLE   *Correct:*   1000 mg : 1 g = 2000 mg : 2 g
                 Incorrect: 1000 mg : 1 g = 2 g : 2000 mg

4. The numbers on the ends of a proportion are called the **extremes**, and the numbers in the middle of the proportion are known as the **means**. In this example, the means consist of 1 g and 2000 mg, and the extremes are 1000 mg and 2 g.

EXAMPLE   1000 mg : 1 g = 2000 mg : 2g
                      └──── means ────┘
                 └──────── extremes ────────┘

5. The product of the means equals the product of the extremes. The calculation of the product of the means in the example is 1 × 2000 = 2000. The calculation of the product of the extremes is 1000 × 2 = 2000. The product of the means equals the product of the extremes or 2000 = 2000.

EXAMPLE   1000 mg : 1 g = 2000 mg : 2 g
                 $1 \times 2000 = 1000 \times 2$
                 $2000 = 2000$

6. In setting up a proportion, one side of the equation consists of the known quantities, and the other side of the equation consists of the unknown quantity. The letter x is commonly used to express the unknown quantity. To be consistent, the known quantities are indicated on the left side of the equation, and the unknown quantity is indicated on the right side of the equation. Using the previous proportion example, but inserting an unknown quantity, or x, the equation is set up as follows:

EXAMPLE   1000 mg : 1 g   = x mg : 2 g
                 (known quantities)   (unknown quantity)

Ratio and Proportion: Practice Problems

Answer the following questions.

1. What is a ratio? _____

_____

2. In the space provided, place a check mark next to each correct example of a ratio.

_____ a. 15 drops : 15 minims : 1 mL

_____ b. 1000 mL = 1 L

_____ c. 1 ounce : 8 drams

_____ d. 60 minims/1 fluid dram

_____ e. 1 dram : 60 grains

_____ f. 1 mL : 1 cc

Chapter **26** **Administration of Medication and Intravenous Therapy**

3. What is a proportion?

_____

_____

_____

4. In the space provided, place a check mark next to each correct example of a proportion.

    _____ a. 1 mL : 1 cc

    _____ b. 1 grain : 60 mg = 4 grains : 240 mg

    _____ c. 2x = 60 mg

    _____ d. 1000 mL : 1 L = 500 mL : 0.5 L

    _____ e. 1000 mg : 1 grain = 1000 mL : 1 L

5. In the space provided, place a check mark next to each proportion that has correct sequencing for the units of measurement.

    _____ a. 1000 g : 1 kg = 1500 g : 1.5 kg

    _____ b. 60 grains : 1 dram = 2 drams : 120 grains

    _____ c. 1000 mg : 1 g = 2000 mg : x g

6. Circle the means and underline the extremes in each of the following proportions:

    a. 1000 mg : 1 g = 500 mg : 0.5 g

    b. 2 pints : 1 quart = 4 pints : 2 quarts

    c. 1 mL : 1 cc = 2 mL : 2 cc

7. In each of the following proportions, what is the product of the means, and what is the product of the extremes?

    a. 1000 g : 1 kg = 1500 g : 1.5 kg

        _____ product of the means

        _____ product of the extremes

    b. 60 minims : 1 fluid dram = 120 minims : 2 fluid drams

        _____ product of the means

        _____ product of the extremes

    c. 60 mg : 1 grain = 300 mg : 5 grains

        _____ product of the means

        _____ product of the extremes

8. In each of the following proportions, circle the known quantities and underline the unknown quantity.

    a. 1000 mg : 1 g = 500 mg : x g

    b. 1 g : 15 grains = 2 g : x grains

    c. 8 drams : 1 ounce = x drams : 4 ounces

B. Converting Units Using Ratio and Proportion

Units can be converted using ratio and proportion.

> METHOD OF CONVERSION: To convert a unit of measurement using ratio and proportion, use the following steps:
> a. Look at the appropriate conversion table at the end of this chapter to determine what is known about the two units of measurement (equivalent value).
> b. State the known quantities as a ratio.
> c. Determine the unknown quantity.
> d. State the unknown quantity as a ratio.
> e. Set up the proportion with the known quantities on the left side and the unknown quantity on the right side of the equation.
> f. To solve the equation, multiply the product of the means and the product of the extremes. Divide the equation by the numbers before the x.
> g. Include the unit of measure corresponding to x in the original equation with the answer.

EXAMPLES

PROBLEM $2\,g = $ _____ mg

a. Look at Table 26-1 (Metric Conversion) to determine what is known about the two units of measurement:

$1000\,mg = 1\,g$

b. State the known quantities as a ratio:

$1000\,mg : 1\,g$

c. Determine the unknown quantity:

$2\,g = x\,mg$

d. State the unknown quantity as a ratio using the correct unit of measurement sequencing:

$x\,mg : 2\,g$

e. Set up the proportion with the known quantities on the left side and the unknown quantity on the right side of the equation:

$1000\,mg : 1\,g = x\,mg : 2\,g$

f. Solve the equation by multiplying the product of the means and the product of the extremes and dividing the equation by the number before the x:

$1000\,mg : 1\,g = x\,mg : 2\,g$
$1 \times x = 1000 \times 2$
$1x = 2000$
$x = 2000$

g. Include the unit of measure corresponding to x in the original equation with the answer:

$x = 2000\,mg$

> **Answer** $2\,g = 2000\,mg$

PROBLEM
$300\,mg = $ _____ grains

The steps previously outlined are followed here. However, they are combined as they would be in working an actual conversion problem.

$60\,mg : 1\,grain = 300\,mg : x\,grains$
$1 \times 300 = 60 \times x$
$300 = 60\,x$
$300 \div 60 = 60\,x \div 60$
$x = 5\,grains$

> **Answer** $300\,mg = 5\,grains$

Converting Units Using Ratio and Proportion: Practice Problems

Directions: Use ratio and proportion to convert among the apothecary, metric, and household systems by completing the problems below. In the space at the right, indicate what is known regarding the two units of measurement.

			ANSWER	**KNOWN QUANTITIES**
1. 30 minims	=	_____ mL		_____
2. 4 kg	=	_____ pounds		_____
3. 90 mL	=	_____ fluid ounces		_____
4. 30 mg	=	_____ grains		_____
5. 60 mg	=	_____ ounces		_____
6. 250 mL	=	_____ pints		_____
7. 6 g	=	_____ drams		_____
8. ½ quart	=	_____ mL		_____
9. 3 g	=	_____ grains		_____
10. 5 fluid drams	=	_____ mL		_____
11. 80 pounds	=	_____ kg		_____
12. 500 mL	=	_____ quarts		_____
13. 8 mL	=	_____ teaspoons		_____
14. 4 grains	=	_____ mg		_____
15. 32 mL	=	_____ fluid drams		_____
16. 120 mg	=	_____ grains		_____
17. 30 mL	=	_____ tablespoons		_____
18. 60 drops	=	_____ mL		_____
19. ½ fluid ounce	=	_____ tablespoons		_____
20. ½ fluid ounce	=	_____ mL		_____

UNIT 7: DETERMINING DRUG DOSE

A. Oral Administration

Dose refers to the amount of medication to be administered to the patient. Each medication has a certain dose range or range of quantities that produce therapeutic effects. It is important to administer the exact drug dose. If the dose is too small, it will not produce a therapeutic effect, whereas too large a dose could harm or even kill the patient. The steps to follow in determining drug dose depend on the unit of measurement in which the drug is ordered and the unit of measurement of the drug you have available, or the dose on hand.

1. If the dose on hand is the same as that ordered, no calculation is required. In this example, the dose ordered and the dose on hand are in the same unit of measurement, and one tablet is administered to the patient.

   EXAMPLE   The physician orders 50 mg of a medication po.
              The drug label reads 50 mg/tablet.

2. If the dose ordered is in the same unit of measurement as that indicated on the medication label, only one calculation step is required. In this example, the dose ordered and the dose on hand are in the same unit of measurement, or grains. The calculation determines the number of tablets to administer to the patient.

   EXAMPLE   The physician orders gr $\overline{v}$ of a medication po.
              The drug label reads gr $\overline{x}$ tablet.

3. If the dose ordered is in a different unit of measurement than indicated on the drug label, two calculation steps are required to determine the amount of medication to administer to the patient. In this example, the dose ordered and the dose on hand are stated in different units of measurement, or in grams and milligrams. The first step requires conversion of the dose ordered to the unit of measurement of the dose on hand; in this example, grams must be converted to milligrams. The second step is to determine the number of tablets to administer to the patient.

EXAMPLE   The physician orders 1 g of a medication po.
           The drug label reads 500 mg/tablet.

A detailed discussion of determining drug dose for administration of oral medication follows. The method used to calculate drug dose when the units of measurement are the same is presented first, followed by the method used when the units of measurement are different.

Determining Drug Dose with the Same Units of Measurement

Determining the correct drug dose to be administered when the units of measurement are the same requires the use of a drug dose formula.

DRUG DOSE FORMULA

$$\frac{D \ (dose \ ordered)}{H \ (on \ hand)} \times V \ (vehicle) = x \ (\text{Amount of medication to be administered})$$

D (*dose ordered*): This is the amount of medication ordered by the physician.

H (*drug strength on hand*): This is the dose strength available as indicated on the medication label or the dose on hand.

V (*vehicle*): The vehicle refers to the type of preparation containing the dose on hand (e.g., tablet, capsule, liquid).

x: The letter *x* is used to express the unknown quantity or the amount of medication to be administered.

GUIDELINES

1. The units of measurement must be included when setting up the problem.
2. The values for D and H must be in the same unit of measurement.
3. The value of *x* is expressed in the same unit as V.
4. When determining the drug dose for oral liquid medication, the vehicle must also include the amount of liquid in which the available drug is contained. For example, if the medication label reads 250 mg/5 mL, the value of V is 5 mL.

The method to follow to determine drug dose using this formula is outlined in the following examples. The first problem illustrates determining dose for solid medication taken orally.

EXAMPLES

PROBLEM   *Oral* solid medication:
           The physician orders 50 mg of a medication po.
           The medication label reads 25 mg/tablet.
           How much medication should be administered to the patient?

Drug dose formula:

$$\frac{D}{V} \times V = x$$

a. Identify the dose ordered.
   D = 50 mg

b. Identify the strength of the drug on hand.
   H = 25 mg

c. Determine the vehicle containing the dose on hand.
   V = 1 tablet

Chapter **26**   **Administration of Medication and Intravenous Therapy**

d. Calculate the amount of medication to administer to the patient. The units of measurement must be included when setting up the problem, and the values for D and H must be in the same unit of measurement. The value of x is expressed in the same unit as V; in this problem V = 1 tablet.

$$\frac{50\,mg}{25\,mg} \times 1\ tablet = x$$

$(50 \div 25 = 2) \times 1\ tablet = x$

$2 \times 1\ tablet = x$

$x = 2\ tablets$

> ***Answer***   2 tablets administered to the patient

The next problem illustrates the determination of drug dose for liquid medication taken orally. The steps previously outlined are followed; however, they are combined as should be done when working out drug dose problems. Remember, with oral liquid medication, the vehicle must also include the amount of liquid in which the available drug is contained; in the following problem, V = 5 mL.

PROBLEM   *Oral liquid medication*:
The physician orders 500 mg of a medication.
The medication label reads 250 mg/5 mL.
How much medication should be administered to the patient?

$$\frac{D}{V} \times 1\ tablet = x$$

$$\frac{500\,mg}{250\,mg} \times 1\ tablet = x$$

$(500 \div 250 = 2) \times 5\,mL = x$

$2 \times 5\,mL = x$

$x = 10\,mL$

> ***Answer***   A dose of 10 mL of medication is administered to the patient.

Determining Drug Dose with Different Units of Measurement

Sometimes, the medication ordered is in a different unit of measurement than indicated on the drug label. In this case, the desired dose quantity must be converted to the unit of measurement of the dose on hand before the drug dose is determined. The method chosen to convert a unit of measurement is based on personal preference. Refer to Units 5 and 6 to review methods of conversion before completing this section.

> The following steps are required to determine drug dose when the units of measurement are different:
>
> *Step 1:* Convert the dose quantities to the same unit of measurement. For consistency, it is best to convert to the unit of measurement of the drug on hand.
>
> *Step 2:* Determine the amount of medication to administer to the patient, using the drug dose formula.

EXAMPLES

PROBLEM   *Oral solid medication*:
The physician orders gr $\overline{x}$ of medication po.
The medication label reads 300 mg/tablet.
How much medication should be administered to the patient?

Step 1: The dose ordered must be converted to the unit of measurement of the medication on hand. In this problem, 10 grains must be converted to milligrams. The ratio and proportion method of conversion is used to make the conversion.

gr $\overline{x}$ = _____ mg

1 grain : 60 mg = 10 grains : x mg

$600 = 1\ x$

$x = 600\,mg$

> ***Answer***   gr $\overline{x}$ = 600 mg

672

The medication ordered is in the same unit of measurement as the medication on hand.

Step 2: Determine the amount of medication to administer to the patient using the drug dose formula.

$$\frac{D}{H} \times V = x$$

$$\frac{600\,mg}{300\,mg} \times 1 \text{ tablet}$$

$(600 \div 300 = 2) \times 1 \text{ tablet} = x$

$2 \times 1 \text{ tablet} = x$

$x = 2 \text{ tablets}$

> **Answer**   A dose of 2 tablets is administered to the patient.

PROBLEM   *Oral liquid medication:*

The physician orders gr $\overline{xv}$ of a medication po.
The medication label reads 300 mg/fluid dram.
How much medication should be administered to the patient?

Step 1: Convert 15 grains to milligrams using ratio and proportion:

gr $\overline{xv}$ = _____ mg

$60\,mg : 1 \text{ grain} = x\,mg : 15 \text{ grains}$

$1\,x = 900\,mg$

$x = 900\,mg$

> **Answer**   gr $\overline{xv}$ = 900 mg

Step 2: Determine the amount of medication to administer to the patient using the drug dose formula.

$$\frac{D}{H} \times V = x$$

$$\frac{900\,mg}{300\,mg} \times 1 \text{ fluid dram} = x$$

$(900 \div 300 = 3) \times 1 \text{ fluid dram} = x$

$3 \times 1 \text{ fluid dram} = x$

$x = 3 \text{ fluid drams}$

> **Answer**   A dose of 3 fluid drams of medication is administered to the patient.

Oral Administration: Practice Problems

Directions: Determine the drug dose to be administered for each of the following oral medication orders, and record your answer below. In the space provided, indicate the drug category based on action for each medication using a drug reference.

Oral Solid Medications

1. The physician orders Inderal 160 mg po.
   Medication label:

   | Inderal |
   | propranolol |
   | 80 mg/capsule |

   How much medication should be administered? _____

   Drug category: _____

2. The physician orders Tagamet gr $\overline{v}$ po.
Medication label:

> Tagamet
> cimetidine
>
> 300 mg/tablet

How much medication should be administered? _____

Drug category: _____

3. The physician orders Amoxil 0.5 g po.
Medication label:

> Amoxil
> amoxicillin
>
> 250 mg/capsule

How much medication should be administered? _____

Drug category: _____

4. The physician orders Lasix 80 mg po.
Medication label:

> Lasix
> furosemide
>
> 40 mg/tablet

How much medication should be administered? _____

Drug category: _____

5. The physician orders Lomotil 5 mg po.
Medication label:

> Lomotil
> diphenoxylate/atropine
>
> 2.5 mg/tablet

How much medication should be administered? _____

Drug category: _____

6. The physician orders Zithromax 0.5 g po.
Medication label:

> Zithromax
> azithromycin
>
> 250 mg/tablet

How much medication should be administered? _____

Drug category: _____

7. The physician orders Calan gr ii po.
   Medication label:

   | Calan |
   | verapamil |
   | 40 mg/tablet |

   How much medication should be administered? _____

   Drug category: _____

8. The physician orders Xanax 0.5 mg po.
   Medication label:

   | Xanax |
   | alprazolam |
   | 0.25 mg/tablet |

   How much medication should be administered? _____

   Drug category: _____

9. The physician orders Phenergan 25 mg po.
   Medication label:

   | Phenergan |
   | promethazine |
   | 12.5 mg/tablet |

   How much medication should be administered? _____

   Drug category: _____

10. The physician orders Procardia XL gr s̄s̄ po.
    Medication label:

    | Procardia |
    | nifedipine |
    | 10 mg/tablet |

    How much medication should be administered? _____

    Drug category: _____

Oral Liquid Medications

1. The physician orders Sumycin Suspension 250 mg po.
   Medication label:

   | Sumycin Suspension |
   | tetracycline |
   | 125 mg/5 mL |

   How much medication should be administered? _____

   Drug category: _____

2. The physician orders Tagamet liquid 300 mg po.
   Medication label:

   > Tagamet
   > Cimetidine liquid
   >
   > 300 mg/5 mL

   How much medication should be administered? _____

   Drug category: _____

3. The physician orders Tylenol Elixir 60 mg po.
   Medication label:

   > Tylenol Elixir
   > acetaminophen
   >
   > 120 mg/5 mL

   How much medication should be administered? _____

   Drug category: _____

4. The physician orders Amoxil Suspension 0.5 g po.
   Medication label:

   > Amoxil Suspension
   > amoxicillin
   >
   > 125 mg/5 mL

   How much medication should be administered? _____

   Drug category: _____

5. The physician orders Gantanol Suspension 1 g po.
   Medication label:

   > Gantanol Suspension
   > sulfamethoxazole
   >
   > 500 mg/5 mL

   How much medication should be administered? _____

   Drug category: _____

B. Parenteral Administration

Medications for parenteral administration must be suspended in solution. The medication label indicates the amount of the drug contained in each milliliter of solution. For example, if a medication label reads 10 mg/mL, there are 10 mg of medication for each 1 mL of liquid volume. Some medications, such as penicillin, insulin, and heparin, are ordered and measured in *units* (e.g., 300,000 units/mL). This refers to their biologic activity in animal tests or the amount of the drug that is required to produce a particular response.

Parenteral medication is available in several dispensing forms, including ampules, single-dose vials, and multiple-dose vials. After the proper drug dose has been determined, the medication is drawn into a syringe from the dispensing unit. Most syringes are calibrated in milliliters (mL).

Determining drug dose for parenteral administration is calculated in a similar manner as that for oral liquid medication. The first problem illustrates the determination of drug dose when the medication is ordered in a different unit of measurement from the dose on hand, requiring two calculation steps.

EXAMPLES

PROBLEM   The physician orders 0.5 g of a medication IM.
The medication label reads 250 mg/2 mL.
How much medication should be administered?

Step 1: Convert 0.5 gram to milligrams.

$0.5\,g = mg$

$1000\,mg : 1\,g = x\,mg : 0.5\,g$

$1\,x = 500$

$x = 500\,mg$

> **Answer** $0.5\,mg = 500\,mg$

Step 2: Determine the amount of medication to administer to the patient:

$$\frac{D}{H} \times V = x$$

$$\frac{500\,mg}{250\,mg} \times 2\,mL = x$$

$(500 \div 250 = 2) \times 2\,mL = x$

$2 \times 2\,mL = x$

$x = 4\,mL$

> **Answer**   A dose of 4 mL of medication is administered to the patient

The next problem illustrates the determination of drug dose with a medication ordered in units. Notice that the dose ordered and the dose on hand are in the same unit of measurement; therefore, conversion of units of measurement is not necessary.

PROBLEM   The physician orders 600,000 units of a medication IM.
The medication label reads 300,000 units/mL.
How much medication should be administered?

$$\frac{D}{H} \times V = x$$

$$\frac{6000,000\text{ units}}{300,000\text{ units}} \times 1\,mL = x$$

$(600,000 \div 300,000 = 2) \times 1\,mL = x$

$x = 2\,mL$

> **Answer**   A dose of 2 mL of medication is administered to the patient.

Parenteral Administration: Practice Problems

Determine the drug dose to be administered for each of the following parenteral medication orders, and record your answer. In the space provided, indicate the drug category based on action using a drug reference.

1. The physician orders Vistaril 75 mg IM.
   Medication label:

Vistaril
hydroxyzine injection
50 mg/mL

   How much medication should be administered? _____

   Drug category: _____

677

2. The physician orders Cobex (vitamin B_{12}) 200 mcg IM.
   Medication label:

   > Cobex
   > cyanocobalamin injection
   >
   > 100 mcg/mL

   How much medication should be administered? _____

   Drug category: _____

3. The physician orders Depo-Medrol 40 mg IM.
   Medication label:

   > Depo-Medrol
   > methylprednisolone injection
   >
   > 80 mg/mL

   How much medication should be administered? _____

   Drug category: _____

4. The physician orders Wycillin 600,000 units IM.
   Medication label:

   > Wycillin
   > porcine penicillin G injection
   >
   > 300,000 units/mL

   How much medication should be administered? _____

   Drug category: _____

5. The physician orders Rocephin 1000 mg IM.
   Medication label:

   > Rocephin
   > ceftriaxone injection
   >
   > 1 g/mL

   How much medication should be administered? _____

   Drug category: _____

6. The physician orders INFeD 100 mg IM.
   Medication label:

   > INFeD
   > iron dextran injection
   >
   > 50 mg/mL

   How much medication should be administered? _____

   Drug category: _____

7. The physician orders Bicillin 1.2 million units IM.
   Medication label:

   > Bicillin
   > benzathine penicillin G injection
   >
   > 600,000 units/mL

   How much medication should be administered? _____

   Drug category: _____

8. The physician orders Depo-Provera 150 mg IM.
   Medication label:

   > Depo-Provera
   > medroxyprogesterone
   >
   > 150 mg/mL

   How much medication should be administered? _____

   Drug category: _____

9. The physician orders Pronestyl 0.25 g IM.
   Medication label:

   > Pronestyl
   > procainamide injection
   >
   > 500 mg/mL

   How much medication should be administered? _____

   Drug category: _____

10. The physician orders Compazine 7 mg IM.
    Medication label:

    > Compazine
    > prochlorperazine injection
    >
    > 5 mg/mL

    How much medication should be administered? _____

    Drug category: _____

Table 26-1. Metric System Conversion of Equivalent Values

WEIGHT
1000 micrograms = 1 milligram
1000 milligrams = 1 gram
1000 grams = 1 kilogram

VOLUME
1000 milliliters = 1 liter
1000 liters = 1 kiloliter
1 milliliter = 1 cubic centimeter

Table 26-2. Apothecary System: Conversion of Equivalent Values

WEIGHT
60 grains = 1 dram
8 drams = 1 ounce
12 ounces = 1 pound

VOLUME
60 minims = 1 fluid dram
8 fluid drams = 1 fluid ounce
16 fluid ounces = 1 pint
2 pints = 1 quart
4 quarts = 1 gallon

Table 26-3. Household System: Conversion of Equivalent Values

ABBREVIATIONS
drop: gtt
teaspoon: tsp
tablespoon: T
ounce: oz
cup: c

VOLUME
60 drops = 1 teaspoon
3 teaspoons = 1 tablespoon
6 teaspoons = 1 ounce
2 tablespoons = 1 ounce
6 ounces = 1 teacup
8 ounces = 1 glass
8 ounces = 1 cup

Table 26-4. Conversion Chart for Metric and Apothecary Systems (Commonly Used Approximate Equivalents)

Metric System to Apothecary System	Apothecary System to Metric System
WEIGHT 60 mg = 1 grain 1 g = 15 grains 4 g = 1 dram 30 mg = 1 ounce 1 kg = 2.2 pounds **VOLUME** 0.06 mL = 1 minim 1 mL (cc) = 15 minims 4 mL = 1 fluid dram 30 mL = 1 fluid ounce 500 mL = 1 pint 1000 mL (1 L) = 1 quart	**WEIGHT** 15 grains = 1000 mg (1 g) 10 grains = 600 mg 7.5 grains = 500 mg 5 grains = 300 mg 3 grains = 200 mg 1.5 grains = 100 mg 1 grain = 60 mg ¾ grain = 50 mg ½ grain = 30 mg ¼ grain = 15 mg ⅙ grain = 10 mg ⅛ grain = 8 mg 1/12 grain = 5 mg 1/15 grain = 4 mg 1/20 grain = 3 mg 1/30 grain = 2 mg 1/40 grain = 1.5 mg 1/50 grain = 1.2 mg 1/60 grain = 1 mg 1/100 grain = 0.6 mg 1/120 grain = 0.5 mg 1/150 grain = 0.4 mg 1/200 grain = 0.3 mg 1/300 grain = 0.2 mg 1/600 grain = 0.1 mg

Table 26-5. Conversion Chart for Apothecary and Metric Equivalents of Household Measures (Volume)

Household	Apothecary	Metric
1 drop	= 1 minim	= 0.06 mL
15 drops	= 15 minims	= 1 mL (cc)
1 teaspoon	= 1 fluid dram	= 5 (4) mL
1 tablespoon	= 4 fluid drams	= 15 mL
2 tablespoons	= 1 fluid ounce	= 30 mL
1 ounce	= 1 fluid ounce	= 30 mL
1 teacup	= 6 fluid ounces	= 180 mL
1 glass	= 8 fluid ounces	= 240 mL

Notes

27 Cardiopulmonary Procedures

CHAPTER ASSIGNMENTS

√ After Completing	Date Due	Textbook Pages	TEXTBOOK ASSIGNMENTS	Possible Points	Points You Earned
		619-650	Read Chapter 27: Cardiopulmonary Procedures		
		627 648	Read Case Study 1 Case Study 1 questions	5	
		638 648	Read Case Study 2 Case Study 2 questions	5	
			TOTAL POINTS		

√ After Completing	Date Due	Study Guide Pages	STUDY GUIDE ASSIGNMENTS (CTA = Critical Thinking Activity)	Possible Points	Points You Earned
		687	Pretest	10	
		688 689	Term Key Term Assessment A. Definitions B. Word Parts (Add 1 point for each medical term)	21 15	
		690-696	Evaluation of Learning questions	48	
		696	CTA A: Chest Leads	5	
			Evolve Activity: Find That Lead (Record points earned)		
		696	CTA B: ECG Cycle	10	
		698-703	CTA C: GO TO! Game (Record points earned)		
			Evolve Site: It's a Cycle (Record points earned)		
			Evolve Site: It's an Artifact (Record points earned)		
		704-706	CTA D: Myocardial Infarction	20	
		707	CTA E: Crossword Puzzle	22	

√ After Completing	Date Due	Study Guide Pages	STUDY GUIDE ASSIGNMENTS (CTA = Critical Thinking Activity)	Possible Points	Points You Earned
			Evolve Site: Animations	20	
			Evolve Site: Apply Your Knowledge questions	10	
			Evolve Site: Video Evaluation	33	
		687	Posttest	10	
			ADDITIONAL ASSIGNMENTS		
			TOTAL POINTS		

√ When Assigned By Your Instructor	Study Guide Pages	Practices Required	LABORATORY ASSIGNMENTS (Procedure Number and Name)	Score*
	708-709	3	**Practice for Competency** 27-1: Running a 12-Lead, Three-Channel Electrocardiogram Textbook reference: pp. 632-635	
	711-713		**Evaluation of Competency** 27-1: Running a 12-Lead, Three-Channel Electrocardiogram	*
	708-709	3	**Practice for Competency** 27-A: Spirometry Testing Textbook reference: pp. 637-638	
	715-717		**Evaluation of Competency** 27-A: Spirometry Testing	*
	708-709	3	**Practice for Competency** 27-2: Measuring Peak Flow Rate Textbook reference: pp. 642-644	
	719-721		**Evaluation of Competency** 27-2: Measuring Peak Flow Rate	*
			ADDITIONAL ASSIGNMENTS	

Notes

Procedure 27-A: Spirometry Testing

Name: _____   Date: _____

Evaluated by: _____   Score: _____

Performance Objective

Outcome:	Perform a spirometry test.
Conditions:	Using a spirometer.
	Given the following: disposable tubing, disposable mouthpiece, disposable nose clips, waste container.
Standards:	Time: 20 minutes. Student completed procedure in _____ minutes.
	Accuracy: Satisfactory score on the Performance Evaluation Checklist.

Performance Evaluation Checklist

Trial 1	Trial 2	Point Value	Performance Standards
		●	Sanitized hands.
		●	Assembled and prepared equipment.
		●	Calibrated the spirometer.
		▷	Stated the reason for calibrating the spirometer.
		●	Applied a disposable mouthpiece to the mouthpiece holder.
		●	Greeted the patient and introduced yourself.
		●	Identified the patient and explained the procedure.
		●	Asked the patient if he or she prepared properly.
		●	Asked the patient to remove heavy or restrictive clothing, to loosen tight clothing, and to discard gum.
		▷	Explained why tight clothing should be loosened.
		●	Measured the patient's weight and height.
		▷	Explained the reason for measuring weight and height.
		●	Asked the patient to sit near the machine.
		●	Entered patient's data into the computer database of the spirometer.
			Described and demonstrated the breathing maneuver:
		●	Relax and take the deepest breath possible.
		●	Place the mouthpiece in your mouth and seal your lips tightly around it.
		●	Blow out as hard as you can for as long as possible.

715

Trial 1	Trial 2	Point Value	Performance Standards
		●	Do not block the opening of the mouthpiece with your tongue.
		●	Remove the mouthpiece from your mouth.
		▷	Explained why the lips should be tightly sealed around the mouthpiece.
		●	Told the patient the instructions would be repeated during the test.
		●	Encouraged the patient to remain calm.
		●	Gently applied the nose clips.
		▷	Stated the purpose of the nose clips.
		●	Handed mouthpiece to patient.
		●	Began the test and actively coached the patient.
		●	Informed patient of modifications needed if breathing maneuver was not performed correctly.
		●	Continued the test until three acceptable efforts were obtained.
		●	Gently removed the nose clips from patient's nose.
		●	Removed the mouthpiece from its holder.
		●	Disposed of nose clips and mouthpiece in a waste container.
		●	Allowed the patient to remain seated for a few minutes.
		●	Sanitized your hands.
		●	Printed the report and labeled it.
		●	Charted the procedure correctly.
		●	Placed the spirometry report in appropriate location for review by the physician.
		●	Cleaned the spirometer according to the manufacturer's instructions.
		★	Completed the procedure within 20 minutes.
			TOTALS
			CHART
Date			

716

Evaluation of Student Performance

EVALUATION CRITERIA			COMMENTS
Symbol	**Category**	**Point Value**	
✱	Critical Step	16 points	
●	Essential Step	6 points	
▷	Theory Question	2 points	

Score calculation: 100 points

           −   points missed

                        ____ Score

Satisfactory score: 85 or above

CAAHEP Competencies Achieved

Psychomotor (Skills)
☑ I. 4. Perform pulmonary function testing.
☑ I. 11. Perform quality control measures.

Affective (Behavior)
☑ I. 2. Use language/verbal skills that enable patients' understanding.

ABHES Competencies Achieved

☑ 8. cc. Communicate on the recipient's level of comprehension.
☑ 9. o. Perform: (2) Respiratory testing.

Notes

Procedure 27-2: Measuring Peak Flow Rate

Name: _____   Date: _____

Evaluated by: _____   Score: _____

Performance Objective

Outcome:	Measure a patient's peak flow rate.
Conditions:	Using a spirometer.
	Given the following: disposable mouthpiece, waste container.
Standards:	Time: 15 minutes. Student completed procedure in _____ minutes.
	Accuracy: Satisfactory score on the Performance Evaluation Checklist.

Performance Evaluation Checklist

Trial 1	Trial 2	Point Value	Performance Standards
		●	Sanitized hands.
		●	Assembled and prepared equipment.
		●	Moved the sliding indicator to the bottom of the scale.
		▷	Stated why the indicator must be moved to the bottom of the scale.
		●	Applied a disposable mouthpiece to the mouthpiece holder.
		▷	Stated the purpose of the disposable mouthpiece.
		●	Greeted the patient and introduced yourself.
		●	Identified the patient and explained the procedure.
		●	Asked the patient to remove heavy or restrictive clothing, to loosen tight clothing, and to discard any gum.
			Described and demonstrated the breathing maneuver:
		●	Relax and take the deepest breath possible.
		●	Place the mouthpiece in your mouth and seal your lips tightly around it.
		●	Blow out as hard and fast as you can.
		●	Try to move the marker as high as you can on the scale.
		●	Do not block the opening of the mouthpiece with your tongue.
		●	Remove the mouthpiece from your mouth.

			●	Told the patient the instructions would be repeated during the test.
			●	Encouraged the patient to remain calm during the procedure.
			▷	Explained why the patient should remain calm.
			●	Placed a new disposable mouthpiece on the peak flow meter.
			●	Slid the marker to the bottom of the numbered scale.
			●	Handed the peak flow meter to patient.
			●	Instructed patient to stand up straight and look straight ahead.
			●	Began the test and actively coached the patient.
			●	Noted the number where the indicator stopped on the scale and jotted it down on a piece of paper.
			●	Informed patient of modifications needed if breathing maneuver was not performed correctly.
			●	Continued the test until three acceptable efforts were obtained.
			▷	Explained why three acceptable efforts must be obtained.
			●	The numbers from the three tests were about the same.
			▷	Stated the significance of the three numbers being about the same.
			●	Took the peak flow meter from the patient.
			●	Removed the mouthpiece from its holder and discarded it in a waste container.
			●	Sanitized your hands.
			●	Noted the highest of the three peak flow measurements.
			●	Charted the procedure correctly.
			●	Cleaned the peak flow meter.
			▷	Explained how to clean the peak flow meter.
			✳	Completed the procedure within 15 minutes.
				TOTALS
		CHART		
	Date			

Evaluation of Student Performance

EVALUATION CRITERIA			COMMENTS
Symbol	Category	Point Value	
✱	Critical Step	16 points	
●	Essential Step	6 points	
▷	Theory Question	2 points	

Score calculation: 100 points

       −   points missed

             Score

Satisfactory score: 85 or above

CAAHEP Competencies Achieved

Psychomotor (Skills)
☑ I. 4. Perform pulmonary function testing.

Affective (Behavior)
☑ I. 2. Use language/verbal skills that enable patients' understanding.

ABHES Competencies Achieved

☑ 8. cc. Communicate on the recipient's level of comprehension.
☑ 9. o. Perform: (2) Respiratory testing.

Notes

28 Specialty Examinations and Procedures: Colon Procedures, Male Reproductive Health, and Radiology and Diagnostic Imaging

CHAPTER ASSIGNMENTS

√ After Completing	Date Due	Textbook Pages	TEXTBOOK ASSIGNMENTS	Possible Points	Points You Earned
		651-683	Read Chapter 28: Specialty Examinations and Procedures		
		656 680	Read Case Study 1 Case Study 1 questions	5	
		667 680-681	Read Case Study 2 Case Study 2 questions	5	
		677 681	Read Case Study 3 Case Study 3 questions	5	
			TOTAL POINTS		

√ After Completing	Date Due	Study Guide Pages	STUDY GUIDE ASSIGNMENTS (CTA = Critical Thinking Activity)	Possible Points	Points You Earned
		727	? Pretest	10	
		728 728-729	Term Key Term Assessment A. Definitions B. Word Parts (Add 1 point for each medical term)	23 23	
		729-737	Evaluation of Learning questions	76	
		737	CTA A: FOBT Patient Preparation	10	
		738	CTA B: Capsule Endoscopy	25	
		738-739	CTA C: Dear Gabby	10	
		739	CTA D: Lower Gastrointestinal Tract	5	
		739-740	CTA E: Intravenous Pyelogram	5	
		740	CTA F: Magnetic Resonance Imaging	7	
		741	CTA G: Crossword Puzzle	27	
			e Evolve Site: Animations	20	
			e Evolve Site: Apply Your Knowledge questions	12	

√ After Completing	Date Due	Study Guide Pages	STUDY GUIDE ASSIGNMENTS (CTA = Critical Thinking Activity)	Possible Points	Points You Earned
			Evolve Site: Video Evaluation	18	
		727	Posttest	10	
			ADDITIONAL ASSIGNMENTS		
			TOTAL POINTS		

√ When Assigned By Your Instructor	Study Guide Pages	Practices Required	LABORATORY ASSIGNMENTS (Procedure Number and Name)	Score*
	743	5	**Practice for Competency** 28-1 and 28-2: Fecal Occult Blood Testing: Guaiac Slide Test Method and Developing the Hemoccult Slide Test Textbook reference: pp. 657-659 and 660-661	
	745-748		**Evaluation of Competency** 28-1 and 28-2: Fecal Occult Blood Testing: Guaiac Slide Test Method and Developing the Hemoccult Slide Test	*
	743	5	**Practice for Competency** 28-A: Testicular Self-Examination Instructions Textbook reference: pp. 667-668	
	749-750		**Evaluation of Competency** 28-A: Testicular Self-Examination Instructions	*
	744	3	**Practice for Competency** 28-B: Preparation for Radiology Examinations Textbook reference: pp. 668-674	
	751-752		**Evaluation of Competency** 28-B: Preparation for Radiology Examinations	*
	744	3	**Practice for Competency** 28-C: Preparation for Diagnostic Imaging Procedures Textbook reference: pp. 674-675	
	753-754		**Evaluation of Competency** 28-C: Preparation for Diagnostic Imaging Procedures	*
			ADDITIONAL ASSIGNMENTS	

Notes

Procedures 28-1 and 28-2: Fecal Occult Blood Testing: Guaiac Slide Test Method and Developing the Hemoccult Slide Test

Name: _____   Date: _____

Evaluated by: _____   Score: _____

Performance Objective

Outcome:	Instruct an individual in the specimen collection procedure for a Hemoccult slide test and develop the test.
Conditions:	Given the following: Hemoccult slide testing kit, disposable gloves, developing solution, reference card, and a waste container.
Standards:	Time: 15 minutes. Student completed procedures in _____ minutes.
	Accuracy: Satisfactory score in the Performance Evaluation Checklist.

Performance Evaluation Checklist

Trial 1	Trial 2	Point Value	Performance Standards
			Instructions for the Hemoccult slide test
		●	Obtained the Hemoccult slide testing kit.
		●	Checked expiration date on the slides.
		▷	Described what may occur if the slides are outdated.
		●	Greeted the patient and introduced yourself.
		●	Identified the patient and explained purpose of the test.
		●	Informed patient when the test should not be performed.
		●	Instructed patient in the proper preparation required for the test.
		●	Encouraged patient to adhere to the diet modifications.
		▷	Explained why the patient should follow the diet modifications.
		●	Provided patient with the Hemoccult slide test kit.
		●	Instructed patient in completion of the information on the front flap of each card.
		●	Provided instructions on the proper care and storage of the slides.
		▷	Explained why the slides must be stored properly.
			Instructed the patient in the initiation of the test
		●	Began the diet modifications.
		●	Collected a stool specimen from the first bowel movement after the 3-day preparatory period.

Trial 1	Trial 2	Point Value	Performance Standards
			Instructed the patient in the collection of the stool specimen
		●	Filled in the collection date on the front flap.
		●	Used a clean dry container to collect the stool specimen.
		●	Collected the stool sample before it came in contact with toilet bowel water.
		●	Used the wooden applicator to obtain specimen from one part of the stool.
		●	Opened the front flap of the first cardboard slide.
		●	Spread a thin smear of the specimen over the filter paper in the square labeled A.
		●	Obtained another specimen from a different area of the stool, using the other end of the applicator.
		●	Spread a thin smear of the specimen over the filter paper in the square labeled B.
		●	Closed the front flap of the cardboard slide and filled in the date.
		●	Discarded the applicator in a waste container.
		▷	Explained why a sample is collected from two different parts of the stool.
		●	Instructed patient to place slides in a regular envelope to air-dry overnight.
		●	Instructed the patient to continue the testing period on 3 different days until all three specimens have been obtained.
		●	Instructed patient to place the cardboard slides in the foil envelope and return them to the medical office.
		●	Provided patient with an opportunity to ask questions.
		●	Made sure the patient understood the instructions.
		●	Charted the procedure correctly.
			Developing the Hemoccult slide test
		●	Assembled equipment.
		●	Checked expiration date on the developing solution bottle.
		▷	Explained how the solution should be stored.
		●	Sanitized hands and applied gloves.
		●	Opened the back flap of the cardboard slides.
		●	Applied 2 drops of the developing solution to the guaiac test paper underlying the back of each smear.

746

Trial 1	Trial 2	Point Value	Performance Standards
		●	Did not allow the developing solution to come in contact with skin or eyes.
		●	Read results within 60 seconds.
		✱	Results were identical to the evaluator's results.
		▷	Explained why the slides should be read within 60 seconds.
		●	Performed the quality control procedure on each slide.
		●	Read the quality control results after 10 seconds.
		▷	Described what is observed during a normal positive and negative control reaction.
		▷	Stated the purpose of the quality control procedure.
		●	Properly disposed of the slides in a regular waste container.
		●	Removed gloves and sanitized hands.
		●	Charted the results correctly.
		✱	Completed the procedure within 15 minutes.
			TOTALS
CHART			
Date			

Evaluation of Student Performance

EVALUATION CRITERIA			COMMENTS
Symbol	Category	Point Value	
✱	Critical Step	16 points	
●	Essential Step	6 points	
▷	Theory Question	2 points	
Score calculation: 100 points			

Score calculation: 100 points

− _____ points missed

_____ Score

Satisfactory score: 85 or above

CAAHEP Competencies Achieved

Psychomotor (Skills)
☑ I. 11. Perform quality control measures.
☑ IV. 5. Instruct patients according to their needs to promote health maintenance and disease prevention.

Affective (Behavior)
☑ III. 1. Display sensitivity to patient rights and feelings in collecting specimens.

ABHES Competencies Achieved

☑ 8. cc. Communicate on the recipient's level of comprehension.
☑ 10. b. Perform selected CLIA-waived test that assist with diagnosis and treatment: (6) kit testing.
☑ 10. f. Instruct patients in the collection of a fecal specimen.

Procedure 28-A: Testicular Self-Examination Instructions

Name: _____ Date: _____

Evaluated by: _____ Score: _____

Performance Objective

Outcome:	Instruct an individual in the procedure for performing a testicular self-examination (TSE).
Conditions:	None.
Standards:	Time: 10 minutes. Student completed procedure in _____ minutes.
	Accuracy: Satisfactory score on the Performance Evaluation Checklist.

Performance Evaluation Checklist

Trial 1	Trial 2	Point Value	Performance Standards
		●	Greeted the patient and introduced yourself.
		●	Identified patient and explained that you will be instructing the patient in a TSE.
		●	Explained purpose of the examination and when to perform it.
			Instructed the patient as follows:
		●	Take a warm bath or shower.
		●	Stand in front of a mirror.
		●	Inspect for any swelling of the skin of the scrotum.
		●	Place the index and middle fingers of both hands on the underside of one testicle and the thumbs on top of the testicle.
		●	Apply a small amount of pressure, and gently roll the testicle between the thumb and fingers of both hands.
		●	Palpate for lumps, swelling, or any change in the size, shape, or consistency of the testicle.
		▷	Stated the normal characteristics of a testicle.
		●	Locate the epididymis so that you do not confuse it with a lump.
		▷	Stated the characteristics and function of the epididymis.
		●	Repeated the examination on the other testicle.
		●	Report any abnormalities to the physician.
		▷	Stated examples of abnormalities that should be reported.
		●	Charted the procedure correctly.

Trial 1	Trial 2	Point Value	Performance Standards
		✷	Completed the procedure within 10 minutes.
			TOTALS
CHART			
Date			

Evaluation of Student Performance

EVALUATION CRITERIA			COMMENTS
Symbol	**Category**	**Point Value**	
✷	Critical Step	16 points	
●	Essential Step	6 points	
▷	Theory Question	2 points	

Score calculation: 100 points

−   _____ points missed

_____ Score

Satisfactory score: 85 or above

CAAHEP Competencies Achieved

Psychomotor (Skills)
☑ IV. 5. Instruct patients according to their needs to promote health maintenance and disease prevention.
☑ IV. 9. Document patient education.

Affective (Behavior)
☑ I. 2. Use language/verbal skills that enable patients' understanding.
☑ IV. 3. Use appropriate body language and other nonverbal skills in communicating with patients, family, and staff.

ABHES Competencies Achieved

☑ 8. e. Locate resources and information for patients and employers.
☑ 8. cc. Communicate on the recipient's level of comprehension.
☑ 8. ii. Recognize and respond to verbal and nonverbal communication.
☑ 9. r. Teach patients methods of health promotion and disease prevention.

Procedure 28-B: Preparation for Radiology Examinations

Name: _____ Date: _____

Evaluated by: _____ Score: _____

Performance Objective

Outcome:	Instruct a patient in the proper preparation required for each of the following radiographic examinations: mammogram, upper GI, lower GI, and intravenous pyelogram.
Conditions:	Given the following: a patient instruction sheet for each radiographic examination.
Standards:	Time: 15 minutes. Student completed procedure in _____ minutes.
	Accuracy: Satisfactory score in the Performance Evaluation Checklist.

Performance Evaluation Checklist

Trial 1	Trial 2	Point Value	Performance Standards
		●	Greeted and identified patient.
		●	Introduced yourself.
			Instructed patient in the proper preparation for each of the following radiographic examinations:
		●	Mammogram
		●	Bone density scan
		●	Upper GI
		●	Lower GI
		●	Intravenous pyelogram
		●	Charted the procedure correctly.
		✱	Completed the procedure within 15 minutes.
			TOTALS
CHART			
Date			

Evaluation of Student Performance

EVALUATION CRITERIA			COMMENTS
Symbol	Category	Point Value	
✱	Critical Step	16 points	
●	Essential Step	6 points	
▷	Theory Question	2 points	

Score calculation: 100 points

     –   points missed

        Score

Satisfactory score: 85 or above

CAAHEP Competencies Achieved

Psychomotor (Skills)
☑ IV. 6. Prepare a patient for procedures and/or treatments.

Affective (Behavior)
☑ I. 2. Use language/verbal skills that enable patient's understanding.

ABHES Competencies Achieved

☑ 8. cc. Communicate on the recipient's level of communication.
☑ 9. l. Prepare the patient for examinations and treatments.

Procedure 28-C: Preparation for Diagnostic Imaging Procedures

Name: _____ Date: _____

Evaluated by: _____ Score: _____

Performance Objective

Outcome:	Instruct a patient in the proper preparation required for each of the following diagnostic imaging procedures: ultrasonography, computed tomography, magnetic resonance imaging, and nuclear medicine.
Conditions:	Given the following: a patient instruction sheet for each diagnostic imaging procedure.
Standards:	Time: 15 minutes. Student completed procedure in _____ minutes.
	Accuracy: Satisfactory score in the Performance Evaluation Checklist.

Performance Evaluation Checklist

Trial 1	Trial 2	Point Value	Performance Standards
		●	Greeted and identified patient.
		●	Introduced yourself.
			Instructed patient in the proper preparation for each of the following diagnostic imaging procedures:
		●	Ultrasonography
		●	Computed tomography
		●	Magnetic resonance imaging
		●	Nuclear medicine
		●	Charted the procedure correctly.
		★	Completed the procedure within 15 minutes.
		TOTALS	
CHART			
Date			

753

Evaluation of Student Performance

EVALUATION CRITERIA			COMMENTS
Symbol	**Category**	**Point Value**	
✱	Critical Step	16 points	
●	Essential Step	6 points	
▷	Theory Question	2 points	

Score calculation: 100 points

    −   _____ points missed

       _____ Score

Satisfactory score: 85 or above

CAAHEP Competencies Achieved

Psychomotor (Skills)
☑ IV. 6. Prepare a patient for procedures and/or treatments.

Affective (Behavior)
☑ I. 2. Use language/verbal skills that enable patient's understanding.

ABHES Competencies Achieved

☑ 8. cc. Communicate on the recipient's level of communication.
☑ 9. l. Prepare patient for examinations and treatments.

Introduction to the Clinical Laboratory

CHAPTER ASSIGNMENTS

√ After Completing	Date Due	Textbook Pages	TEXTBOOK ASSIGNMENTS	Possible Points	Points You Earned
		684-716	Read Chapter 29: Introduction to the Clinical Laboratory		
		695 714	Read Case Study 1 Case Study 1 questions	5	
		700 714	Read Case Study 2 Case Study 2 questions	5	
		700 715	Read Case Study 3 Case Study 3 questions	5	
			TOTAL POINTS		
√ After Completing	**Date Due**	**Study Guide Pages**	**STUDY GUIDE ASSIGNMENTS (CTA = Critical Thinking Activity)**	**Possible Points**	**Points You Earned**
		757	Pretest	10	
		758	Term Key Term Assessment	22	
		759-764	Evaluation of Learning questions	43	
		764	CTA A: Laboratory Directory Information	10	
		764-765	CTA B: Specimen Requirements	15	
		765	CTA C: Identifying Abnormal Values	10	
		765-766	CTA D: Laboratory Report	25	
		766	CTA E: Laboratory Directory	9	
		767-768	CTA F: Testing Kit Product Insert (3 points for each section)	42	
		769	CTA G: Crossword Puzzle	29	
			Evolve Site: Apply Your Knowledge questions	10	
		757	Posttest	10	

√ After Completing	Date Due	Study Guide Pages	STUDY GUIDE ASSIGNMENTS (CTA = Critical Thinking Activity)	Possible Points	Points You Earned
			ADDITIONAL ASSIGNMENTS		
			TOTAL POINTS		

√ When Assigned By Your Instructor	Study Guide Page	Practices Required	LABORATORY ASSIGNMENTS (Procedure Number and Name)	Score*
	761	3	Practice for Competency 29-A: Laboratory Requisition Form Textbook reference: pp. 691-695	

Name _____ Date _____

True or False

_____ 1. When the body is in homeostasis, an imbalance exists in the body.

_____ 2. A routine test is performed to assist in the early detection of disease.

_____ 3. The laboratory request form provides the outside laboratory with information needed to test the specimen.

_____ 4. The clinical diagnosis is indicated on a laboratory request to correlate laboratory data with the needs of the physician.

_____ 5. The purpose of a laboratory report is to indicate the patient's diagnosis.

_____ 6. A patient who is fasting in preparation for a laboratory test is permitted to drink diet soda.

_____ 7. A small sample taken from the body to represent the nature of the whole is known as a *specimen*.

_____ 8. A laboratory report marked QNS means that the patient did not prepare properly.

_____ 9. Fecal occult blood testing is an example of a CLIA-waived test.

_____ 10. The purpose of quality control is to prevent accidents in the laboratory.

? POSTTEST

True or False

_____ 1. Laboratory tests are most frequently ordered by the physician to assist in the diagnosis of pathologic conditions.

_____ 2. A laboratory directory indicates the patient preparation required for laboratory tests.

_____ 3. Laboratory tests called *profiles* contain a number of different tests.

_____ 4. A lipid profile includes a test for glucose.

_____ 5. The purpose of patient preparation for a laboratory test is to ensure the test results fall within the reference range.

_____ 6. A comprehensive metabolic profile requires that the patient fast.

_____ 7. Antibiotics taken by the patient before the collection of a throat specimen for culture may produce a false-positive result.

_____ 8. The purpose of CLIA is to prevent exposure of employees to bloodborne pathogens.

_____ 9. If a POL is performing moderate-complexity tests, CLIA requires that two levels of controls be run daily.

_____ 10. *In vitro* means occurring in the living body.

Chapter **29** **Introduction to the Clinical Laboratory**

Directions: Match each medical term with its definition.

_____ 1. Analyte

_____ 2. Calibration

_____ 3. Clinical diagnosis

_____ 4. Control

_____ 5. Fasting

_____ 6. Homeostasis

_____ 7. In vivo

_____ 8. Laboratory test

_____ 9. Nonwaived test

_____ 10. Plasma

_____ 11. Product insert

_____ 12. Profile

_____ 13. Qualitative test

_____ 14. Quality control

_____ 15. Quantitative test

_____ 16. Reagent

_____ 17. Reference range

_____ 18. Routine test

_____ 19. Serum

_____ 20. Specimen

_____ 21. Test system

_____ 22. Waived test

A. Liquid part of the blood, consisting of a clear, yellowish fluid that comprises approximately 55% of the total blood volume

B. State in which body systems are functioning normally and the internal environment of the body is in equilibrium; the body is in a healthy state

C. Array of laboratory tests for identifying a disease state or evaluating a particular organ or organ system

D. Printed document supplied by the manufacturer with a laboratory test product that contains information on the proper storage and use of the product

E. Solution that is used to monitor a test system to ensure the reliability and accuracy of the test results

F. Test that indicates whether a substance is present in the specimen being tested and provides an approximate indication of the amount of the substance present

G. Application of methods to ensure that test results are reliable and valid and that errors are detected and eliminated

H. Occurring in the living body or organism

I. Test that indicates the exact amount of a chemical substance that is present in the body, with the results being reported in measurable units

J. Substance that is being identified or measured in a laboratory test

K. Substance that produces a reaction with a patient specimen that allows detection or measurement of the substance by the test system

L. A certain established and acceptable parameter of reference range within which the laboratory test results of a healthy individual are expected to fall

M. Tentative diagnosis of a patient's condition obtained through the evaluation of the health history and the physical examination, without the benefit of laboratory or diagnostic tests

N. Abstaining from food or fluids (except water) for a specified amount of time before the collection of a specimen

O. Laboratory test that meets the CLIA criteria for being a simple procedure that is easy to perform and has a low risk of erroneous test results

P. Laboratory test performed routinely on apparently healthy patients to assist in the early detection of disease

Q. Clear, straw-colored part of the blood (plasma) that remains after the solid elements and the clotting factor fibrinogen have been separated from it

R. Mechanism to check the precision and accuracy of a test system, such as an automated analyzer

S. Small sample of something taken to show the nature of the whole

T. Clinical analysis and study of materials, fluids, or tissues obtained from patients to assist in diagnosis and treatment of disease

U. Setup that includes all of the test components required to perform a laboratory test such as testing devices, controls, and testing reagents

V. Complex laboratory test that does not meet the CLIA criteria for waiver and is subject to the CLIA regulations

Directions: Fill in each blank with the correct answer.

1. What is the general purpose of a laboratory test?

_____

_____

_____

2. List five specific uses of laboratory test results.

_____

_____

_____

_____

_____

3. What is the purpose of performing a routine test?

_____

_____

4. What is the purpose of CLIA?

_____

_____

5. What requirements must be followed regarding a refrigerator used to store specimens and testing components?

_____

_____

6. What temperature is usually required for storing testing materials and performing laboratory tests?

_____

7. What information is included in a laboratory directory?

_____

_____

_____

8. What is the purpose of a laboratory request?

_____

_____

9. What is the reason for indicating the following information on the laboratory request form?

   a. Patient's age and gender:

_____

_____

   b. Date and time of collection of the specimen:

_____

_____

   c. Source of the specimen:

_____

_____

   d. Physician's clinical diagnosis:

_____

_____

   e. Medications the patient is taking:

_____

_____

10. How does a laboratory report the results when a laboratory request is marked STAT?

_____

_____

_____

11. What tests are included in the following profiles?

   a. Comprehensive metabolic profile:

_____

_____

   b. Hepatic function profile:

_____

_____

   c. Prenatal profile:

_____

_____

12. What information is included on laboratory reports?

_____

_____

_____

_____

13. Why must the test results of specimens tested by an outside laboratory be compared with the reference ranges supplied by the laboratory?

_____

_____

_____

14. How are laboratory reports delivered to the medical office?

_____

_____

15. If a laboratory request form is completed on a computer, how is it transmitted to the laboratory?

_____

_____

_____

16. Why do some laboratory tests require advance patient preparation?

_____

_____

_____

17. Why is it important to explain the reason for the advance preparation to the patient?

_____

_____

18. Why are fasting specimens usually collected in the morning?

_____

_____

_____

19. What is a specimen?

_____

_____

20. List 10 examples of specimens.

_____

_____

_____

_____

_____

21. What reference source should be used to locate the specimen collection and handling requirements for the following?

    a. Specimen transported to an outside laboratory:

    _____

    b. Specimen tested in the medical office:

    _____

22. Why must the appropriate container be used to collect a specimen?

    _____

    _____

23. What is a unique identifier?

    _____

    _____

24. What two methods can be used to label a specimen?

    _____

    _____

25. Why is it important to properly identify a patient?

    _____

26. Why must a specimen be properly handled and stored?

    _____

    _____

27. List the CLIA-waived tests that are most frequently performed in the medical office.

    _____

    _____

    _____

    _____

28. What is included in a laboratory testing kit?

    _____

    _____

29. What may occur if a testing kit is outdated?

    _____

    _____

30. What is a unitized testing device?

    _____

    _____

31. Describe a CLIA-waived automated analyzer.

_____

_____

32. What is the purpose of quality control?

_____

_____

33. What are the storage requirements for most testing systems?

_____

_____

34. What should be written on the label of a control that is stable only for a certain period of time after opening it?

_____

_____

35. What is an internal control?

_____

36. An internal control checks for what conditions?

_____

_____

37. What is the purpose of an external control?

_____

_____

38. What types of results are produced by the following controls?

    a. Low-level control:

    _____

    b. High-level control:

    _____

39. What may cause a control to fail to produce expected results?

_____

_____

40. What may cause invalid test results to occur when testing a specimen with a testing kit?

_____

_____

41. What is the difference between qualitative test results and quantitative test results?

_____

_____

42. List 10 laboratory safety guidelines that should be followed in the medical office to prevent accidents from occurring.

_____

_____

_____

_____

_____

CRITICAL THINKING ACTIVITIES

A. Laboratory Directory Information
Look at a laboratory directory (from an outside medical laboratory), and list the categories of information included in it (e.g., normal range of laboratory tests).

_____

_____

_____

_____

_____

_____

B. Specimen Requirements
Refer to Table 29-1 in your textbook, and list the specimen requirements for each of the following tests:

1. ALT _____

2. Bilirubin, total _____

3. Blood group (ABO) and Rh Type _____

4. BUN, serum _____

5. Calcium_____

6. CBC (with differential) _____

7. CRP _____

8. Glucose, plasma _____

9. LD _____

10. PT/INR _____

11. RPR _____

12. Sedimentation rate (ESR) _____

764

13. Thyroxine (T$_4$) _____

14. Triglycerides _____

15. Urinalysis _____

C. Identifying Abnormal Values

Refer to the laboratory report in your textbook (Figure 29-5), and circle any abnormal values using a red pen.

D. Laboratory Report

Refer to the laboratory report in your textbook (Figure 29-5). Using the normal values listed on this report, determine whether the following tests fall within normal ranges or whether they are high or low. Mark each test according to the following: **N** = normal, **H** = high, **L** = low. Your patient is an adult female.

1. Glucose: 140 mg/dL _____

2. BUN: 15 mg/dL _____

3. Creatinine: 1.7 mg/dL _____

4. Calcium: 10.2 mg/dL _____

5. Magnesium: 0.4 mmol/L _____

6. Sodium: 156 mmol/L _____

7. Potassium: 5.5 mmol/L _____

8. Chloride: 84 mmol/L _____

9. Carbon dioxide: 18 mmol/L _____

10. Uric acid: 5.2 mg/dL _____

11. Total protein: 4.0 g/dL _____

12. Albumin: 3.5 g/dL _____

13. Total bilirubin: 0.8 mg/dL _____

14. Alkaline phosphatase: 80 U/L _____

15. LD: 132 U/L _____

16. AST: 24 U/L _____

17. ALT: 44 U/L _____

18. Total cholesterol: 260 mg/dL _____

19. HDL cholesterol: 57 mg/dL _____

20. LDL cholesterol: 165 mg/dL _____

21. WBC: 15.5 ($\times 10^3$/mm^3) _____

22. Hemoglobin: 10.4 g/dL _____

23. Hematocrit: 34% _____

24. Prothrombin time: 10 seconds _____

25. Neutrophils: 84% _____

E. Laboratory Directory

Your physician has ordered a triglyceride test on a patient that will be analyzed at an outside laboratory. You are required to collect the specimen and prepare it for transport to the outside laboratory. Using Figure 29-9 in your textbook as a reference, respond to the following questions in the space provided.

1. What is the amount and type of specimen required for this test?

_____

2. What patient preparation is required for this test?

_____

_____

3. What collection supplies are required for this test?

_____

4. What collection techniques must be performed after collecting the specimen?

_____

_____

5. How should you store the specimen while awaiting pickup by the laboratory?

_____

_____

6. What would cause the laboratory to reject the specimen?

_____

_____

7. What are the limitations of this test?

_____

_____

_____

8. When would be the best time to collect this specimen (AM or PM)? Explain the reason for your answer.

_____

_____

_____

9. When the laboratory report is returned, the triglyceride test results are 250 mg/dL. How is this interpreted: desirable, borderline high, high, or very high?

_____

F. Testing Kit Product Insert

Obtain a product insert from a CLIA-waived testing kit. The product insert can be obtained from an actual testing kit or from a Google search on the Internet. Provide a brief description of the information included in each section of the product insert in the space provided. Examples of brand names of CLIA-waived testing kits include the following:

Hemoccult fecal occult blood test

ColoScreen fecal occult blood test

Seracult fecal occult blood test

Hemoccult ICT test

QuickVue iFOB test

OSOM Mono test

Clearview Mono Test

QuickVue hCG pregnancy test

OSOM hCG urine pregnancy test

ICON hCG urine pregnancy test

QuickVue In-Line Strep A test

OSOM Ultra Strep A test

ICON DS Strep A test

Acceava Strep A test

Name of Testing Kit: _____

Section	Brief description of information included in this section of the product insert
Intended use	
Summary and explanation	
Principles of the procedure	
Precautions and warnings	
Reagents and materials provided	
Materials not provided	
Storage and stability	
Specimen collection and handling	
Test procedure	
Interpretation and reading results	
Quality control	
Limitations of the procedure	
Expected values	
Performance characteristics	

G. Crossword Puzzle: Introduction to the Clinical Laboratory

Directions: Complete the crossword puzzle using the clues provided.

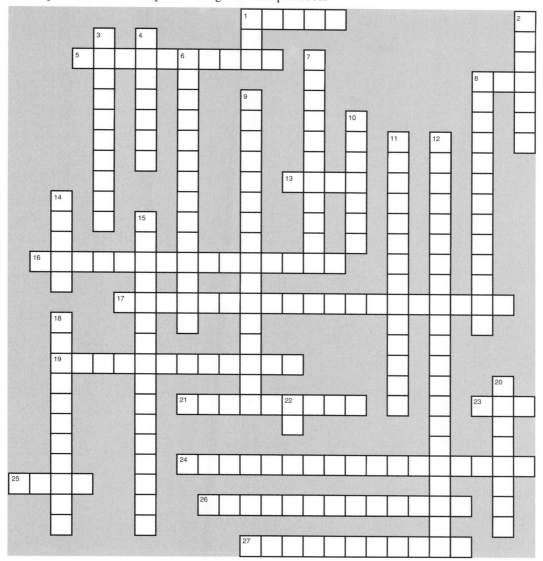

Across

1 For documenting control results
5 Order a laboratory test
8 In-house laboratory
13 As soon as possible
16 Approximate amount of substance present
17 Outside lab reference source
19 Determines CAD risk
21 What are the results?
23 Microscopic analysis of urine (ex)
24 Tentative diagnosis
25 To improve quality of lab testing
26 Complex lab test
27 Detects disease early

Down

1 Not enough specimen?
2 A substance being identified
3 Has a low risk of erroneous test results
4 More than one lab test
6 Accurate and reliable test results
7 Healthy body
8 Provides info on performing lab test
9 Is that you?
10 No food or fluid
11 Where healthy test results should fall
12 Which disease is it?
14 Plasma minus fibrinogen
15 A cause of abnormal control results
18 Test system working ok?
20 Sample of the body
22 CLIA requires 3 times per year

769

Notes

Procedure 29-A: Laboratory Requisition Form. Complete the Laboratory Request form below using a classmate as a patient. The tests that have been ordered by the physician include the following: CBC (with differential), total cholesterol, HDL cholesterol, and plasma glucose.

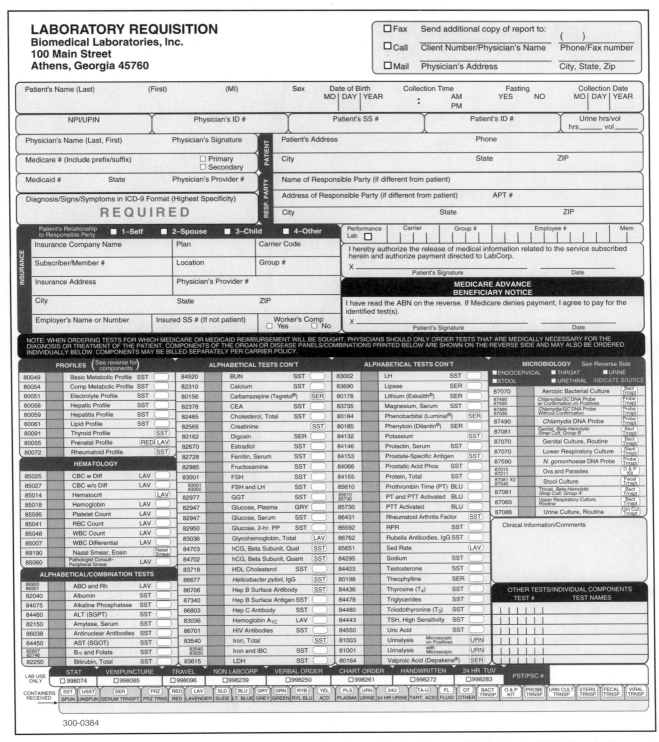

(From Bonewit-West K: *Study guide for clinical procedures for medical assistants.* ed 8, St. Louis, 2011, Saunders)

Notes

30 Urinalysis

CHAPTER ASSIGNMENTS

√ After Completing	Date Due	Textbook Pages	TEXTBOOK ASSIGNMENTS	Possible Points	Points You Earned
		717-744	Read Chapter 30: Urinalysis		
		719 741-742	Read Case Study 1 Case Study 1 questions	5	
		724 742	Read Case Study 2 Case Study 2 questions	5	
		740 742	Read Case Study 3 Case Study 3 questions	5	
			TOTAL POINTS		

√ After Completing	Date Due	Study Guide Pages	STUDY GUIDE ASSIGNMENTS (CTA = Critical Thinking Activity)	Possible Points	Points You Earned
		777	Pretest	10	
		778 778-779	Key Term Assessment A. Definitions B. Word Parts (Add 1 point for each medical term)	23 16	
		779-782	Evaluation of Learning questions	42	
		782	CTA A: First-Voided Specimen	2	
		782	CTA B: Clean-Catch Specimen	4	
		783	CTA C: Urine Testing Kit Instructions	6	
			Evolve Site: Chemical Testing of Urine (Record points earned)		
		784	CTA D: Crossword Puzzle	20	
			Evolve Site: Road to Recovery: Urinalysis Terminology (Record points earned)		
			Evolve Site: Animations	20	
			Evolve Site: Apply Your Knowledge questions	10	

√ After Completing	Date Due	Study Guide Pages	STUDY GUIDE ASSIGNMENTS (CTA = Critical Thinking Activity)	Possible Points	Points You Earned
			e Evolve Site: Video Evaluation	25	
		777	[?] Posttest	10	
			ADDITIONAL ASSIGNMENTS		
			TOTAL POINTS		

√ When Assigned By Your Instructor	Study Guide Pages	Practices Required	LABORATORY ASSIGNMENTS (Procedure Number and Name)	Score*
	785-786	3	**Practice for Competency** 30-1: Clean-Catch Midstream Specimen Collection Instructions Textbook reference: pp. 721-722	
	789-791		**Evaluation of Competency** 30-1: Clean-Catch Midstream Specimen Collection Instructions	*
	785-786	5	**Practice for Competency** 30-A: Assessing Color and Appearance of a Urine Specimen Textbook reference: pp. 722-728	
	793-794		**Evaluation of Competency** 30-A: Assessing Color and Appearance of a Urine Specimen	*
	785-787	5	**Practice for Competency** 30-2: Chemical Testing of Urine with the Multistix 10 SG Reagent Strip Textbook reference: pp. 728-730	
	795-798		**Evaluation of Competency** 30-2: Chemical Testing of Urine with the Multistix 10 SG Reagent Strip	*
	785-786	2	**Practice for Competency** 30-3: Prepare a Urine Specimen for Microscopic Examination: Kova Method Textbook reference: pp. 735-737	
	799-881		**Evaluation of Competency** 30-3: Prepare a Urine Specimen for Microscopic Examination: Kova Method	*
	785-786	2	**Practice for Competency** 30-4: Performing a Urine Pregnancy Test Textbook reference: pp. 740-741	
	803-804		**Evaluation of Competency** 30-4: Performing a Urine Pregnancy Test	*
			ADDITIONAL ASSIGNMENTS	

Notes

Procedure 30-1: Clean-Catch Midstream Specimen Collection Instructions

Name: _____ Date: _____

Evaluated by: _____ Score: _____

Performance Objective

Outcome:	Instruct a patient in the procedure for collecting a clean-catch midstream urine specimen.
Conditions:	Given the following: sterile specimen container, personal antiseptic towelettes, and tissues.
Standards:	Time: 10 minutes. Student completed procedure in _____ minutes.
	Accuracy: Satisfactory score on the Performance Evaluation Checklist.

Performance Evaluation Checklist

Trial 1	Trial 2	Point Value	Performance Standards
		●	Sanitized hands.
		●	Greeted the patient and introduced yourself.
		●	Identified the patient and explained the procedure.
		●	Assembled equipment.
		●	Labeled specimen container.
			Instructed the female patient by telling her to
		●	Wash hands and open antiseptic towelettes.
		●	Remove lid from specimen container without touching inside of container or lid.
		●	Pull down undergarments and sit on the toilet.
		●	Expose the urinary meatus by spreading the labia apart with one hand.
		●	Cleanse each side of the urinary meatus with a front-to-back motion using a separate towelette on each side of the meatus.
		▷	Explained why a front-to-back motion should be used.
		●	After use, discard each towelette into toilet.
		●	Cleanse directly across the meatus using a third towelette and discard it.
		●	Void a small amount of urine into the toilet, while continuing to hold the labia apart.

Trial 1	Trial 2	Point Value	Performance Standards
		▷	Explained the purpose of voiding into the toilet.
		●	Without stopping the urine flow, collect the next amount of urine by voiding into the sterile container.
		●	Fill container approximately half full with urine without touching the inside of the container.
		▷	Stated why the inside of the container should not be touched.
		●	Void the last amount of urine into the toilet.
		●	Replace specimen container lid.
		●	Wipe area dry with a tissue, flush the toilet, and wash hands.
			Instructed the male patient by telling him to
		●	Wash hands and open antiseptic towelettes, and remove lid from specimen container.
		●	Pull down undergarments and stand in front of toilet.
		●	Retract the foreskin of the penis if uncircumcised.
		●	Cleanse area around the meatus and the urethral opening by wiping each side of the meatus with a separate antiseptic towelette.
		●	Cleanse directly across the meatus using a third antiseptic towelette.
		●	Discard each towelette into the toilet after use.
		●	Void a small amount of urine into the toilet.
		●	Collect the next amount of urine by voiding into the sterile container without touching the inside of the container.
		●	Fill container approximately half full with urine.
		●	Void the last amount of urine into the toilet.
		●	Replace lid on specimen container.
		●	Wipe area dry with a tissue, flush the toilet, and wash hands.
			Performed the following:
		●	Provided patient with instructions on what to do with specimen.
		●	Charted the procedure correctly.

Trial 1	Trial 2	Point Value	Performance Standards
		●	Tested specimen or prepared it for transport to an outside laboratory.
		✶	Completed the procedure within 10 minutes.
			TOTALS

CHART	
Date	

Evaluation of Student Performance

EVALUATION CRITERIA			COMMENTS
Symbol	**Category**	**Point Value**	
✶	Critical Step	16 points	
●	Essential Step	6 points	
▷	Theory Question	2 points	

Score calculation: 100 points

    −   _____ points missed

          _____ Score

Satisfactory score: 85 or above

CAAHEP Competencies Achieved

Psychomotor (Skills)
☑ IV. 2. Report relevant information to others succinctly and accurately.

Affective (Behavior)
☑ III. 1. Display sensitivity to patient rights and feelings in collecting specimens.
☑ III. 2. Explain the rationale for performance of a procedure to the patient.

ABHES Competencies Achieved

☑ 8. cc. Communicate on the recipient's level of comprehension.
☑ 10. e. Instruct patients in the collection of a clean-catch midstream urine specimen.

Notes

Procedure 30-A: Assessing Color and Appearance of a Urine Specimen

Name: _____ Date: _____

Evaluated by: _____ Score: _____

Performance Objective

Outcome:	Assess the color and appearance of a urine specimen.
Conditions:	Given a transparent container and a urine specimen.
Standards:	Time: 5 minutes. Student completed procedure in _____ minutes.
	Accuracy: Satisfactory score on the Performance Evaluation Checklist.

Performance Evaluation Checklist

Trial 1	Trial 2	Point Value	Performance Standards
			Color
		●	Sanitized hands and applied gloves.
		●	Transferred urine specimen to a transparent container.
		●	Assessed the color of the urine specimen.
		✱	The assessment was identical to the evaluator's assessment.
		●	Charted the results correctly.
			Appearance
		●	Assessed the appearance of the urine specimen in the transparent container.
		✱	The assessment was identical to the evaluator's assessment.
		●	Charted the results correctly.
		●	Properly disposed of urine specimen.
		●	Sanitized hands and removed gloves.
		✱	Completed the procedure within 5 minutes.
			Totals
		CHART	
Date			

793

Evaluation of Student Performance

EVALUATION CRITERIA			COMMENTS
Symbol	**Category**	**Point Value**	
✱	Critical Step	16 points	
●	Essential Step	6 points	
▷	Theory Question	2 points	

Score calculation: 100 points

− ____ points missed

_____

___ Score

Satisfactory score: 85 or above

CAAHEP Competencies Achieved

Psychomotor (Skills)
☑ I. 14. Perform urinalysis.

Affective (Behavior)
☑ II. 2. Distinguish between normal and abnormal test results.

ABHES Competencies Achieved

☑ 10. b. Perform selected CLIA-waived tests that assist with diagnosis and treatment; (1) urinalysis.

EVALUATION OF COMPETENCY

Procedure 30-2: Chemical Testing of Urine with the Multistix 10 SG Reagent Strip

Name: _____ Date: _____

Evaluated by: _____ Score: _____

Performance Objective

Outcome:	Perform a chemical assessment of a urine specimen.
Conditions:	Given the following: disposable gloves, Multistix 10 SG reagent strips, urine container, laboratory report form, and a waste container.
Standards:	Time: 5 minutes. Student completed procedure in _____ minutes.
	Accuracy: Satisfactory score on the performance evaluation checklist.

Performance Evaluation Checklist

Trial 1	Trial 2	Point Value	Performance Standards
		●	If necessary, performed a quality control testing procedure.
		▷	Stated when a quality control procedure should be performed.
		●	Obtained a freshly voided urine specimen from patient.
		▷	Explained why the container used to collect the specimen should be clean.
		●	Sanitized hands.
		●	Assembled equipment.
		●	Checked expiration date of the reagent strips.
		▷	Stated why expiration date should be checked.
		●	Applied gloves.
		●	Removed a reagent strip from container and recapped immediately.
		▷	Explained why container should be recapped immediately.
		●	Did not touch the test areas with fingers.
		▷	Explained why the test areas should not be touched with fingers.
		●	Mixed the urine specimen thoroughly.
		●	Removed the lid and completely immersed the reagent strip in urine specimen.
		●	Removed the strip immediately and ran the edge against the rim of urine container. Started the timer.
		▷	Explained why excess urine should be removed from the strip.

Trial 1	Trial 2	Point Value	Performance Standards
		●	Held the reagent strip in a horizontal position and placed it as close as possible to the corresponding color blocks on color chart.
		▷	Explained why the strip should be held in a horizontal position.
		●	Read the results at the exact reading times specified on the color chart.
		▷	Explained why the results must be read at specified times.
		✱	The results were identical to the evaluator's results.
		●	Disposed of the strip in a regular waste container.
		●	Removed gloves and sanitized hands.
		●	Charted the results correctly.
		✱	Completed the procedure within 5 minutes.
			TOTALS
			CHART
Date			

Evaluation of Student Performance

EVALUATION CRITERIA			COMMENTS
Symbol	**Category**	**Point Value**	
✱	Critical Step	16 points	
●	Essential Step	6 points	
▷	Theory Question	2 points	

Score calculation: 100 points

  −   points missed
  _____
  ___ Score

Satisfactory score: 85 or above

Multistix® *10 SG Reageant Strips for Urinalysis*

PATIENT

DATE   TIME

LEUKOCYTES	NEGATIVE ☐		TRACE ☐	SMALL ☐ +	MODERATE ☐ ++	LARGE ☐ +++	
NITRITE	NEGATIVE ☐		POSITIVE ☐	POSITIVE ☐	(Any degree of uniform pink color is found)		
UROBILINOGEN	NORMAL ☐ 0.2	NORMAL ☐ 1	mg/dL ☐ 2	4 ☐	8 ☐ (1mg = approx. 1 BU)		
PROTEIN	NEGATIVE ☐	TRACE ☐	mg/dL ☐ 30 *	100 ☐ ++	300 ☐ +++	2000 OR MORE ☐	
pH	5.0 ☐	6.0 ☐	6.5 ☐	7.0 ☐	7.5 ☐	8.0 ☐	8.5 ☐
BLOOD	NEGATIVE ☐	NON-HEMOLYZED ☐ TRACE	NON-HEMOLYZED ☐ MODERATE	HEMOLYZED ☐ TRACE	SMALL ☐ +	MODERATE ☐ ++	LARGE ☐ +++
SPECIFIC GRAVITY	1.000 ☐	1.006 ☐	1.010 ☐	1.015 ☐	1.020 ☐	1.025 ☐	1.030 ☐
KETONE	NEGATIVE ☐	mg/dL	TRACE ☐ 5	SMALL ☐ 15	MODERATE ☐ 40	LARGE ☐ 80	LARGE ☐ 160
BILIRUBIN	NEGATIVE ☐		SMALL ☐ +	MODERATE ☐ ++	LARGE ☐ +++		
GLUCOSE	NEGATIVE ☐	g/L (%) mg/dL	1/10 tr.) ☐ 100	1/6 ☐ 250	1/2 ☐ 500	1 ☐ 1000	2 or more ☐ 2000 or more

(Modified and printed by permission of Siemens Healthcare Diagnostics, Deerfield, Ill, 60015.)

Multistix® 10 SG Reageant Strips for Urinalysis

PATIENT

DATE   TIME

LEUKOCYTES	NEGATIVE ☐		TRACE ☐	SMALL + ☐	MODERATE ☐ ++	LARGE +++ ☐	
NITRITE	NEGATIVE ☐		POSITIVE ☐	POSITIVE ☐	(Any degree of uniform pink color is found)		
UROBILINOGEN	NORMAL 0.2 ☐	NORMAL 1 ☐	mg/dL 2 ☐	4 ☐	8 ☐ (1mg = approx. 1 BU)		
PROTEIN	NEGATIVE ☐	TRACE ☐	mg/dL 30 * ☐	100 ++ ☐	300 +++ ☐	2000 OR MORE ☐	
pH	5.0 ☐	6.0 ☐	6.5 ☐	7.0 ☐	7.5 ☐	8.0 ☐	8.5 ☐
BLOOD	NEGATIVE ☐	NON-HEMOLYZED TRACE ☐	NON-HEMOLYZED MODERATE ☐	HEMOLYZED TRACE ☐	SMALL + ☐	MODERATE ++ ☐	LARGE +++ ☐
SPECIFIC GRAVITY	1.000 ☐	1.006 ☐	1.010 ☐	1.015 ☐	1.020 ☐	1.025 ☐	1.030 ☐
KETONE	NEGATIVE ☐	mg/dL	TRACE 5 ☐	SMALL 15 ☐	MODERATE 40 ☐	LARGE 80 ☐	LARGE 160 ☐
BILIRUBIN	NEGATIVE ☐		SMALL + ☐	MODERATE ++ ☐	LARGE +++ ☐		
GLUCOSE	NEGATIVE ☐	g/L (%) mg/dL	1/10 tr.) 100 ☐	1/6 250 ☐	1/2 500 ☐	1 1000 ☐	2 or more 2000 or more ☐

(Modified and printed by permission of Siemens Healthcare Diagnostics, Deerfield, III, 60015.)

EVALUATION OF COMPETENCY

Procedure 30-3: Prepare a Urine Specimen for Microscopic Examination of Urine: Kova Method

Name: _____   Date: _____

Evaluated by: _____   Score: _____

Performance Objective

Outcome:	Prepare a urine specimen for microscopic analysis by the physician.
Conditions:	Given the following: disposable gloves; first-voided morning urine specimen; Kova urine centrifuge tube, cap, pipet, slide, and stain; test tube rack; urine centrifuge; mechanical stage microscope; and waste container.
Standards:	Time: 15 minutes. Student completed procedure in _____ minutes.
	Accuracy: Satisfactory score on the Performance Evaluation Checklist.

Performance Evaluation Checklist

Trial 1	Trial 2	Point Value	Performance Standards
		●	Sanitized hands.
		●	Assembled equipment.
		●	Applied gloves.
		●	Mixed urine specimen with pipet.
		▷	Stated the purpose of mixing the specimen.
		●	Poured urine specimen into urine centrifuge tube to the 12-mL mark.
		●	Capped the tube.
		●	Centrifuged specimen for 5 minutes.
		▷	Stated the purpose of centrifuging the specimen.
		●	Removed the tube from the centrifuge without disturbing the sediment.
		●	Removed the cap.
		●	Inserted Kova pipet into the urine tube and seated it firmly.
		●	Poured off the supernatant fluid.
		●	Removed pipet from the tube.
		●	Added one drop of Kova stain to the tube.
		▷	Stated the purpose of the stain.
		●	Placed pipet back in tube and mixed specimen thoroughly.
		●	Placed urine tube in test tube rack.
		●	Transferred a sample of the specimen to the Kova slide.

Trial 1	Trial 2	Point Value	Performance Standards
		●	Did not overfill or underfill the well of the Kova slide.
		●	Placed pipet in the urine tube.
		●	Allowed specimen to sit for 1 minute.
		▷	Explained the purpose of allowing the specimen to sit 1 minute.
		●	Properly focused the specimen under low power.
		●	Placed the slide on the stage of the microscope.
		●	Properly focused the specimen for the physician.
		●	Removed the slide from the stage when the physician is finished examining the specimen.
		●	Disposed of the slide and pipet in a regular waste container.
		●	Rinsed the remaining urine down the sink.
		●	Capped the empty urine tube and disposed of it in a regular waste container.
		●	Removed gloves and sanitized hands.
		★	Completed the procedure within 15 minutes.
			TOTALS
			CHART
Date			

Evaluation of Student Performance

EVALUATION CRITERIA			COMMENTS
Symbol	**Category**	**Point Value**	
✶	Critical Step	16 points	
●	Essential Step	6 points	
▷	Theory Question	2 points	

Score calculation: 100 points

         −   points missed

              Score

Satisfactory score: 85 or above

CAAHEP Competencies Achieved

Psychomotor (Skills)
☑ I. 11. Perform quality control measures.
☑ I. 14. Perform urinalysis.

Affective (Behavior)
☑ III. 2. Explain the rationale for performance of a procedure to the patient.

ABHES Competencies Achieved

☑ 10. a. Practice quality control.
☑ 10. b. Perform selected CLIA-waived tests that assist with diagnosis and treatment: (1) Urinalysis.

Notes

Procedure 30-4: Performing a Urine Pregnancy Test

Name: _____   Date: _____

Evaluated by: _____   Score: _____

Performance Objective

Outcome:	Perform a urine pregnancy test.
Conditions:	Given the following: disposable gloves, urine pregnancy testing kit, first-voided morning urine specimen, waste container.
Standards:	Time: 5 minutes. Student completed procedure in _____ minutes.
	Accuracy: Satisfactory score on the Performance Evaluation Checklist.

Performance Evaluation Checklist

Trial 1	Trial 2	Point Value	Performance Standards
		●	Sanitized hands.
		●	Assembled equipment.
		●	Checked the expiration date on the pregnancy test.
		▷	Explained why the expiration date should be checked.
		●	If necessary, ran controls on the pregnancy test.
		▷	Stated when controls should be run.
		●	Applied gloves.
		●	Mixed the urine specimen.
		●	Removed the test cassette from its pouch.
		●	Placed the test cassette on a clean, dry, level surface.
		●	Added 3 drops of urine to the well on the test cassette.
		●	Disposed of the pipet in a regular waste container.
		●	Waited 3 minutes and read the results.
		●	Interpreted the test results.
		★	The results were identical to the evaluator's results.
		▷	Described the appearance of a positive and a negative test result.

Trial 1	Trial 2	Point Value	Performance Standards
		▷	Explained what should be done if a blue control line does not appear.
		●	Disposed of the test cassette in a regular waste container.
		●	Removed gloves and sanitized hands.
		●	Charted the results correctly.
		✶	Completed the procedure within 5 minutes.
			TOTALS

CHART	
Date	

Evaluation of Student Performance

EVALUATION CRITERIA			COMMENTS
Symbol	**Category**	**Point Value**	
✶	Critical Step	16 points	
●	Essential Step	6 points	
▷	Theory Question	2 points	

Score calculation: 100 points

     −   _____ points missed

         ___ Score

Satisfactory score: 85 or above

CAAHEP Competencies Achieved

Psychomotor (Skills)
☑ I. 11. Perform quality control measures.
☑ I. 16. Screen test results.

Affective (Behavior)
☑ II. 2. Distinguish between normal and abnormal test results.

ABHES Competencies Achieved

☑ 10. a. Practice quality control.
☑ 10. b. Perform selected CLIA-waived tests that assist with diagnosis and treatment: (6) kit testing (a) pregnancy.

31 Phlebotomy

CHAPTER ASSIGNMENTS

√ After Completing	Date Due	Textbook Pages	TEXTBOOK ASSIGNMENTS	Possible Points	Points You Earned
		745-783	Read Chapter 31: Phlebotomy		
		755 781	Read Case Study 1 Case Study 1 questions	5	
		759 781-782	Read Case Study 2 Case Study 2 questions	5	
		771 782	Read Case Study 3 Case Study 3 questions	5	
			TOTAL POINTS		

√ After Completing	Date Due	Study Guide Pages	STUDY GUIDE ASSIGNMENTS (CTA = Critical Thinking Activity)	Possible Points	Points You Earned
		809	Pretest	10	
		810	Key Term Assessment A. Definitions B. Word Parts (Add 1 point for each medical term)	16 13	
		811-815	Evaluation of Learning questions	41	
		815	CTA A: Antecubital Veins	5	
			Evolve Site: Got Blood? (Record points earned)		
		816-817	CTA B: Venipuncture-Vacuum Tube Method	15	
		817-818	CTA C: Venipuncture Situations	7	
		818	CTA D: Skin Puncture	8	
		819	CTA E: Crossword Puzzle	29	
			Evolve Site: Apply Your Knowledge questions	10	
			Evolve Site: Video Evaluation	42	
		809	Posttest	10	

√ After Completing	Date Due	Study Guide Pages	STUDY GUIDE ASSIGNMENTS (CTA = Critical Thinking Activity)	Possible Points	Points You Earned
			ADDITIONAL ASSIGNMENTS		
			TOTAL POINTS		

√ When Assigned By Your Instructor	Study Guide Pages	Practices Required	LABORATORY ASSIGNMENTS (Procedure Number and Name)	Score*
	821-822	5	**Practice for Competency** 31-1: Venipuncture—Vacuum Tube Method Textbook reference: pp. 760-765	
	823-826		**Evaluation of Competency** 31-1: Venipuncture—Vacuum Tube Method	*
	821-822	5	**Practice for Competency** 31-2: Venipuncture—Butterfly Method Textbook reference: pp. 767-771	
	827-830		**Evaluation of Competency** 31-2: Venipuncture— Butterfly Method	*
	821-822	3	**Practice for Competency** 31-3: Skin Puncture— Disposable Semiautomatic Lancet Device Textbook reference: pp. 779-781	
	831-833		**Evaluation of Competency** 31-3: Skin Puncture— Disposable Semiautomatic Lancet Device	*
	821-822	3	**Practice for Competency** 31-A: Skin Puncture— Reusable Semiautomatic Lancet Device Textbook reference: pp. 776-779	
	835-837		**Evaluation of Competency** 31-A: Skin Puncture— Reusable Semiautomatic Lancet Device	*
			ADDITIONAL ASSIGNMENTS	

Notes

Name _____   Date _____

True or False

_____ 1. An individual who collects blood specimens is known as a vampire.

_____ 2. The purpose of applying a tourniquet when performing venipuncture is to make the patient's veins stand out.

_____ 3. The tourniquet should be left on the patient's arm for at least 2 minutes before performing a venipuncture.

_____ 4. Serum is obtained from whole blood that has been centrifuged.

_____ 5. A 25-gauge needle is recommended for performing venipuncture.

_____ 6. The size of the evacuated tube used to obtain a venous blood specimen depends on the size of the patient's veins.

_____ 7. A correct order of draw for the vacuum tube method of venipuncture is red, lavender, gray, and green.

_____ 8. Veins are most likely to collapse in patients with large veins and thick walls.

_____ 9. Hemolysis of a blood specimen results in inaccurate test results.

_____ 10. When obtaining a capillary specimen, the first drop of blood should be used for the test.

?≡ **POSTTEST**

True or False

_____ 1. Venous reflux can be prevented by filling the evacuated tube to the exhaustion of the vacuum.

_____ 2. If the tourniquet is applied too tightly, inaccurate test results may occur.

_____ 3. The median cubital vein is the best vein to use for venipuncture.

_____ 4. On standing, a blood specimen to which an anticoagulant has been added separates into plasma, buffy coat, and blood cells.

_____ 5. Whole blood is obtained by using a tube containing an anticoagulant.

_____ 6. An evacuated glass tube with a lavender stopper contains EDTA.

_____ 7. A red-stoppered tube is used to collect a blood specimen for most blood chemistries.

_____ 8. Not filling a tube to the exhaustion of the vacuum can result in hemolysis of the blood specimen.

_____ 9. If the needle is removed from the arm before removing the tourniquet, the evacuated tube will not fill completely.

_____ 10. If a fibrin clot forms in the serum layer of a blood specimen, it will lead to inaccurate test results.

A. Definitions

Directions: Match each medical term with its definition.

_____ 1. Antecubital space

_____ 2. Anticoagulant

_____ 3. Buffy coat

_____ 4. Evacuated tube

_____ 5. Hematoma

_____ 6. Hemoconcentration

_____ 7. Hemolysis

_____ 8. Osteochondritis

_____ 9. Osteomyelitis

_____ 10. Phlebotomist

_____ 11. Phlebotomy

_____ 12. Plasma

_____ 13. Serum

_____ 14. Venipuncture

_____ 15. Venous reflux

_____ 16. Venous stasis

A. The liquid part of blood, consisting of a clear, straw-colored fluid that makes up approximately 55% of the blood volume

B. A substance that inhibits blood clotting

C. Health professional trained in the collection of blood specimens

D. The breakdown of blood cells

E. A closed glass or plastic tube that contains a premeasured vacuum

F. The temporary cessation or slowing of the venous blood flow

G. A thin, light-colored layer of white blood cells and platelets that lies between a top layer of plasma and a bottom layer of red blood cells when an anticoagulant has been added to a blood specimen

H. The surface of the arm in front of the elbow

I. Inflammation of bone and cartilage

J. An increase in the concentration of the nonfilterable blood components

K. Plasma from which the clotting factor fibrinogen has been removed

L. Incision of a vein for the removal of blood

M. Inflammation of the bone or bone marrow as a result of bacterial infection

N. A swelling or mass of coagulated blood caused by a break in a blood vessel

O. Puncturing of a vein

P. The backflow of blood (from an evacuated tube) into the patient's vein

B. Word Parts

Directions: Indicate the meaning of each word part in the space provided. List as many medical terms as possible that incorporate the word part in the space provided.

Word Part	Meaning of Word Part	Medical Terms That Incorporate Word Part
1. ante-		
2. anti-		
3. hemat/o		
4. -oma		
5. hem/o		
6. lysis		
7. oste/o		
8. myel/o		
9. -itis		
10. phleb/o		
11. -otomy		
12. ven/o		
13. -ous		

810

Directions: Fill in each blank with the correct answer.

1. List the three major areas of blood collection included in phlebotomy.

2. What is the purpose of performing a venipuncture?

3. List methods that can be used to perform a venipuncture.

4. What are the advantages of using the vacuum tube method of venipuncture?

5. When would the butterfly method of venipuncture be preferred over the vacuum tube method?

6. What reference source should be consulted for collection and handling requirements in the following situations?

    a. The specimen is being transported to an outside laboratory for testing:

    b. The specimen is being tested in the medical office:

7. Why should a patient be identified using two forms of identification?

8. What is a unique identifier?

9. Explain how to prevent venous reflux.

10. What is the purpose of the tourniquet?

_____

_____

11. Why are the antecubital veins preferred for performing a venipuncture?

_____

_____

_____

12. After locating a suitable vein for venipuncture, what three qualities should be determined with respect to the vein?

_____

_____

_____

13. List four techniques that can be used to make veins more prominent.

_____

_____

_____

_____

14. Why should the veins of the hand be used only as a last resort when performing a venipuncture?

_____

_____

_____

15. How is a serum specimen obtained?

_____

_____

16. How is a whole blood specimen obtained?

_____

_____

17. List the three layers into which blood separates when it is mixed with an anticoagulant.

_____

_____

18. List the layers into which blood separates when an anticoagulant is not added to it.

_____

_____

19. List six OSHA safety precautions that must be followed when performing a venipuncture and separating serum or plasma from whole blood.

_____

_____

_____

_____

20. What are the ranges for the gauge and length of the needle used for the vacuum tube method of venipuncture?

_____

_____

21. What is the purpose of the flange on the plastic holder of the vacuum tube system?

_____

_____

22. What type of additive is present in each of the following evacuated tubes?

Red _____

Red/gray speckled _____

Lavender _____

Light blue _____

Green _____

Gray_____

Royal blue _____

23. What color stopper must be used to collect the blood specimen for each of the tests listed?

Complete blood count _____

Prothrombin time _____

Glucose tolerance test _____

Most blood chemistry tests _____

Blood gas determinations _____

Lead testing _____

24. Why is it important to use the correct order of draw when performing a venipuncture?

_____

_____

25. Why is it important to mix a tube containing an anticoagulant immediately after drawing it?

_____

_____

26. What are the ranges for the gauge and length of needle used for the butterfly method of venipuncture?

_____

_____

27. How can a vein be prevented from rolling when performing a venipuncture on the cephalic or basic veins?

_____

_____

28. What is typically observed when performing a venipuncture on a vein that collapses?

_____

_____

29. What are three ways in which a hematoma may occur?

_____

_____

_____

30. List four ways to prevent a blood specimen from becoming hemolyzed.

_____

_____

_____

_____

31. List examples of substances dissolved in the serum of blood.

_____

_____

_____

32. What is the purpose of performing laboratory tests on serum?

_____

_____

_____

33. List the proper size tube that must be used to obtain the following serum specimens:

2 mL of serum_____

6 mL of serum_____

4 mL of serum_____

34. What is a fibrin clot, and why should it be avoided in a serum specimen?

_____

_____

_____

35. How does a serum separator tube function in the collection of a serum specimen?

_____

_____

_____

36. What is the preferred site for a skin puncture for the following individuals?

    a. Adult _____

    b. Infant _____

37. Why is it important not to penetrate the skin too deeply when performing a skin puncture?

_____

_____

38. How does the medical assistant determine the blade length to use to perform a skin puncture?

_____

_____

39. What are two examples of microcollection devices?

_____

_____

40. Why should a finger puncture not be performed on the index finger?

_____

_____

41. Why should the first drop of blood be wiped away when performing a finger puncture?

_____

_____

CRITICAL THINKING ACTIVITIES

A. Antecubital Veins

Practice palpating the antecubital veins on at least five classmates. Use a tourniquet applied to each person's arm, and ask the individual to clench his or her fist. Record the individual's name and which vein would be considered the best to use on each person when performing venipuncture.

NAME	SUITABLE VEIN
1. _____	_____
2. _____	_____
3. _____	_____
4. _____	_____
5. _____	_____

B. Venipuncture—Vacuum Tube Method

Using the principles outlined in the vacuum tube venipuncture procedure, state what can happen under the following circumstances:

1. An evacuated tube is used that is past its expiration date.

   _____

   _____

2. The vacuum tube is not labeled.

   _____

   _____

3. The tourniquet is not applied tightly enough.

   _____

   _____

4. The tourniquet is left on for more than 1 minute.

   _____

   _____

5. The area that has just been cleansed with an antiseptic is not allowed to dry before the venipuncture is made.

   _____

   _____

6. The evacuated tube is inserted past the indentation in the plastic holder before the vein is entered.

   _____

   _____

7. An angle of less than 15 degrees is used when performing venipuncture.

   _____

   _____

8. An angle of more than 15 degrees is used when performing venipuncture.

   _____

   _____

9. The needle is moved after inserting it.

   _____

   _____

10. Venous reflux occurs when using an EDTA evacuated tube.

    _____

    _____

11. The vacuum tube is removed before it has filled to the exhaustion of the vacuum.

_____

_____

12. The needle is removed from the arm before the tourniquet has been removed.

_____

_____

13. A gauze pad is not placed slightly above the puncture site before removing the needle.

_____

_____

14. The patient bends the arm at the elbow after the needle is removed.

_____

_____

15. The patient lifts a heavy object after the procedure.

_____

_____

C. Venipuncture Situations

You are responsible for performing the venipunctures in your medical office. In the space provided, explain what you would do in each of the following situations:

1. The patient asks you if the venipuncture will hurt.

_____

_____

2. On palpating the patient's vein, you find that it feels stiff and hard.

_____

_____

3. You have attempted one venipuncture in a patient with small veins using the vacuum tube method of venipuncture; however, the vein collapsed, and you were unable to obtain blood.

_____

_____

4. The patient moves during the procedure, causing the needle to come out of his or her arm.

_____

_____

5. You have inserted the needle in the vein but notice a sudden swelling around the puncture site.

_____

_____

6. You inadvertently puncture the brachial artery after inserting the needle.

_____

_____

7. The patient begins to sweat and tells you that he or she feels warm and light-headed.

_____

_____

D. Skin Puncture

The medical assistant is performing a skin puncture on an adult patient to obtain a capillary blood specimen for a hemoglobin test. For each of the following situations, write **C** if the technique is correct and **I** if the technique is incorrect. If the technique is correct, explain the rationale for performing it that way; if incorrect, explain what might happen if the technique were performed in the incorrect manner.

_____ 1. Before making the puncture, the medical assistant asks the patient to rinse his or her hand in warm water.

_____

_____

_____ 2. The puncture is made with the patient in a standing position.

_____

_____

_____ 3. The site is allowed to dry thoroughly after it is cleansed with an antiseptic wipe.

_____

_____

_____ 4. The specimen is collected from the lateral part of the tip of the ring finger.

_____

_____

_____ 5. The puncture is made perpendicular to the lines of the fingerprint.

_____

_____

_____ 6. The depth of the puncture is 4 mm.

_____

_____

_____ 7. The first drop of blood is wiped away.

_____

_____

_____ 8. The puncture site is squeezed to obtain the blood specimen.

_____

_____

E. Crossword Puzzle: Phlebotomy

Directions: Complete the crossword puzzle using the clues provided.

Across

1 What BP does during fainting
3 Makes RBCs clot quicker
6 Rolling vein
8 Best VP vein
9 Inflammation of bone and cartilage
10 Outdated tube problem
11 Inhibits blood clotting
13 Faint position
14 PT tube
18 EDTA tube
19 Backflow of blood
21 For small veins
23 Broken RBCs
24 Bad bruise
25 No additive tube
26 Based on size of pt's finger

Down

2 In front of the elbow
3 Select lavender tube for this test
4 Collects blood
5 First drop of capillary blood?
7 Contains a "separating" gel
9 Time limit for tourniquet
12 Do not use for skin puncture
15 Fluoride/oxalate tube
16 Don't use to palpate vein
17 WBCs and platelets
20 Fainting warning signal
22 Color of serum
23 Last choice veins

Notes

Procedure 31-1: Venipuncture Vacuum Tube Method. Practice the procedure for collecting a venous blood specimen using the vacuum tube method. Record the procedure in the chart provided.

Procedure 31-2: Venipuncture Butterfly Method. Practice the procedure for collecting a venous blood specimen using the butterfly method. Record the procedure in the chart provided.

Procedure 31-3: Disposable Lancet. Obtain a capillary blood specimen using a disposable semiautomatic lancet device.

Procedure 31-A: Reusable Lancet. Obtain a capillary blood specimen using a reusable semiautomatic lancet.

CHART	
Date	

821

CHART	
Date	

Chapter **31**   **Phlebotomy**

Procedure 31-1: Venipuncture—Vacuum Tube Method

Name: _____ Date: _____

Evaluated by: _____ Score: _____

Performance Objective

Outcome:	Perform a venipuncture using the vacuum tube method.
Conditions:	Given the following: disposable gloves, tourniquet, antiseptic wipe, double-pointed needle, plastic holder, evacuated tubes with labels, gauze pad, adhesive bandage, biohazard sharps container, biohazard specimen bag, and a laboratory request form.
Standards:	Time: 10 minutes. Student completed procedure in _____ minutes.
	Accuracy: Satisfactory score on the Performance Evaluation Checklist.

Performance Evaluation Checklist

Trial 1	Trial 2	Point Value	Performance Standards
		●	Reviewed requirements for collecting and handling the blood specimen.
		●	Sanitized hands.
		●	Greeted the patient and introduced yourself.
		●	Identified the patient.
		●	Asked patient if he or she prepared properly.
			Prepared the equipment
		●	Assembled equipment.
		●	Selected the proper evacuated tubes.
		●	Checked the expiration date of the tubes.
		▷	Stated the purpose of checking the expiration date.
		●	Labeled the evacuated tubes.
		●	Completed a laboratory request form, if necessary.
		●	Screwed the plastic holder onto the Luer adapter and tightened securely.
		●	Opened the gauze packet.
		●	Positioned the evacuated tubes in the correct order of draw.
		●	Tapped evacuated tubes with a powdered additive below the stopper.
		▷	Stated the purpose for tapping the tube.
		●	Placed the first tube loosely in the plastic holder.

Trial 1	Trial 2	Point Value	Performance Standards
			Prepared the patient
		●	Explained the procedure to the patient and reassured patient.
		●	Performed a preliminary assessment of both arms.
		●	Correctly applied the tourniquet.
		●	Asked patient to clench fist.
		▷	Stated the purpose of the tourniquet and clenched fist.
		●	Assessed the veins of both arms.
		●	Determined the best vein to use.
		●	Positioned the patient's arm correctly.
		●	Thoroughly palpated the selected vein.
		●	Did not leave the tourniquet on for more than 1 minute.
		▷	Explained why the tourniquet should not be left on for more than 1 minute.
		●	Removed tourniquet and cleansed the puncture site.
		●	Allowed puncture site to air dry.
		▷	Explained why the site should be allowed to air dry.
		●	Did not touch the site after cleansing.
		●	Placed supplies within comfortable reach of the nondominant hand.
		●	Reapplied tourniquet and applied gloves.
			Performed the venipuncture
		●	Correctly positioned safety shield and removed cap from the needle.
		●	Properly held the venipuncture setup (bevel up) with the dominant hand.
		●	Positioned the tube with the label facing downward.
		▷	Explained why the label should face downward.
		●	Grasped the patient's arm and anchored the vein correctly.
		●	Positioned the venipuncture setup at a 15-degree angle to the arm, with the needle pointing in the same direction as the vein to be entered.
		●	Positioned the needle approximately $1/8$ inch below the place where the vein is to be entered.
		●	Told the patient that a small stick will be felt.

824

Trial 1	Trial 2	Point Value	Performance Standards
		●	With one continuous motion, entered the skin and then the vein.
		●	Stabilized the vacuum tube setup.
		▷	Stated why the vacuum tube setup should be stabilized.
		●	Pushed the tube forward slowly to the end of the holder using the flange.
		●	Allowed evacuated tube to fill to the exhaustion of the vacuum.
		▷	Explained why the tube should be allowed to fill to the exhaustion of the vacuum.
		●	Removed the tube from the plastic holder using the flange.
		●	Immediately and gently inverted tube 5 times if it contained a clot activator and 8 to 10 times if it contained an anticoagulant.
		●	Inserted the next tube into the holder using the flange.
		●	Continued until the last tube was filled.
		✱	Removed the tourniquet and asked the patient to unclench fist.
		●	Removed the last tube from the holder.
		▷	Stated why the last tube should be removed.
		●	Placed gauze pad slightly above puncture site and withdrew the needle slowly and at the same angle as that for penetration.
		●	Immediately moved gauze over puncture site and applied pressure.
		●	Pushed safety shield forward with thumb until audible click is heard.
		●	Properly disposed of holder and needle in a biohazard sharps container.
		●	Instructed patient to apply pressure with the gauze pad for 1 to 2 minutes.
		▷	Stated why pressure should be applied.
		●	Applied adhesive bandage to puncture site.
		●	Placed tube in an upright position in a test tube rack.
		●	Removed gloves and sanitized hands.
		●	Charted the procedure correctly.

Trial 1	Trial 2	Point Value	Performance Standards
		●	Tested specimen or prepared specimen for transport according to medical office policy.
		✷	Completed the procedure within 10 minutes.
			TOTALS
			CHART
Date		

Evaluation of Student Performance

EVALUATION CRITERIA			COMMENTS
Symbol	**Category**	**Point Value**	
✷	Critical Step	16 points	
●	Essential Step	6 points	
▷	Theory Question	2 points	

Score calculation: 100 points

       −   points missed

           ___ Score

Satisfactory score: 85 or above

CAAHEP Competencies Achieved

Psychomotor (Skills)
☑ I. 2. Perform venipuncture.

Affective (Behavior)
☑ I. 1. Apply critical thinking skills in performing patient assessment and care.
☑ IV. I. Demonstrate empathy in communicating with patients, family, and staff.

ABHES Competencies Achieved

☑ 8. bb. Are impartial and show empathy when dealing with patients.
☑ 10. c. Dispose of biohazardous materials.
☑ 10. d. Collect, label, and process specimens: (1) perform venipuncture.

Procedure 31-2: Venipuncture—Butterfly Method

Name: _____   Date: _____

Evaluated by: _____   Score: _____

Performance Objective

Outcome:	Perform a venipuncture using the butterfly method.
Conditions:	Given the following: disposable gloves, tourniquet, antiseptic wipe, winged infusion set, plastic holder, evacuated tubes with labels, gauze pad, adhesive bandage, biohazard sharps container, biohazard specimen bag, and a laboratory request form.
Standards:	Time: 10 minutes. Student completed procedure in _____ minutes.
	Accuracy: Satisfactory score on the Performance Evaluation Checklist.

Performance Evaluation Checklist

Trial 1	Trial 2	Point Value	Performance Standards
		●	Reviewed requirements for collecting and handling the blood specimen.
		●	Sanitized hands.
		●	Greeted the patient and introduced yourself.
		●	Identified patient.
		▷	Stated why the patient must be correctly identified.
		●	Asked patient if he or she prepared properly.
		▷	Explained why it is important for the patient to prepare properly.
			Prepared the equipment
		●	Assembled equipment.
		●	Selected the proper evacuated tubes.
		●	Checked the expiration date of the tubes.
		●	Labeled the evacuated tubes.
		●	Completed a laboratory request form, if necessary.
		●	Removed the winged infusion set from its package.
		●	Extended the tubing to its full length and stretched it.
		▷	Explained why the tubing should be extended and stretched.
		●	Screwed the plastic holder onto the Luer adapter and tightened it securely.
		●	Opened the gauze packet.

827

Trial 1	Trial 2	Point Value	Performance Standards
		●	Positioned the evacuated tubes in the correct order of draw.
		●	Tapped evacuated tubes with a powdered additive below the stopper.
		▷	Stated why tubes with powdered additives must be tapped.
		●	Placed the first tube loosely in the plastic holder with the label facing downward.
		▷	Explained why the label should be facing downward.
			Prepared the patient
		●	Explained the procedure to the patient and reassured patient.
		●	Performed a preliminary assessment of both arms.
		●	Correctly applied the tourniquet and asked patient to clench fist.
		●	Assessed the veins of both arms.
		●	Determined the best vein to use.
		●	Positioned the patient's arm correctly.
		▷	Stated why arm must be positioned correctly.
		●	Thoroughly palpated the selected vein.
		▷	Stated the purpose of palpating the vein.
		●	Did not leave the tourniquet on for more than 1 minute.
		●	Removed tourniquet and cleansed puncture site.
		●	Allowed puncture site to air dry.
		●	Did not touch the site after cleansing.
		●	Placed supplies within comfortable reach.
		●	Reapplied tourniquet and applied gloves.
			Performed the venipuncture
		●	Grasped the winged infusion set correctly.
		●	Removed the protective shield.
		●	Positioned the needle with the bevel up.
		▷	Explained why the bevel should be up.
		●	Grasped patient's arm and anchored the vein correctly.
		●	Positioned the needle at a 15-degree angle to arm, with needle pointing in the same direction as the vein to be entered.
		●	Positioned the needle approximately $1/8$ inch below the place where the vein is to be entered.

828

Trial 1	Trial 2	Point Value	Performance Standards
		●	Told the patient that a small stick will be felt.
		●	With one continuous motion, entered the skin and then the vein.
		▷	Explained why a continuous motion should be used.
		●	Decreased the angle of the needle to 5 degrees.
		●	Seated the needle.
		▷	Stated the purpose of seating the needle.
		●	Opened the butterfly wings and rested them flat against the skin.
		●	Kept the tube and holder in a downward position.
		●	Slowly pushed the tube forward to the end of the plastic holder.
		●	Allowed evacuated tube to fill to the exhaustion of the vacuum.
		▷	Explained why the tube should be filled to the exhaustion of the vacuum.
		●	Removed the tube from the plastic holder.
		●	Immediately and gently inverted evacuated tube 5 times if it contained a clot activator and 8 to 10 times if it contained an anticoagulant.
		▷	Explained why a tube with an anticoagulant must be inverted immediately.
		●	Inserted the next tube into the holder.
		●	Continued until the last tube was filled.
		✳	Removed the tourniquet and asked the patient to unclench fist.
		▷	Stated why the tourniquet must be removed before the needle.
		●	Removed the last tube from the holder.
		●	Placed gauze pad slightly above puncture site. Grasped the setup just below the wings and withdrew the needle slowly and at the same angle as that for penetration.
		●	Immediately moved gauze over puncture site and applied pressure.
		●	Instructed the patient to apply pressure with the gauze.
		●	Activated the safety shield on the needle.
		●	Properly disposed of the winged infusion set and plastic holder in a biohazard sharps container.
		●	Continued to apply pressure for 1 to 2 minutes.
		●	Applied adhesive bandage.

Trial 1	Trial 2	Point Value	Performance Standards
		●	Placed the tubes in an upright position in a test tube rack.
		●	Removed gloves and sanitized hands.
		●	Charted the procedure correctly.
		●	Tested specimen or prepared specimen for transport according to medical office policy.
		✷	Completed the procedure within 10 minutes.
			TOTALS

CHART

Date	

Evaluation of Student Performance

EVALUATION CRITERIA			COMMENTS
Symbol	**Category**	**Point Value**	
✷	Critical Step	16 points	
●	Essential Step	6 points	
▷	Theory Question	2 points	

Score calculation: 100 points

  −   points missed
  _____
  ____ Score

Satisfactory score: 85 or above

CAAHEP Competencies Achieved

Psychomotor (Skills)
☑ I. 2. Perform venipuncture.

Affective (Behavior)
☑ I. 1. Apply critical thinking skills in performing patient assessment and care.
☑ IV. I. Demonstrate empathy in communicating with patients, family, and staff.

ABHES Competencies Achieved

☑ 8. bb. Are impartial and show empathy when dealing with patients.
☑ 10. c. Dispose of biohazardous materials.
☑ 10. d. Collect, label, and process specimens: (1) perform Venipuncture

Procedure 31-3: Skin Puncture—Disposable Semiautomatic Lancet Device

Name: _____ Date: _____

Evaluated by: _____ Score: _____

Performance Objective

Outcome:	Obtain a capillary blood specimen.
Conditions:	Given the following: disposable gloves, antiseptic wipe, CoaguChek lancet, gauze pad, and a biohazard sharps container.
Standards:	Time: 5 minutes. Student completed procedure in _____ minutes.
	Accuracy: Satisfactory score on the Performance Evaluation Checklist.

Performance Evaluation Checklist

Trial 1	Trial 2	Point Value	Performance Standards
		●	Sanitized hands.
		●	Greeted the patient and introduced yourself.
		●	Identified the patient.
		●	Asked patient if he or she prepared properly.
		●	Assembled equipment.
		●	Opened sterile gauze packet.
		●	Explained the procedure to the patient and reassured patient.
		●	Seated patient in chair.
		●	Extended the palmar surface of patient's hand facing up.
		●	Selected a puncture site.
		●	Warmed site if needed.
		▷	Explained why the site should be warmed.
		●	Cleansed puncture site and allowed it to air dry.
		▷	Explained why the site should be allowed to air dry.
		●	Did not touch the site after cleansing.
		●	Applied gloves.
		●	Firmly grasped patient's finger.
		●	Positioned the lancet firmly on the fingertip slightly to the side of center.
		●	Depressed the activation button without moving the lancet or finger.

Trial 1	Trial 2	Point Value	Performance Standards
		▷	Stated why the lancet and finger should not be moved.
		●	Disposed of lancet in biohazard sharps container.
		●	Waited a few seconds to allow blood flow to begin.
		●	Wiped away the first drop of blood with a gauze pad.
		▷	Stated why the first drop of blood should be wiped away.
		●	Allowed a second large, well-rounded drop of blood to form.
		●	Did not squeeze finger to obtain blood.
		●	Collected the blood specimen on a test strip or in the appropriate microcollection device.
		●	Instructed patient to hold a gauze pad over puncture site with pressure.
		●	Remained with patient until bleeding stopped.
		●	Applied an adhesive bandage if needed.
		●	Tested the blood specimen following the manufacturer's instructions.
		●	Removed gloves.
		●	Sanitized hands.
		✱	Completed the procedure within 5 minutes.
			TOTALS

Evaluation of Student Performance

EVALUATION CRITERIA			COMMENTS
Symbol	**Category**	**Point Value**	
✱	Critical Step	16 points	
●	Essential Step	6 points	
▷	Theory Question	2 points	

Score calculation: 100 points

　　　　　　－　　　 points missed
　　　　　　　　 _____
　　　　　　　　 ___ Score

Satisfactory score: 85 or above

Notes

Procedure 31-A: Skin Puncture—Reusable Semiautomatic Lancet Device

Name: _____ Date: _____

Evaluated by: _____ Score: _____

Performance objective

Outcome:	Obtain a capillary blood specimen.
Conditions:	Given the following: disposable gloves, antiseptic wipe, Glucolet II lancet device, sterile lancet/endcap, gauze pad, and a biohazard sharps container.
Standards:	Time: 10 minutes. Student completed procedure in _____ minutes.
	Accuracy: Satisfactory score on the Performance Evaluation Checklist.

Performance Evaluation Checklist

Trial 1	Trial 2	Point Value	Performance Standards
		●	Sanitized hands.
		●	Greeted the patient and introduced yourself.
		●	Identified patient.
		●	Asked patient if he or she prepared properly.
		●	Assembled equipment.
		●	Pushed the transparent barrel toward the release button until it clicked into place.
		●	Inserted lancet/endcap onto the lancet device.
		●	Opened sterile gauze packet.
		●	Explained the procedure to the patient and reassured patient.
		●	Seated patient in chair.
		●	Extended the palmar surface of patient's hand facing up.
		●	Selected a puncture site.
		●	Warmed site if needed.
		▷	Explained how patient's finger can be warmed.
		●	Cleansed puncture site and allowed it to air dry.
		●	Applied gloves.
		●	Twisted off plastic post from the endcap.
		●	Firmly grasped patient's finger.
		●	Placed the endcap firmly on the fingertip slightly to the side of center.

Trial 1	Trial 2	Point Value	Performance Standards
		●	Depressed the activation button without moving the Glucolet or finger.
		●	Wiped away the first drop of blood with a gauze pad.
		●	Allowed a second large, well-rounded drop of blood to form.
		▷	Explained why the finger should not be squeezed.
		●	Collected the blood specimen on a test strip or in the appropriate microcollection device.
		●	Instructed patient to hold a gauze pad over puncture site with pressure.
		●	Remained with patient until bleeding stopped.
		●	Applied an adhesive bandage if needed.
		●	Removed the endcap from the lancet device.
		●	Discarded the endcap in a biohazard waste container.
		●	Tested the blood specimen following the manufacturer's instructions.
		●	Removed gloves.
		●	Sanitized hands.
		●	Sanitized and disinfected the Glucolet.
		●	Stored Glucolet in its resting position.
		✶	Completed the procedure within 5 minutes.
			TOTALS

Evaluation of Student Performance

EVALUATION CRITERIA			COMMENTS
Symbol	**Category**	**Point Value**	
✶	Critical Step	16 points	
●	Essential Step	6 points	
▷	Theory Question	2 points	

Score calculation: 100 points

− _____ points missed

_____ Score

Satisfactory score: 85 or above

Notes

32 Hematology

CHAPTER ASSIGNMENTS

√ After Completing	Date Due	Textbook Pages	TEXTBOOK ASSIGNMENTS	Possible Points	Points You Earned
		784-799	Read Chapter 32: Hematology		
		787 797	Read Case Study 1 Case Study 1 questions	5	
		791 797	Read Case Study 2 Case Study 2 questions	5	
		792 798	Read Case Study 3 Case Study 3 questions	5	
			TOTAL POINTS		

√ After Completing	Date Due	Study Guide Pages	STUDY GUIDE ASSIGNMENTS (CTA = Critical Thinking Activity)	Possible Points	Points You Earned
		843	Pretest	10	
		844	Term Key Term Assessment A. Definitions B. Word Parts (Add 1 point for each medical term)	7 10	
		845-847	Evaluation of Learning questions	26	
		847-850	CTA A: Diseases	40	
		851	CTA B: Hematocrit	5	
		851	CTA C: Iron Content of Food	10	
		852	CTA D: Iron Deficiency Anemia	20	
		852	CTA E: Dear Gabby	10	
		853	CTA F: Crossword Puzzle	27	
			Evolve Site: Animations	20	
			Evolve Site: Apply Your Knowledge questions	10	
			Evolve Site: Video Evaluation	38	
		843	Posttest	10	
			ADDITIONAL ASSIGNMENTS		
			TOTAL POINTS		

Notes

√ When Assigned By Your Instructor	Study Guide Pages	Practices Required	LABORATORY ASSIGNMENTS (Procedure Number and Name)	Score*
	855-857	3	**Practice for Competency** 32-A: Hemoglobin Determination Textbook reference: pp. 785-787	
	859-861		**Evaluation of Competency** 32-A: Hemoglobin Determination	*
	855-856	3	**Practice for Competency** 32-1: Hematocrit Determination Textbook reference: pp. 788-789	
	863-865		**Evaluation of Competency** 32-1: Hematocrit Determination	*
	855-856	10	**Practice for Competency** 32-2: Preparation of a Blood Smear for a Differential Cell Count Textbook reference: pp. 793-794	
	867-869		**Evaluation of Competency** 32-2: Preparation of a Blood Smear for a Differential Cell Count	*
			ADDITIONAL ASSIGNMENTS	

Notes

Name _____ Date _____

True or False

_____ 1. The study of blood is known as *serology*.

_____ 2. The function of hemoglobin is to assist in blood clotting.

_____ 3. The normal hemoglobin range for a female is 12 to 16 g/dL.

_____ 4. A low hemoglobin reading occurs with polycythemia.

_____ 5. The normal hematocrit range for a female is 40% to 54%.

_____ 6. Leukocytosis is an abnormal increase in the number of leukocytes.

_____ 7. Strenuous exercise can result in an increase in the white blood cell count.

_____ 8. Leukemia can cause a decrease in the red blood cell count.

_____ 9. The normal range for neutrophils is 50% to 70%.

_____ 10. The PT test measures how long it takes for an individual's blood to form a clot.

? POSTTEST

True or False

_____ 1. Red and white blood counts are included in a CBC.

_____ 2. The normal range for hemoglobin for an adult male is 14 to 18 g/dL.

_____ 3. An increase in the hemoglobin level occurs with CHF.

_____ 4. The term *hematocrit* means "to separate blood."

_____ 5. The buffy coat consists of red blood cells.

_____ 6. Hematocrit test results should be read at the top of the red blood cell column.

_____ 7. The normal adult range for a white blood cell count is 4500 to 11,000.

_____ 8. Leukopenia occurs when a patient has appendicitis.

_____ 9. The normal range for a red blood cell count for a woman is 4 to 5.5 million.

_____ 10. The function of warfarin is to inhibit the growth of bacteria in the body.

A. Definitions

Directions: Match each medical term with its definition.

_____ 1. Anemia

_____ 2. Anticoagulant

_____ 3. Hematology

_____ 4. Hemoglobin

_____ 5. Leukocytosis

_____ 6. Leukopenia

_____ 7. Polycythemia

A. An abnormal decrease in the number of white blood cells (less than 4500 per cubic millimeter of blood)

B. A disorder in which there is an increase in the red blood cell mass

C. A condition in which there is a decrease in the number of erythrocytes or in the amount of hemoglobin in the blood

D. The study of blood and blood-forming tissues

E. An abnormal increase in the number of white blood cells (greater than 11,000 per cubic millimeter of blood)

F. The protein- and iron-containing pigment of erythrocytes that transports oxygen in the body

G. A substance that inhibits blood clotting

B. Word Parts

Directions: Indicate the meaning of each word part in the space provided. List as many medical terms as possible that incorporate the word part in the space provided.

Word Part	Meaning of Word Part	Medical Terms That Incorporate Word Part
1. cyt/o		
2. -ia		
3. -osis		
4. anti-		
5. coagulant		
6. hemato/o		
7. -ology		
8. leuk/o		
9. -penia		
10. poly-		

Directions: Fill in each blank with the correct answer.

1. List the tests generally included in a complete blood cell count (CBC).

   _____

   _____

2. What is the normal hemoglobin range?

   a. Adult female: _____

   b. Adult male: _____

3. List five conditions that cause a decrease in the hemoglobin level.

   _____ _____

   _____

   _____

4. What is the purpose of the hematocrit?

   _____

   _____

5. What is the normal hematocrit range?

   a. Adult female: _____

   b. Adult male: _____

6. What is the normal range for the white blood count for an adult?

   _____

7. List examples of conditions that may result in leukocytosis.

   _____

   _____

8. What is the normal range for the red blood count for an adult?

   a. Adult female: _____

   b. Adult male: _____

9. List the five types of white blood cells and the normal adult range for each.

   _____

   _____

   _____

10. What are the red blood cell indices?

    _____

    _____

11. What information is provided by the RBC indices?

_____

_____

12. What are the advantages of the following methods for performing a differential cell count?

   a. Automatic method: _____

   b. Manual: _____

13. Why must the white blood cells be stained when performing a manual differential cell count?

_____

_____

14. List the abbreviation for each of the following tests:

   a. Hematocrit _____

   b. Hemoglobin _____

   c. Differential cell count _____

   d. White blood cell count _____

   e. Red blood cell count _____

15. What does the PT test measure?

_____

16. What is the PT adult reference range?

_____

17. What is the purpose of performing an INR on a PT test?

_____

_____

18. What is the range for a PT/INR result of a healthy individual with a normal clotting ability?

_____

19. What is the function of warfarin?

_____

20. What are the most common conditions for which warfarin is prescribed?

_____

_____

21. What is the usual desired PT/INR range for a patient who is on warfarin therapy for a heart attack or stroke?

_____

22. What is the goal of warfarin therapy?

_____

_____

23. How often should a patient on warfarin therapy have a PT/INR test performed?

_____

24. What color-stopped tube should be used to collect a specimen for a PT/INR test?

_____

25. Why is it important to fill the blood tube for a PT/INR test to the exhaustion of the vacuum?

_____

_____

26. What are the advantages of PT/INR home testing?

_____

_____

CRITICAL THINKING ACTIVITIES

A. Diseases

1. You and your classmates work at a large clinic. It is National Disease Awareness Week. The physicians at your clinic ask you to develop informative, creative, and colorful brochures for patients about various diseases. Choose a condition from the list, and design a brochure using the blank Frequently Asked Questions (FAQ) brochure provided on the following page. Each student in the class should select a different disease. On a separate sheet of paper, write three true or false questions relating to the information in your brochure.

2. Present your brochure to the class. After all the brochures have been presented, each student should ask three questions to the entire class to see how well the class understands the diseases that were presented. (*Note:* Students can take notes during the presentations and refer to them when answering the questions.)

Conditions

1. Addison's disease
2. Amyotrophic lateral sclerosis
3. Aplastic anemia
4. Bell's palsy
5. Cirrhosis
6. Crohn's disease
7. Cushing's syndrome
8. Cystic fibrosis
9. Degenerative disc disease
10. Epilepsy
11. Hemolytic anemia
12. Hemophilia
13. Hernia
14. Hodgkin's disease
15. Hyperthyroidism
16. Hypothyroidism
17. Leukemia
18. Lupus erythematosus
19. Multiple sclerosis
20. Muscular dystrophy
21. Parkinson's disease
22. Peptic ulcer
23. Pernicious anemia
24. Polycythemia
25. Sickle-cell anemia
26. Ulcerative colitis

Notes

FAQ on:

Q:

A:

Q:

A:

Q:

A:

Q:

A:

Q:

A:

Q:

A:

Illustration

Q:

A:

Q:

A:

B. Hematocrit

Label the layers of this microhematocrit capillary tube that has been centrifuged. Place an arrow at the point where you would take the hematocrit reading.

Sealing compound

(From Bonewit-West K: *Study guide for clinical procedures for medical assistants,* ed 8, St. Louis, 2011, Saunders.)

C. Iron Content of Food

Consuming food that is high in iron helps to prevent iron deficiency anemia. To become familiar with foods that are high in iron content and foods that contain little or no iron, plan the following two meals. One meal should be as high as possible in iron content and the other meal should not contain any iron at all.

Meal 1

_____

_____

_____

_____

_____

Meal 2

_____

_____

_____

_____

_____

D. Iron Deficiency Anemia

Create a profile of an individual who has iron deficiency anemia following these guidelines:

1. Using a blank piece of paper, colored pencils, crayons, or markers, draw a figure of an individual exhibiting iron deficiency anemia. Be as creative as possible.

2. Do not use any text on your drawing other than to label items you have drawn in your picture. (A picture is worth a thousand words!)

3. Try to include all of the symptoms of iron deficiency anemia in your drawing. The Iron Deficiency Anemia Patient Teaching Box on p. 790 in your textbook can be used as a reference source.

4. In the classroom, find a partner and trade drawings. Identify the symptoms of iron deficiency anemia in your partner's drawing. With your partner, discuss what treatment is recommended and also what this person could do to prevent iron deficiency anemia.

E. Dear Gabby

Gabby is attending her class reunion and wants you to fill in for her. In the space provided, respond to the following letter.

Dear Gabby,

I am a housewife with two adorable children, ages 2 and 4. I have been feeling rundown and tired lately, so I bought some vitamin pills at the drug store. They came individually packaged in foil and plastic. They are hard to open, so I cut each package and transferred the iron pills to a little plastic baggie. When I told my mother about what I thought was a great idea, she got very upset. She told me that I could possibly be putting my children at danger. She said that iron is poisonous to children and that I should not do that. Gabby, my mom has always been overprotective. Is this just another one of her episodes?

Signed,

Curious in Kansas

_____

_____

_____

_____

_____

_____

_____

_____

_____

_____

F. Crossword Puzzle: Hematology

Directions: Complete the crossword puzzle using the clues provided.

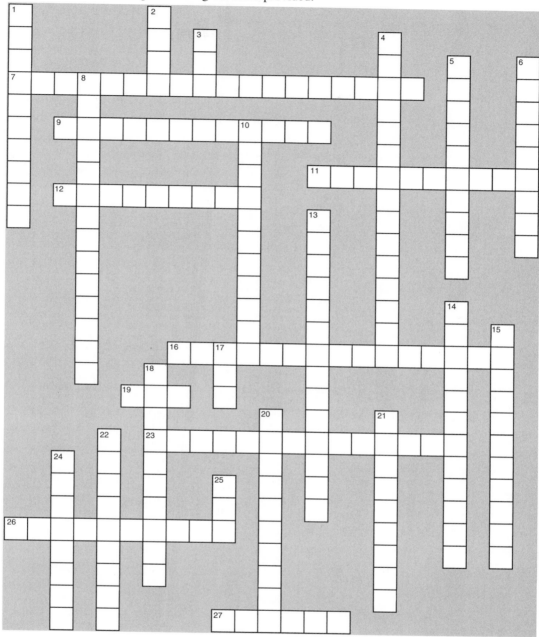

Across

- **7** Cause of blood pooling in heart
- **9** Condition of too many RBCs
- **11** Carries oxygen
- **12** Platelets and WBCs
- **16** Causes inaccurate PT/INR results
- **19** Common hematology test
- **23** Common cause of anemia
- **26** To separate blood
- **27** Liquid part of the blood

Down

- **1** Study of blood
- **2** Differential WBC count abbreviation
- **3** Hemoglobin abbreviation
- **4** Blood clotting test
- **5** Most numerous WBC
- **6** Symptom of anemia
- **8** Causes black stool
- **10** Red blood cell
- **13** May affect PT/INR test results
- **14** Above 11,000 WBCs
- **15** Indication for warfarin
- **17** aka thrombophlebitis
- **18** Calculations on CBC tests
- **20** Below 4500 WBCs
- **21** White blood cell
- **22** Color tube for PT/INR
- **24** Warfarin brand name
- **25** Hematocrit abbreviation

Notes

Procedure 32-A: Hemoglobin Determination.

a. Run controls on a CLIA-waived hemoglobin analyzer, and record results on the quality control log on p. 857.

b. Perform a hemoglobin determination on a patient using a CLIA-waived hemoglobin analyzer, and record results in the chart provided. Circle any values that fall outside the normal range.

Procedure 32-1: Hematocrit Determination. Perform a hematocrit determination in duplicate, and record results in the chart provided. Circle any values that fall outside the normal range.

Procedure 32-2: Preparation of a Blood Smear for a Differential Cell Count. Prepare a blood smear for a differential white blood cell count.

CHART	
Date	

855

CHART	
Date	

QUALITY CONTROL HEMOGLOBIN LOG SHEET

Name of Meter _____   Control Lot Number: _____

Low-Level Range: _____   Control Exp. Date: _____

High-Level Range: _____

Date	Test Cards: Lot # and Expiration	Low-Level Value	Accept	Reject	High-Level Value	Accept	Reject	Technician

Chapter **32** **Hematology**

Notes

Procedure 32-A: Hemoglobin Determination

Name: _____ Date: _____

Evaluated by: _____ Score: _____

Performance Objective

Outcome:	Perform a hemoglobin determination.
Conditions:	Using a hemoglobin meter and operating manual and given the following: disposable gloves, antiseptic wipe, lancet, gauze pad, test cards, cod key, control solutions, quality control log, and a biohazard sharps container.
Standards:	Time: 10 minutes. Student completed procedure in _____ minutes.
	Accuracy: Satisfactory score on the Performance Evaluation Checklist.

Performance Evaluation Checklist

Trial 1	Trial 2	Point Value	Performance Standards
		●	Sanitized hands.
		●	Assembled equipment.
		●	Checked expiration date of test cards.
		●	Calibrated the hemoglobin meter.
		▷	Stated the purpose of calibrating the meter.
		●	Checked expiration date of control solution.
		●	Applied gloves and ran a low and high control.
		▷	Stated the purpose of running controls.
		●	Removed gloves and sanitized hands.
		●	Recorded control results in the quality control log.
		●	Greeted the patient and introduced yourself.
		●	Identified the patient and explained the procedure.
		●	Turned on the hemoglobin meter and checked the code number.
		●	Inserted a test card into the meter.
		●	Opened gauze packet.
		●	Cleansed puncture site and allowed it to air-dry.
		▷	Stated what happens to the blood drop if the site is not dry.

Trial 1	Trial 2	Point Value	Performance Standards
		●	Applied gloves and performed a finger puncture.
		●	Wiped away the first drop of blood.
		●	Collected the blood specimen.
		●	Placed a gauze pad over puncture site and applied pressure.
		●	Applied blood specimen to test card.
		●	Waited while hemoglobin meter analyzed the blood specimen.
		●	Read results on the display screen.
		▷	Stated the normal hemoglobin range for a female (12 to 16 g/dL) and a male (14 to 18 g/dL).
		●	Removed test card from meter.
		●	Properly disposed of test card in a biohazard waste container.
		●	Checked puncture site and applied adhesive bandage, if needed.
		●	Removed gloves and sanitized hands.
		●	Charted the test results correctly.
		✶	Hemoglobin recording was identical to the reading on the digital display screen.
		✶	Completed the procedure within 10 minutes.
			TOTALS

CHART

Date	

Evaluation of Student Performance

EVALUATION CRITERIA			COMMENTS
Symbol	**Category**	**Point Value**	
✶	Critical Step	16 points	
●	Essential Step	6 points	
▷	Theory Question	2 points	

Score calculation: 100 points

−   points missed

———

___ Score

Satisfactory score: 85 or above

Notes

Name: _____   Date: _____

Evaluated by: _____   Score: _____

Performance Objective

Outcome:	Perform a hematocrit determination.
Conditions:	Given the following: microhematocrit centrifuge, disposable gloves, lancet, antiseptic wipe, gauze pad, capillary tubes, sealing compound, and a biohazard sharps container.
Standards:	Time: 10 minutes. Student completed procedure in _____ minutes. Accuracy: Satisfactory score on the Performance Evaluation Checklist.

Performance Evaluation Checklist

Trial 1	Trial 2	Point Value	Performance Standards
		●	Sanitized hands.
		●	Greeted the patient and introduced yourself.
		●	Identified the patient and explained the procedure.
		●	Assembled equipment.
		●	Opened gauze packet.
		●	Cleansed site with an antiseptic wipe and allowed it to air-dry.
		●	Applied gloves.
		●	Performed a finger puncture and discarded the lancet in a biohazard sharps container.
		●	Wiped away the first drop of blood.
		●	Massaged finger until large blood drop formed.
		●	Held one end of capillary tube horizontally but slightly downward next to the free-flowing puncture.
		●	Kept the tip of the pipet in the blood but did not allow it to press against the skin of the patient's finger.
		▷	Explained why the capillary tube should be kept in the blood specimen.
		●	Filled capillary tube (calibrated tubes filled to the calibration line; uncalibrated tubes filled approximately three-fourths full).
		▷	Explained why a tube with air bubbles is unacceptable.
		●	Filled a second capillary tube.
		▷	Stated why 2 capillary tubes must be filled.
		●	Placed gauze pad over puncture site and applied pressure.
		●	Sealed the dry end of each capillary tube.

863

Trial 1	Trial 2	Point Value	Performance Standards
		●	Checked puncture site and applied adhesive bandage, if needed.
		●	Placed capillary tubes in the microhematocrit centrifuge with the sealed end facing toward the outside.
		▷	Explained why the sealed end must face toward the outside.
		●	Balanced one tube with the other tube placed opposite it.
		●	Placed the cover over the capillary tubes and locked it securely.
		●	Centrifuged blood specimen for 3 to 5 minutes.
		▷	Explained the reason for centrifuging the blood specimen.
		●	Allowed centrifuge to come to a complete stop.
		●	Removed the protective cover from the capillary tubes.
		●	Read the results using the appropriate reading device.
		●	Determined if the results agreed within 4 percentage points.
		▷	Explained what to do if the results are not within 4 percentage points.
		●	Averaged the values of the two tubes together to derive the test results.
		✶	Results were within ±1% of the evaluator's results.
		▷	Stated the normal hematocrit range for a female (37% to 47%) and a male (40% to 54%).
		●	Properly disposed of capillary tubes in a biohazard sharps container.
		●	Removed gloves and sanitized hands.
		●	Charted the test results correctly.
		●	Returned equipment.
		✶	Completed the procedure within 10 minutes.
			TOTALS

	CHART	
Date		

EVALUATION CRITERIA			COMMENTS
Symbol	**Category**	**Point Value**	
✳	Critical Step	16 points	
●	Essential Step	6 points	
▷	Theory Question	2 points	

Score calculation: 100 points

      −   _____ points missed

           _____ Score

Satisfactory score: 85 or above

CAAHEP Competencies Achieved

Psychomotor (Skills)
☑ I. 11. Perform quality control measures.
☑ I. 12. Perform hematology testing.

Affective (Behavior)
☑ II. 2. Distinguish between normal and abnormal test results.

ABHES Competencies Achieved

☑ 10. a. Practice quality control.
☑ 10. b. Perform selected CLIA-waived tests that assist with diagnosis and treatment: (2) hematology testing.
☑ 10. c. Dispose of biohazardous materials.

Notes

Procedure 32-2: Preparation of a Blood Smear for a Differential Cell Count

Name: _____ Date: _____

Evaluated by: _____ Score: _____

Performance Objective

Outcome:	Prepare a blood smear for a differential white blood cell count.
Conditions:	Given the following: disposable gloves, supplies to perform a finger puncture or venipuncture, slides with a frosted edge, slide container, biohazard specimen bag, laboratory request form, and a biohazard sharps container.
Standards:	Time: 10 minutes. Student completed procedure in _____ minutes.
	Accuracy: Satisfactory score on the Performance Evaluation Checklist.

Performance Evaluation Checklist

Trial 1	Trial 2	Point Value	Performance Standards
		●	Sanitized hands.
		●	Greeted the patient and introduced yourself.
		●	Identified the patient and explained the procedure.
		●	Assembled equipment.
		●	Labeled slides.
		●	Opened the gauze packet.
		●	Cleansed puncture site.
		●	Applied gloves.
		●	Performed a venipuncture or finger puncture.
		●	Placed a drop of blood in the middle of each slide approximately ¼ inch from the frosted edge of the slide.
		●	Held a spreader slide at a 30-degree angle to first slide in front of the drop of blood.
		▷	Stated what occurs if the angle is more than 30 degrees or less than 30 degrees.
		●	Moved the spreader slide until it touched the drop of blood.
		●	Spread the blood thinly and evenly across slide using the spreader slide.
		●	Prepared the second blood smear.
		●	Disposed of the spreader slide in a biohazard sharps container.
		●	Laid the blood smears on a flat surface and allowed them to dry.
		▷	Explained why the blood smears should be dried immediately.

Trial 1	Trial 2	Point Value	Performance Standards
		●	The length of the smear was approximately 1½ inches.
		●	The smear was smooth and even, with no ridges, holes, lines, streaks, or clumps.
		●	The smear was not too thick or too thin.
		●	There was a feathered edge at the thin end of the smear.
		●	There was a margin on all sides of the smear.
		●	Placed the slides in a protective slide container.
		●	Placed lavender-stoppered tube and slide container in a biohazard specimen bag.
		●	Removed gloves and sanitized hands.
		●	Completed a laboratory request form.
		●	Placed lab request in outside pocket of specimen bag.
		●	Charted the procedure correctly.
		●	Filed copy of lab request in patient's chart.
		●	Placed specimen bag in appropriate location for pickup by lab courier.
		●	Charted the procedure correctly.
		✶	Completed the procedure within 10 minutes.
			TOTALS

CHART

	Date	

Evaluation of Student Performance

EVALUATION CRITERIA			COMMENTS
Symbol	Category	Point Value	
★	Critical Step	16 points	
●	Essential Step	6 points	
▷	Theory Question	2 points	

Score calculation: 100 points

– _____ points missed

_____ Score

Satisfactory score: 85 or above

CAAHEP Competencies Achieved

Psychomotor (Skills)
☑ I. 11. Perform quality control measures.

Affective (Behavior)
☑ I. 1. Apply critical thinking skills in performing patient assessment and care.

ABHES Competencies Achieved

☑ 10. a. Practice quality control
☑ 10. d. Collect, label, and process specimens.

Notes

33 Blood Chemistry and Immunology

CHAPTER ASSIGNMENTS

√ After Completing	Date Due	Textbook Pages	TEXTBOOK ASSIGNMENTS	Possible Points	Points You Earned
		800-824	Read Chapter 33: Blood Chemistry and Immunology		
		806 823	Read Case Study 1 Case Study 1 questions	5	
		809 823	Read Case Study 2 Case Study 2 questions	5	
		818 823	Read Case Study 3 Case Study 3 questions	5	
			TOTAL POINTS		
√ After Completing	Date Due	Study Guide Pages	STUDY GUIDE ASSIGNMENTS (CTA = Critical Thinking Activity)	Possible Points	Points You Earned
		875	Pretest	10	
		876	Term Key Term Assessment	10	
		876-881	Evaluation of Learning questions	47	
		881-884	CTA A: Type 2 Diabetes	40	
		885	CTA B: Oral Glucose Tolerance Test (2 points each)	10	
		885	CTA C: Coronary Artery Disease	20	
		885-886	CTA D: Cholesterol and Saturated Fat (5 points each)	15	
			Evolve Site: The Right Chemistry (Record points earned)		
		886	CTA E: Rh Incompatibility (5 points each)	20	
		887	CTA F: Crossword Puzzle	22	
			Evolve Site: Immunologic Tests (Record points earned)		
			Evolve Site: Animations	20	
			Evolve Site: Apply Your Knowledge questions	10	

√ After Completing	Date Due	Study Guide Pages	STUDY GUIDE ASSIGNMENTS (CTA = Critical Thinking Activity)	Possible Points	Points You Earned
			Evolve Site: Video Evaluation	16	
		875	Posttest	10	
			ADDITIONAL ASSIGNMENTS		
			TOTAL POINTS		

√ When Assigned By Your Instructor	Study Guide Pages	Practices Required	LABORATORY ASSIGNMENTS (Procedure Number and Name)	Score*
	889-890	3	**Practice for Competency** 33-A: Performing a Blood Chemistry Test Textbook reference: pp. 801-802	
	893-894		**Evaluation of Competency** 33-A: Performing a Blood Chemistry Test	*
	889-891	3	**Practice for Competency** 33-1: Blood Glucose Measurement Using the Accu-Chek Advantage Glucose Meter Textbook reference: pp. 812-815	
	895-897		**Evaluation of Competency** 33-1: Blood Glucose Measurement Using the Accu-Chek Advantage Glucose Meter	*
	889-892	3	**Practice for Competency** 33-B: Rapid Mononucleosis Testing (QuickVue + Mono Test) Textbook reference: pp. 820-822	
	899-900		**Evaluation of Competency** 33-B: Rapid Mononucleosis Testing (QuickVue + Mono Test)	*
			ADDITIONAL ASSIGNMENTS	

Notes

Name _____   Date _____

True or False

_____ 1. The function of glucose in the body is to build and repair tissue.

_____ 2. Insulin is required for normal use of glucose in the body.

_____ 3. An abnormally low level of glucose in the body is known as *hypoglycemia.*

_____ 4. The hemoglobin A_{1C} test measures the average amount of blood glucose over a 3-month period.

_____ 5. Most of the cholesterol found in the blood comes from the intake of dietary cholesterol.

_____ 6. The primary use of the cholesterol test is to screen for the presence of coronary artery disease.

_____ 7. LDL picks up cholesterol from ingested fats and the liver and carries it to the cells.

_____ 8. An antibody is a substance that is capable of combining with an antigen.

_____ 9. Mononucleosis is transmitted through coughing and sneezing.

_____ 10. Symptoms of infectious mononucleosis include severe fatigue, fever, and sore throat.

POSTTEST

True or False

_____ 1. Serum is required for most blood chemistry tests.

_____ 2. The normal range for a fasting blood glucose level is 120 to 160 mg/dL.

_____ 3. The oral glucose tolerance test is used to assist in the diagnosis of diabetes mellitus.

_____ 4. Before meals, it is recommended that the blood glucose level for a diabetic patient be 60 to 80 mg/dL.

_____ 5. The recommended hemoglobin A_{1C} level for a patient with diabetes is 4% to 6%.

_____ 6. The buildup of plaque (due to high cholesterol) on the walls of arteries is known as thrombophlebitis.

_____ 7. An HDL cholesterol level greater than 50 mg/dL is a risk factor for coronary artery disease.

_____ 8. The triglyceride test requires that the patient not eat or drink for 12 hours before the test.

_____ 9. The RPR test is a screening test for syphilis.

_____ 10. The varicella virus causes infectious mononucleosis.

Directions: Match each medical term with its definition.

_____ 1. Agglutination

_____ 2. Analyte

_____ 3. Antibody

_____ 4. Antigen

_____ 5. Glycogen

_____ 6. HDL cholesterol

_____ 7. Hyperglycemia

_____ 8. Hypoglycemia

_____ 9. LDL cholesterol

_____ 10. Lipoprotein

A. An abnormally high level of glucose in the blood

B. A complex molecule consisting of protein and a lipid fraction such as cholesterol

C. The form in which carbohydrate is stored in the body

D. A lipoprotein consisting of protein and cholesterol that removes excess cholesterol from the cells

E. An abnormally low level of glucose in the blood

F. A lipoprotein, consisting of protein and cholesterol, that picks up cholesterol and delivers it to the cells

G. A substance that is capable of combining with an antigen resulting in an antigen-antibody reaction

H. Substance capable of stimulating the formation of antibodies

I. A substance that is being identified or measured in a laboratory test.

J. Clumping of blood cells

EVALUATION OF LEARNING

Directions: Fill in each blank with the correct answer.

1. What type of specimen is required for most blood chemistry tests?

_____

2. What is the purpose of quality control?

_____

_____

3. What is the purpose of calibrating a blood chemistry analyzer?

_____

_____

4. At a minimum, when should a calibration check be performed on a blood chemistry analyzer?

_____

5. What is the purpose of running a control on a blood chemistry analyzer?

_____

_____

6. List three reasons why a control may not produce expected results.

_____

_____

7. When running controls on a blood chemistry analyzer, what should be done if the controls do not perform as expected?

_____

8. What is the function of glucose in the body?

_____

_____

9. Explain the function of insulin in the body.

_____

_____

10. List the abbreviation for each of the following tests:

   a. Fasting blood glucose _____

   b. Two-hour postprandial blood glucose _____

   c. Oral glucose tolerance test _____

11. What type of patient preparation is required for a fasting blood glucose test?

_____

_____

12. List two reasons for performing a fasting blood glucose test.

_____

13. What is prediabetes?

_____

_____

14. What are the values recommended by the American Diabetes Association for interpreting fasting blood glucose results?

   a. Normal _____

   b. Prediabetes_____

   c. Diabetes_____

15. What type of patient preparation is required for a 2-hour postprandial blood glucose test?

_____

_____

16. Describe the procedure for performing a 2-hour postprandial blood glucose test.

_____

_____

17. What is the purpose of an oral glucose tolerance test?

_____

_____

Chapter **33** **Blood Chemistry and Immunology**

18. What type of patient preparation is required for an oral glucose tolerance test?

_____

_____

19. Describe the procedure for an oral glucose tolerance test.

_____

_____

20. Define hypoglycemia and list three conditions that may cause it to occur.

_____

_____

21. Why is it important for an insulin-dependent diabetic to perform self-monitoring of blood glucose (SMBG)?

_____

_____

22. What is the ideal insulin testing schedule for SMBG?

_____

_____

23. What type of damage can occur to the body from prolonged high glucose levels in blood?

_____

_____

24. List three advantages of blood glucose monitoring at home.

_____

_____

_____

25. What is the recommended blood glucose level for a diabetic during the following times of the day:

a. Before meals _____

b. One to 2 hours after meals _____

c. At bedtime _____

26. What information is provided by a hemoglobin A_{1C} test?

_____

_____

27. What is the normal A_{1C} range for an individual without diabetes?

_____

28. What is the recommended A_{1C} percentage for an individual with diabetes?

_____

_____

878

29. What are the storage requirements for blood glucose reagent test strips?

_____

_____

30. When should the calibration (coding) procedure be performed on a glucose meter?

_____

31. What is cholesterol?

_____

_____

32. List the two main sources of cholesterol in the blood.

_____

_____

33. What is atherosclerosis, and why is it a health risk?

_____

_____

34. Why is LDL cholesterol referred to as *bad cholesterol* and HDL referred to as *good cholesterol*?

_____

_____

_____

_____

35. What does a total cholesterol test measure?

_____

_____

36. List the ranges for each of the following cholesterol categories:

   a. Desirable cholesterol level _____

   b. Borderline cholesterol level _____

   c. High cholesterol level _____

37. At what level is HDL cholesterol considered a risk factor for coronary heart disease?

_____

_____

38. What is the primary use of the cholesterol test?

_____

_____

39. What type of patient preparation is required for a triglyceride test?

_____

_____

40. List the ranges for each of the following triglyceride categories:

    a. Normal _____

    b. Borderline high _____

    c. High _____

    d. Very high _____

41. What conditions result in elevated blood triglycerides?

_____

_____

_____

42. What is the purpose of performing a BUN?

_____

_____

43. What is the definition of immunology?

_____

_____

_____

44. List three examples of antigens.

_____

_____

45. What is the purpose of performing each of the following serologic tests?

    a. Rheumatoid factor

_____

_____

    b. Antistreptolysin test

_____

_____

    c. C-reactive protein

_____

_____

    d. ABO and Rh blood typing

_____

_____

46. How is infectious mononucleosis transmitted?

_____

_____

47. What are the symptoms of infectious mononucleosis?

_____

_____

CRITICAL THINKING ACTIVITIES

A. Type 2 Diabetes

You are working for a physician specializing in internal medicine. The physician is concerned about the increased numbers of patients developing type 2 diabetes mellitus. He asks you to design a colorful, creative, and informative brochure on type 2 diabetes using the brochure format provided on the next page. This brochure will be published and placed in the waiting room to provide patients with education on type 2 diabetes. The diabetes Internet sites listed under **On the Web** at the end of Chapter 33 in your textbook can be used to complete this activity.

Notes

FAQ
ON:

Q: A:

Q: A:

Q: A:

Q: A:

Q:

A:

Q:

A:

Illustration

Q:

A:

Q:

A:

B. Oral Glucose Tolerance Test

Marty Wolf has arrived at your office for an oral glucose tolerance test. What should you tell her regarding the following subjects? Explain the reason for each answer.

1. Consumption of food and fluid

_____

_____

2. Water consumption

_____

_____

3. Smoking

_____

_____

4. Leaving the test site

_____

_____

5. Activity

_____

_____

C. Coronary Artery Disease

Create a profile of an individual who is at risk for coronary artery disease (CAD) following these guidelines:

1. Using a blank piece of paper, colored pencils, crayons, or markers, draw a figure of an individual exhibiting risk factors for CAD. Be as creative as possible.
2. Do not use any text on your drawing other than to label items you have drawn in your picture. (A picture is worth a thousand words!)
3. Try to include at least eight risk factors for CAD in your drawing. The *Highlight on Coronary Heart Disease with a Focus on Coronary Artery Disease* box on p. 816 in your textbook can be used as a reference source.
4. In the classroom, find a partner and trade drawings. Identify the risk factors for CAD in your partner's drawing. With your partner, discuss what this person could do to lower his or her chances of developing CAD.

D. Cholesterol and Saturated Fat

Using a reference source, complete the following activities:

1. Create a dinner meal that is as high as possible in saturated fat and cholesterol.

_____

_____

_____

_____

_____

2. Create a dinner meal that is as low as possible in saturated fat and cholesterol.

_____

_____

_____

_____

_____

3. Choose a fast-food restaurant, and plan a meal that is as low as possible in saturated fat and cholesterol.

_____

_____

_____

_____

_____

E. Rh Incompatibility

Erythroblastosis fetalis is a blood disorder of the newborn. It usually is caused by incompatibility between the infant's blood and the mother's blood. Using a reference source, answer the following questions regarding this condition in the space provided.

1. Explain how Rh incompatibility between the mother and her infant can cause this condition to occur.

_____

_____

_____

_____

_____

2. Describe the symptoms associated with erythroblastosis fetalis.

_____

_____

_____

3. Explain the treatment used for this condition.

_____

_____

_____

4. How can this condition be prevented?

_____

_____

_____

F. Crossword Puzzle: Blood Chemistry and Immunology

Directions: Complete the crossword puzzle using the clues provided.

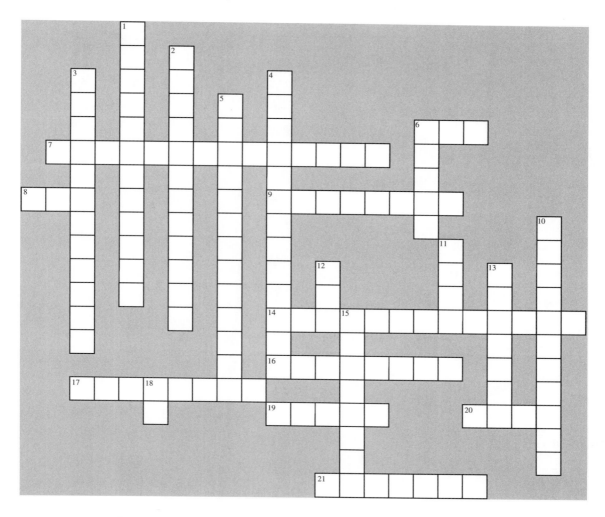

Across

6 Bad cholesterol
7 Cholesterol: 200-239
8 Good cholesterol
9 Stored glucose
14 Kissing disease
16 Combines with an antigen
17 Increases HDL cholesterol
19 Keep diabetic A_{1c} below this
20 Series of glucose tests
21 Provides energy for body

Down

1 #1 killer in the U.S.
2 Raises cholesterol level
3 Low BG
4 High BG
5 Desirable: <150 mg/dL
6 Makes cholesterol
10 FBG: 100-125 mg/dL
11 Syphilis test
12 Detects renal disease
13 Risk factor for CAD
15 Unsaturated fat (ex)
18 Rheumatoid arthritis test

Notes

Procedure 33-A: Blood Chemistry Test. Perform a blood chemistry test, and record results in the chart provided. Examples of blood chemistry tests: cholesterol, triglycerides, and BUN.

Procedure 33-1: Blood Glucose Measurement.
a. Run controls on a CLIA-waived glucose meter, and record results on the quality control log on p. 891.
b. Perform a fasting blood glucose test, and record results in the chart provided.

Procedure 33-B: Rapid Mononucleosis Test.
a. Run controls on a CLIA-waived mono, and record results on the quality control log on p. 892.
b. Perform a rapid mononucleosis test, and record results in the chart provided.

CHART	
Date	

CHART	
Date	

QUALITY CONTROL LOG
BLOOD GLUCOSE

NAME OF METER		CONTROLS
Test Strips:		**Low-Level Control:**
Lot Number: _____		Lot Number: _____
Exp Date: _____		Exp Date: _____
Code Number: _____		Expected Range: _____
		High-Level Control:
		Lot Number: _____
		Exp Date: _____
		Expected Range: _____

Date	Low-Level Control	Accept	Reject	High-Level Control	Accept	Reject	Technician

QUALITY CONTROL LOG

MONONUCLEOSIS TEST

Date	Name of Test	Control Lot #	Control Expiration Date	External Positive Control	External Negative Control	Technician

Chapter **33** **Blood Chemistry and Immunology**

Procedure 33-A: Performing a Blood Chemistry Test

Name: _____ Date: _____

Evaluated by: _____ Score: _____

Performance Objective

Outcome:	Perform a fasting blood glucose test.
Conditions:	Given the following: disposable gloves, an antiseptic wipe, a lancet, gauze pad, quality control log, and a biohazard sharps container. Using an automated blood chemistry analyzer and operating manual.
Standards:	Time: 10 minutes. Student completed procedure in _____ minutes.
	Accuracy: Satisfactory score on the Performance Evaluation Checklist.

Performance Evaluation Checklist

Trial 1	Trial 2	Point Value	Performance Standards
		●	Sanitized hands.
		●	Assembled equipment.
		●	Calibrated the blood chemistry analyzer.
		●	Applied gloves and ran controls.
		●	Recorded results in the quality control log.
		●	Sanitized hands.
		●	Greeted the patient and introduced yourself.
		●	Identified patient and explained the procedure.
		●	Applied gloves.
		●	Performed a finger puncture.
		●	Collected the specimen according to manufacturer's instructions.
		●	Placed a gauze pad over the puncture site and applied pressure.
		●	Inserted the specimen into blood chemistry analyzer according to manufacturer's instructions.
		●	Operated the blood chemistry analyzer according to manufacturer's instructions.
		●	Read the results on digital display screen.
		●	Properly disposed of used materials.
		●	Checked puncture site and applied adhesive bandage if needed.
		●	Removed gloves.
		●	Sanitized hands.

893

Trial 1	Trial 2	Point Value	Performance Standards
		●	Charted the test results correctly.
		✷	The recording was identical to the reading on the digital display screen.
		✷	Completed the procedure within 10 minutes.
			TOTALS
			CHART
Date			

Evaluation of Student Performance

EVALUATION CRITERIA			COMMENTS
Symbol	**Category**	**Point Value**	
✷	Critical Step	16 points	
●	Essential Step	6 points	
▷	Theory Question	2 points	

Score calculation:　　100 points

　　　　−　＿＿ points missed

　　　　＿＿＿ Score

Satisfactory score: 85 or above

CAAHEP Competencies Achieved

Psychomotor (Skills)
☑ I. 11. Perform quality control measures.
☑ I. 13. Perform chemistry testing.
☑ II. 2. Maintain laboratory test results using flow sheets.

Affective (Behavior)
☑ II. 2. Distinguish between normal and abnormal test results.

ABHES Competencies Achieved

☑ 10. a. Practice quality control.
☑ 10. b. Perform selected CLIA-waived tests that assist with diagnosis and treatment: (3) chemistry testing.

Procedure 33-1: Blood Glucose Measurement Using the Accu-Chek Advantage Glucose Meter

Name: _____ Date: _____

Evaluated by: _____ Score: _____

Performance Objective

Outcome:	Perform a fasting blood glucose test.
Conditions:	Given the following: disposable gloves, Accu-Chek Advantage glucose meter, reagent test strips, check strip, code key, control solutions, lancet, antiseptic wipe, gauze pad, quality control log, and a biohazard sharps container.
Standards:	Time: 10 minutes. Student completed procedure in _____ minutes. Accuracy: Satisfactory score on the Performance Evaluation Checklist.

Performance Evaluation Checklist

Trial 1	Trial 2	Point Value	Performance Standards
		•	Sanitized hands.
		•	Assembled equipment.
		•	Checked the expiration date on container of test strips.
		•	Calibrated the meter using the code key.
		▷	Stated the purpose of calibrating the meter.
		•	Ran a low and high control.
		▷	Stated the purpose for running controls.
		•	Recorded results in the quality control log.
		•	Sanitized hands.
		•	Greeted the patient and introduced yourself.
		•	Identified the patient and explained the procedure.
		•	Asked the patient if he or she prepared properly.
		▷	Stated the preparation required for a fasting blood glucose test.
		•	Removed a test strip from the container.
		•	Immediately replaced the lid of the container.
		▷	Explained why the lid should be replaced immediately.
		•	Gently inserted the test strip into the test strip guide.
		•	Checked that the code number matches the code number on the test strip container.
		•	Opened gauze packet.
		•	Cleansed the puncture site with an antiseptic wipe and allowed it to dry.

Trial 1	Trial 2	Point Value	Performance Standards
		●	Applied gloves.
		●	Performed a finger puncture.
		●	Disposed of the lancet in the biohazard sharps container.
		●	Wiped away the first drop of blood with a gauze pad.
		▷	Explained why the first drop of blood should be wiped away.
		●	Placed the patient's hand in a dependent position and gently massaged finger until a large drop of blood formed.
		●	Applied the drop of blood to the yellow target area of the test strip.
		●	Completely filled the yellow target area with blood.
		▷	Explained what to do if the yellow area is not completely covered with blood.
		●	Placed a gauze pad over puncture site and applied pressure.
		●	Observed the digital display of the test results.
		▷	Stated the normal range for a fasting blood glucose level (70 to 99 mg/dL).
		●	Removed the test strip from the meter and discarded it in a biohazard waste container.
		●	Turned off the meter.
		●	Checked puncture site and applied adhesive bandage, if needed.
		●	Removed gloves and sanitized hands.
		●	Charted the test results correctly.
		✳	The recording was identical to the reading on the digital display screen.
		●	Properly stored the glucose meter.
		✳	Completed the procedure within 10 minutes.
			TOTALS

Evaluation of Student Performance

EVALUATION CRITERIA			COMMENTS
Symbol	**Category**	**Point Value**	
✱	Critical Step	16 points	
●	Essential Step	6 points	
▷	Theory Question	2 points	

Score calculation: 100 points

       −   _____ points missed

           ___ Score

Satisfactory score: 85 or above

CAAHEP Competencies Achieved

Psychomotor (Skills)

☑ I. 11. Perform quality control measures.
☑ I. 13. Perform chemistry testing.
☑ II. 2. Maintain laboratory test results using flow sheets.

Affective (Behavior)

☑ II. 2. Distinguish between normal and abnormal test results.

ABHES Competencies Achieved

☑ 10. a. Practice quality control.
☑ 10. b. Perform selected CLIA-waived tests that assist with diagnosis and treatment: (3) chemistry testing.

Chapter **33**   **Blood Chemistry and Immunology**

Notes

Procedure 33-B: Rapid Mononucleosis Testing (QuickVue + Mono Test)

Name: _____   Date: _____

Evaluated by: _____   Score: _____

Performance Objective

Outcome:	Perform a rapid mononucleosis test.
Conditions:	Given the following: disposable gloves, the supplies needed to perform a finger puncture, a mononucleosis testing kit, and a biohazard container.
Standards:	Time: 10 minutes. Student completed procedure in _____ minutes.
	Accuracy: Satisfactory score on the Performance Evaluation Checklist.

Performance Evaluation Checklist

Trial 1	Trial 2	Point Value	Performance Standards
		●	Sanitized hands.
		●	Assembled equipment.
		●	Checked the expiration date on the testing kit.
		●	Applied gloves and ran a positive and a negative control, if necessary.
		●	Removed gloves and recorded results in the quality control log.
		●	Greeted the patient and introduced yourself.
		●	Identified the patient and explained the procedure.
		●	Cleansed the puncture site and allowed it to air dry.
		●	Applied gloves.
		●	Performed a finger puncture.
		●	Disposed of the lancet in a biohazard sharps container.
		●	Wiped away the first drop of blood.
		●	Collected the blood specimen with a capillary tube.
		●	Placed a gauze pad over puncture site and applied pressure.
		●	Dispensed the blood specimen into the add well on the test cassette.
		●	Added 5 drops of developing solution to the add well.
		●	Waited 5 minutes and read the results.
		▷	Described the appearance of a positive and negative test result.
		●	Disposed of the test cassette in a biohazard waste container.
		●	Checked puncture site and applied adhesive bandage, if needed.

899

Chapter **33 Blood Chemistry and Immunology**

Trial 1	Trial 2	Point Value	Performance Standards
		•	Removed gloves.
		•	Sanitized hands.
		•	Charted the results correctly.
		•	The results were identical to the evaluator's results.
		✲	Completed the procedure within 10 minutes.
			TOTALS

			CHART
Date			

Evaluation of Student Performance

EVALUATION CRITERIA			COMMENTS
Symbol	**Category**	**Point Value**	
✲	Critical Step	16 points	
•	Essential Step	6 points	
▷	Theory Question	2 points	

Score calculation: 100 points

− _____ points missed

___ Score

Satisfactory score: 85 or above

CAAHEP Competencies Achieved

Psychomotor (Skills)

☑ I. 11. Perform quality control measures.
☑ I. 13. Perform immunology testing.

Affective (Behavior)

☑ II. 2. Distinguish between normal and abnormal test results.

ABHES Competencies Achieved

☑ 10. a. Practice quality control.
☑ 10. b. Perform selected CLIA-waived tests that assist with diagnosis and treatment (4) immunology testing.

34 Medical Microbiology

CHAPTER ASSIGNMENTS

√ After Completing	Date Due	Textbook Pages	TEXTBOOK ASSIGNMENTS	Possible Points	Points You Earned
		825-843	Read Chapter 34: Medical Microbiology		
		828 841-842	Read Case Study 1 Case Study 1 questions	5	
		836 842	Read Case Study 2 Case Study 2 questions	5	
		840 842	Read Case Study 3 Case Study 3 questions	5	
			TOTAL POINTS		
√ After Completing	**Date Due**	**Study Guide Pages**	**STUDY GUIDE ASSIGNMENTS (CTA = Critical Thinking Activity)**	**Possible Points**	**Points You Earned**
		905	Pretest	10	
		906	Term Key Term Assessment	15	
		906-909	Evaluation of Learning questions	27	
		910	CTA A: Stages of an Infectious Disease	20	
			Evolve Site: Microscope Identification (Record points earned)		
		911	CTA B: Disease and Infection Control	10	
		911	CTA C: Sensitivity Testing	12	
		912	CTA D: Crossword Puzzle	21	
			Evolve Site: Animations	20	
			Evolve Site: Apply Your Knowledge questions	10	
			Evolve Site: Video Evaluation	15	
		905	Posttest	10	

√ After Completing	Date Due	Study Guide Pages	STUDY GUIDE ASSIGNMENTS (CTA = Critical Thinking Activity)	Possible Points	Points You Earned
			ADDITIONAL ASSIGNMENTS		
			TOTAL POINTS		

√ When Assigned By Your Instructor	Study Guide Pages	Practices Required	LABORATORY ASSIGNMENTS (Procedure Number and Name)	Score*
	913-914	3	**Practice for Competency** 34-1: Using the Microscope Textbook reference: pp. 832-834	
	915-917		**Evaluation of Competency** 34-1: Using the Microscope	*
	913-914	3	**Practice for Competency** 34-2: Collecting a Throat Specimen Textbook reference: p. 837	
	919-922		**Evaluation of Competency** 34-2: Collecting a Throat Specimen	*
	913-914	3	**Practice for Competency** 34-A: Rapid Strep Testing Textbook reference: pp. 838-839	
	923-925		**Evaluation of Competency** 34-A: Rapid Strep Testing	*
			ADDITIONAL ASSIGNMENTS	

Notes

Name _____   Date _____

True or False

_____ 1. Microbiology is the scientific study of microorganisms and their activities.

_____ 2. A disease that can be spread from one person to another is known as an *infectious disease*.

_____ 3. Droplet infection is the transfer of pathogens from a fine spray emitted from a person already infected with the disease.

_____ 4. Streptococci are round bacteria that grow in pairs.

_____ 5. Chickenpox is caused by a virus.

_____ 6. The course adjustment on a microscope is used to obtain precise focusing of an object.

_____ 7. The purpose of transport media is to provide nutrients for the multiplication of the specimen.

_____ 8. A throat specimen should be collected from the tonsillar area and posterior pharynx.

_____ 9. A wet mount is used to examine microorganisms in the living state.

_____ 10. A smear is material spread on a slide for microscopic examination.

[?] **POSTTEST**

True or False

_____ 1. Microorganisms that reside in the body but do not cause disease are known as *transient flora*.

_____ 2. The invasion of the body by a pathogenic microorganism is known as *infection*.

_____ 3. The interval of time between the invasion by a pathogen and the first symptoms of disease is known as the *prodromal period*.

_____ 4. Staphylococcal infections usually result in pus formation.

_____ 5. *Escherichia coli* normally reside in the urinary tract.

_____ 6. The high-power objective has a magnification of 40×.

_____ 7. Examination of urine sediment requires the use of the oil immersion objective.

_____ 8. A sequela to streptococcal sore throat is rheumatic fever.

_____ 9. The purpose of sensitivity testing is to identify the type of microorganism present.

_____ 10. When viewed under a microscope, gram-positive bacteria appear pink or red.

Directions: Match each medical term with its definition.

_____ 1. Bacilli

_____ 2. Cocci

_____ 3. Contagious

_____ 4. Culture

_____ 5. Culture medium

_____ 6. Incubate

_____ 7. Incubation period

_____ 8. Infectious disease

_____ 9. Inoculate

_____ 10. Microbiology

_____ 11. Normal flora

_____ 12. Sequelae

_____ 13. Smear

_____ 14. Specimen

_____ 15. Spirilla

A. A disease caused by a pathogen that produces harmful effects on its host

B. Capable of being transmitted directly or indirectly from one person to another

C. To introduce microorganisms into a culture medium for growth and multiplication

D. Bacteria that have a round shape

E. The scientific study of microorganisms and their activities

F. Material spread on a slide for microscopic examination

G. Morbid (secondary) condition occurring as a result of a less serious primary infection

H. A mixture of nutrients in which microorganisms are grown in the laboratory

I. The interval of time between invasion by a pathogenic microorganism and the appearance of the first symptoms of the disease

J. Bacteria that have a spiral or curved shape

K. Harmless, nonpathogenic microorganisms that normally reside in many parts of the body but do not cause disease

L. Bacteria that have a rod shape

M. The propagation of a mass of microorganisms in a laboratory culture medium

N. In microbiology, the act of placing a culture in a chamber that provides optimal growth requirements for the multiplication of the organisms, such as the proper temperature, humidity, and darkness

O. A small sample or part taken from the body to show the nature of the whole

EVALUATION OF LEARNING

Directions: Fill in each blank with the correct answer.

1. What occurs when pathogens invade the body, and what is the response of the body to the invasion?

_____

_____

2. What is droplet infection?

_____

_____

3. What is the prodromal period of an infectious disease?

_____

_____

4. List three infectious diseases caused by *Staphylococcus aureus*.

_____

_____

Chapter **34** *Medical Microbiology*

5. List three infectious diseases caused by different types of streptococci.

_____

_____

6. List three infectious diseases caused by different types of bacilli.

_____

_____

7. In what part of the body do *E. coli* bacteria normally reside?

_____

8. List four infectious diseases caused by different viruses.

_____

_____

9. Explain the purpose of each of the following parts of a microscope:

Stage

_____

_____

Substage condenser

_____

_____

Iris diaphragm

_____

_____

Coarse adjustment

_____

_____

Fine adjustment

_____

_____

Ocular lens

_____

_____

10. Describe the function of each of the following objective lenses:

Low power

_____

_____

High power

_____

_____

Oil immersion

_____

_____

11. What is the purpose of using oil with the oil-immersion objective?

_____

_____

12. List five guidelines that should be followed for proper care of the microscope.

_____

_____

_____

_____

13. List five common areas of the body from which a microbiologic specimen may be obtained.

_____

_____

14. List two ways to prevent contamination of a specimen with extraneous microorganisms.

_____

_____

15. List two precautions a medical assistant should take to prevent infecting herself or himself with a microbiologic specimen.

_____

_____

16. Why should a specimen be processed as soon as possible after it is collected?

_____

17. What is the purpose of a transport medium?

_____

_____

18. How should a collection and transport system be stored?

_____

_____

19. Describe the procedure for collecting a wound specimen.

_____

_____

20. A throat specimen is used to perform tests that assist in the diagnosis of what conditions?

_____

_____

21. Why is it important to diagnose and treat streptococcal pharyngitis as early as possible?

_____

_____

22. What type of reaction is used to identify streptococci with the direct antigen identification test?

_____

23. What is the advantage of using the direct antigen identification test to diagnose streptococci compared with a culture test?

_____

_____

24. What is the purpose of performing a sensitivity test on a bacterial culture?

_____

25. List two reasons for examining a microorganism in the living state.

_____

_____

26. What is the purpose of staining a smear?

_____

_____

27. What color do the following bacteria exhibit in a Gram-stained smear?

Gram-positive bacteria: _____

Gram-negative bacteria: _____

A. Stages of an Infectious Disease

Your physician wants you to design a poster to hang in the office that outlines the stages of an infectious disease. Complete this project using the following diagram in your study guide.

STAGES OF INFECTIOUS DISEASE

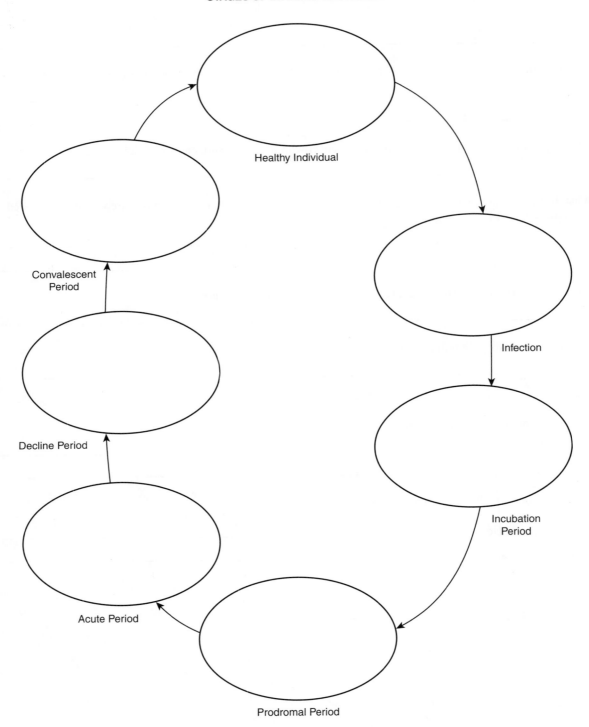

(From Bonewit-West K: *Study guide for clinical procedures for medical assistants,* ed 8, St. Louis, 2011, Saunders.)

B. Disease and Infection Control

Obtain a current journal article on disease and infection control. The Internet sites listed under **On the Web** at the end of Chapter 34 in your textbook can be used to locate an article. List the important parts of your article below.

_____

_____

_____

_____

_____

_____

_____

_____

_____

C. Sensitivity Testing

Refer to Figure 34-7 of the textbook. Place a check mark next to each antibiotic that is effective against the pathogen growing on the culture medium in the Petri plate.

_____ 1. azithromycin

_____ 2. cephalothin

_____ 3. ciprofloxacin

_____ 4. cefprozil

_____ 5. clarithromycin

_____ 6. doxycycline

_____ 7. erythromycin

_____ 8. nitrofurantoin

_____ 9. norfloxacin

_____ 10. penicillin

_____ 11. sulfisoxazole

_____ 12. tetracycline

D. Crossword Puzzle: Medical Microbiology

Directions: Complete the crossword puzzle using the clues provided.

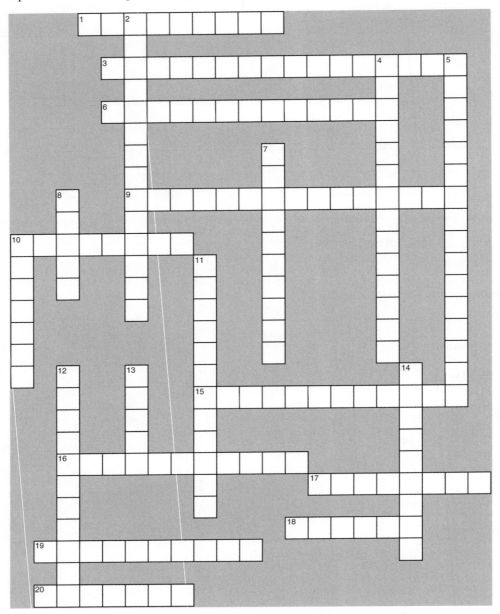

Across

1 Invasion by pathogens
3 Between invasion and first symptoms
6 Absent when present
9 Which antibiotic?
10 Sample of the body
15 Body's protective response
16 Treatment for strep throat
17 Disease-producing MO
18 Color of gram-positive bacteria
19 Can catch it!
20 Rod-shaped bacteria

Down

2 For precise focusing
4 Sequela to strep throat
5 Way to transmit pathogens
7 It's everywhere!
8 Material spread on a slide
10 Secondary condition
11 Study of microorganisms
12 Harmless MOs residing in body
13 Round bacteria
14 Magnifies 40x

Procedure 34-1: Using the Microscope. Practice using a microscope.

Procedure 34-2: Collecting a Throat Specimen. Obtain a throat specimen using a sterile cotton swab or a collection and transport system. Record the procedure in the chart provided.

Procedure 34-A: Rapid Strep Testing. Perform a strep test using a rapid strep testing kit, and record results in the chart provided.

	CHART
Date	

CHART	
Date	

Procedure 34-1: Using the Microscope

Name: _____   Date: _____

Evaluated by: _____   Score: _____

Performance Objective

Outcome:	Use a microscope.
Conditions:	Given a microscope, lens paper, specimen slide, tissue or gauze, immersion oil, xylene, and a soft cloth.
Standards:	Time: 15 minutes. Student completed procedure in _____ minutes.
	Accuracy: Satisfactory score on the Performance Evaluation Checklist.

Performance Evaluation Checklist

Trial 1	Trial 2	Point Value	Performance Standards
		●	Cleaned the ocular and objective lenses with lens paper.
		●	Turned on the light source.
		●	Rotated the nosepiece to the low-power objective.
		●	Used the coarse adjustment to provide sufficient working space for placing the slide on the stage.
		●	Placed the slide on the stage, specimen side up, and secured it.
		●	Positioned the low-power objective until it almost touched the slide using the coarse adjustment.
		●	Observed this step.
		▷	Explained why this step should be observed.
		●	Looked through the ocular lens.
		●	Brought the specimen into coarse focus using the coarse adjustment knob.
		●	Observed the specimen until it came into coarse focus.
		●	Used the fine-adjustment knob to bring the specimen into sharp, clear focus.
		●	Adjusted the light as needed using the iris diaphragm.
		●	Rotated the nosepiece to the high-power objective.
		●	Used the fine-adjustment knob to bring the specimen into a precise focus.
		●	Did not use the coarse-adjustment knob to focus the high-power objective.

Trial 1	Trial 2	Point Value	Performance Standards
		▷	Explained why the coarse-adjustment knob should not be used for focusing at this point.
		●	Examined the specimen as required by the test or procedure being performed.
		●	Turned off the light after use.
		●	Removed the slide from the stage.
		●	Cleaned the stage with a tissue or gauze.
		●	Properly cared for and stored the microscope.
			Using the oil-immersion objective:
		●	Rotated the nosepiece to the oil-immersion objective.
		●	Placed the objective to one side.
		●	Placed a drop of immersion oil on the slide directly over the center opening in the stage.
		●	Moved the oil-immersion objective into place.
		●	Made sure the objective did not touch the stage or slide.
		●	Used the coarse adjustment to position the oil-immersion objective.
		●	Brought the objective down until the lens touched the oil but did not come in contact with the slide.
		●	Looked through the eyepiece.
		●	Focused slowly using the coarse objective until the object was visible.
		●	Used the fine adjustment to bring the object into sharp focus.
		●	Adjusted the light as needed using the iris diaphragm.
		●	Examined the specimen as required by the test or procedure being performed.
		●	Turned off the light after use.
		●	Removed the slide from the stage.
		●	Cleaned the oil-immersion objective with lens paper.
		▷	Explained why the lens must be cleaned immediately.
		●	Cleaned the oil from the slide by immersing it in xylene and wiping it with a soft cloth.
		✶	Completed the procedure within 15 minutes.
			TOTALS

Evaluation of Student Performance

EVALUATION CRITERIA			COMMENTS
Symbol	Category	Point Value	
★	Critical Step	16 points	
●	Essential Step	6 points	
▷	Theory Question	2 points	

Score calculation: 100 points

–   points missed

_____

___ Score

Satisfactory score: 85 or above

CAAHEP Competencies Achieved

Psychomotor (Skills)
☑ I. 10. Assist physician with patient care.

ABHES Competencies Achieved

☑ 9. m. Assist physician with routine and specialty examinations and treatments.

Notes

Procedure 34-2: Collecting a Throat Specimen

Name: _____ Date: _____

Evaluated by: _____ Score: _____

Performance Objective

Outcome:	Collect a throat specimen.
Conditions:	Given the following: disposable gloves, tongue depressor, sterile swab, collection and transport system, laboratory request form, and a biohazard specimen bag.
Standards:	Time: 5 minutes. Student completed procedure in _____ minutes.
	Accuracy: Satisfactory score on the Performance Evaluation Checklist.

Performance Evaluation Checklist

Trial 1	Trial 2	Point Value	Performance Standards
			Throat specimen—sterile swab for strep testing in medical office
		●	Sanitized hands.
		●	Assembled equipment.
		●	Greeted the patient and introduced yourself.
		●	Identified the patient and explained the procedure.
		●	Positioned patient and adjusted light.
		●	Applied gloves.
		●	Removed the sterile swab from its peel-apart package, being careful not to contaminate it.
		●	Depressed patient's tongue with tongue depressor.
		●	Placed swab at the back of patient's throat and firmly rubbed it over lesions or white or inflamed areas of the tonsillar area and posterior pharynx.
		▷	Explained why swab should be rubbed over suspicious looking areas.
		●	Constantly rotated swab as the specimen was being obtained.
		▷	Described why a rotating motion should be used.
		●	Did not allow swab to touch any area other than throat.
		▷	Explained why swab should not be allowed to touch any areas other than throat.
		●	Kept patient's tongue depressed and withdrew swab and removed tongue depressor.

919

Trial 1	Trial 2	Point Value	Performance Standards
		●	Disposed of the tongue depressor.
		●	Performed the rapid strep test according to the directions accompanying the rapid strep testing kit.
		●	Removed gloves and sanitized hands.
		●	Charted the test results correctly.
		★	Completed the procedure within 5 minutes.
			Throat specimen—collection and transport system
		●	Sanitized hands.
		●	Greeted the patient and introduced yourself.
		●	Identified the patient and explained the procedure.
		●	Positioned patient and adjusted light.
		●	Applied gloves.
		●	Checked the expiration date on the peel-apart package.
		●	Peeled open the package and removed the cap from the collection tube.
		●	Removed the cap/swab unit from the peel-apart package.
		●	Depressed the patient's tongue with tongue depressor.
		●	Placed swab at the back of patient's throat and firmly rubbed it over lesions or white or inflamed areas of the tonsillar area and posterior pharynx.
		●	Constantly rotated swab as the specimen was being obtained.
		●	Did not allow swab to touch any area other than the collection site.
		●	Kept patient's tongue depressed and withdrew swab and removed tongue depressor.
		●	Disposed of the tongue depressor.
		●	Inserted swab into the collection tube.
		●	Pushed cap or swab in as far as it will go.
		●	Made sure the cap was tightly in place.
		●	Removed gloves and sanitized hands.
		●	Labeled tube.
		●	Completed a laboratory request form.
		●	Placed tube in a biohazard specimen transport bag.
		●	Placed laboratory request in outside pocket of bag.
		●	Charted the procedure.

Trial 1	Trial 2	Point Value	Performance Standards
		●	Transported specimen to the laboratory within 24 hours.
		▷	Explained why the specimen must be transported within 24 hours.
		★	Completed the procedure within 5 minutes.
			TOTALS

	CHART
Date	

Evaluation of Student Performance

EVALUATION CRITERIA			COMMENTS
Symbol	Category	Point Value	
★	Critical Step	16 points	
●	Essential Step	6 points	
▷	Theory Question	2 points	

Score calculation: 100 points

− _____ points missed

_____ Score

Satisfactory score: 85 or above

Chapter **34** **Medical Microbiology**

Procedure 34-A: Rapid Strep Testing

Name: _____   Date: _____

Evaluated by: _____   Score: _____

Performance Objective

Outcome:	Perform a rapid strep test.
Conditions:	Given the following: disposable gloves, tongue blade, a QuickVue rapid strep testing kit, controls, manufacturer's instructions, quality control log, and a biohazard sharps container.
Standards:	Time: 10 minutes. Student completed procedure in _____ minutes.
	Accuracy: Satisfactory score on the Performance Evaluation Checklist.

Performance Evaluation Checklist

Trial 1	Trial 2	Point Value	Performance Standards
		●	Sanitized hands.
		●	Assembled equipment.
		●	Checked the expiration date on the testing kit.
		●	Applied gloves and ran a positive and negative control, if needed.
		▷	Stated when controls should be run.
		●	Disposed of test cassettes and swabs in a biohazard waste container.
		●	Removed gloves and sanitized hands.
		●	Recorded results in the quality control log.
		●	Greeted the patient and introduced yourself.
		●	Identified the patient and explained the procedure.
		●	Positioned patient and adjusted light.
		●	Sanitized hands and applied gloves.
		●	Removed test cassette from its foil pouch, and placed it on a clean, dry, level surface.
		●	Removed the sterile swab from its peel-apart package.
		●	Depressed patient's tongue with tongue depressor.
		●	Placed swab at the back of patient's throat and firmly rubbed it over lesions or white or inflamed areas of the tonsillar area and posterior pharynx.
		●	Constantly rotated swab as the specimen was being obtained.

Trial 1	Trial 2	Point Value	Performance Standards
		▷	Stated why the swab should be rotated.
		●	Did not allow swab to touch any area other than throat.
		●	Kept patient's tongue depressed and withdrew swab.
		●	Removed tongue depressor and discarded it.
		●	Inserted the swab completely into the swab chamber.
		●	Squeezed the extraction bottle once to break the glass ampule.
		●	Vigorously shook the extraction bottle five times.
		●	Filled the swab chamber to the rim.
		●	Started the timer.
		●	Waited 5 minutes and read the results.
		▷	Described the appearance of a positive and negative result.
		▷	Described the appearance of an invalid result.
		▷	Explained what to do if an invalid result occurs.
		✶	The results were identical to the evaluator's results.
		●	Disposed of the test cassette and swab in a biohazard waste container.
		●	Removed gloves and sanitized hands.
		●	Recorded results in patient's chart.
		✶	Completed the procedure within 10 minutes.
			TOTALS

CHART	
Date	

Evaluation of Student Performance

EVALUATION CRITERIA			COMMENTS
Symbol	Category	Point Value	
✱	Critical Step	16 points	
●	Essential Step	6 points	
▷	Theory Question	2 points	

Score calculation: 100 points

      − _____ points missed

           ___ Score

Satisfactory score: 85 or above

CAAHEP Competencies Achieved

Psychomotor (Skills)
☑ I. 11. Perform quality control measures.
☑ III. 7. Obtain specimens for microbiological testing.
☑ III. 8. Perform CLIA-waived microbiology testing.

Affective (Behavior)
☑ II. 2. Distinguish between normal and abnormal test results.
☑ III. 1. Display sensitivity to patient rights and feelings in collecting specimens.
☑ III. 3. Show awareness of patients' concerns regarding their perceptions related to the procedures being
      performed.

ABHES Competencies Achieved

☑ 10. a. Practice quality control.
☑ 10. b. Perform selected CLIA-waived tests that assist with diagnosis and treatment: (2) microbiology testing (6)
      kit testing (b) quick strep.
☑ 10. c. Dispose of biohazardous materials.

Notes

Emergency Medical Procedures

√ After Completing	Date Due	Textbook Pages	TEXTBOOK ASSIGNMENTS	Possible Points	Points You Earned
		844-867	Read Chapter 35: Emergency Medical Procedures		
		859 865	Read Case Study 1 Case Study 1 questions	5	
		860 866	Read Case Study 2 Case Study 2 questions	5	
		863 866	Read Case Study 3 Case Study 3 questions	5	
			TOTAL POINTS		
√ After Completing	**Date Due**	**Study Guide Pages**	**STUDY GUIDE ASSIGNMENTS (CTA = Critical Thinking Activity)**	**Possible Points**	**Points You Earned**
		929	Pretest	10	
		930	Key Term Assessment	16	
		931-935	Evaluation of Learning questions	27	
		936	CTA A: First-Aid Kit	10	
		936	CTA B: EMD Information	5	
		936	CTA C: Emergency Care (2 points each)	6	
		937-938	CTA D: Emergency Situations (3 points each)	33	
		929	Posttest	10	
			ADDITIONAL ASSIGNMENTS		
			TOTAL POINTS		

Notes

Name _____   Date _____

True or False

_____ 1. A specially equipped cart for holding and transporting medications, equipment, and supplies needed in an emergency is known as a *crash cart*.

_____ 2. Symptoms of an asthmatic attack include dyspnea and wheezing.

_____ 3. Symptoms of a heart attack include sudden weakness on one side of the body.

_____ 4. Another name for a stroke is a *coronary occlusion*.

_____ 5. Arterial bleeding is characterized by a slow and steady flow of blood that is dark red.

_____ 6. A laceration is an example of a closed wound.

_____ 7. Symptoms of a fracture include pain, swelling, deformity, and loss of function.

_____ 8. A sprain is a tearing of ligaments at a joint.

_____ 9. Heat stroke is a life-threatening emergency.

_____ 10. Insulin enables glucose to enter the body's cells and be converted to energy.

📄 POSTTEST

True or False

_____ 1. When providing emergency care, you should obtain information about what happened from bystanders.

_____ 2. Emphysema is a progressive lung disorder in which there is a loss of elasticity of the alveoli of the lungs.

_____ 3. Symptoms that may occur with hyperventilation include rapid and deep respirations and tachycardia.

_____ 4. The first priority for hypovolemic shock is to control bleeding.

_____ 5. Status asthmaticus is the type of shock caused by a reaction of the body to a substance to which an individual is highly allergic.

_____ 6. Another name for a nosebleed is epistaxis.

_____ 7. The type of fracture in which the broken ends of the bone are forcefully jammed together is a greenstick fracture.

_____ 8. The type of seizure in which the abnormal electrical activity is localized into very specific areas of the brain is a tonic-clonic seizure.

_____ 9. Chipmunks have a high incidence of rabies.

_____ 10. Emergency care for insulin shock is to give the patient sugar immediately.

Directions: Match each medical term with its definition.

_____ 1. Burn

_____ 2. Crash cart

_____ 3. Crepitus

_____ 4. Dislocation

_____ 5. Emergency medical services

_____ 6. First aid

_____ 7. Fracture

_____ 8. Hypothermia

_____ 9. Poison

_____ 10. Pressure point

_____ 11. Seizure

_____ 12. Shock

_____ 13. Splint

_____ 14. Sprain

_____ 15. Strain

_____ 16. Wound

A. A network of community resources, equipment, and personnel that provides care to victims of injury or sudden illness
B. Any substance that causes illness, injury, or death if it enters the body
C. An injury to the tissues caused by exposure to thermal, chemical, electrical, or radioactive agents
D. Any device that immobilizes a body part
E. A grating sensation caused by fractured bone fragments rubbing against each other
F. A sudden episode of involuntary muscular contractions and relaxation, often accompanied by changes in sensation, behavior, and level of consciousness
G. A stretching or tearing of muscles or tendons caused by trauma
H. The immediate care that is administered to an individual who is injured or suddenly becomes ill before complete medical care can be obtained
I. A break in the continuity of an external or internal surface caused by physical means
J. A specially equipped cart for holding and transporting medications, equipment, and supplies needed for performing lifesaving procedures in an emergency
K. Any break in a bone
L. The failure of the cardiovascular system to deliver enough blood to all the vital organs of the body
M. An injury in which one end of a bone making up a joint is separated or displaced from its normal anatomic position
N. A life-threatening condition in which the temperature of the entire body falls to a dangerously low level
O. A site on the body where an artery lies close to the surface of the skin and can be compressed against an underlying bone to control bleeding
P. Trauma to a joint that causes tearing of ligaments

Directions: Fill in each blank with the correct answer.

1. What is the purpose of first aid?

   _____

   _____

   _____

   _____

2. What is the purpose of the office crash cart?

   _____

   _____

   _____

   _____

3. What is the difference between an EMT-basic and an EMT-paramedic?

   _____

   _____

   _____

4. What are the responsibilities of an emergency medical dispatcher?

   _____

   _____

   _____

5. List five OSHA Standards that should be followed when administering first aid.

   _____

   _____

   _____

   _____

6. What is the reason for performing each of the following during an emergency situation?

   a. Remaining calm and speaking in a normal tone of voice

   _____

   _____

   b. Making sure it is safe before approaching the patient

   _____

   _____

c. Following OSHA Standards when providing emergency care

_____

_____

d. Activating the emergency medical services

_____

_____

e. Not moving the patient unnecessarily

_____

_____

f. Checking the patient for a medical alert tag

_____

_____

7. What are the symptoms of asthma?

_____

_____

8. What is emphysema?

_____

_____

9. What are the symptoms of hyperventilation?

_____

_____

10. What are the symptoms of a heart attack?

_____

_____

11. What are the symptoms of a stroke?

_____

_____

12. What is the cause of the following types of shock?

a. Hypovolemic

_____

_____

b. Cardiogenic

_____

_____

c. Neurogenic

_____

_____

d. Anaphylactic

_____

_____

e. Psychogenic

_____

_____

13. What are the characteristics of each of the following types of external bleeding?

a. Capillary

_____

_____

b. Venous

_____

_____

c. Arterial

_____

_____

14. What is the difference between an open wound and a closed wound?

_____

_____

15. What are the signs and symptoms of a fracture?

_____

_____

16. What are the characteristics of each of the following types of fractures?

a. Impacted

_____

_____

b. Greenstick

_____

_____

c. Transverse

_____

_____

d. Oblique

_____

_____

e. Comminuted

_____

_____

f. Spiral

_____

_____

17. What are the characteristics of each of the following types of burns?

a. Superficial

_____

_____

b. Partial thickness

_____

_____

c. Full thickness

_____

_____

18. What is the difference between a partial seizure and a generalized seizure?

_____

_____

19. List two examples of each of the following types of poisoning:

a. Ingested

_____

_____

b. Inhaled

_____

_____

c. Absorbed

_____

_____

d. Injected

_____

_____

20. What spiders (found in the United States) have bites that can result in serious or life-threatening reactions?

_____

_____

21. What species of snakes (found in the United States) are poisonous?

_____

_____

22. What animals tend to have a high incidence of rabies?

_____

_____

23. What factors place an individual at higher risk for developing heat- and cold-related injuries?

_____

_____

24. What areas of the body are most susceptible to frostbite?

_____

_____

25. What is the difference between type 1 diabetes and type 2 diabetes?

_____

_____

26. What is insulin shock, and what causes it to occur?

_____

_____

27. What is a diabetic coma, and what causes it to occur?

_____

_____

CRITICAL THINKING ACTIVITIES

A. First-Aid Kit
You are assembling a first-aid kit. What supplies should be included in your kit? Identify one use for each of the supplies you list.

_____

_____

_____

_____

_____

_____

_____

_____

_____

_____

B. EMD Information
Jeff Stickler suddenly develops weakness in his left arm and leg, has difficulty speaking, and has a severe headache and dizziness. You immediately call the Emergency Medical Services (EMS). What information should you be prepared to relay to the emergency medical dispatcher (EMD)?

_____

_____

_____

_____

C. Emergency Care
In which of the following emergency situations would you be legally permitted to administer first aid? Explain your answers.

1. A patient is unconscious and bleeding profusely.

   _____

   _____

2. You identify yourself and state your level of training and what you plan to do. You ask the patient if it is alright to administer emergency care. The patient responds by saying, "Yes, please help me."

   _____

   _____

3. You ask the patient if you can administer emergency care, but the patient refuses your help.

   _____

   _____

D. Emergency Situations

Explain what you would do in each of the following situations.

1. Holly Murphy falls while roller skating. She comes down hard on her left arm, which begins to swell and discolor. Holly guards her arm and complains of intense pain.

_____

_____

_____

_____

2. John Phillips is mowing the grass and mows over a yellow jacket nest. He is stung twice and soon starts complaining of intense itching and exhibits erythema and hives on his arms, torso, and face.

_____

_____

_____

_____

3. Steve Williams complains of severe indigestion and squeezing pain in the chest. He is short of breath and perspiring profusely.

_____

_____

_____

_____

4. Clara Miller is playing basketball and is accidentally hit in the face with the ball. Her nose begins bleeding profusely.

_____

_____

_____

_____

5. Debbie Carter, age 4 years, finds some children's chewable vitamins that have been left open on a table. She eats about 10 of them.

_____

_____

_____

_____

6. Rita Preston accidentally cuts her finger with a knife while preparing dinner. Her finger begins bleeding profusely.

_____

_____

_____

_____

7. Jose Perez is jogging on a cinder track. He falls and scrapes his left knee on the cinders.

_____

_____

_____

_____

8. Charlotte Lambert is getting ready to perform a piano recital for her entire church congregation. Suddenly she starts breathing very rapidly and deeply and complains that she feels light-headed and dizzy.

_____

_____

_____

_____

9. Bruce Jones is a diabetic. He is in a hurry and forgets to eat breakfast. He begins exhibiting behavior similar to that of someone who is intoxicated.

_____

_____

_____

_____

10. Debra Murray is delivering newspapers and is bitten by a strange dog. The bite causes several puncture marks and slight bleeding.

_____

_____

_____

_____

11. Tanya Howe is playing tennis on a hot and humid day and begins to feel weak and nauseous. Her skin feels cold and clammy, and she is sweating profusely and complains of dizziness.

_____

_____

_____

_____

36 The Medical Record

CHAPTER ASSIGNMENTS

√ After Completing	Date Due	Textbook Pages	TEXTBOOK ASSIGNMENTS	Possible Points	Points You Earned
		869-914	Read Chapter 36: The Medical Record		
		874 912	Read Case Study 1 Case Study 1 questions	5	
		893 912	Read Case Study 2 Case Study 2 questions	5	
		899 912	Read Case Study 3 Case Study 3 questions	5	
			TOTAL POINTS		

√ After Completing	Date Due	Study Guide Pages	STUDY GUIDE ASSIGNMENTS (CTA = Critical Thinking Activity)	Possible Points	Points You Earned
		943	Pretest	10	
		944	Term Key Term Assessment	20	
		944-949	Evaluation of Learning questions	50	
		950	CTA A: Medication Administration Record	4	
		950	CTA B: Consultation Report	4	
		950	CTA C: Radiology Report	3	
		950	CTA D: Diagnostic Imaging Report	4	
		951	CTA E: Discharge Summary Report	5	
		951	CTA F: Release of Medical Information	4	
		951-952	CTA G: Chief Complaint	6	
		952	CTA H: Crossword Puzzle	23	
			Evolve Site: Road to Recovery: Medical Abbreviations (Record points earned)		
		970-976	Taking Patient Symptoms: Supplemental Education for Chapter 36 (10 points for each problem)	60	
			Evolve Site: Apply Your Knowledge questions	10	

√ After Completing	Date Due	Study Guide Pages	STUDY GUIDE ASSIGNMENTS (CTA Critical Thinking Activity)	Possible Points	Points You Earned
			Evolve Site: Video Evaluation	12	
		943	Posttest	10	
			ADDITIONAL ASSIGNMENTS		
			TOTAL POINTS		

√ When Assigned By Your Instructor	Study Guide Pages	Practices Required	LABORATORY ASSIGNMENTS (Procedure Number and Name)	Score*
	953-955	1	**Practice for Competency** Health History Form Textbook reference: pp. 900-902	
	956	1	**Practice for Competency** 36-1: Completion of a Consent to Treatment Form Textbook reference: p. 890	
	959-960		**Evaluation of Competency** 36-1: Completion of a Consent to Treatment Form	*
	957	1	**Practice for Competency** 36-2: Release of Medical Information Textbook reference: p. 891	
	961-963		**Evaluation of Competency** 36-2: Release of Medical Information	*
	958	2	**Practice for Competency** 36-3: Preparing a Medical Record Textbook reference: pp. 897-898	
	965-966		**Evaluation of Competency** 36-3: Preparing a Medical Record	*
	958	5	**Practice for Competency** 36-4: Obtaining and Recording Patient Symptoms Textbook reference: pp. 908-909	
	967-969		**Evaluation of Competency** 36-4: Obtaining and Recording Patient Symptoms	*
			ADDITIONAL ASSIGNMENTS	

Notes

Name _____   Date _____

True or False

_____ 1. The medical record serves as a legal document.

_____ 2. The purpose of progress notes is to update the medical record with new information.

_____ 3. The patient registration record consists of a list of the problems associated with the patient's illness.

_____ 4. All OTC medications taken by the patient should be charted on the medication record form.

_____ 5. A consultation report is a narrative report of a clinical opinion about a patient's condition by a practitioner other than the primary physician.

_____ 6. A report of the analysis of body specimens is known as a diagnostic report.

_____ 7. Medical impressions are conclusions drawn from an interpretation of data.

_____ 8. A consent to treatment form is required for tuberculin skin testing.

_____ 9. Diabetes mellitus is an example of a familial disease.

_____ 10. Pain is an example of an objective symptom.

⁉ POSTTEST

True or False

_____ 1. The purpose of HIPAA is to provide patients with more control over the use and disclosure of their health information.

_____ 2. The health history provides subjective data about a patient to assist the physician in arriving at a diagnosis.

_____ 3. Physical therapy helps a patient with a disability learn new skills to perform the activities of daily living.

_____ 4. A copy of the patient's emergency room report is sent to the patient's family physician.

_____ 5. When a medical assistant (MA) witnesses a patient's signature on a form, it means that the MA is verifying that the patient understands the information on the form.

_____ 6. SOAP is the acronym for the format used to organize POR progress notes.

_____ 7. The chief complaint is the symptom causing the patient the most trouble.

_____ 8. The social history includes information on the patient's lifestyle, such as health habits and living environment.

_____ 9. The patient's name must be included at the beginning of each entry charted in the patient's medical record.

_____ 10. A decrease in the amount of water in the body is known as edema.

Directions: Match each medical term with its definition.

_____ 1. Attending physician

_____ 2. Charting

_____ 3. Consultation report

_____ 4. Diagnosis

_____ 5. Diagnostic procedure

_____ 6. Discharge summary report

_____ 7. Electronic medical record

_____ 8. Familial

_____ 9. Health history report

_____ 10. Informed consent

_____ 11. Inpatient

_____ 12. Medical impressions

_____ 13. Medical record

_____ 14. Objective symptom

_____ 15. Patient

_____ 16. Physical examination report

_____ 17. Problem

_____ 18. Prognosis

_____ 19. Subjective symptom

_____ 20. Symptom

A. A collection of subjective data about a patient
B. A narrative report of an opinion about a patient's condition by a practitioner other than the attending physician
C. Any condition that requires further observation, diagnosis, management, or patient education
D. A symptom felt by the patient but not observed by an examiner
E. The process of making written entries about a patient in the medical record
F. The consent given by a patient for a medical procedure after being informed of the procedure
G. Any change in the body or its functioning that indicates the presence of disease
H. Conclusions drawn by the physician from an interpretation of data
I. A medical record that is stored on a computer
J. A brief summary of the significant events of a patient's hospitalization
K. A written record of the important information regarding a patient
L. A symptom that can be observed by an examiner
M. The probable course and outcome of a disease and the prospects for recovery
N. The scientific method of determining and identifying a patient's condition
O. A report of the objective findings from the physician's assessment of each body system
P. Occurring or affecting members of a family more frequently than would be expected by chance
Q. The physician responsible for the care of a hospitalized patient
R. A procedure performed to assist in the diagnosis, management, or treatment of a patient's condition
S. A patient who has been admitted to the hospital for at least one overnight stay
T. An individual receiving medical care

EVALUATION OF LEARNING

Directions: Fill in each blank with the correct answer.

1. List three functions of the medical record.

_____

2. What is the meaning of the acronym HIPAA?

_____

3. What is the purpose of the HIPAA privacy rule?

_____

4. Who must comply with HIPAA?

_____

5. What is a Notice of Privacy Practices (NPP)?

_____

6. List examples of when HIPAA does not require written consent for the use or disclosure of a patient's health information in the following categories:

    a.   Treatment: _____

    b.   Payment: _____

    c.   Health care operations: _____

7. What two general categories of information are included on a patient registration record?

_____

8. List three uses of the health history.

_____

_____

_____

9. What is the purpose of the physical examination?

_____

_____

10. What is the purpose of progress notes?

_____

_____

11. List three categories of medication that may be included in a medication record.

_____

_____

12. What is the purpose of home health care?

_____

_____

13. List five examples of home health services.

_____

_____

_____

_____

14. What is the purpose of a laboratory report?

_____

_____

945

15. List five examples of diagnostic procedure reports.

_____

_____

16. What is the purpose of a therapeutic service report?

_____

_____

17. What is the difference between physical therapy and occupational therapy?

_____

_____

_____

18. List examples of physical agents used in physical therapy?

_____

_____

19. What is speech therapy?

_____

_____

20. What is the purpose of an operative report?

_____

_____

21. What is the purpose of the discharge summary report?

_____

_____

22. What is included in a pathology report?

_____

_____

23. Why is a copy of the emergency room report sent to the patient's family physician?

_____

_____

24. When is a consent to treatment form required?

_____

_____

25. What is the purpose of a consent to treatment form?

_____

_____

26. What information must the patient receive before signing a consent to treatment form?

_____

_____

27. What does *witnessing a signature* mean? What does it not mean?

_____

_____

_____

28. When must a patient complete a release of medical information form?

_____

_____

29. When does a release of medical information form not have to be completed?

_____

_____

30. What is the difference between a PPR and an EMR?

_____

_____

31. What functions are performed by an EMR software program?

_____

_____

32. How are documents organized in a source-oriented medical record?

_____

_____

33. What is reverse chronological order?

_____

_____

34. How are documents organized in a problem-oriented medical record (POR)?

_____

_____

35. List and describe the four parts of a POR.

_____

_____

_____

_____

36. List and describe the format used to organize progress notes in a POR.

_____

_____

37. How can a health history be entered into the EMR?

_____

_____

_____

38. What are the seven parts of the health history?

_____

_____

_____

_____

_____

_____

_____

39. What is a chief complaint?

_____

40. What guidelines should be followed in recording the chief complaint?

_____

_____

_____

41. What is the current illness, and how is this information obtained?

_____

_____

42. List five examples of information included in the past medical history.

_____

_____

_____

_____

_____

43. List three examples of familial diseases.

_____

_____

_____

44. Explain the importance of the social history.

_____

_____

45. What is the purpose of the review of systems (ROS)?

_____

_____

46. List the guidelines that should be followed to ensure accurate and concise charting.

_____

_____

_____

_____

47. List three examples of subjective symptoms.

_____

_____

_____

48. List three examples of objective symptoms.

_____

_____

_____

49. What is the difference between a productive and a nonproductive cough?

_____

_____

50. Why should the following be charted in the patient's medical record?

   a. Procedures performed on the patient

_____

_____

   b. Specimens collected from the patient

_____

_____

   c. Laboratory tests ordered for the patient

_____

_____

   d. Instructions given to the patient regarding medical care

_____

_____

CRITICAL THINKING ACTIVITIES

A. Medication Administration Record

Refer to the medication administration record (see Figure 36-2) in your textbook, and answer the following questions.

1. Does Kristen Antle have any allergies?

   _____

2. How much Rocephin was administered to Kristen?

   _____

3. What was the route of administration of the Rocephin injection, and where was it administered?

   _____

4. What is the name of the company that manufactures Rocephin?

   _____

B. Consultation Report

Refer to the consultation report (see Figure 36-3) in your textbook, and identify the following information using the corresponding numbers (1, 2, 3, or 4).

1. Documentation that the consultant reviewed the patient's health history

2. Documentation that the consultant examined the patient

3. A report of the consultants' impressions

4. A report of the consultants' recommendations

C. Radiology Report

Refer to the radiology report (see Figure 36-5) in your textbook, and answer the following questions.

1. What type of radiologic examination was performed on Rose Baker?

   _____

2. Were the lungs clear? _____

3. Were any abnormal masses noted in the abdomen? _____

D. Diagnostic Imaging Report

Refer to the diagnostic imaging report (see Figure 36-6) in your textbook, and answer the following questions.

1. What type of diagnostic imaging procedure was performed on Vera Ruth?

   _____

2. Which vertebrae of the spine were scanned?

   _____

3. What problem may affect L4-5?

   _____

4. What additional tests might be scheduled for Vera Ruth?

   _____

950

Chapter **36**   **The Medical Record**

E. Discharge Summary Report

Refer to the discharge summary report (see Figure 36-10) in your textbook, and answer the following questions.

1. How long was Susan Brennan hospitalized?

   _____

2. What was her hemoglobin level at admission?

   _____

3. What was the reason for the hospitalization?

   _____

4. Was Susan pregnant?

   _____

5. What was the discharge diagnosis?

   _____

F. Release of Medical Information

Refer to the release of medical information form (see Figure 36-14) in your textbook, and answer the following questions.

1. What medical information is protected by law and cannot be released unless specifically authorized by the patient?

   _____

   _____

2. List three reasons why a patient may authorize the release of his or her medical information.

   _____

   _____

   _____

3. After this form is completed and signed, how long is it valid before it expires?

   _____

4. What must the patient do if he or she wants to revoke the authorization?

   _____

   _____

G. Chief Complaint

Indicate whether each of the following statements is an incorrect (**I**) or correct (**C**) example of recording a chief complaint (CC). If the example is incorrect, explain which recording guideline is not being followed.

_____ 1. CC: Low back pain _____

_____ 2. CC: Sore throat and fever for the past 2 days _____

_____ 3. CC: Dyspnea, paleness, and fatigue, similar to that associated with anemia, which have lasted for 2 weeks

   _____

_____ 4. CC: Poor health for the past several months _____

_____ 5. CC: Weakness and fatigue related to poor eating habits and lack of exercise

_____

_____

_____ 6. CC: Heart palpitations occurring after drinking coffee in the morning before work

_____

_____

H. Crossword Puzzle: The Medical Record

Directions: Complete the crossword puzzle using the clues provided.

(From Bonewit-West K: *Study guide for clinical procedures for medical assitants,* ed 8, St. Louis, 2011, Saunders.)

Across
2 Stool is hard and dry
4 Blue skin due to lack of O_2
5 Nosebleed
10 Skin eruption
11 Dizziness
14 No appetite
15 Yellow skin
18 Severe itching
19 Involuntary contractions of muscles
20 Gas
21 Head pain

Down
1 Fast pulse rate
2 Shivering
3 May be productive or nonproductive
5 Fluid retention
6 Ejection of stomach contents
7 Decreased H_2O levels in the body
8 Red face
9 Elevated temp
12 Bad all over
13 Loose, watery stools
16 Sensation of stomach discomfort
17 Feeling of distress or suffering

Health History Form. Complete the health history form (pp. 953 to 955) using yourself as the patient.

PATIENT HEALTH HISTORY

A   **IDENTIFICATION DATA**   Please print the following information.

Today's date _____

Name _____   ___ Male ___ Female

Address _____   ___ Married ___ Separated ___ Divorced ___ Widowed ___ Single

_____   Date of Birth _____

Telephone _____ _____

B   **PAST HISTORY**

Have you ever had the following: (Circle "no" or "yes", leave blank if uncertain)

Measles _____ no yes	Heart Disease _____ no yes	Diabetes _____ no yes	Hemorrhoids _____ no yes
Mumps _____ no yes	Arthritis _____ no yes	Cancer _____ no yes	Asthma _____ no yes
Chickenpox _____ no yes	Sexually Transmitted _ no yes Disease	Polio _____ no yes	Allergies _____ no yes
Whooping Cough ___ no yes	Anemia _____ no yes	Glaucoma _____ no yes	Eczema _____ no yes
Scarlet Fever _____ no yes	Bladder Infections ___ no yes	Hernia _____ no yes	AIDS or HIV+ _____ no yes
Diphtheria _____ no yes	Epilepsy _____ no yes	Blood or Plasma ____ no yes Transfusions	Infectious Mono ____ no yes
Pneumonia _____ no yes	Migraine Headaches __ no yes	Back Trouble _____ no yes	Bronchitis _____ no yes
Rheumatic Fever ____ no yes	Tuberculosis _____ no yes	High Blood _____ no yes Pressure	Mitral Valve Prolapse no yes
Stroke _____ no yes	Ulcer _____ no yes	Thyroid Disease ____ no yes	Any other disease ___ no yes Please list: _____
Hepatitis. _____ no yes	Kidney Disease _____ no yes	Bleeding Tendency __ no yes	_____

MAJOR HOSPITALIZATIONS: If you have ever been hospitalized for any major medical illness or operation, write in your most recent hospitalizations below.

Hospitalizations	Year	Operation or illness	Name of hospital	City and state
1st Hospitalization				
2nd Hospitalization				
3rd Hospitalization				
4th Hospitalization				

TESTS AND IMMUNIZATIONS: Mark an X next to those that you have had.

Tests: Immunizations:

☐ TB Test   ☐ Electrocardiogram   ☐ Influenza

☐ Rectal/Hemoccult   ☐ Chest X-ray   ☐ Hepatitis B

☐ Sigmoidoscopy   ☐ Mammogram   ☐ Tetanus

☐ Colonoscopy   ☐ Pap Test   ☐ MMR

☐ Polio

ALLERGIES: List all allergies (foods, drugs, environment). ☐ None

_____
_____
_____
_____

CURRENT MEDICATIONS: List the following that you are currently taking: Prescription medications, over-the-counter (OTC) medications, vitamin supplements, and herbal supplements. ☐ None

Medication	Frequency

ACCIDENTS/ INJURIES: Describe all serious accidents, severe injuries, head injury, or fractrures. Include the date each occurred. ☐ None

Accident/Injury: Date:

_____
_____
_____

(From Bonewit-West K: *Study guide for clinical procedures for medical assistants,* ed 8, St. Louis, 2011, Saunders.)

C FAMILY HISTORY

For each member of your family, follow the purple or blue line across the page and check boxes for:
1. Their present state of health
2. Any illnesses they have had

	Good Health	Poor Health	Deceased	If deceased, write in age and cause of death.	Allergies or Asthma	Diabetes	Heart Disease	Stroke	Cancer	High Blood Pressure	Glaucoma	Arthritis	Ulcer	Kidney Disease	Mental Health Problems	Alcohol/Drug Abuse	Obesity	High Cholesterol	Thyroid Disease
Father:																			
Mother:																			
Brothers/Sisters:																			

D SOCIAL HISTORY

EDUCATION _____ High school _____ College _____ Post graduate

Occupation _____ Years _____

Previous occupations _____ Years _____

_____ Years _____

Have you ever been exposed to any of the following in your environment?

☐ Excess dust (coal, lime, rock) ☐ Cleaning fluids/solvents ☐ Radiation ☐ Other toxic materials
☐ Sand ☐ Hair spray ☐ Insecticides
☐ Chemicals ☐ Smoke or auto exhaust fumes ☐ Paints

Please answer the follwing questions by placing an X in the box in front of the word Yes or No, except where you are asked for specific information. This information is obviously highly confidential and will be released to other health professionals or insurance carriers ONLY with your consent.

DIET:

Do you eat a good breakfast?	☐ Yes	☐ No
Do you snack between meals (soft drinks, chips, candy bars)?	☐ Yes	☐ No
Do you eat fresh fruits and vegetables each day?	☐ Yes	☐ No
Do you eat whole grain breads and cereals?	☐ Yes	☐ No
Is your diet high in fat content?	☐ Yes	☐ No
Is your diet high in cholesterol content?	☐ Yes	☐ No
Is your diet high in salt content?	☐ Yes	☐ No
Are you allergic to any foods?	☐ Yes	☐ No

How many glasses of water do you drink each day? _____

How would you describe your overall eating habits? ☐ Excellent ☐ Good ☐ Fair ☐ Poor

PERSONAL HISTORY:

Do you find it hard to make decisions?	☐ Yes	☐ No
Do you find it hard to concentrate or remember?	☐ Yes	☐ No
Do you feel depressed?	☐ Yes	☐ No
Do you have difficulty relaxing?	☐ Yes	☐ No
Do you have a tendency to worry a lot?	☐ Yes	☐ No
Have you gained or lost much weight recently?	☐ Yes	☐ No
Do you lose your temper often?	☐ Yes	☐ No
Are you disturbed by any work or family problems?	☐ Yes	☐ No
Are you having sexual difficulties?	☐ Yes	☐ No
Have you ever considered committing suicide?	☐ Yes	☐ No
Have you ever desired or sought psychiatric help?	☐ Yes	☐ No

EXERCISE:

Do you exercise on a regular basis?	☐ Yes	☐ No
Does your job require strenuous, sustained physical work?	☐ Yes	☐ No

SLEEP PATTERNS:

Do you seem to feel exhausted or fatigued most of the time?	☐ Yes	☐ No
Do you have difficulty either falling asleep or staying asleep?	☐ Yes	☐ No

USE OF TOBACCO/ALCOHOL/CAFFEINE/DRUGS:

Amt:

How much do you smoke per day? ☐ Cigarettes ___ ☐ Don't smoke ☐ Cigars/pipes ___

Do you take two or more alcoholic drinks per day?	☐ Yes	☐ No
Do you drink six or more cups of coffee or tea per day?	☐ Yes	☐ No
Are you a regular user of sleeping pills, marijuana, tranquilizers, pain killers, etc?	☐ Yes	☐ No
Have you ever used heroin, cocaine, LSD, PCP, etc?	☐ Yes	☐ No

List any country outside the USA you have visited in the past six months? _____

When did you have your last physical examination? _____

(From Bonewit-West K: *Study guide for clinical procedures for medical assistants,* ed 8, St. Louis, 2011, Saunders.)

E REVIEW OF SYSTEMS

HEAD AND NECK
- _____ Frequent headaches
- _____ Neck pain
- _____ Neck lumps or swelling

EYES
- _____ Wears glasses
- _____ Blurry vision
- _____ Eyesight worsening
- _____ Sees double
- _____ Sees halo
- _____ Eye pain or itching
- _____ Watering eyes
- _____ Eye trouble

EARS
- _____ Hearing difficulties
- _____ Earaches
- _____ Running ears
- _____ Buzzing in ears
- _____ Motion sickness

MOUTH
- _____ Dental problems
- _____ Swellings on gums or jaws
- _____ Sore tongue
- _____ Taste changes

NOSE AND THROAT
- _____ Congested nose
- _____ Running nose
- _____ Sneezing spells
- _____ Headcolds
- _____ Nose bleeds
- _____ Sore throat
- _____ Enlarged tonsils
- _____ Hoarse voice

RESPIRATORY
- _____ Wheezes or gasps
- _____ Coughing spells
- _____ Coughs up phlegm
- _____ Coughed up blood
- _____ Chest colds
- _____ Excessive sweating, night sweats

CARDIOVASCULAR
- _____ High blood pressure
- _____ Racing heart
- _____ Chest pains
- _____ Dizzy spells
- _____ Shortness of breath
- _____ Shortness of breath at night
- _____ More pillows to breathe
- _____ Swollen feet or ankles
- _____ Leg cramps
- _____ Heart murmur

DIGESTIVE
- _____ Heartburn
- _____ Bloated stomach
- _____ Belching
- _____ Stomach pains
- _____ Nausea
- _____ Vomited blood
- _____ Difficulty swallowing
- _____ Constipation
- _____ Loose bowels
- _____ Black stools
- _____ Grey stools
- _____ Pain in rectum
- _____ Rectal bleeding

URINARY
- _____ Night frequency
- _____ Day frequency
- _____ Wets pants or bed
- _____ Burning on urination
- _____ Brown, black, or bloody urine
- _____ Difficulty starting urine
- _____ Urgency

MALE GENITAL
- _____ Weak urine stream
- _____ Prostate trouble
- _____ Burning or discharge
- _____ Lumps on testicles
- _____ Painful testicles

FEMALE GENITAL
- _/_/_ Last menstrual period
- _/_/_ Last Pap test
- _____ Post-menopausal or hysterectomy
- _____ Noticed vaginal bleeding
- _____ Abnormal LMP
- _____ Heavy bleeding during periods
- _____ Bleeding between periods
- _____ Bleeding after intercourse
- _____ Recent vaginal itching/ discharge
- _____ No monthly breast exam
- _____ Lump or pain in breasts
- _____ Complications with birth control

OBSTETRIC HISTORY
- _____ Gravida
- _____ Para
- _____ Pre-term
- _____ Miscarriages
- _____ Still births
- _____ Has had an abortion

MUSCULOSKELETAL
- _____ Aching muscles
- _____ Swollen joints
- _____ Back or shoulder pains
- _____ Painful feet
- _____ Disability

SKIN
- _____ Skin problems
- _____ Itching or burning skin
- _____ Bleeds easily
- _____ Bruises easily

NEUROLOGICAL
- _____ Faintness
- _____ Numbness
- _____ Convulsions
- _____ Change in handwriting
- _____ Trembles

F PROGRESS NOTES

Date	

(From Bonewit-West K: *Study guide for clinical procedures for medical assistants,* ed 8, St. Louis, 2011, Saunders.)

Procedure 36-1: Consent to Treatment. Complete the consent to treatment form using a classmate as the patient.

(attach label or complete blanks)

First name: _____   Last name: _____

Date of Birth: _____ Month _____ Day _____ Year

Account Number: _____

Procedure Consent Form

I, _____, hereby consent to have

Dr. _____, perform _____.

I have been fully informed of the following by my physician:

  1. The nature of my condition.
  2. The nature and purpose of the procedure.
  3. An explanation of risks involved with the procedure.
  4. Alternative treatments or procedures available.
  5. The likely results of the procedure.
  6. The risks involved with declining or delaying the procedure.

My physician has offered to answer all questions concerning the proposed procedure.

I am aware that the practice of medicine and surgery is not an exact science, and I acknowledge that no guarantees have been made to me about the results of the procedure.

Patient _____   Date _____
              (or guardian and relationship)

Witnessed _____   Date _____

(From Bonewit-West K: *Study guide for clinical procedures for medical assistants,* ed 8, St. Louis, 2011, Saunders.)

Procedure 36-2: Release of Medical Information. Complete the release of medical information form using a classmate as the patient.

RELEASE OF MEDICAL INFORMATION

All information contained in the medical record is confidential and the release of information is closely controlled. A properly completed and signed authorization is required for the release of the following information.

PATIENT INFORMATION

Patient Name _____

Address _____

City _____ State _____ ZIP _____   Social Security # _____

Phone (Home) _____ Work _____   Birthdate _____ / _____ / _____

RELEASE FROM:

Name _____

Address _____

City _____ State _____ ZIP _____

RELEASE TO:

Name _____

Address _____

City _____ State _____ ZIP _____

INFORMATION TO BE RELEASED:

1. GENERAL RELEASE:

_____ Entire Medical Record (excluding protected information)
_____ Hospital Records only (specify) _____
_____ Lab Results only (specify) _____
_____ X-ray Reports only (specify) _____
_____ Other Records (specify) _____

2. INFORMATION PROTECTED BY STATE/FEDERAL LAW:
If indicated below, I hereby authorize the disclosure and release of information regarding:

_____ Drug Abuse Diagnosis/Treatment
_____ Alcoholism Diagnosis/Treatment
_____ Mental Health Diagnosis/Treatment
_____ Sexually Transmitted Disease

PURPOSE/NEED FOR INFORMATION:

_____ Taking records to another doctor
_____ Moving
_____ Legal purposes
_____ Insurance purposes
_____ Workman's Compensation
_____ Other/Explain: _____

METHOD OF RELEASE:

_____ US Mail

_____ Fax

_____ Telephone

_____ To Patient

PATIENT AUTHORIZATION TO RELEASE INFORMATION:

Authorization is valid for 60 days only from the date of my signature. I reserve the right to revoke this authorization at any time prior to 60 days (except for action that has already been taken) by notifying the medical office in writing.

I understand that my records are protected under HIPAA (Health Insurance Portability and Accountability Act) Standards for Privacy of Individually Identifiable Information (45 CFR Parts 160 and 164) unless otherwise permitted by federal law. Any information released or received shall not be further relayed to any other facility or person without my written authorization. I also understand that such information will not be given, sold, transferred or in any way relayed to any other person or party not specified above without my further written authorization.

I hereby grant authorization to release the information listed above. I certify that this request has been made voluntarily and that the information given above is accurate to the best of my knowledge.

_____   _____
Signature of Patient/Legally Responsible Party   Date

_____   _____
Witness Signature   Date

OFFICE USE ONLY

Information indicated above released on _____
                                        Date

Explanation of information released: _____

_____

Signature and credentials of individual releasing information: _____

(From Bonewit-West K: *Study guide for clinical procedures for medical assistants*, ed 8, St. Louis, 2011, Saunders.)

Procedure 36-3: Preparing a Medical Record. Prepare a medical record.
Procedure 36-4: Obtaining and Recording Patient Symptoms. Practice obtaining patient symptoms by completing Taking Patient Symptoms: Supplemental Education for Chapter 36 (pp. 970 to 976 in this study guide).

Procedure 36-1: Completion of a Consent to Treatment Form

Name: _____   Date: _____

Evaluated by: _____   Score: _____

Performance Objective

Outcome:	Complete a consent to treatment form.
Conditions:	Given a consent to treatment form.
Standards:	Time: 10 minutes. Student completed procedure in _____ minutes.
	Accuracy: Satisfactory score on the Performance Evaluation Checklist.

Performance Evaluation Checklist

Trial 1	Trial 2	Point Value	Performance Standards
		●	Typed or printed required information on the consent to treatment form.
		●	Confirmed that the physician discussed the procedure with the patient.
		▷	Explained why the procedure should be discussed with the patient before the form is signed.
		●	Greeted the patient and introduced yourself.
		▷	Explained the purpose of the form to the patient.
		●	Gave the consent form to the patient to read.
		●	Asked if the patient had any questions.
		●	Asked the patient to sign the form.
		●	Witnessed the patient's signature and dated the form.
		▷	Explained what *witnessing a signature* means.
		●	Provided the patient with a copy of the completed form.
		∗	Filed the original form in the patient's medical record.
		▷	Explained why the form must be filed in the medical record.
		∗	Completed the procedure within 10 minutes.
			TOTALS

Evaluation of Student Performance

EVALUATION CRITERIA			COMMENTS
Symbol	**Category**	**Point Value**	
∗	Critical Step	16 points	
●	Essential Step	6 points	
▷	Theory Question	2 points	
Score calculation: 100 points			
− _____ points missed			
_____ Score			
Satisfactory score: 85 or above			

CAAHEP Competencies Achieved

Psychomotor (Skills)
☑ IV. 2. Report relevant information to others succinctly and accurately.
☑ IX. 7. Document accurately in the patient record.

Affective (Behavior)
☑ IV. 2. Apply active listening skills.
☑ IV. 7. Demonstrate recognition of the patient's level of understanding in communications.
☑ IV. 8. Analyze communications in providing appropriate responses or feedback.

ABHES Competencies Achieved

☑ 4. a. Document accurately.
☑ 8. aa. Are attentive, listen, and learn.
☑ 8. cc. Communicate on the recipient's level of comprehension.
☑ 8. dd. Serve as liaison between physician and others.

Procedure 36-2: Release of Medical Information

Name: _____   Date: _____

Evaluated by: _____   Score: _____

Performance Objective

Outcome:	1. Assist a patient in the completion of a release of medical information form.
	2. Release information according to a completed release of medical information form.
Conditions:	Given a release of medical information form and the patient's medical record.
Standards:	Time: 15 minutes. Student completed procedure in _____ minutes.
	Accuracy: Satisfactory score on the Performance Evaluation Checklist.

Performance Evaluation Checklist

Trial 1	Trial 2	Point Value	Performance Standards
			Completion of a release of information form
		●	Greeted the patient and introduced yourself.
		●	Identified the patient by full name and date of birth.
		▷	Explained the procedure to follow if you do not recognize the patient.
		●	Explained the purpose of the form to the patient.
		●	Provided the patient with a release of medical information form.
		●	Asked the patient to complete the form.
		●	Provided assistance if needed.
		●	Checked to make sure all information was completed.
		●	Asked the patient to sign the form.
		●	Witnessed the patient's signature and dated the form.

		•	Provided the patient with a copy of the completed form.	
		•	Copied the medical information requested on the form.	
		✳	Released only the information requested.	
		•	Included a copy of the completed form with the medical information.	
		•	Documented what information was released along with the date of release.	
		•	Signed the release form with your name and credentials verifying you were the individual releasing the information.	
		✳	Filed the original document and the release form in the patient's medical record.	
		▷	Explained the reason for filing the form.	
		•	Sent the medical information according to the medical office policy.	
			Mailed or faxed requests	
		•	Checked the expiration date on the release of medical information form.	
		▷	Explained the procedure to follow if the form is expired.	
		•	Verified the signature on the form.	
		▷	Stated what to do if in doubt regarding the authenticity of the signature.	
		•	Copied the information requested on the form.	
		✳	Released only the information requested.	
		•	Documented what information was released along with the date of release.	
		•	Signed the document with your name and credentials.	
		•	Filed the original document and the release form in the patient's medical record.	
		•	Sent the medical information according to the medical office policy.	
		✳	Completed the procedure within 15 minutes.	
			TOTALS	

Evaluation of Student Performance

EVALUATION CRITERIA			COMMENTS
Symbol	Category	Point Value	
✳	Critical Step	16 points	
●	Essential Step	6 points	
▷	Theory Question	2 points	

Score calculation: 100 points

     −   _____ points missed

          _____ Score

Satisfactory score: 85 or above

CAAHEP Competencies Achieved

Psychomotor (Skills)
☑ IV. 2. Report relevant information to others succinctly and accurately.
☑ IV. 4. Explain general office policies.
☑ IX. 1. Respond to issues of confidentiality.
☑ IX. 2. Perform within scope of practice.
☑ IX. 3. Apply HIPAA rules in regard to privacy/release of information.
☑ IX. 7. Document accurately in the patient record.
☑ IX. 8. Apply local, state, and federal health care legislation and regulation appropriate to the medical assisting practice setting.

Affective (Behavior)
☑ IX. 1. Demonstrate sensitivity to patient rights.
☑ IX. 3. Recognize the importance of local, state, and federal legislation and regulations in the practice setting.

ABHES Competencies Achieved

☑ 4. a. Document accurately.
☑ 4. b. Institute federal and state guidelines when releasing medical records or information.
☑ 4. f. Comply with federal, state, and local health laws and regulations.
☑ 8. dd. Serve as liaison between physician and others.
☑ 8. hh. Receive, organize, prioritize, and transmit information expediently.
☑ 9. p. Advise patients of office policies and procedures.

Notes

🔵 **Procedure 36-3: Preparing a Medical Record**

Name: _____   Date: _____

Evaluated by: _____   Score: _____

Performance Objective

Outcome:	Prepare a medical record for a new patient.
Conditions:	Given the following: patient registration form, Notice of Privacy Practices and acknowledgment form, file folder, metal fasteners, name labels, alphabetic labels, miscellaneous chart labels, chart dividers, preprinted forms, and a two-hole punch.
Standards:	Time: 10 minutes. Student completed procedure in _____ minutes.
	Accuracy: Satisfactory score on the Performance Evaluation Checklist.

Performance Evaluation Checklist

Trial 1	Trial 2	Point Value	Performance Standards
		●	Greeted the patient and introduced yourself.
		●	Identified the patient and verified that the patient was a new patient.
		●	Asked the patient to complete a patient registration form, read an NPP, and sign an acknowledgment form.
		●	Offered to answer questions.
		●	Checked the registration form for accuracy and legibility.
		●	Copied the patient's insurance card.
		▷	Stated the purpose of copying the card.
		●	Entered the data on the completed registration form into the computer.
		●	Assembled supplies needed to prepare the medical record.
			Typed the patient's full name on the name label
		●	The patient's name was in transposed order.
		●	The name was typed using correct spacing.
		●	The patient's name was spelled correctly.
		●	Attached appropriate color-coded labels to the side tab.
		●	Attached the labels using the indentations on the tab.
		●	Attached the name label immediately above the alphabetical label.
		●	Attached additional labels to the folder as required.
		●	Inserted chart dividers onto the metal fasteners.
		●	Placed the original registration form in front of the medical record.
		●	Placed the signed NPP acknowledgment form in the record.

965

Trial 1	Trial 2	Point Value	Performance Standards
		•	Placed the insurance card (copy) in the appropriate section of the record.
		•	Labeled preprinted forms with required information.
		▷	Stated examples of preprinted forms included in the medical record.
		•	Punched holes into the forms if required.
		•	Inserted each form under its proper chart divider.
		•	Checked the medical record to make sure it was prepared properly.
		✳	Completed the procedure within 10 minutes.
			TOTALS

Evaluation of Student Performance

EVALUATION CRITERIA			COMMENTS
Symbol	**Category**	**Point Value**	
✳	Critical Step	16 points	
•	Essential Step	6 points	
▷	Theory Question	2 points	

Score calculation: 100 points

− _____ points missed

_____ Score

Satisfactory score: 85 or above

CAAHEP Competencies Achieved

Psychomotor (Skills)

☑ IV. 2. Report relevant information to others succinctly and accurately.
☑ IV. 4. Explain general office policies.
☑ V. 3. Organize a patient's medical record.
☑ V. 5. Execute data management using electronic health care records such as the EMR.
☑ V. 6. Use office hardware and software to maintain office systems.
☑ V. 8. Maintain organization by filing.
☑ IX. 3. Apply HIPAA rules in regard to privacy/release of information.
☑ IX. 8. Apply local, state, and federal health care legislation and regulation appropriate to the medical assisting practice setting.

Affective (Behavior)

☑ IV. 2. Apply active listening skills.
☑ IV. 8. Analyze communications in providing appropriate responses or feedback.
☑ IV. 9. Recognize and protect personal boundaries in communicating with others.
☑ IX. 3. Recognize the importance of local, state, and federal legislation and regulations in the practice setting.

ABHES Competencies Achieved

☑ 4. a. Document accurately.
☑ 4. b. Institute federal and state guidelines when releasing medical records or information.
☑ 4. c. Follow established policies when initiating or terminating medical treatment.
☑ 4. f. Comply with federal, state, and local health laws and regulations.
☑ 8. b. Prepare and maintain medical records.
☑ 8. aa. Are attentive, listen, and learn.
☑ 8. ll. Apply electronic technology.

Procedure 36-4: Obtaining and Recording Patient Symptoms

Name: _____   Date: _____

Evaluated by: _____   Score: _____

Performance Objective

Outcome:	Obtain and record patient symptoms.
Conditions:	Given the following: medical record of the patient to be interviewed and a black ink pen.
Standards:	Time: 10 minutes. Student completed procedure in _____ minutes.
	Accuracy: Satisfactory score on the Performance Evaluation Checklist.

Performance Evaluation Checklist

Trial 1	Trial 2	Point Value	Performance Standards
		●	Assembled equipment.
		●	Made sure the correct patient record was obtained.
		●	Went to the waiting room and asked the patient to come back.
		●	Escorted the patient to a quiet room.
		●	In a calm and friendly manner, greeted the patient and introduced yourself.
		●	Identified the patient by full name and date of birth.
		●	Asked the patient to be seated.
		●	Seated yourself facing the patient at a distance of 3 to 4 feet.
		▷	Explained the purpose of this seating arrangement.
			Used good communication skills
		●	Used the patient's name of choice.
		●	Demonstrated genuine interest and concern for the patient.
		●	Maintained appropriate eye contact.
		●	Used terminology the patient could understand.
		●	Listened carefully and attentively to the patient.
		●	Paid attention to the patient's nonverbal messages.
		●	Avoided judgmental comments.
		●	Avoided rushing the patient.
		●	Located the progress note sheet in the medical record.
		●	Charted the date, time, and CC abbreviation

967

Trial 1	Trial 2	Point Value	Performance Standards
		●	Used an open-ended question to obtain the chief complaint.
		▷	Explained why an open-ended question should be used.
			Charted the chief complaint
		●	Limited the CC to one or two symptoms.
		●	Referred to a specific rather than a vague symptom.
		●	Charted concisely and briefly.
		●	Used the patient's own words as much as possible.
		●	Included the duration of the symptom.
		●	Avoided using names of diseases.
		●	Obtained additional information regarding the chief complaint using what, when, and where questions.
		●	Thanked the patient and proceeded to the next step in the patient workup.
		●	Informed the patient that the physician will be in soon.
		●	Placed the medical record in the appropriate location for review by the physician.
		✱	Completed the procedure within 10 minutes.
			TOTALS
			CHART
	Date		

Evaluation of Student Performance

EVALUATION CRITERIA			COMMENTS
Symbol	**Category**	**Point Value**	
✱	Critical Step	16 points	
●	Essential Step	6 points	
▷	Theory Question	2 points	

Score calculation: 100 points

− _____ points missed

_____ Score

Satisfactory score: 85 or above

CAAHEP Competencies Achieved

Psychomotor (Skills)

☑ IV. 1. Use reflection, restatement, and clarification techniques to obtain a patient history.

☑ IV. 3. Use medical terminology, pronouncing medical terms correctly, to communicate information, patient history, data, and observations.

☑ IV. 7. Demonstrate telephone techniques.

☑ IV. 11. Respond to nonverbal communication.

☑ IX. 7. Document accurately in the patient record.

☑ X. 2. Develop a plan for separation of personal and professional ethics.

Affective (Behavior)

☑ IV. 2. Apply active listening skills.

☑ IV. 3. Use appropriate body language and other nonverbal skills in communicating with parents, family, and staff.

☑ IV. 4. Demonstrate awareness of the territorial boundaries of the person with whom communicating.

☑ IV. 9. Recognize and protect personal boundaries in communicating with others.

☑ IV. 10. Demonstrate respect for individual diversity, incorporating awareness of one's own biases in areas including gender, race, religion, age, and economic status.

ABHES Competencies Achieved

☑ 3. d. Recognize and identify acceptable medical abbreviations.

☑ 4. a. Document accurately.

☑ 5. b. Identify and respond appropriately when working/caring for patients with special needs.

☑ 8. aa. Are attentive, listen, and learn.

☑ 8. bb. Are impartial and show empathy when dealing with patients.

☑ 8. cc. Communicate on the recipient's level of comprehension.

☑ 8. ee. Use proper telephone techniques.

☑ 8. ff. Interview effectively.

☑ 8. gg. Use pertinent medical terminology.

☑ 8. ii. Recognize and respond to verbal and nonverbal communication.

☑ 8. jj. Perform fundamental writing skills including correct grammar, spelling, and formatting techniques when writing prescriptions, documenting medical records, etc.

☑ 8. kk. Adapt to individualized needs.

☑ 9. a. Obtain chief complaint, recording patient history.

Taking a patient's symptoms is a frequent and important responsibility of the medical assistant, who must have a thorough knowledge of symptoms and related terminology. A **symptom** is defined as any change in the body or its functioning that indicates the presence of disease. The medical assistant can observe **objective symptoms** presented by the patient, such as coughing, rash, and swelling. The medical assistant must rely on information relayed by the patient to obtain data on **subjective symptoms**. Examples of subjective symptoms include pain, pruritus, and vertigo.

This section is designed as supplemental education for Chapter 36 (The Medical Record) in your textbook. Completion of the exercises in this section can assist you in recording a patient's symptoms effectively and thoroughly, which is essential to an accurate diagnosis by the physician.

Learning Objectives

After completing this chapter, you should be able to do the following:
1. Explain the purpose of analyzing a symptom.
2. State the seven basic types of information that must be obtained to analyze a symptom.
3. Analyze a symptom by using direct questions.

Analysis of a Symptom

Before a symptom can be analyzed, the **chief complaint** (CC) must first be identified. The chief complaint is the patient's reason for seeking care or the symptom causing the patient the most trouble. An open-ended question should be used to elicit the chief complaint from the patient, and it should be charted following the charting guidelines presented in your textbook (pp. 903-907). The next step is to analyze the chief complaint in detail from the time of its onset. The purpose of this is to provide a complete description of the current status of the chief complaint.

Analyzing the chief complaint requires a combination of good listening and writing skills. The medical assistant must know what information should be recorded for each symptom and the questions to ask the patient to obtain this information. A list of symptoms, explanation of the information required for each symptom, and examples of questions to ask the patient are provided.

Type of Information Required

The following information is needed for each symptom to provide a full description of the current status of the chief complaint:

1. Location of the symptom. This refers to the specific area of the body where the symptom is located. Locating the symptom is the first step in determining the cause of the patient's disease. The patient may refer to the location in general terms, such as the head, arm, stomach, or back. The medical assistant must be more specific than this and determine the exact location using descriptions, such as "occurs in the lower back" or "occurs under the sternum." Several questions can assist in accomplishing this.
   - Where exactly does it hurt?
   - Can you show me where it hurts?
   - Do you feel it anywhere else?

2. Quality of the symptom. The quality of the symptom includes a complete and concise description of the symptom. The medical assistant should use informative terms to describe the character of each symptom. For example, if the patient complains of pain, the character of the pain must be included. Several terms can be used to describe pain.
   - Burning
   - Aching
   - Sharp
   - Dull
   - Throbbing
   - Cramplike
   - Squeezing

   If the patient has vomited, the medical assistant should indicate the color, odor, and consistency of the vomitus. If the patient has a cough, the medical assistant should indicate if it is productive or nonproductive and whether blood is present. Refer to the table of terms on pages 975 and 976 of this manual, which can assist in describing symptoms. Specific examples of questions that are helpful in determining the quality of the symptom are as follows:
   - Describe it (the symptom) to me as fully as possible.
   - What is it (the symptom) like?

970

3. Severity of the symptom. Severity refers to the quantitative aspect of the symptom. It includes the following:
   - Intensity of the symptom (e.g., mild, moderate, severe)
   - Number (e.g., of convulsions, of nosebleeds)
   - Volume (e.g., of vomitus, of blood, of mucus)
   - Size or extent (e.g., of the rash, edema, lumps, or masses)

   This information assists the physician in determining the extensiveness or seriousness of the illness. Questions to determine severity are often specific to that symptom. For example, if the patient has a productive cough, the medical assistant should determine how much phlegm is being coughed up (e.g., teaspoon, half of a cup). At first, this area may appear difficult, but as you practice taking symptoms, you will learn what questions to ask the patient, and it eventually it will become automatic. The examples at the end of this section and the student practice problems provide guidance in developing skill in this area. Some examples of general questions that can be used to determine the severity of a symptom are as follows:
   - How bad is it (the symptom)?
   - Does it (the symptom) limit your normal activities?

4. Chronology and timing of the symptom. Chronology and timing include a sequential account of the symptom up to the time the patient came to the medical office for treatment. This information is important in determining the duration of the symptom and change in it since it first occurred. Chronology and timing include the following four areas:
   a. Date of onset: The date of onset of the symptom should be indicated, if possible, as a calendar date and clock time. The patient may need some time to recall this information. Examples of questions that help obtain this information are as follows:
      - When did you experience this (the symptom) for the first time?
      - Exactly when did this begin?
   b. Duration: The duration of the symptom refers to how long the symptom lasts after it occurs; for example: 10 minutes, 2 hours, continuously. Examples of questions to obtain this information are as follows:
      - How long does it last after occurring?
      - For what length of time do you experience this symptom?
   c. Frequency: The frequency of the symptom refers to how often the symptom occurs, such as twice daily or a single attack every 2 weeks. Examples of questions to obtain this information are as follows:
      - How often does it occur?
      - How often has the symptom recurred?
   d. Change over time: This area refers to any change in the symptom since it first occurred. A change in a symptom reflects the nature of the underlying disease, which assists the physician in making a diagnosis. Examples of questions to obtain this information are as follows:
      - Has the symptom changed since it first occurred?
      - Is it (the symptom) getting better, worse, or staying the same?

5. Manner of onset. The manner of onset refers to what the patient was doing when the symptom first occurred and exactly what was experienced by the patient when the symptom began. These data help provide information on the pathologic process responsible for the symptom. For example, the patient might have been lifting a heavy object before experiencing low back pain. This information helps the physician in making an accurate diagnosis. Examples of questions that are helpful in determining the manner of onset are as follows:
   - What exactly did you experience when it (the symptom) first occurred?
   - What was the first thing you noticed?
   - Did it (the symptom) come on suddenly or gradually?
   - What were you doing when it (the symptom) began?
   - Where were you when this happened?
   - How were you feeling before it (the symptom) began?

6. Modifying factors. Symptoms are often influenced by activities or physiologic processes, such as physical exercise, change in weather, bodily functions (e.g., bowel movements, eating, coughing), pregnancy, emotional states, and fatigue. Some activities may aggravate the symptom while others may alleviate it. These influences may help to determine what is causing the problem. For example, pain that becomes worse after the patient eats but is relieved after taking an antacid assists the physician in focusing on gastrointestinal disorders. Questions to assist in determining modifying factors are as follows:
   - Does anything make it (the symptom) better?
   - Does anything make it worse?

- What have you done to make it better?
- What did you do to help it?
- Are you taking any medication for it? Did it help?

7. Associated symptoms. There is usually more than one symptom associated with a disease process. Determining these additional symptoms gives the physician a complete picture of the illness. Examples of questions that help to identify the presence of additional symptoms are as follows:
   - Are you having any other symptoms?
   - What other problems have you noticed since you became ill?

Examples

The following examples illustrate how to analyze a symptom. The chief complaint is listed first, followed by questions to ask the patient from the seven basic categories of information.

> *Example: Chief complaint: Headaches that began 2 months ago*

1. Using your finger, point to the location of the headache.

2. Describe the pain. Is it sharp, dull, throbbing?

3. Are you able to carry on normal activities when you have a headache?

4. Is it sometimes more severe than usual?

5. When exactly did your headaches begin?

6. How long does your headache last when it occurs?

7. How often do you get a headache?

8. Since your headaches began, have they gotten better or worse, or have they stayed the same?

9. What were you doing the first time you experienced a headache?

10. What was your health status before your headaches began?

11. Do you get a headache before, during, or after a particular activity, such as reading or watching TV?

12. Does anything make your headache better?

13. Are you taking any medication for your headache? Does it help?

14. Have you had any other problems since your headaches began, such as nausea, vomiting, dizziness, or problems with vision?

> *Example: Chief complaint: The patient has been coughing for the past 3 days.*

1. Does it hurt when you cough? Where? Show me with one of your fingers.

2. What is the cough like?

3. Can you cough for me?

4. Do you bring up any phlegm when you cough? What color is it? Is blood present?

5. Describe the pain. Is it sharp, dull, squeezing?

6. Do you become exhausted when you cough?

7. How much phlegm do you bring up? A teaspoon? Half a cup?

8. How much blood is present in the phlegm?

9. When did your cough first begin?

10. Does it seem like an attack? How long does the attack last?

11. How often do you get a coughing attack?

12. Does your cough seem to be getting better or worse?

13. What was the first thing you noticed when you became ill?

14. How were you feeling before your symptoms began?

15. Is there anything that makes your cough better?

16. Is there anything that makes your cough worse?

17. Do you cough more at night or during the day?

18. Are you taking any medication for it? Does it help?

19. Are you having any other problems?

Practice Problems

In the space provided, indicate examples of direct questions to ask the patient to obtain the necessary information for the symptoms presented in the chief complaint.

Problem 1

> **Chief complaint:** *Earache and fever for the past 2 days*

Questions:

_____

_____

_____

_____

_____

_____

_____

_____

_____

_____

Problem 2

| Chief complaint: *Rash with itching that began 3 days ago* |

Questions:

_____

_____

_____

_____

_____

_____

_____

_____

_____

_____

_____

Problem 3

| Chief complaint: *Pain during urination that began yesterday* |

Questions:

_____

_____

_____

_____

_____

_____

_____

_____

_____

_____

_____

Problem 4

| Chief complaint: *Low back pain for the past 3 months* |

Questions:

_____

_____

_____

_____

_____

_____

_____

_____

_____

_____

Problem 5

| Chief complaint: *Sore throat and fever for the past 24 hours* |

Questions:

_____

_____

_____

_____

_____

_____

_____

Problem 6

| Chief complaint: *Chest pain that occurred this morning* |

Questions:

_____

_____

_____

_____

_____

_____

_____

_____

Terms for Describing Symptoms

Pain

    Burning, aching, sharp, dull, throbbing, cramping, squeezing

    Radiating, transient, constant

    Localized, superficial, deep

Respirations

    Rapid, irregular, shallow, deep, labored, gasping, noisy, wheezing

    Apnea, dyspnea, orthopnea

    Discomfort, pain, cyanosis, cough

Cough

    Nonproductive, productive

    Persistent, dry, hacking, barking, spasmodic

    Phlegm: color, consistency, presence or absence of blood

    Exhausting or painful

Cardiovascular System

    Pain, palpitations

    Sharp, radiating

    Dyspnea, orthopnea

    Cyanosis

Gastrointestinal System

    Abdomen: flaccid, rigid, distended

    Appetite: anorexia, intolerance to foods

    Heartburn, pain after eating, belching, nausea, vomiting, flatulence, change in bowel habits, constipation, diarrhea, black stools

Urine or Stool

    Abnormality: color, odor, consistency, frequency

    Contents: sediment, mucus, blood

    Elimination: urgency, nocturia, pain, burning

Skin

    Rash: pruritus, red, swelling, distribution

    Lesions: color, character, distribution

    Pallor: flushing, jaundice, warm, dry, cold, clammy

    Ecchymosis, petechiae, cyanosis, edema

    Pruritus, sweating, change in color, bruises easily

Ears

    Pain, loss of hearing, tinnitus, vertigo

    Discharge, infection

Eyes

    Itching, burning, blurry vision, seeing double, photophobia

    Discharge, watering, infection

37 Patient Reception

CHAPTER ASSIGNMENTS

√ After Completing	Date Due	Textbook Pages	TEXTBOOK ASSIGNMENTS	Possible Points	Points You Earned
		915-928	Read Chapter 37: Patient Reception		
		921 927	Read Case Study 1 Case Study 1 questions	5	
		923 927	Read Case Study 2 Case Study 2 questions	5	
		925 927	Read Case Study 3 Case Study 3 questions	5	
			TOTAL POINTS		

√ After Completing	Date Due	Study Guide Pages	STUDY GUIDE ASSIGNMENTS (CTA = Critical Thinking Activity)	Possible Points	Points You Earned
		979	Pretest	10	
		980	Term Key Term Assessment	5	
		980-982	Evaluation of Learning questions	18	
		982	CTA A: Privacy Practices	5	
		982	CTA B: Verifying Insurance and Referrals	8	
		983	CTA C: Patient Informational Material	20	
			Evolve Site: Apply Your Knowledge questions	10	
			Evolve Site: Video Evaluation	8	
		979	Posttest	10	
			ADDITIONAL ASSIGNMENTS		
			TOTAL POINTS		

√ When Assigned By Your Instructor	Study Guide Pages	Practices Required	LABORATORY ASSIGNMENTS (Procedure Number and Name)	Score*
	985	3	**Practice for Competency** 37-1: Opening the Medical Office Textbook reference: pp. 917-918	
	989-990		**Evaluation of Competency** 37-1: Opening the Medical Office	*
	985	3	**Practice for Competency** 37-2: Closing the Medical Office Textbook reference: p. 918	
	991-992		**Evaluation of Competency** 37-2: Closing the Medical Office	*
	986-987	3	**Practice for Competency** 37-3: Obtaining New Patient Information Textbook reference: p. 924	
	993-994		**Evaluation of Competency** 37-3: Obtaining New Patient Information	*
	987	3	**Practice for Competency** 37-4: Explaining Office Policies and Procedures Textbook reference: p. 926	
	995-996		**Evaluation of Competency** 37-4: Explaining Office Policies and Procedures	*
			ADDITIONAL ASSIGNMENTS	

Name _____   Date _____

True or False

_____ 1. The first thing the medical assistant (MA) does when opening the office is to unlock the file cabinets, medical record files, and medicine cabinets.

_____ 2. After opening the office, the MA should be sure that the telephones are switched to the day message or call the answering service.

_____ 3. An electronic task system consists of a folder for each month and a folder for each day.

_____ 4. Paper medical records are usually pulled the evening before the appointment.

_____ 5. A radio, CD player, television, or DVD player is usually turned on in the morning before patients arrive.

_____ 6. The autoclave is often run just before closing the medical office so that instruments can dry overnight.

_____ 7. Only one person at a time should be permitted to stand at the reception desk to check in.

_____ 8. A new patient must sign a form acknowledging receipt of HIPAA privacy practices.

_____ 9. Only the top side of the insurance card must be photocopied.

_____ 10. If a patient has managed care insurance, a referral form may be required to see a physician other than the primary care provider.

? POSTTEST

True or False

_____ 1. As soon as the MA has opened the office, he or she usually runs the autoclave.

_____ 2. After opening the office, the MA should check the fax machine for faxes that may have arrived overnight.

_____ 3. A tickler file is used to remind the MA of tasks to be done on a specific day.

_____ 4. If paper medical records are used, the first major task for the MA in the morning is to pull the medical records for all patients to be seen that day.

_____ 5. Holders for patient information brochures are often located in the waiting room.

_____ 6. The MA turns off all equipment as the last thing when closing the office.

_____ 7. A sliding glass window between the waiting room and reception desk helps maintain patient confidentiality.

_____ 8. A new patient must sign a form providing consent for treatment and release of information.

_____ 9. Insurance companies usually require authorization every time the patient sees the primary care physician.

_____ 10. If the patient has a copayment, it is usually collected before the patient sees the physician.

Directions: Match each medical term with its definition.

_____ 1. Assignment of benefits

_____ 2. Call-in times

_____ 3. Copayment

_____ 4. Medicaid

_____ 5. Tickler file

A. A fixed amount of money that the patient is responsible to pay at each visit

B. A chronological file containing reminders of things to be done

C. Authorization given by the patient to allow the insurance company to make payments directly to the health care provider

D. Blocks of time when a physician accepts telephone calls from patients

E. A federal and state insurance program for low-income patients

EVALUATION OF LEARNING

Directions: Fill in each blank with the correct answer.

1. List five activities that the MA must perform to open the office.

_____

_____

2. How does the MA prepare the telephone system for patient calls at the beginning of the day?

_____

_____

3. How should the MA prepare for the day's activities in the medical office?

_____

_____

4. If an office uses paper medical records, how are they prepared before patients arrive?

_____

_____

_____

5. What should the MA do to be sure the waiting room is ready for patients?

_____

_____

6. How does the MA check equipment and prepare supplies at the beginning of the day?

_____

_____

_____

7. List seven tasks that the MA should perform when closing the medical office.

_____

_____

_____

8. How does the medical office identify which patients have arrived for appointments?

_____

_____

9. What is the function of a sliding glass window between the reception desk and the patient waiting area?

_____

10. Identify at least three statements or forms that a new patient must sign before being examined by the physician.

_____

_____

11. What is required by the HIPAA legislation related to notifying patients about privacy practices?

_____

_____

12. How does the MA verify a patient's identity and insurance information?

_____

_____

_____

_____

13. When does a patient need a written or electronic referral form?

_____

14. What information is included in a written or electronic referral form?

_____

_____

15. What information must be obtained from an established patient who is checking in?

_____

_____

16. What is a copayment, and when is a copayment usually collected?

_____

17. What are at least eight pieces of information about a medical practice that might be found on a website or in an informational brochure?

_____

_____

_____

_____

_____

18. What are three reasons that a physician might not be accepting new patients?

_____

_____

CRITICAL THINKING ACTIVITIES

A. Privacy Practices

Obtain a printed sample Notice of Privacy Practices from a medical office either from your own physician or from the Internet. Many organizations post their privacy statements on their websites. Using the copy of the privacy practices statement, highlight the sections where the following required content is included. Then write a brief statement stating whether your example contains all required information or not.

1. How the medical office may use and disclose protected health information about an individual.

2. The individual's rights with respect to the information and how the individual may exercise these rights, including how the individual may complain to the medical office.

3. The medical office's legal duties with respect to the information, including a statement that the medical office is required by law to maintain the privacy of protected health information.

4. How individuals can obtain further information about the medical office's privacy policies.

5. The effective date of the Notice of Privacy Practices.

B. Verifying Insurance and Referrals

Based on information in the chapter, choose the following methods necessary to verify that the patient's insurance will cover charges and that the patient has a completed referral form if necessary. Enter the letter(s) of the correct step(s) the MA must take when a patient checks in. Some situations require more than one answer.

   a. Ask to see the patient's insurance card (or card of the insured party).

   b. Ask to see *and* make a photocopy of the patient's insurance card (or card of the insured party).

   c. Check that the patient has current insurance using a card reader, fax, computer, or telephone.

   d. Use a telephone or computer to verify insurance coverage and/or obtain preauthorization.

   e. Check to see that there is a completed referral form.

   f. Explain that the patient will be responsible for the bill because insurance will not cover the service(s).

1. An established patient has an appointment with his or her primary care physician. _____

2. A new patient has an appointment with a primary care physician. _____

3. A new patient with managed care insurance has an appointment with a cardiologist. _____

4. An established patient with Medicaid has an appointment for a blood pressure check. _____

5. An established patient tells the MA that she has changed insurance since the last visit. _____

6. A new patient with managed care insurance visits a dermatologist for a minor surgical procedure. _____

7. A mother brings an infant to the pediatrician for his or her first well-baby checkup. _____

8. An established patient is being scheduled for a cosmetic laser procedure. _____

C. Patient Informational Material

1. Create a patient information brochure or use a word processing program to create two or more web pages for a physician in private practice. Assume that the location of the office is at the same address as your medical assisting school. Include the following information:
   - Physician's name, credentials, and specialty
   - Brief statement of the physician's philosophy of patient care
   - Directions to the office, parking, and access to public transportation, if any
   - General statement that most insurance is accepted and that copayments are expected at the time of the visit
   - Policy regarding cancellation of appointments
   - Name of a local hospital that the physician is affiliated with
   - Description of how medication refills are handled

2. Compare your patient informational material with that of at least two of your classmates and discuss how this material could be used by the medical office.

Notes

PRACTICE FOR COMPETENCY

Procedure 37-1: Opening the Medical Office. Practice opening the office.

A. Make a list of tasks to open the office:

_____

_____

_____

_____

_____

_____

Procedure 37-2: Closing the Medical Office. Practice closing the office.

A. Make a list of tasks to close the office:

_____

_____

_____

_____

_____

_____

New Patient Information Form. Complete the new patient information form using yourself as the patient. Use the form to practice Procedure 37-3.

REGISTRATION
(PLEASE PRINT)

Home Phone: _____   Today's Date: _____

PATIENT INFORMATION

Name _____ Soc. Sec.# _____
       Last Name   First Name   Initial

Address _____

City _____ State _____ Zip _____

Single ___ Married ___ Widowed ___ Separated ___ Divorced ___ Sex M___ F___ Age ___ Birthdate _____

Patient Employed by _____ Occupation _____

Business Address _____ Business Phone _____

By whom were you referred? _____

In case of emergency who should be notified? _____ Phone _____
                                  Last Name   Relationship to Patient

PRIMARY INSURANCE

Person Responsible for Account _____
                       Last Name   First Name   Initial

Relation to Patient _____ Birthdate _____ Soc. Sec.# _____

Address (if different from patient's) _____ Phone _____

City _____ State _____ Zip _____

Person Responsible Employed by _____ Occupation _____

Business Address _____ Business Phone _____

Insurance Company _____

Contract # _____ Group # _____ Subscriber # _____

Name of other dependents covered under this plan _____

ADDITIONAL INSURANCE

Is patient covered by additional insurance? ___ Yes ___ No

Subscriber Name _____ Relationship to Patient _____ Birthdate _____

Address (if different from patient's) _____ Phone _____

City _____ State _____ Zip _____

Subscriber Employed by _____ Business Phone _____

Insurance Company _____

Contract # _____ Group # _____ Subscriber # _____

Name of other dependents covered under this plan _____

ASSIGNMENT AND RELEASE

I, the undersigned, certify that I (or my dependent) have insurance coverage with _____
                                                          Name of Insurance Company(ies)

and assign directly to Dr. _____ insurance benefits, if any, otherwise payable to me for services rendered. I understand that I am financially responsible for all charges whether or not paid by insurance. I hereby authorize the doctor to release all information necessary to secure the payment of benefits. I authorize the use of this signature on all insurance submissions.

_____   _____   _____
   Responsible Party Signature   Relationship   Date

ORDER# 58-8426 • © 1996 BIBBERO SYSTEMS, INC. • PETALUMA, CALIFORNIA • TO REORDER CALL TOLL FREE: (800) 242-9330

(Courtesy Bibbero Systems, Inc., Petaluma, Calif. [800] 242-2376; Fax [800] 242-9330; *www.bibbero.com*.)

Acknowledgment of Receipt of Notice of HIPAA Privacy Practices Form. Complete the Acknowledgment of Receipt of Notice of HIPAA Privacy Practices Form using yourself as the patient. Use the form to practice Procedure 37-3.

Acknowledgment of Receipt of the Notice of Privacy Practices

Please Review Carefully

The Notice of Privacy Practices tells you how [**Practice Name**] uses and discloses information about you. Not all situations will be described. We are required to give you a notice of our privacy practices for the information we collect and keep about you. We reserve the right to revise this notice, and you can obtain a copy of any revision upon written request.

I, _____, have been given a copy of the **Notice of Privacy Practices.**

_____   _____   _____
Patient or Legal Guardian's Signature   Date   Relationship to Patient

_____   _____
Print Patient's Name   Print Name of Legal Guardian (if any)

_____   _____
Signature of Witness (If signed with an "X" or mark)   Date

Effective Date: April 14, 2003

Procedure 37-3: Obtaining New Patient Information. Practice obtaining new patient information from classmates using the forms they completed above.

Procedure 37-4: Explaining Office Policies and Procedures. Using the patient information brochure prepared for Critical Thinking Activity C, practice orienting classmates (as simulated new patients) to office policies and procedures.

Notes

Procedure 37-1: Opening the Medical Office

Name: _____ Date: _____

Evaluated By: _____ Score: _____

Performance Objective

Outcome:	Open the medical office.
Conditions:	In a medical office.
Standards:	Time: 15 minutes. Student completed procedure in _____ minutes.
	Accuracy: Satisfactory score on the Performance Evaluation Checklist.

Performance Evaluation Checklist

Trial 1	Trial 2	Point Value	Performance Standards
		●	Entered the office and disarmed any alarm system.
		●	Turned on the lights.
		●	Adjusted heat or air conditioning to a comfortable setting.
		●	Unlocked the door for patients and visitors to enter.
		●	Turned on computers, printers, copier, and/or other machines.
		●	Called answering service for messages or listened to messages from voice mail or office answering machine.
		●	Wrote down complete message information on message forms.
		●	Arranged messages in order of importance.
		●	Dealt with urgent messages or calls.
		●	Pulled paper medical records for routine messages about patients.
		●	Clipped each message about a patient to the correct medical record.
		●	Placed routine messages in appropriate location(s) for office staff to review.
		●	Reviewed the day's activities and noted any special tasks.
		●	Counted the money in the cash drawer and recorded the amount.
		●	Checked the office for safety hazards.
		●	Straightened up the waiting room and turned on radio, television, or DVD player.
		●	Refilled holder of patient information brochures as needed.
		●	Printed appointment lists as needed.

989

Trial 1	Trial 2	Point Value	Performance Standards
		●	Pulled medical records as needed for the day's appointments.
		●	Arranged paper medical records in order of appointments.
		●	Printed or stamped the date on progress notes of paper medical records as needed.
		●	Printed any necessary paperwork required by an electronic medical record system.
		●	Prepared charge slips and clipped to patient records, if office policy.
		●	Checked biohazard waste containers and changed or discarded properly.
		●	Ran or emptied the autoclave as needed.
		★	Completed the procedure within 15 minutes.
			TOTALS

Evaluation of Student Performance

EVALUATION CRITERIA			COMMENTS
Symbol	**Category**	**Point Value**	
★	Critical Step	16 points	
●	Essential Step	6 points	
▷	Theory Question	2 points	

Score calculation: 100 points

      −   _____ points missed

           _____ Score

Satisfactory score: 85 or above

CAAHEP Competencies Achieved

Psychomotor (Skills)
☑ V. 9. Perform routine maintenance of office equipment with documentation.
☑ XI. 2. Evaluate the work environment to identify safe vs. unsafe working conditions.

Affective (Behavior)
☑ V. 2. Implement time management principles to maintain effective office function.

ABHES Competencies Achieved

☑ 8. a. Perform basic clerical functions.
☑ 8. x. Maintain medical facility.
☑ 8. y. Perform routine maintenance of administrative and clinical equipment.

Procedure 37-2: Closing the Medical Office

Name: _____   Date: _____

Evaluated by: _____   Score: _____

Performance Objective

Outcome:	Open the medical office.
Conditions:	In a medical office.
Standards:	Time: 15 minutes. Student completed procedure in _____ minutes.
	Accuracy: Satisfactory score on the Performance Evaluation Checklist.

Performance Evaluation Checklist

Trial 1	Trial 2	Point Value	Performance Standards
		●	Made sure examination rooms were clean and contained all necessary supplies.
		●	Ran the autoclave if needed.
		●	Printed a patient schedule for the next day.
		●	Pulled paper medical records for the next day.
		●	Printed charge slips and clipped to the medical records, if office policy.
		●	Made sure cabinets or rooms containing medical records were locked.
		●	Balanced the cash drawer and prepared the bank deposit. Made bank deposit at the end of the day.
		●	Locked the cash drawer or placed the cash fund in the office safe.
		●	Activated the night telephone system by switching telephone message or calling the answering service.
		●	Turned off office machines including computers, printers, and photocopier.
		●	Unplugged coffee pot, toaster, or other machines that might pose a fire hazard.
		●	Locked door used for patients and visitors.
		●	Turned heat or air conditioning to night setting.
		●	Turned off the lights.
		●	Armed the security system.
		●	Made sure that staff exit door was locked securely.
		★	Completed the procedure within 15 minutes.
		TOTALS	

Evaluation of Student Performance

EVALUATION CRITERIA			COMMENTS
Symbol	**Category**	**Point Value**	
✶	Critical Step	16 points	
●	Essential Step	6 points	
▷	Theory Question	2 points	

Score calculation: 100 points

− _____ points missed

_____

_____ Score

Satisfactory score: 85 or above

CAAHEP Competency Achieved

Affective (Behavior)

☑ V. 2. Implement time management principles to maintain effective office function.

ABHES Competency Achieved

☑ 8. a. Perform basic clerical functions.

☑ 8. x. Maintain medical facility.

Procedure 37-3: Obtaining New Patient Information

Name: _____   Date: _____

Evaluated by: _____   Score: _____

Performance Objective

Outcome:	Obtain new patient information, obtain consents, and validate insurance coverage.
Conditions:	Given the following: clipboard, pen, new patient information form, Notice of Privacy Practices form, receipt of Notice of Privacy Practices form, consent for release of protected health information (optional), photocopier, insurance card reader (optional), telephone, medical record, computer, scanner.
Standards:	Time: 10 minutes. Student completed procedure in _____ minutes.

Accuracy: Satisfactory score on the Performance Evaluation Checklist. |

Performance Evaluation Checklist

Trial 1	Trial 2	Point Value	Performance Standards
		●	Placed a new patient information form on a clipboard with a pen.
		●	Asked a new patient to complete the form and return it.
		●	Verified that the form was complete and signed by the patient or authorized representative.
		●	Asked to see the insurance card of the patient or insured individual.
		●	Photocopied both sides of the insurance card.
		●	Placed the photocopy of the insurance card in the patient's medical record.
		●	Confirmed patient eligibility for insurance as needed using a card reader, computer or telephone.
		●	Verified that there was a completed referral form as needed.
		●	Verified patient's identification using a photo ID or two other forms of identification (if it is office policy)
		●	Discussed the patient's financial responsibility, if the visit would not be completely covered by insurance, in a private area.
		●	Gave the patient a copy of the Notice of Privacy Practices or made it available for the patient to read.
		✴	Asked the patient to sign the form indicating receipt of the Notice of Privacy Practices.
		●	Signed the Notice of Privacy Practices form as a witness.
		●	Asked the patient to read and sign any consent for release of personal health information used by the office.

993

Trial 1	Trial 2	Point Value	Performance Standards
		●	Inserted new forms into the paper medical record.
		●	Placed the medical record (or other paperwork) and charge slip to indicate that the patient has been checked in.
		●	Asked the patient to have a seat and indicate the probable wait time.
		●	Entered new patient information into the computer or validated patient information.
		●	Scanned patient forms according to office policy (if the office uses an electronic medical record).
		✱	Completed the procedure within 10 minutes.
			TOTALS

Evaluation of Student Performance

EVALUATION CRITERIA			COMMENTS
Symbol	**Category**	**Point Value**	
✱	Critical Step	16 points	
●	Essential Step	6 points	
▷	Theory Question	2 points	

Score calculation: 100 points

− _____ points missed

_____ Score

Satisfactory score: 85 or above

CAAHEP Competency Achieved

Psychomotor (Skills)
☑ VII. 1. Apply both managed care policies and procedures.
☑ VII. 2. Apply third party guidelines.
☑ VII. 6. Verify eligibility for managed care services.
☑ IX. 1. Respond to issues of confidentiality.
☑ IX. 3. Apply HIPAA rules in regard to the privacy/release of information.

Affective (Behavior)
☑ IV. 2. Apply active listening skills.
☑ IX. 1. Demonstrate sensitivity to patient rights.
☑ IX. 3. Recognize the importance of local, state, and federal legislation and regulations in the practice setting.

ABHES Competency Achieved

☑ 4. c. Follow established policies when initiating or terminating medical treatment.
☑ 4. f. Comply with federal, state and local health laws and regulations.
☑ 8. r. Apply third party guidelines.
☑ 8. y. Perform routine maintenance of administrative and clinical equipment.
☑ 8. ff. Interview effectively.

Procedure 37-4: Explaining Office Policies and Procedures

Name: _____   Date: _____

Evaluated by: _____   Score: _____

Performance Objective

Outcome:	Orient a new patient to the medical office.
Conditions:	Given the following: patient information booklet, map, list of points to cover.
Standards:	Time: 10 minutes. Student completed procedure in _____ minutes.
	Accuracy: Satisfactory score on the Performance Evaluation Checklist.

Performance Evaluation Checklist

Trial 1	Trial 2	Point Value	Performance Standards
		●	Offered to give or send a patient information booklet if one is available.
		●	Identified the name, credentials, and specialty of each physician who would accept new patients.
		●	Offered information as required about languages spoken in the office and any additional services that would be available.
		●	Identified the location of the office, gave directions, and discussed parking as needed.
		●	Told the patient if the office accepted his or her medical insurance plan.
		●	Discussed expectations for payment of the patient's bill.
		●	Described how far in advance to make and/or cancel appointments.
		●	Told the patient how to contact the office.
		●	Informed the patient if the physician had specific call-in times.
		●	Explained how prescription refills would be handled.
		●	Identified hospital affiliation(s) of the office physician(s).
		●	Asked if there were other questions and responded appropriately.
		✱	Completed the procedure within 10 minutes.
			TOTALS

EVALUATION CRITERIA			COMMENTS
Symbol	Category	Point Value	
✳	Critical Step	16 points	
●	Essential Step	6 points	
▷	Theory Question	2 points	

Score calculation: 100 points

− _____ points missed

___ Score

Satisfactory score: 85 or above

CAAHEP Competency Achieved

Psychomotor (Skills)
☑ IV. 4. Explain general office policies.

Affective (Behavior)
☑ IV. 2. Apply active listening skills.
☑ IV. 7. Demonstrate recognition of the patient's level of understanding in communication.
☑ VII. 3. Communicate in language the patient can understand regarding managed care and insurance plans.

ABHES Competency Achieved

☑ 8. cc. Communicate on the recipient's level of understanding.
☑ 8. ii. Recognize and respond to verbal and nonverbal communication.

38 Medical Office Computerization

CHAPTER ASSIGNMENTS

√ After Completing	Date Due	Textbook Pages	TEXTBOOK ASSIGNMENTS	Possible Points	Points You Earned
		929-957	Read Chapter 38: Medical Office Computerization		
		946 954	Read Case Study 1 Case Study 1 questions	5	
		947 954	Read Case Study 2 Case Study 2 questions	5	
		953 954-955	Read Case Study 3 Case Study 3 questions	5	
			TOTAL POINTS		

√ After Completing	Date Due	Study Guide Pages	STUDY GUIDE ASSIGNMENTS (CTA = Critical Thinking Activity)	Possible Points	Points You Earned
		999	Pretest	10	
		1000	Key Term Assessment	30	
		1001-1007	Evaluation of Learning questions	76	
		1008	CTA A: Computer System	7	
		1008-1009	CTA B: Computer Monitor	6	
		1009	CTA C: Medical Practice Management Program	22	
		1010	CTA D: Crossword Puzzle	29	
			Evolve Site: Road to Recovery Game: Computer Terminology (Record points earned)		
			Evolve Site: Apply Your Knowledge questions	10	
		999	Posttest	10	
			ADDITIONAL ASSIGNMENTS		
			TOTAL POINTS		

Notes

Name _____ Date _____

True or False

_____ 1. Computers that are linked together are known as a *network*.

_____ 2. The transfer of data to the computer for processing is known as *input*.

_____ 3. Spreadsheet software consists of an electronic ledger designed to perform mathematical calculations quickly.

_____ 4. RAM (random access memory) determines how fast a computer can process information.

_____ 5. Screen size of a monitor refers to the measurement from one side of the screen horizontally to the other side.

_____ 6. A microfiber cloth can be used to clean the screen of a monitor.

_____ 7. Printed output from a computer is known as *hard copy*.

_____ 8. A USB flash drive stores information in the form of magnetized particles.

_____ 9. The posting transactions system is used to post patient charges and payments.

_____ 10. Paper documents are entered into a patient's EMR by scanning them into the computer.

[?≡] POSTTEST

True or False

_____ 1. A program that consists of raw, unorganized facts about subject matter is entered into the computer for processing.

_____ 2. An operating system assists the computer in carrying out its tasks.

_____ 3. The mainboard directs the step-by-step operation of all the processing functions.

_____ 4. One gigabyte is equal to 1000 MB.

_____ 5. The screen size of a typical desktop monitor is larger than the screen size of a laptop computer.

_____ 6. The monitor should be placed so that the top of the monitor is about 4 inches below eye level.

_____ 7. Grime can be removed from a computer keyboard using a can of compressed inert gas.

_____ 8. When a computer is turned off, all the information in RAM is lost.

_____ 9. The reports system allows the user to customize a medical management program to meet the specific requirements of a medical office.

_____ 10. Software designed to penetrate a computer or network without consent is known as a *computer virus*.

Directions: Match each computer term with its definition.

_____ 1. Computer

_____ 2. Computer system

_____ 3. CPU (central processing unit)

_____ 4. Data

_____ 5. Data processing

_____ 6. Documentation

_____ 7. Electronic medical record (EMR)

_____ 8. Firewall

_____ 9. Hard disk

_____ 10. Hardcopy

_____ 11. Hardware

_____ 12. Input

_____ 13. Input device

_____ 14. Medical practice management program

_____ 15. Microcomputer

_____ 16. Operating system

_____ 17. Optical disc

_____ 18. Optical drive

_____ 19. Output

_____ 20. Output device

_____ 21. Printing speed

_____ 22. Processing

_____ 23. Program

_____ 24. RAM (random-access memory)

_____ 25. Server

_____ 26. Software

_____ 27. Storage capacity

_____ 28. Storage device

_____ 29. User

_____ 30. Video card

A. A circuit board connected to the mainboard that converts computer video output into electronic signals

B. A computerized record of the important health information regarding a patient including the care of that individual and the progress of the patient's condition

C. A device for entering data into the computer (e.g., keyboard, mouse, scanner)

D. A device installed in a drive bay on the main computer unit that uses a laser to read an optical disc or write onto (burn) an optical disc

E. A device that permanently stores information for later retrieval by the computer

F. A device that transfers processed data to the user (e.g., computer monitor and printer)

G. A general term for the programs or instructions that tell a computer what to do

H. A program that provides instructions to the computer for performing medical practice management procedures

I. A set of instructions organized in a logical step-by-step sequence, which tells the computer how to perform a specific function

J. A small general purpose computer that relies on a tiny microprocessor chip to perform its processing functions

K. A storage device consisting of a flat, round, portable disk that stores data using laser technology

L. A storage device consisting of one or more rigid, nonflexible platters coated with a magnetically sensitive material and encased in a permanently sealed, air-tight container

M. A system that protects a computer network from unauthorized access by users on its own network or another network, such as the Internet

N. A type of system software that performs tasks required by the computer to operate itself

O. A written set of instructions accompanying an application program, designed to assist the user in understanding how to operate the program

P. All of the hardware and software components making up the computer

Q. An electronic machine that has the ability to process data according to a program in order to produce a desired result

R. Printed output from a computer

S. Raw, unorganized facts about subject matter presented to the computer for processing.

T. The "brain" of the computer housed in the main unit that interprets and executes the instructions that operate the computer

U. The changing of raw facts or data into usable information following a three-part sequence: input, processing, output

V. The individual using the computer

W. The main computer memory of a microcomputer, which is used to temporarily store items until needed by the computer for processing

X. The manipulation and reorganization of data according to the instructions in a program

Y. The maximum amount of information that a device can hold, measured in bytes

Z. The number of pages per minute (ppm) generated by a printer

AA. The physical devices making up a computer system (e.g., main computer unit, keyboard, monitor, printer)

BB. The transfer of data to the computer for processing

CC. The transfer of processed data back to the user

DD. A large computer that stores data and manages tasks for other computers on a network

Directions: Fill in each blank with the correct answer.

Computer Concepts

1. What are the principal advantages of using a computer to perform administrative procedures in the medical office?

_____

_____

2. What is a computer network?

_____

3. What are the three phases included in the data processing sequence?

_____

4. Why must data be converted into an electronic code before being processed by the computer?

_____

5. What are four examples of input devices?

_____

6. List two examples of output devices.

_____

7. What is the difference between system software and application software?

_____

_____

8. What is the function of an operating system?

_____

_____

9. What tasks are performed by the word processing program included in a medical practice management program?

_____

10. What is spreadsheet software?

_____

_____

11. What is the function of the spreadsheet software included in a practice management program?

_____

12. What are the functions of the telecommunications software included in a practice management program?

_____

13. What is database management?

_____

14. What functions can be performed by database management software?

_____

_____

15. What are examples of documentation?

_____

16. What computer hardware is necessary to perform administrative procedures in the medical office?

_____

_____

17. What is the function of the mainboard?

_____

_____

18. What is the function of the CPU (central processing unit)?

_____

19. What is the difference in processing speed between a CPU with a 3-GHz chip and one with a 1.5-GHz chip?

_____

20. What is the function of main memory (RAM)?

_____

_____

21. What items are commonly held in RAM?

_____

_____

22. What is the difference between random access and sequential access?

_____

_____

23. What happens to items in RAM when a computer is turned off?

_____

24. One byte is equivalent to how many characters?

_____

25. How many bytes are in a kilobyte (KB)? Kilobytes in a megabyte (MB)? Megabytes in a gigabyte (GB)? Gigabytes in a terabyte (TB)?

_____

_____

26. Explain how to prevent overheating of the computer.

_____

_____

27. What is the primary cause of improper functioning of the computer?

_____

28. What can happen if a liquid spills into the main computer unit?

_____

29. What is the function of the computer monitor?

_____

30. What are the advantages and disadvantages of a liquid crystal display (LCD) flat panel monitor?

_____

_____

31. How is the screen size of a computer monitor measured?

_____

32. Monitor resolution is measured in what type of units?

_____

33. How should the monitor be positioned to prevent back and neck tension?

_____

34. What can be done to prevent eye strain when working with a computer monitor?

_____

_____

35. What is the difference between a glare filter and a privacy filter?

_____

_____

36. What are the functions and examples of the following special keys?
    a. Modifier keys

_____

_____

    b. Lock keys

_____

_____

c. Navigation keys

_____

_____

37. How should the computer keyboard be positioned to prevent muscle fatigue?

_____

38. How should the following parts of a keyboard be cleaned?

a. Surface of the keyboard: _____

b. Interior of the keyboard: _____

39. What should be done if water spills into the keyboard?

_____

_____

_____

40. What types of printers are most commonly used in the medical office?

_____

41. What are the advantages and disadvantages of an inkjet printer?

_____

_____

42. What are the advantages and disadvantages of a laser printer?

_____

_____

43. How should the outside casing of a printer be cleaned?

_____

44. Where should you look to find information on cleaning the inside of the printer?

_____

45. List examples of storage devices used with a microcomputer.

_____

46. What method or organization is used to store and retrieve information from a hard disk?

_____

47. What is the storage capacity range for a hard disk?

_____

48. How does an optical disc store data?

_____

49. Which type of optical disc holds more information, a CD or a DVD?

_____

50. What makes up a USB (universal serial bus) flash drive?

_____

Medical Office Computerization

1. What are the advantages of medical office computerization?

_____

_____

_____

2. What is an audit trail?

_____

3. What are the disadvantages of computerization of the medical office?

_____

_____

4. How does a medical office minimize the effects of a computer system malfunction?

_____

5. What measures should be taken to promote the efficient running of a computerized medical office?

_____

_____

6. What is the function of each of the following systems included in a medical practice management program?

   a. Patient registration system: _____

   b. Appointment system: _____

   c. Posting transactions system: _____

   d. Patient billing system: _____

   e. Insurance billing system: _____

   f. Reports system: _____

   g. File maintenance system: _____

7. Give three examples of specific tasks that access the information previously entered into the patient registration system.

_____

_____

8. What are examples of start-up tasks?

_____

_____

9. What functions can be performed by an electronic medical record (EMR) program?

_____

_____

10. What are advantages of the EMR?

_____

_____

11. How are paper documents entered into a patient's EMR?

_____

12. How can a health history be entered into the EMR?

_____

_____

13. How does an EMR alleviate the need for medical transcription?

_____

_____

14. What is provided by the program for entering data into an EMR?

_____

15. What functions are performed by an EMR prescription program?

_____

_____

_____

16. How can an EMR program send a prescription to the pharmacy?

_____

17. What laboratory functions can be performed by an EMR program?

_____

_____

18. What are the advantages of having a diagnostic image available as a digital image?

_____

19. How do modern systems connect computers or networks to the Internet?

_____

20. What is clinical messaging and why is it more secure than e-mail?

_____

_____

21. What is encryption, and what standard is required as of January 1, 2012, to transmit patient health information electronically?

_____

_____

22. What is an advantage of transmitting prescriptions electronically?

_____

_____

23. What procedures typically are performed by a medical assistant using an EMR?

_____

_____

_____

24. Describe the following measures that maintain the security of the EMR.

a. Authentication: _____

_____

b. Levels of authorization: _____

_____

c. Automatic logoff: _____

_____

d. Audit controls: _____

_____

e. Antiviral software: _____

_____

f. Firewall:_____

_____

25. List two ways in which backups are performed in the medical office.

_____

_____

26. What are three important aspects of maintaing a computer system?

_____

_____

_____

CRITICAL THINKING ACTIVITIES

A. Computer System

Observe a computer system, and complete the following questions.

1. What is the brand name of the computer?

   _____

2. What hardware is included with this computer system?

   _____

   _____

3. What application software is installed on this computer system?

   _____

   _____

4. What operating system is being used with this computer?

   _____

5. What input devices are included with this computer system?

   _____

6. What output devices are included with this computer system?

   _____

7. How many optical drives does this computer have?

   _____

B. Computer Monitor

Observe a computer monitor, and complete the following questions.

1. Is this a CRT (cathode ray tube) monitor or an LCD flat panel monitor?

   _____

2. What is the screen size (in inches) of this monitor?

   _____

   _____

3. What controls are present on the monitor? If there is a menu, what menu options are present?

   _____

   _____

4. Position the monitor correctly to prevent back and neck tension. Explain what steps you took to do this.

   _____

   _____

5. Adjust the brightness or contrast to determine the setting that works best for your viewing comfort. Explain what you did to accomplish this.

_____

_____

_____

C. Medical Practice Management Program

Indicate which system you would use to perform the following using a medical practice management program.

A. Patient registration system
B. Appointments system
C. Posting transactions system
D. Patient billing system
E. Insurance billing system
F. Reports system
G. File maintenance system

_____ 1. Assign a user password

_____ 2. Change a patient's address

_____ 3. Reschedule a patient's appointment

_____ 4. Change a patient's insurance carrier and policy number

_____ 5. Electronically submit insurance claims

_____ 6. Enter a new insurance carrier

_____ 7. Enter demographic and insurance information for a new patient

_____ 8. Make an appointment

_____ 9. Post a charge for an allergy injection

_____ 10. Look up a patient's telephone number

_____ 11. Post an insurance payment

_____ 12. Prepare and print out a practice analysis report

_____ 13. Prepare bills for processing

_____ 14. Prepare insurance forms

_____ 15. Print billing statements

_____ 16. Print out a patient receipt

_____ 17. Print out a patient reminder card

_____ 18. Enter a new referring physician

_____ 19. Print out an appointment log

_____ 20. Change a patient's last name

_____ 21. Enter a new diagnosis code

_____ 22. Post a copayment made by a patient

D. Crossword Puzzle: Computer Terminology

Directions: Complete the crossword puzzle using the clues provided.

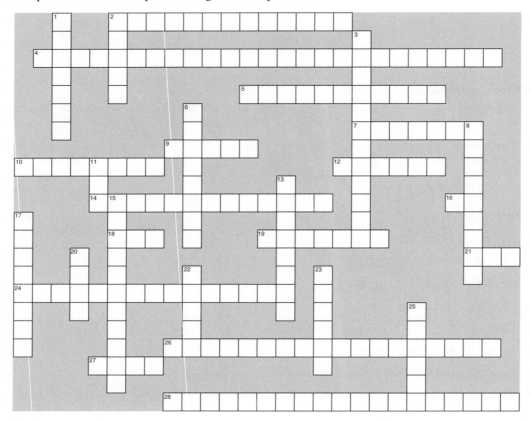

Across

2 Destroys computer information without consent
4 Main unit's worst enemy
5 Removes unneeded files
7 Step-by-step computer instructions
9 Transfer of information from RAM to a hard disk
10 Monitor's visual display
12 Dot locations on computer screen
14 Small circuit board storage device
16 1000 MB
18 Computerized medical record
19 Linked together computers
21 Temporarily stores information
24 Adjusts screen for viewing comfort
26 Computer talking to another computer
27 One character
28 Stores files closer together on hard drive

Down

1 Example of an OS
2 Read-only optical disc
3 Uses toner powder
6 Computer's physical devices
8 Computer's nervous system
11 Computer's brain
13 Protects computer from unauthorized access
15 Keys that issue commands
17 Printed output
20 Raw facts
22 Point and click device
23 Duplicate copy of computer information
25 Back at you

39 Telephone Techniques

CHAPTER ASSIGNMENTS

√After Completing	Date Due	Textbook Pages	TEXTBOOK ASSIGNMENTS	Possible Points	Points You Earned
		958-972	Read Chapter 39: Telephone Techniques		
		963 971	Read Case Study 1 Case Study 1 questions	5	
		964 971-972	Read Case Study 2 Case Study 2 questions	5	
		969 972	Read Case Study 3 Case Study 3 questions	5	
			TOTAL POINTS		

√After Completing	Date Due	Study Guide Pages	STUDY GUIDE ASSIGNMENTS (CTA = Critical Thinking Activity)	Possible Points	Points You Earned
		1015	Pretest	10	
		1016	Term Key Term Assessment	5	
		1016-1019	Evaluation of Learning questions	26	
		1019	CTA A: Screening Telephone Calls	8	
		1019-1020	CTA B: Follow-up Questions	5	
		1020	CTA C: Telephone Messages When the Office is Closed	10	
		1020	CTA D: Outgoing Calls	4	
			Evolve Site: Taking a Telephone Message	10	
			Evolve Site: Apply Your Knowledge questions	10	
			Evolve Site: Video Evaluation	10	
		1015	Posttest	10	

√After Completing	Date Due	Study Guide Pages	STUDY GUIDE ASSIGNMENTS (CTA = Critical Thinking Activity)	Possible Points	Points You Earned
			ADDITIONAL ASSIGNMENTS		
			TOTAL POINTS		

Chapter **39** **Telephone Techniques**

√When Assigned By Your Instructor	Study Guide Pages	Practices Required	LABORATORY ASSIGNMENTS (Procedure Number and Name)	Score*
	1021	3	**Practice for Competency** 39-1: Performing Telephone Screening Textbook reference: p. 966	
	1025-1026		**Evaluation of Competency** 39-1: Performing Telephone Screening	*
	1021-1023	3	**Practice for Competency** 39-2: Taking a Telephone Message Textbook reference: p. 967	
	1027-1028		**Evaluation of Competency** 39-2: Taking a Telephone Message	*
	1021-1024	3	**Practice for Competency** 39-3: Taking Requests for Medication or Prescription Refills Textbook reference: p. 968	
	1029-1030		**Evaluation of Competency** 39-3: Taking Requests for Medication or Prescription Refills	*
	1021-1024	3	**Practice for Competency** 39-4: Telephoning a Patient for Follow-up Textbook reference: p. 970	
	1031-1032		**Evaluation of Competency** 39-4: Telephoning a Patient for Follow-up	*
			ADDITIONAL ASSIGNMENTS	

Notes

Name _____   Date _____

True or False

_____ 1. The medical assistant (MA) should obtain a caller's name before placing the caller on hold.

_____ 2. A caller will not be able to pick up nonverbal cues during a telephone call with the medical office.

_____ 3. Call forwarding sends telephone calls to a different extension or telephone number.

_____ 4. Most medical offices rely only on voice mail during the night and weekends.

_____ 5. When taking a message about a patient, the medical assistant should include the patient's age or date of birth.

_____ 6. Physicians should not be contacted when out of the office using cell phones or pagers.

_____ 7. A telephone electronic routing system avoids placing incoming calls on hold.

_____ 8. A physician will accept a call from another physician, even if it interrupts a patient examination.

_____ 9. The MA may not take a message from a laboratory that includes the results of diagnostic tests.

_____ 10. If a patient requests a prescription refill, the MA should ask for the pharmacy name and telephone number.

? POSTTEST

True or False

_____ 1. If a call is on hold, the MA should check back with the caller at least every 30 seconds.

_____ 2. When answering the telephone, the MA should first identify the practice and himself or herself.

_____ 3. Call park places a call on hold so that it can be retrieved from a different telephone.

_____ 4. Voice mail mailboxes each have a separate extension.

_____ 5. Medical assistants should transfer all calls from patients requesting medication refills to a licensed professional.

_____ 6. Physicians may have access to e-mail using their smartphones.

_____ 7. A telephone electronic routing system saves the expense of designating one person to answer incoming telephone calls.

_____ 8. Most physicians take calls from patients while they are seeing other patients.

_____ 9. Medical assistants routinely give patients the results of normal diagnostic tests over the telephone.

_____ 10. The MA may take a message if a patient wants a referral or a diagnostic test.

Directions: Match each medical term with its definition.

_____ 1. Enunciation

_____ 2. Pager

_____ 3. PDA (personal digital assistant)

_____ 4. Smartphone

_____ 5. Voice mail

A. A portable hand-held computing device with access to various reference tools

B. A method for delivery, storage, and retrieval of telephone messages that is built into the telephone system

C. An electronic device that notifies the recipient to receive a message or return a telephone call

D. The act of speaking clearly and concisely

E. A cell phone with computer capabilities

EVALUATION OF LEARNING

Directions: Fill in each blank with the correct answer.

1. Give examples of three ways the MA can display courtesy when answering the telephone in the medical office.

_____

_____

_____

2. How can the MA project a pleasing telephone personality when talking to callers in the medical office?

_____

_____

_____

3. How should the MA answer the office telephone?

_____

_____

4. Identify three ways to maintain proper body mechanics and avoid muscle strain when spending several minutes on the telephone.

_____

_____

_____

5. How does the MA handle a second call when speaking to a caller on a multiline telephone?

_____

_____

_____

6. Identify and describe four features of most telephone systems.

_____

_____

_____

7. How is voicemail used in the medical office?

_____

_____

_____

8. How can patients get assistance for an urgent situation that occurs when the office is closed?

_____

_____

9. What are two devices that may be used to maintain contact with the physician when he or she is not in the medical office?

_____

10. What is an electronic routing system for incoming telephone calls?

_____

_____

11. When answering incoming calls, what three types of calls take priority over other telephone calls?

_____

_____

12. Identify four types of calls that are usually handled by the MA.

_____

_____

_____

13. List nine pieces of information that should be included if the MA takes a telephone message.

_____

_____

_____

_____

14. What are two ways an MA might take a message using a computer?

_____

_____

15. How should the MA handle a telephone call requesting test results?

_____

_____

_____

16. If a patient or pharmacy calls with a request to have a prescription refilled or renewed, what specific information should the MA record on a telephone message?

_____

_____

_____

17. How should the MA handle a call if the caller has a medical question?

_____

_____

18. How should the MA handle a call from another physician?

_____

_____

19. How should the MA handle a telephone call about a serious emergency?

_____

_____

_____

20. If a telephone call concerns a possible case of poisoning, where should the caller be referred?

_____

_____

21. What should the MA do if a caller's condition does not seem to be a serious emergency, but the MA is not sure how urgent the problem is?

_____

_____

22. How should the MA handle a call if the caller asks for the physician but will not identify himself or herself?

_____

_____

_____

23. How should the MA handle a call if the caller has a complaint about service received in the medical office?

_____

_____

24. What guidelines should the MA follow when calling a patient?

_____

_____

1018

25. How is the telephone used to remind patients about appointments?

_____

_____

_____

26. What guidelines should the MA follow related to his or her own personal telephone calls?

_____

_____

CRITICAL THINKING ACTIVITIES

A. Screening Telephone Calls

For each of the following telephone calls, choose the best action for the MA from the following options. Assume that Dr. Warner is in the office seeing patients and a registered nurse is also in the office.

a. Transfer the call to Dr. Warner

b. Transfer the call to a licensed professional, such as one of the physicians or a nurse

c. Handle the call

d. Tell the caller that Dr. Warner is seeing patients, and offer to take a message

_____ 1. The caller identifies himself as Dr. Stephen Miller and asks to speak to Dr. Warner.

_____ 2. The caller asks for Dr. Warner and states that she wants the results of an MRI done last week.

_____ 3. The caller says that she has a question about her bill.

_____ 4. The caller asks for an appointment because the practice has been recommended to her.

_____ 5. The caller says that her daughter, a patient of Dr. Warner, fell off a swing and screams when anyone touches her left arm.

_____ 6. The caller identifies herself as a pharmacist and asks for Dr. Warner.

_____ 7. The caller says that she is calling to get results of a blood test done that morning.

_____ 8. The caller asks for an appointment because she has a sore throat and fever of 101°F.

B. Follow-Up Questions

If you were the MA taking a message in each of the following examples, identify two questions you would ask the patient to complete the message.

1. Maria Reyes, a 38-year-old patient of Dr. Gomez, is calling because she wants to know the results of blood tests that were done for her 6-year-old daughter the previous week. She tells you her daughter's date of birth. She tells you that she is at work, and the best time to call is after 2:00 PM.

_____

_____

2. John Dalton, a 24-year-old patient of Dr. Hughes, is calling to get a refill of his cholesterol medication. He takes Lipitor 20 mg every morning. He tells you his date of birth. He only has two tablets left. He gives you his home telephone number and says that it is his day off.

_____

_____

1019

3. A nurse calls from the hospital and says that she would like to obtain an order for a stronger pain medication for Angela White, a hospitalized patient. She tells you the patient's date of birth and gives you the telephone number of the nurse's station. She will be available until the end of the shift at 4:00 PM.

_____

_____

4. Melissa Sanders calls about her daughter who fell at school and twisted her ankle. Mrs. Sanders picked her daughter up from school, and she would like to discuss the injury with Dr. Warner. She gives you her home telephone number and cell phone number and says she will be available at any time.

_____

_____

5. A caller identifies himself as Robert Warner. He says that Dr. Gomez contacted him to obtain information about purchasing new examination tables. He gives you his office telephone number and cell phone number.

_____

_____

C. Telephone Message When the Office is Closed

Create a telephone message for Western Medical Center to be used when the office is closed. The message should include instructions for an emergency, instructions if the caller needs medical advice, and instructions to leave a nonurgent message. If the caller wants a prescription refill, he or she should be referred to a different specific number to leave a detailed message.

_____

_____

_____

_____

_____

D. Outgoing Calls

Explain the procedure for each of the following:

1. Calling a patient for an appointment reminder

_____

_____

2. Calling a pharmacy with a prescription refill

_____

_____

3. Placing a telephone call from a physician in the office to another physician

_____

_____

PRACTICE FOR COMPETENCY

Procedure 39-1: Performing Telephone Screening. Practice the procedure with a classmate as if you are an MA at Western Medical Center. When you are the caller, choose one of the scenarios below without preparing your classmate ahead of time.

1. Pretend to be another physician calling to speak to Dr. Warner.
2. Pretend to be a patient calling for results of a laboratory or diagnostic test for your husband or mother.
3. Pretend to be a patient who wants directions to the office or who has questions about public transportation to the office.
4. Pretend to be a relative of Dr. Warner who wants to speak to the physician.
5. Pretend to be a patient experiencing severe chest pain or bleeding.

Procedure 39-2: Taking a Telephone Message. Practice the procedure with a classmate as if you are an MA at Western Medical Center. When you are the caller, choose one of the scenarios below without telling your classmate ahead of time. One person should answer the calls for Dr. Gomez, and the other should answer the calls for Dr. Warner. When you are the caller, provide a simulated telephone number or other information if the MA requests it. When you are the MA, inform the caller that the doctor is with a patient, offer to take a message, and complete a telephone message form making sure to ask for all necessary information.

1. You are calling from the Admitting Department at Memorial Hospital to get admitting orders from Dr. Warner for Diane Walters, DOB 1/22/1972. The patient is in the admitting department.
2. You are calling from the Nuclear Medicine Department at Memorial Hospital. You want to speak to Dr. Gomez about a test you just did on John Perkins. You are concerned about the test because the results seem to be very abnormal.
3. You are calling to find out the results of a thyroid scan that you had at Memorial Hospital yesterday. Your physician is Dr. Warner.
4. You are calling to find out the results of a complete blood count and chemistry screen that were done at the laboratory 2 days ago. Your physician is Dr. Gomez.
5. You cut your left hand with a knife, and you are a patient of Dr. Warner. It is a deep cut, about ¾ inch long. It does not bleed if you put pressure on it, but it does start to bleed again if you take the gauze square off. You want to know if you should come to the office or go to the emergency room.
6. A neighbor's child told you she saw your 3-year-old daughter eat several berries from a plant in the yard. The child does not seem ill, but you want to ask her doctor, Dr. Gomez, what to do. Should you bring her to the office or take her to the emergency room? Can the doctor call you back?

Procedure 39-3: Taking Requests for Medication or Prescription Refills. Practice this procedure with a classmate. Use information from the following simulated prescription labels to call for prescription refills. If the medication is an antibiotic or analgesic, ask for symptoms that require the refill. Document in the medical record.

Furosemide 20 mg tab Generic equivalent for: Lasix Take 1 tablet daily West Street Pharmacy Pharmacy telephone: (490) 555-2211	Indomethacin 25 mg cap Take 1-2 capsules with food up to three times daily for moderate to severe pain Best Pharmacy Pharmacy telephone: (490) 555-6155
Tetracycline 250 mg cap Take 1 capsule twice daily Twelve Oaks Pharmacy Pharmacy telephone: (490) 555-8719	Lipitor 20 mg tab Take 1 tablet every day Wide River Pharmacy Pharmacy telephone: (490) 555-1981
Crestor 10 mg tab Take 1 tablet by mouth every day Best Pharmacy Pharmacy telephone: (490) 555-6155	Atenolol 50 mg tab Take 1 tablet by mouth daily West Street Pharmacy Pharmacy telephone: (490) 555-2211

MESSAGE FROM

For Dr.	Name of Caller	Ref. to pt.	Patient	Pt. Age	Pt. Temp.	Message Date /	Message Time AM PM	Urgent ☐ Yes ☐ No

Message:					Allergies

Respond to Phone #	Best Time to Call AM PM	Pharmacy Name / #	Patient's Chart Attached ☐ Yes ☐ No	Patient's chart #	Initials

DOCTOR - STAFF RESPONSE

Doctor's / Staff Orders / Follow-up Action

	Call Back ☐ Yes ☐ No	Chart. Mes. ☐ Yes ☐ No	Follow-up Date / /	Follow-up Completed-Date/Time / /	AM PM	Response By:

Product # 78-9156-Pkg, #78-9157-Pads, Bibbero Systems, Inc., Petaluma, CA. To order, call toll free 800-BIBBERO (800 242-2376) OR FAX 800-242-9330.

MESSAGE FROM

For Dr.	Name of Caller	Ref. to pt.	Patient	Pt. Age	Pt. Temp.	Message Date /	Message Time AM PM	Urgent ☐ Yes ☐ No

Message:					Allergies

Respond to Phone #	Best Time to Call AM PM	Pharmacy Name / #	Patient's Chart Attached ☐ Yes ☐ No	Patient's chart #	Initials

DOCTOR - STAFF RESPONSE

Doctor's / Staff Orders / Follow-up Action

	Call Back ☐ Yes ☐ No	Chart. Mes. ☐ Yes ☐ No	Follow-up Date / /	Follow-up Completed-Date/Time / /	AM PM	Response By:

Product # 78-9156-Pkg, #78-9157-Pads, Bibbero Systems, Inc., Petaluma, CA. To order, call toll free 800-BIBBERO (800 242-2376) OR FAX 800-242-9330.

MESSAGE FROM

For Dr.	Name of Caller	Ref. to pt.	Patient	Pt. Age	Pt. Temp.	Message Date /	Message Time AM PM	Urgent ☐ Yes ☐ No

Message:					Allergies

Respond to Phone #	Best Time to Call AM PM	Pharmacy Name / #	Patient's Chart Attached ☐ Yes ☐ No	Patient's chart #	Initials

DOCTOR - STAFF RESPONSE

Doctor's / Staff Orders / Follow-up Action

	Call Back ☐ Yes ☐ No	Chart. Mes. ☐ Yes ☐ No	Follow-up Date / /	Follow-up Completed-Date/Time / /	AM PM	Response By:

Product # 78-9156-Pkg, #78-9157-Pads, Bibbero Systems, Inc., Petaluma, CA. To order, call toll free 800-BIBBERO (800 242-2376) OR FAX 800-242-9330.

(Courtesy Bibbero Systems, Inc., Petaluma, Calif. [800] 242-2376; Fax [800] 242-9330; www.bibbero.com.)

MESSAGE FROM

For Dr.	Name of Caller	Ref. to pt.	Patient	Pt. Age	Pt. Temp.	Message Date	Message Time	Urgent
						/	AM PM	☐ Yes ☐ No

Message:

Allergies

Respond to Phone #	Best Time to Call AM PM	Pharmacy Name / #	Patient's Chart Attached ☐ Yes ☐ No	Patient's chart #	Initials

DOCTOR - STAFF RESPONSE

Doctor's / Staff Orders / Follow-up Action

Call Back ☐ Yes ☐ No	Chart. Mes. ☐ Yes ☐ No	Follow-up Date / /	Follow-up Completed-Date/Time / / AM PM	Response By:

Product # 78-9156-Pkg, #78-9157-Pads, Bibbero Systems, Inc., Petaluma, CA. To order, call toll free 800-BIBBERO (800 242-2376) OR FAX 800-242-9330.

MESSAGE FROM

For Dr.	Name of Caller	Ref. to pt.	Patient	Pt. Age	Pt. Temp.	Message Date	Message Time	Urgent
						/	AM PM	☐ Yes ☐ No

Message:

Allergies

Respond to Phone #	Best Time to Call AM PM	Pharmacy Name / #	Patient's Chart Attached ☐ Yes ☐ No	Patient's chart #	Initials

DOCTOR - STAFF RESPONSE

Doctor's / Staff Orders / Follow-up Action

Call Back ☐ Yes ☐ No	Chart. Mes. ☐ Yes ☐ No	Follow-up Date / /	Follow-up Completed-Date/Time / / AM PM	Response By:

Product # 78-9156-Pkg, #78-9157-Pads, Bibbero Systems, Inc., Petaluma, CA. To order, call toll free 800-BIBBERO (800 242-2376) OR FAX 800-242-9330.

MESSAGE FROM

For Dr.	Name of Caller	Ref. to pt.	Patient	Pt. Age	Pt. Temp.	Message Date	Message Time	Urgent
						/	AM PM	☐ Yes ☐ No

Message:

Allergies

Respond to Phone #	Best Time to Call AM PM	Pharmacy Name / #	Patient's Chart Attached ☐ Yes ☐ No	Patient's chart #	Initials

DOCTOR - STAFF RESPONSE

Doctor's / Staff Orders / Follow-up Action

Call Back ☐ Yes ☐ No	Chart. Mes. ☐ Yes ☐ No	Follow-up Date / /	Follow-up Completed-Date/Time / / AM PM	Response By:

Product # 78-9156-Pkg, #78-9157-Pads, Bibbero Systems, Inc., Petaluma, CA. To order, call toll free 800-BIBBERO (800 242-2376) OR FAX 800-242-9330.

(Courtesy Bibbero Systems, Inc., Petaluma, Calif. [800] 242-2376; Fax [800] 242-9330; www.bibbero.com.)

Record medication refills or prescriptions in the medical record below.

CHART	
Date	

Procedure 39-4: Telephoning a Patient for Follow-Up. Practice the procedure with a classmate as if you are an MA at Western Medical Center. When you are the caller, choose one of the scenarios below without telling your classmate ahead of time. One person should choose the scenarios for Dr. Gomez, and the other should choose the scenarios for Dr. Warner.

1. Dr. Warner has asked you to call the patient above who had a thyroid san to schedule an appointment to discuss the test results. Give the patient an appointment this week.
2. Dr. Gomez has asked you to call the patient who had a complete blood count and chemistry screen above and instruct the patient to repeat the blood tests in a week. The patient should also make an appointment with Dr. Gomez next week.
3. Dr. Warner has asked you to call the patient who had a knife cut and instruct her to come to the office to be seen. Ask how long it will take her to get to the office, and give her that appointment time.
4. Dr. Gomez has asked you to call the patient whose child was seen eating berries. Ask the mother to get a sample of the plant leaves and berries if possible and call Poison Control. Give her the telephone number of the local Poison Control center.
5. Dr. Warner has asked you to call a patient and tell her that her throat culture is positive for strep, and that he has prescribed an antibiotic. Instruct the patient to pick up the medication at her usual pharmacy.
6. Dr. Gomez has asked you to call a patient and tell him that he is prescribing a new medication for his cholesterol based on his recent blood test. The patient should pick up the medication at the pharmacy and make an appointment to follow up after 3 months.

1024

Procedure 39-1: Performing Telephone Screening

Name: _____   Date: _____

Evaluated by: _____   Score: _____

Performance Objective

Outcome:	Screen telephone calls.
Conditions:	Given the following: telephone, message pad, pen or pencil, appointment book or computer, and clock or watch.
Standards:	Time: 10 minutes. Student completed procedure in _____ minutes.
	Accuracy: Satisfactory score in the Performance Evaluation Checklist.

Performance Evaluation Checklist

Trial 1	Trial 2	Point Value	Performance Standards
		●	Answered the telephone within the first three rings.
		●	Identified the medical office and gave name.
		●	Listened as the caller identified the reason for the call.
		●	Decided promptly if it was a call that should be transferred.
		●	Asked for the caller's name if not given by the caller.
		●	Took a message if appropriate (see Procedure 39-2: Taking a Telephone Message).
		●	If necessary to transfer the call, placed the caller on hold.
		●	Told the person to whom the call would be transferred the caller's name and extension (if necessary).
		●	Asked questions to assess any problem requiring immediate care.
		●	Transferred an urgent call to a physician or licensed professional if possible or followed office guidelines.
		●	Instructed a caller whose health was at risk to call 911.
		●	Monitored calls on hold and returned to a caller on hold within 30–45 seconds if a transferred call was not picked up.
		●	Asked a caller for permission before placing on hold to take a new call.
		●	Gave a second caller the option to be placed on hold or have the call returned before returning to a previous call.
		●	Repeated important information before ending a call.
		●	Ended the call politely.
		★	Completed the procedure within 10 minutes.
			TOTALS

Evaluation of Student Performance

EVALUATION CRITERIA			COMMENTS
Symbol	**Category**	**Point Value**	
✶	Critical Step	16 points	
●	Essential Step	6 points	
▷	Theory Question	2 points	

Score calculation: 100 points

     −   _____ points missed

           _____ Score

Satisfactory score: 85 or above

CAAHEP Competencies Achieved

Psychomotor (Skills)
☑ IV. 7. Demonstrate telephone techniques.
Affective (Behavior)
☑ IV. 2. Apply active listening skills.
☑ IV. 7. Demonstrate recognition of the patient's level of understanding in communication.

ABHES Competencies Achieved

☑ 8. d. Apply concepts for office procedures.
☑ 8. cc. Communicate on the recipient's level of comprehension.
☑ 8. ee. Use proper telephone techniques.
☑ 9.o.(3) Perform telephone and in-person screening.

Procedure 39-2: Taking a Telephone Message

Name: _____   Date: _____

Evaluated by: _____   Score: _____

Performance Objective

Outcome:	Take a telephone message.
Conditions:	Given the following: telephone, message pad, pen or pencil, and clock or watch.
Standards:	Time: 5 minutes. Student completed procedure in _____ minutes.
	Accuracy: Satisfactory score in the Performance Evaluation Checklist.

Performance Evaluation Checklist

Trial 1	Trial 2	Point Value	Performance Standards
		●	Determined that the person being called was not available.
		●	Offered to take a message.
		●	Gave the caller a reason why the person could not take the call.
		●	Filled in complete information legibly on the telephone message pad.
		●	Wrote down the name of the caller.
		●	Wrote down the business affiliation of the caller if appropriate.
		●	Wrote down the date and time of the call.
		●	Wrote down the telephone number of the caller, including area code.
		●	Wrote down the reason for the call and information the caller included in the message.
		●	Initialed the message form.
		●	Left any response section blank for the intended recipient to complete.
		●	Verified information.
		●	Gave caller a time when the call might be returned or told caller that the message would be given to the intended recipient.
		●	Ended the call politely.
		●	Clipped a message related to a patient to the patient's paper medical record.
		●	Placed the message where the intended recipient would expect to find it.
		●	Performed follow up according to office procedure.
		✱	Completed the procedure within 5 minutes.
			TOTALS

1027

Evaluation of Student Performance

EVALUATION CRITERIA			COMMENTS
Symbol	Category	Point Value	
✶	Critical Step	16 points	
●	Essential Step	6 points	
▷	Theory Question	2 points	

Score calculation: 100 points

− _____ points missed

_____ Score

Satisfactory score: 85 or above

CAAHEP Competencies Achieved

Psychomotor (Skills)
☑ IV. 7. Demonstrate telephone techniques.

Affective (Behavior)
☑ IV. 2. Apply active listening skills.
☑ IV. 7. Demonstrate recognition of the patient's level of understanding in communication.

ABHES Competencies Achieved

☑ 8. cc. Communicate on the recipient's level of comprehension.
☑ 8. ee. Use proper telephone techniques.

Procedure 39-3: Taking Requests for Medication or Prescription Refills

Name: _____   Date: _____

Evaluated by: _____   Score: _____

Performance Objective

Outcome:	Take a message requesting medication or a prescription refill.
Conditions:	Given the following: Telephone, message pad, pen or pencil, medical record, and clock or watch.
Standards:	Time: 5 minutes. Student completed procedure in _____ minutes.
	Accuracy: Satisfactory score in the Performance Evaluation Checklist.

Performance Evaluation Checklist

Trial 1	Trial 2	Point Value	Performance Standards
		●	Identified the caller and telephone number.
		●	Identified if the caller was a patient or a pharmacy.
		●	Wrote complete information on the message pad legibly (or entered on computer message form).
		●	Included the name of the medication, dose, and number of times taken daily.
		●	Included the patient's name and telephone number (if the patient was the caller).
		●	Included pharmacy name and telephone number.
		●	If the caller was the pharmacy, gave a time when the physician would be likely to approve the refill.
		●	Ended the call politely.
		●	Clipped the message to the patient's medical record or attached patient medical record to computer message.
		●	Placed the message for review by the physician or forwarded the message electronically.
		●	If the physician was available to take the call, pulled the patient's paper medical record before transferring it.
		●	If instructed by the physician, called the pharmacy with the new medication order.
		●	Read the information exactly as written by the physician.
		●	Documented the refill or prescription in the patient's medical record or filed the message as documentation.
		✱	Completed the procedure within 5 minutes.
			TOTALS

1029

CHART	
Date	

Evaluation of Student Performance

EVALUATION CRITERIA			COMMENTS
Symbol	**Category**	**Point Value**	
✶	Critical Step	16 points	
●	Essential Step	6 points	
▷	Theory Question	2 points	

Score calculation: 100 points

      −   _____ points missed

         _____ Score

Satisfactory score: 85 or above

CAAHEP Competencies Achieved

Psychomotor (Skills)
☑ IV. 7. Demonstrate telephone techniques.

Affective (Behavior)
☑ IV. 2. Apply active listening skills.
☑ IV. 7. Demonstrate recognition of the patient's level of understanding in communication.

ABHES Competencies Achieved

☑ 8. cc. Communicate on the recipient's level of comprehension.
☑ 8. ee. Use proper telephone techniques.

EVALUATION OF COMPETENCY

Procedure 39-4: Telephoning a Patient for Follow-Up

Name: _____   Date: _____

Evaluated by: _____   Score: _____

Performance Objective

Outcome:	Telephone a patient for follow-up.
Conditions:	Given the following: telephone, scratch paper, pen or pencil, telephone book or instructions from the physician, and patient medical record as needed.
Standards:	Time: 5 minutes. Student completed procedure in _____ minutes.
	Accuracy: Satisfactory score in the Performance Evaluation Checklist.

Performance Evaluation Checklist

Trial 1	Trial 2	Point Value	Performance Standards
		●	Organized information that might be necessary during the telephone call.
		●	Wrote down telephone number including area code and country code as needed.
		●	Placed the telephone call.
		●	Asked for the patient or correct individual.
		●	Identified the medical practice and self.
		●	If call was not answered, left message on voicemail or answering machine, including name of medical office, own name, and telephone number.
		●	When speaking to the patient, gave information as instructed by the physician.
		●	Gave the patient only the information authorized by the physician.
		●	Repeated instructions if any were given.
		●	Ended call professionally and said "good-bye."
		✶	Completed the procedure within 5 minutes.
			TOTALS

Evaluation of Student Performance

	EVALUATION CRITERIA		COMMENTS
Symbol	**Category**	**Point Value**	
✶	Critical Step	16 points	
●	Essential Step	6 points	
▷	Theory Question	2 points	

Score calculation: 100 points

− _____ points missed
_____
_____ Score

Satisfactory score: 85 or above

CAAHEP Competencies Achieved

Psychomotor (Skills)
☑ IV. 7. Demonstrate telephone techniques.

Affective (Behavior)
☑ IV. 2. Apply active listening skills.
☑ IV. 7. Demonstrate recognition of the patient's level of understanding in communication.

ABHES Competencies Achieved

☑ 8. cc. Communicate on the recipient's level of comprehension.
☑ 8. ee. Use proper telephone techniques.

1032

40 Scheduling Appointments

CHAPTER ASSIGNMENTS

√ After Completing	Date Due	Textbook Pages	TEXTBOOK ASSIGNMENTS	Possible Points	Points You Earned
		973-991	Read Chapter 40: Scheduling Appointments		
		981 990	Read Case Study 1 / Case Study 1 questions	5	
		983 990	Read Case Study 2 / Case Study 2 questions	5	
		987 990	Read Case Study 3 / Case Study 3 questions	5	
			TOTAL POINTS		

√ After Completing	Date Due	Study Guide Pages	STUDY GUIDE ASSIGNMENTS (CTA = Critical Thinking Activity)	Possible Points	Points You Earned
		1037	Pretest	10	
		1038	Key Term Assessment	15	
		1038-1040	Evaluation of Learning questions	18	
		1041	CTA A: Computer-Generated Appointment Schedule	5	
		1041	CTA B: Methods of Scheduling	5	
		1041	CTA C: Appointment Schedule	5	
		1041-1042	CTA D: Setting Priorities for Appointments	4	
		1042	CTA E: Scheduling Diagnostic Tests and Procedures	5	
			Evolve Site: Guided Practice: Preparing and Maintaining the Appointment Book	10	
			Evolve Site: Guided Practice: Scheduling a New Patient	10	
			Evolve Site: Guided Practice: Scheduling an Outpatient Diagnostic Test	10	

1033

√ After Completing	Date Due	Study Guide Pages	STUDY GUIDE ASSIGNMENTS (CTA = Critical Thinking Activity)	Possible Points	Points You Earned
			e Evolve Site: Guided Practice: Scheduling an Inpatient Admission and an Inpatient Surgical Procedure	10	
			e Evolve Site: Apply Your Knowledge questions	10	
			e Evolve Site: Video Evaluation	16	
		1037	Posttest	10	
			ADDITIONAL ASSIGNMENTS		
			TOTAL POINTS		

√ When Assigned By Your Instructor	Study Guide Pages	Practices Required	LABORATORY ASSIGNMENTS (Procedure Number and Name)	Score*
	1043-1046	3	**Practice for Competency** 40-1: Setting Up the Appointment Schedule Textbook reference: p. 979	
	1053-1054		**Evaluation of Competency** 40-1: Setting Up the Appointment Schedule	*
	1047	3	**Practice for Competency** 40-2: Making an Appointment Textbook reference: p. 982	
	1055-1056	1	**Evaluation of Competency** 40-2: Making an Appointment	*
	1047-1048		**Practice for Competency** 40-3: Managing the Appointment Schedule Textbook reference: pp. 984-985	
	1057-1058		**Evaluation of Competency** 40-3: Managing the Appointment Schedule	*
	1049-1051	1	**Practice for Competency** 40-4: Scheduling Inpatient or Outpatient Diagnostic Tests or Procedures Textbook reference: p. 988	
	1059-1060		**Evaluation of Competency** 40-4: Scheduling Inpatient or Outpatient Diagnostic Tests or Procedures	*
	1051-1052	1	**Practice for Competency** 40-5: Scheduling Inpatient or Outpatient Admissions Textbook reference: p. 989	
	1061-1062		**Evaluation of Competency** 40-5: Scheduling Inpatient or Outpatient Admissions	*
			ADDITIONAL ASSIGNMENTS	

Notes

PRETEST

True or False

_____ 1. For legal purposes, a daily schedule is usually the official record of appointments.

_____ 2. Corrections or changes to the official daily schedule are usually made in pencil.

_____ 3. Most medical offices use some type of time-specified appointment system.

_____ 4. In the stream method of appointment scheduling, each patient is given a different appointment time.

_____ 5. An example of clustering patient appointments is making appointments for new patients.

_____ 6. In the appointment schedule, times when physicians are available to see patients are blocked.

_____ 7. Demographic data for new patients are usually obtained when scheduling the first appointment.

_____ 8. Many medical offices call patients a few days before an appointment as a reminder.

_____ 9. The physician can usually admit a patient to the hospital without insurance preauthorization.

_____ 10. Patients usually call the hospital to schedule their own surgery.

POSTTEST

True or False

_____ 1. A written appointment book must be kept to provide a legal record of appointments.

_____ 2. If a patient fails to call or keep an appointment, the missed appointment should be noted in ink on the official daily schedule.

_____ 3. In wave scheduling, several patients are given the same appointment time.

_____ 4. The method of scheduling appointments with the least waiting time for patients is open hours.

_____ 5. Categorization refers to the practice of scheduling patients with similar problems back to back.

_____ 6. Most medical offices set up the appointment schedule for only the next 2 or 3 months.

_____ 7. If a patient makes an appointment while in the office, he or she should be given a written appointment reminder card.

_____ 8. All patients must obtain a referral from the primary care provider before making an appointment with a specialist.

_____ 9. If a medical assistant (MA) schedules a diagnostic test for a patient, he or she should also provide any written instructions about preparation for the test.

_____ 10. An ECG and blood work are usually required before a patient can have inpatient or outpatient surgery.

Directions: Match each medical term with its definition.

_____ 1. Blocked

_____ 2. Clustering

_____ 3. Double booking

_____ 4. Established patient

_____ 5. Hospice

_____ 6. Matrix

_____ 7. Modified wave scheduling

_____ 8. New patient

_____ 9. No-show

_____ 10. Preadmission testing (PAT)

_____ 11. Preauthorization

_____ 12. Referral

_____ 13. Stream scheduling (single booking)

_____ 14. Triage

_____ 15. Wave scheduling

A. Grouping patients with similar problems or conditions on certain days or at certain times of the day

B. The process of sorting patients according to their need for care

C. Times that are crossed out of the appointment schedule (not available for appointments)

D. A patient who has never been seen by the physician or for billing purposes has not been seen within the past 3 years

E. A scheduling method that uses both fixed appointments and more than one patient scheduled for the same appointment time

F. In managed care, written authorization by the primary care physician for a patient to receive additional services

G. Booking two people into a single time slot

H. Scheduling three or four patients every half hour, who are seen in the order in which they arrive

I. A patient who has been seen by one of the physicians in the practice within the past 3 years

J. A form or arrangement for information, such as appointments

K. An appointment scheduling method where each patient is given a specific appointment time

L. Diagnostic tests that are performed before the patient is admitted for surgery or a diagnostic procedure

M. A person who does not appear for his or her appointment

N. A program or facility that provides care to terminally ill patients

O. Permission from a patient's insurance company for a test, procedure, or surgery

Directions: Fill in each blank with the correct answer.

1. Identify seven guidelines to follow when making appointments.

_____

_____

_____

_____

_____

2. Identify two methods of scheduling appointments.

_____

_____

3. Why must the official daily schedule record any changes in the schedule and/or patients who miss appointments in ink? How is it handled to preserve patient confidentiality?

_____

_____

_____

4. Identify and describe each of the following types of appointment scheduling.

    a. Time-specified (stream) scheduling (single booking)

_____

    b. Wave scheduling

_____

    c. Modified wave scheduling

_____

    d. Double booking

_____

    e. Open booking

_____

    f. Patient self-scheduling

_____

    g. Categorization (clustering)

_____

5. What factors must be considered when setting up the appointment schedule?

_____

_____

_____

6. How are new patients treated differently from established patients when making appointments?

_____

_____

7. Identify eight types of medical problems for which patients would usually be given a same-day appointment.

_____

_____

_____

_____

8. Identify four categories of medical problems that are usually referred to an emergency department.

_____

_____

_____

9. How should the MA handle a patient who comes to the office without an appointment?

_____

_____

10. What should an MA do if an appointment needs to be changed?

_____

_____

11. What should the MA do if a patient who has an appointment does not keep the appointment or call to cancel the appointment?

_____

_____

_____

12. Identify three common methods to help patients remember appointments.

_____

_____

_____

13. What is a referral?

_____

_____

14. How does an MA schedule a diagnostic test at a facility such as the hospital x-ray department?

_____

_____

_____

15. What should the MA document in the patient's medical record after scheduling a diagnostic test for the patient?

_____

_____

16. How should the MA arrange for a patient to be admitted to the hospital?

_____

_____

_____

_____

17. Where will preadmission testing be performed before surgery?

_____

_____

18. If a patient is having inpatient surgery, how should the MA schedule it?

_____

_____

CRITICAL THINKING ACTIVITIES

A. Computer-Generated Appointment Schedule

Refer to the computer-generated appointment schedule (Figure 40-2) in your textbook, and answer the following questions. Note that the stars denote times that are booked for the patient whose name appears above.

1. How many minutes is an appointment with Dr. Warner for a well-baby visit? _____

2. How many minutes is an appointment with Dr. Warner for a recheck? _____

3. What times are blocked in the schedule? _____

4. Who is the first patient scheduled after lunch? _____

5. If the schedule continued, what would be the next available time? _____

B. Methods of Scheduling

Refer to the comparison of single booking, wave scheduling, and modified wave scheduling (Figure 40-3) in your textbook, and answer the following questions.

1. In which method are all patients in the same hour given the same appointment time? _____

2. In which method is each patient given a different appointment time? _____

3. Which method makes it most likely that there will always be a patient waiting even if some patients are delayed or cancel? _____

4. Which method(s) make it easier to work patients in while other patients undress or have diagnostic tests?

_____

5. Which method decreases waiting time for the patient? _____

C. Appointment Schedule

Refer to the manual and computerized appointment schedule (Figure 40-4) in your textbook, and answer the following questions.

1. What is the first available time for patients to have appointments with Dr. Gomez after lunch (computer schedule)?

_____

2. What is the advantage of using color to create the schedule with a computer system? _____

3. How much time has been allowed for lunch (appointment book)? _____

4. If appointments are at least 20 minutes long, what is the last available time for an appointment in Dr. Hughes' schedule (appointment book)? _____

5. From the schedule, what do you assume about scheduling for the satellite clinic? _____

D. Setting Priorities for Appointments

Consider the following four patients who call the office on a day where there are no open appointments. Which patients should be worked into the schedule today, and which patients can be given appointments tomorrow? Give a reason for your answer.

1. Edna Willis, a 64-year-old woman, reports that she has a fever of 100°F and she also had nausea and diarrhea during the previous night.

_____

_____

2. Daniel Jordan, a 32-year-old man, reports that he fell at work that morning, injuring his right arm and shoulder. He can move his right arm and shoulder, but the pain is severe and seems to be getting worse.

_____

_____

3. Mary Anderson, a patient of Dr. Hughes, calls about her father, Lawrence Sheehan, a 72-year-old man who is visiting from out of town. Mr. Sheehan has had angina pectoris for several years, but for the past 2 days he has been having more frequent and more severe episodes of chest pain. He had one episode that morning that was relieved by rest and his usual medication.

_____

_____

4. Linda Jones, a 25-year-old woman, calls complaining of generally feeling tired and without energy for the past 3 weeks. She is concerned because she expected to start feeling better before this.

_____

_____

E. Scheduling Diagnostic Tests and Procedures

Using yourself as a patient, answer the following questions that you might be asked when calling to schedule a diagnostic test or procedure:

1. What is the patient's name? _____

2. What is the patient's date of birth? _____

3. What is the patient's address and telephone number? _____

4. What type of insurance does the patient have? Insurance ID number? _____

5. Who is the patient's employer? _____

Procedure 40-1: Setting Up the Appointment Schedule. Using one of the blank appointment schedule forms, set up the appointment schedule for Blackburn Primary Care Associates.

1. Monday, October 12, 20XX: Dr. Lawler and Dr. Hughes are scheduled for hospital rounds early in the morning and will begin appointments at 9:00 AM. They will take their lunch break at noon. Their first afternoon appointment is at 1:00 PM. Dr. Lawler has a regular Monday meeting from 4:00 PM to 5:00 PM at the hospital. He will not return to the office. Dr. Lopez is scheduled at the satellite office in the morning. His first scheduled appointment will be at 10:30 AM. He will take lunch at 12:30 PM and begin seeing patients again at 1:00 PM. The appointment times from 3:20 PM through 3:30 PM are blocked out for Dr. Hughes and Dr. Lopez as catch-up time.

2. Wednesday, October 14, 20XX: Dr. Lawler, Dr. Hughes, and Dr. Lopez are scheduled for hospital rounds early in the morning and will begin appointments at 9:00 AM. Dr. Lawler and Dr. Lopez will take their lunch break at noon and will see patients in the afternoon from 1:00 PM to 3:00 PM. Dr. Hughes will leave the office at 12:30 PM to attend a conference that will last all afternoon.

3. Friday, October 16, 20XX: Dr. Lawler, Dr. Hughes, and Dr. Lopez are scheduled for hospital rounds early in the morning and will begin appointments at 9:00 AM. They will take their lunch break at noon. They will begin afternoon appointments at 1:00 PM. The appointment times from 2:00 PM to 2:10 PM should be blocked as catch-up time. No appointments should be scheduled after 4:30 PM.

DAY

DATE

8
9
10
11
12
1
2
3
4
5

Bibbero Systems Form 56-7310

(Courtesy Bibbero Systems, Inc., Petaluma, Calif. [800] 242-2376; Fax [800] 242-9330; www.bibbero.com.)

DAY

DATE

8
9
10
11
12
1
2
3
4
5

Bibbero Systems Form 56-7310

(Courtesy Bibbero Systems, Inc., Petaluma, Calif. [800] 242-2376; Fax [800] 242-9330; www.bibbero.com.)

Chapter **40** **Scheduling Appointments**

DAY
DATE

8
9
10
11
12
1
2
3
4
5

(Courtesy Bibbero Systems, Inc., Petaluma, Calif. [800] 242-2376; Fax [800] 242-9330; www.bibbero.com.)

Bibbero Systems Form 56-7310

Procedure 40-2: Making an Appointment. Schedule appointments for the following patients using the first appointment schedule you created for Procedure 40-1. Assume that established patients will be given 20-minute appointments and new patients will be given 30-minute appointments (except for Dr. Lawler, whose new patients are seen for 40 minutes). Use the abbreviation PE for examinations and the abbreviation re √ for patients who are returning for follow-up. Include the patient's day telephone number. All telephone numbers are in area code (555). Make appointments back to back to avoid 10-minute gaps in the schedule. Make appointments in the order that patients call.

1. June St. Cyr, an established patient, calls for an appointment with Dr. Hughes. She is working and wants to come as late as possible. Her telephone number is 648-3333.

2. William Reardon makes a follow-up appointment. He is retired, and his telephone number is 648-9292. He is to see Dr. Lopez as early in the day as possible.

3. Diana Starr telephones for an appointment for an examination. She is a new patient who has recently moved to the area. Her home telephone has not yet been connected, but her work telephone number is 731-1998. She asks to see Dr. Hughes and requests a late afternoon appointment. She works until 5:00 PM.

4. Douglas Wright telephones for an appointment because he has been having dizziness and feeling weak. He has never had an appointment with Dr. Lawler before, but a friend told him that Dr. Lawler is very experienced. He would prefer to come before lunch or as early in the day as possible. His telephone number is 731-8282.

5. Angela Newton needs a follow-up appointment with Dr. Lopez. She is in high school and cannot arrive before 3:00. Her home telephone number is 452-2001.

Procedure 40-3: Managing the Appointment Schedule. Use the computer-generated appointment schedule on the following page to manage appointments for May 30, 20XX. Note that the appointment schedule is full because stars denote times that are booked for the patient whose name appears above. New patients with physical examinations are scheduled for 30 minutes, physical examinations for established patients are 20 minutes, and routine visits for established patients are also scheduled for 20 minutes. Assume that any patient will need 30 minutes to get to the office. Be sure to mark any cancellations who do not reschedule or any no-shows in red. If a patient cancels, you can give his or her appointment to another patient. Double book any patient with an urgent problem who must be seen today.

1. Robert Ricigliano calls at 8:00 AM to cancel his appointment at 9:00 AM. He doesn't want to reschedule at this time.

2. Douglas Wright telephones at 8:15 AM because he has been running a fever of 102°F since yesterday and has been off work. He would like to come as early as possible. His home telephone number is 648-9010. He is a patient of Dr. Warner.

3. Lucille Morena calls at 9:00 AM to reschedule her appointment for next week. She is a new patient.

4. Peter Williams calls at 9:30 AM. He hurt his finger after slamming it in his car door this morning. He has gone to work, but it is hurting more now. It has swollen up, and he can't bend it. He would like to come in to see Dr. Warner. His work telephone number is 932-6554.

5. Maria Santos calls at 10:00 AM to say that she has car trouble and won't be able to arrive by 11:00 AM. She asks if there is any way she could come after lunch.

Western Medical Center

Richard Warner, MD
Schedule for May 30, 20XX

Time	Name	Reason	Home Phone	Work Phone
9:00 AM	ROBERT RICIGLIANO	Physical exam	(490) 459-2811	(490) 459-6217
9:10 AM	*			
9:20 AM	*			
9:30 AM	JUNE ST. JAMES	BP & ECG	(490) 459-5807	(490) 459-9222
9:40 AM	*			
9:50 AM	DARLA SISSLE	Influenza vaccine	(490) 220-1156	
10:00 AM	Catch-up			
10:10 AM	*			
10:20 AM	LLOYD RIDLON	Recheck	(490) 459-4242	(490) 459-0419
10:30 AM	ESTELLE JORDAN	New patient	(490) 459-8249	(490) 459-1062
10:40 AM	*			
10:50 AM	*			
11:00 AM	MARIA SANTOS	Physical exam	(490) 459-0022	
11:10 AM	*			
11:20 AM	THOMAS MAXWELL	Recheck	(490) 459-4123	(490) 459-9201
11:30 AM	*			
11:40 AM	ROBIN SOTO	Well baby	(490) 459-1349	
11:50 AM	*			
12:00 PM	LUNCH			
12:10 PM	*			
12:20 PM	*			
12:30 PM	*			
12:40 PM	*			
12:50 PM	*			
1:00 PM	LUCILLE MORENA	Chem screen	(490) 459-6677	(490) 459-1566
1:10 PM	*			
1:20 PM	*			
1:30 PM	*			

Record the information about the cancelled appointment for Robert Ricigliano in the chart provided.

CHART	
Date	

Procedure 40-4: Scheduling Inpatient or Outpatient Diagnostic Tests or Procedures. Working with a classmate, call the ultrasound department of Memorial Hospital. One student should schedule the diagnostic test, and the other student should ask the questions and record information. Use the New Patient Information sheets for patient information.

Student 1: Schedule the first available time for a computed tomography (CT) scan of the head with contrast for Charles Latham. The patient has never had a procedure done at Memorial Hospital.

Diagnosis: Severe frontal headaches for 1 month. No known allergies.

Preparation for this test: No preparation

Questions to ask: Allergy to iodine or shellfish; ask female if she is pregnant

Student 2: Schedule the first available time for a barium swallow (x-ray) for Darlene Jordan. The patient has never had a procedure done at Memorial Hospital.

Diagnosis: Epigastric pain for two weeks. No known allergies.

Preparation for this test: NPO after midnight

Questions to ask: Ask female if she is pregnant

Record the information about the diagnostic test and instructions given to the patient below.

CHART	
Date	

Questions to ask when scheduling an x-ray or CT scan:

1. What is the test to be scheduled? _____

2. What date and time would the patient prefer? _____

3. What is the patient's name? _____

4. What is the patient's birth date? _____

5. What is the patient's address? _____

6. What city and zip? _____

7. What is the patient's telephone number? _____

8. What is the physician's name? _____

9. What insurance does the patient have? _____

10. Who is the insured? _____

11. What is the group (policy) number? _____

12. What is the ID (subscriber) number? _____

13. What is the diagnosis? _____

14. If female, could the patient be pregnant? _____

15. Does the patient have any allergies to medication or iodine? _____

New Patient Information

(Please Print)   Physician: _Richard Warner, MD_
Home Phone: _(490) 555-3319_   Date: _9/14/20XX_

PATIENT INFORMATION

Last Name _____LATHAM_____ First _____CHARLES_____ Initial _R_
Address _____10971 CLARKWELL ROAD_____
City _____WESTERN_____ State _____OH_____ Zip _44770_
Single ___ Married _X_ Widowed ____ Separated ____ Divorced _____
Sex M _X_ F ____ Age _49_ Birth date _____7/19/1961_____
Employer _____LATHAM PLUMBING_____
Occupation _____PLUMBER_____
In an emergency, who should be notified?
_____ANNA LATHAM_____ (wife) _____ Phone _____(490) 555-3319_____
      Name   Relationship

PRIMARY INSURANCE

Name of insured _____CHARLES LATHAM_____ Responsible Party Yes _X_ No _____
Relation to Patient _____SELF_____ Birth date _____7/19/1961_____
Address (if different from patient)
_____ Phone_____
City _____ State _____ Zip _____

Insured employed by _____LATHAM PLUMBING_____
Occupation _____PLUMBER_____

Business Address _____10971 CLARKWELL ROAD, WESTERN, OH 44770_____
Business Phone _____(490) 555-3320_____

Insurance Company _STANDARD HEALTH INDEMNITY_ ID # _665514281_
Policy (Group) # _544281_

I the undersigned assign directly to Blackburn Primary Care Associates insurance
benefits, if any, otherwise payable to me for services rendered. I understand that
I am financially responsible for all charges whether or not paid by insurance.
I hereby authorize the doctor to release all information necessary to secure the
payment of benefits. I authorize the use of this signature on all insurance
submissions.

_____Charles Latham_____ _____self_____ _____10/25/20XX_____
Responsible party Signature   Relationship   Date

New Patient Information

(Please Print)

Home Phone: _(490) 555-4810_

Physician: _Richard Warner, MD_

Date: _9/14/20XX_

PATIENT INFORMATION

Last Name _____JORDAN_____ First _____DARLENE_____ Initial _L_

Address _617 HILLSIDE ROAD_

City _____WESTERN_____ State ___OH___ Zip _44770_

Single ___ Married _X_ Widowed ___ Separated ___ Divorced _____

Sex M _____ F _X_ Age _30_ Birth date _____4/19/1980_____

Employer _____BEST SUPERMARKET_____

Occupation _____CASHIER_____

In an emergency, who should be notified?

_____EDWARD JORDAN_____ (husband) _____ Phone _____(490) 555-4810_____

    Name   Relationship

PRIMARY INSURANCE

Name of insured _____EDWARD JORDAN_____ Responsible Party Yes _X_ No _____

Relation to Patient _____HUSBAND_____ Birth date _2/24/1978_

Address (if different from patient)

_____ Phone_____

City _____ State _____ Zip _____

Insured employed by _____MEYERS PHARMACY_____

Occupation _____PHARMACIST_____

Business Address _428 MAIN STREET, WESTERN, OH 44770_

Business Phone _____(490) 555-6192_____

Insurance Company _STANDARD HEALTH HMO_ ID # _28621954_

Policy (Group) # _____86190_____

I the undersigned assign directly to Blackburn Primary Care Associates insurance benefits, if any, otherwise payable to me for services rendered. I understand that I am financially responsible for all charges whether or not paid by insurance. I hereby authorize the doctor to release all information necessary to secure the payment of benefits. I authorize the use of this signature on all insurance submissions.

_____Darlene Jordan_____   _self_   _9/14/20XX_

Responsible party Signature   Relationship   Date

Procedure 40-5: Scheduling Inpatient or Outpatient Admissions. Working with a classmate, call Memorial Hospital to schedule an admission for a patient.

Student 1: Schedule an admission for Charles Latham. The patient will be admitted this afternoon, and admission orders will be faxed from the office. His wife will bring him to the hospital. Use the patient information form in Procedure 40-5.

Diagnosis:	Pneumococcal pneumonia.
Insurance precertification number:	M 200068AC

Student 2: Schedule an admission for Darlene Jordan. The patient will be arriving at the hospital by ambulance from home. Admission orders will be faxed from the office. Use the patient information form in Procedure 40-5.

Diagnosis:	Hematemesis; R/O acute peptic ulcer with hemorrhage.
Insurance precertification number:	0011582

Record the information about the hospital admission below.

CHART	
Date	

Questions to ask when the MA is calling for hospital admission (answer telephone as Memorial Hospital Admitting Department):

1. What is the patient's name and address? _____

_____

_____

2. What is the patient's birth date? _____

3. What is the patient's admission diagnosis? _____

4. What type of insurance does the patient have? _____

5. What is/are the patient's insurance number(s)? _____

6. What is the physician's name? _____

7. How is the patient being transported? _____

8. When will the patient be admitted? _____

9. How will the physician's orders be provided? _____

EVALUATION OF COMPETENCY

Procedure 40-1: Setting Up the Appointment Schedule

Name: _____ Date: _____

Evaluated By: _____ Score: _____

Performance Objective

Outcome:	Set up an appointment schedule.
Conditions:	Given the following: appointment book or computer scheduling program, physician schedule, pen, and office calendar.
Standards:	Time: 10 minutes. Student completed procedure in _____ minutes.
	Accuracy: Satisfactory score on the Performance Evaluation Checklist.

Performance Evaluation Checklist

Trial 1	Trial 2	Point Value	Performance Standards
		●	Blocked times when the office would not be open.
		●	Blocked times when each individual physician would not be available to see patients, including lunch and hospital rounds.
		●	Blocked days or parts of days when individual physicians would be away from the office for vacation, conferences, or other scheduled events.
		●	For each physician, marked times scheduled for certain types of examinations or procedures.
		●	Blocked time for same-day appointments, catch-up time, and unexpected needs.
		✱	Completed an accurate appointment schedule.
		✱	Completed the procedure within 10 minutes.
			TOTALS

Evaluation of Student Performance

EVALUATION CRITERIA			COMMENTS
Symbol	**Category**	**Point Value**	
✱	Critical Step	16 points	
●	Essential Step	6 points	
▷	Theory Question	2 points	
Score calculation:	100 points		
	− _____ points missed		
	_____ Score		
Satisfactory score: 85 or above			

Psychomotor (Skills)
☑ V. 1. Manage appointment schedule, using established priorities.

Affective (Behavior)
☑ V. 2. Implement time management principles to maintain effective office function.

ABHES Competencies Achieved

☑ 8. C. Schedule and manage appointments.

EVALUATION OF COMPETENCY

Procedure 40-2: Making an Appointment

Name: _____ Date: _____

Evaluated By: _____ Score: _____

Performance Objective

Outcome:	Make an appointment for a patient.
Conditions:	Given the following: appointment book or computer program, and pencil.
Standards:	Time: 5 minutes. Student completed procedure in _____ minutes.
	Accuracy: Satisfactory score on the Performance Evaluation Checklist.

Performance Evaluation Checklist

Trial 1	Trial 2	Point Value	Performance Standards
		●	Obtained physician name and scheduling preference from the patient.
		●	Found an open appointment of the correct length of time.
		●	Offered the patient a date and time for the appointment.
		●	Kept locating appointments until an acceptable date and time was found.
		●	Entered demographic data into computer for a new patient.
		●	Discussed cost of the visit with a new patient without insurance.
		●	Informed a new patient if a written referral form would be necessary.
		●	Recorded patient name, date of birth, reason for the visit, and daytime telephone number for an established patient or a new patient.
		●	Blocked out correct amount of time based on the reason for the visit. (Used pencil in a manual appointment book.)
		●	Repeated the information to the patient before ending the call.
		●	Offered a new patient directions to the office.
		✱	Completed the procedure within 5 minutes.
			TOTALS

Evaluation of Student Performance

EVALUATION CRITERIA			COMMENTS
Symbol	**Category**	**Point Value**	
✷	Critical Step	16 points	
●	Essential Step	6 points	
▷	Theory Question	2 points	

Score calculation: 100 points

– _____ points missed

_____ Score

Satisfactory score: 85 or above

CAAHEP Competencies Achieved

Psychomotor (Skills)
☑ V. 1. Manage appointment schedule, using established priorities.

Affective (Behavior)
☑ V. 2. Implement time management principles to maintain effective office function.

ABHES Competencies Achieved

☑ 8. c. Schedule and manage appointments.

Procedure 40-3: Managing the Appointment Schedule

Name: _____ Date: _____

Evaluated By: _____ Score: _____

Performance Objective

Outcome:	Review the appointment schedule, cancel an appointment, change an appointment, indicate a missed appointment, and document cancellations and missed appointments.
Conditions:	Given the following: Appointment book or computer scheduling program, printed appointment schedule, and pen.
Standards:	Time: 10 minutes. Student completed procedure in _____ minutes.

Accuracy: Satisfactory score on the Performance Evaluation Checklist. |

Performance Evaluation Checklist

Trial 1	Trial 2	Point Value	Performance Standards
		●	Using the appointment schedule, made sure all medical records and necessary paperwork were prepared.
		●	Checked patients in on the official schedule as they arrived.
		●	Canceled an appointment on the day it was scheduled by drawing a line through the appointment in ink on the official schedule.
		●	Erased the canceled appointment in appointment book.
		●	Offered to make another appointment when a patient cancelled an appointment.
		●	If a patient declined to make another appointment after canceling, documented in the patient's medical record and deleted the appointment in a computer schedule.
		●	If a patient wanted to reschedule, found a new appointment time.
		●	Entered the patient's name and contact information in the new appointment time. In a computer schedule, changed the date and time using the original appointment.
		●	Repeated the new date and time to the patient if using the telephone or filled out an appointment card for a patient in the office.
		●	If the patient missed an appointment without canceling, draw a line through the appointment in ink on the daily schedule and labeled the appointment "No-Show."
		●	Telephoned any patients who missed appointments without canceling if office policy.
		●	Documented the missed appointment in the medical record with any information available.
		✱	Completed the procedure within 10 minutes.
			TOTALS

1057

CHART	
Date	

Evaluation of Student Performance

EVALUATION CRITERIA			COMMENTS
Symbol	**Category**	**Point Value**	
✶	Critical Step	16 points	
●	Essential Step	6 points	
▷	Theory Question	2 points	

Score calculation: 100 points

−   _____ points missed

_____ Score

Satisfactory score: 85 or above

CAAHEP Competencies Achieved

Psychomotor (Skills)
☑ V. 1. Manage appointment schedule, using established priorities.

Affective (Behavior)
☑ V. 2. Implement time management principles to maintain effective office function.

ABHES Competencies Achieved

☑ 8. c. Schedule and manage appointments.

Procedure 40-4: Scheduling Inpatient or Outpatient Diagnostic Tests or Procedures

Name: _____   Date: _____

Evaluated By: _____   Score: _____

Performance Objective

Outcome:	Schedule an inpatient or outpatient diagnostic test or procedure.
Conditions:	Given the following: patient medical record and insurance information, name of test or procedure to be scheduled, telephone, and telephone number of facility and department to schedule the test or procedure.
Standards:	Time: 5 minutes. Student completed procedure in _____ minutes.
	Accuracy: Satisfactory score on the Performance Evaluation Checklist.

Performance Evaluation Checklist

Trial 1	Trial 2	Point Value	Performance Standards
		●	Assembled necessary information about the patient.
		●	Determined the facility and department to call for scheduling using the medical record or a diagnostic test or procedure requisition.
		●	Determined the time frame for scheduling from the physician order.
		●	Asked the patient about preferred days and times for scheduling.
		●	Obtained preauthorization from the patient's insurance if necessary.
		●	Placed a telephone call to the department where the test or procedure would be scheduled and identified the test to be scheduled.
		●	Provided the patient's name and demographic information as needed.
		●	Provided patient insurance information and preauthorization number as needed.
		●	Set up a specific day and time for the procedure.
		●	Informed the patient of the date and time for the test or procedure.
		●	Provided verbal and written instructions about preparation for the test or procedure.
		●	Sent an electronic or paper requisition to the facility or gave a paper requisition to the patient to take to the test.
		●	Documented the scheduled diagnostic test or procedure in the patient's medical record.
		●	Included patient instructions in the documentation.
		★	Completed the procedure within 5 minutes.
			TOTALS

1059

CHART	
Date	

Evaluation of Student Performance

EVALUATION CRITERIA			COMMENTS
Symbol	**Category**	**Point Value**	
★	Critical Step	16 points	
●	Essential Step	6 points	
▷	Theory Question	2 points	

Score calculation: 100 points

         –   points missed

             ____ Score

Satisfactory score: 85 or above

CAAHEP Competencies Achieved

Psychomotor (Skills)

☑ V. 2. Schedule patient admissions and/or procedures.

ABHES Competencies Achieved

☑ 8. c. Schedule and manage appointments.

Procedure 40-5: Scheduling Inpatient or Outpatient Admissions

Name: _____ Date: _____

Evaluated By: _____ Score: _____

Performance Objective

Outcome:	Schedule an inpatient or outpatient admission for a patient
Conditions:	Given the following: patient's medical record and insurance information, reason for admission, telephone, and telephone number of the facility and admitting department.
Standards:	Time: 10 minutes. Student completed procedure in _____ minutes.
	Accuracy: Satisfactory score on the Performance Evaluation Checklist.

Performance Evaluation Checklist

Trial 1	Trial 2	Point Value	Performance Standards
		●	Assembled patient demographic and insurance information.
		●	Determined the reason for the outpatient or inpatient admission.
		●	Determined the time frame for the admission from the physician's orders.
		●	Discussed preferred days and times with the patient.
		●	Obtained preauthorization from the patient's insurance company.
		●	Called the admissions department to schedule the admission.
		●	Provided the patient's name and demographic information as needed.
		●	Provided patient insurance information and preauthorization number.
		●	Provided the patient diagnosis or reason for the admission.
		●	Set up a specific day and time for the admission.
		●	Provided admitting orders as needed and faxed to the admitting department or nursing floor.
		●	If patient was to be admitted directly from the office, arranged transport, obtained consent forms, and prepared a patient transfer form.
		●	If the patient was to be admitted at a future date, informed the patient of the date and time, and provided written instructions for any preoperative needs or procedure.
		●	Documented the admission and instructions given to the patient in the patient's medical record.
		●	For a direct admission from the office, identified any documents sent with the patient.
		✱	Completed the procedure within 10 minutes.
			TOTALS

1061

Date	

EVALUATION CRITERIA			COMMENTS
Symbol	**Category**	**Point Value**	
★	Critical Step	16 points	
●	Essential Step	6 points	
▷	Theory Question	2 points	

Score calculation: 100 points

    –   _____ points missed

           ___ Score

Satisfactory score: 85 or above

CAAHEP Competencies Achieved

Psychomotor (Skills)
☑ V. 2. Schedule patient admissions and/or procedures.

ABHES Competencies Achieved

☑ 8. f. Schedule inpatient and outpatient admissions.

Medical Records Management

√ After Completing	Date Due	Textbook Pages	TEXTBOOK ASSIGNMENTS	Possible Points	Points You Earned
		992-1006	Read Chapter 41: Medical Records Management		
		996 1004	Read Case Study 1 Case Study 1 questions	5	
		998 1004-1005	Read Case Study 2 Case Study 2 questions	5	
		1001 1005	Read Case Study 3 Case Study 3 questions	5	
			TOTAL POINTS		
√ After Completing	**Date Due**	**Study Guide Pages**	**STUDY GUIDE ASSIGNMENTS (CTA = Critical Thinking Activity)**	**Possible Points**	**Points You Earned**
		1067	Pretest	10	
		1068	Term Key Term Assessment	15	
		1068-1071	Evaluation of Learning questions	30	
		1071	CTA A: Filing Units: Alphabetic	10	
		1072	CTA B: Alphabetic Filing	8	
		1072	CTA C: Filing Units: Terminal Digit	8	
		1072	CTA D: Numeric Filing	8	
		1073	CTA E: Filing Reports and Correspondence	8	
			Evolve Site: Filing Medical Records Using the Alphabetic Filing System (Record points earned)		
			Evolve Site: Filing Medical Records Using the Terminal Digit Filing System (Record points earned)		
			Evolve Site: Guided Practice: Adding Supplementary Items to Established Patient File	10	

√ After Completing	Date Due	Study Guide Pages	STUDY GUIDE ASSIGNMENTS (CTA = Critical Thinking Activity)	Possible Points	Points You Earned
			Evolve Site: Apply Your Knowledge questions	10	
			Evolve Site: Video Evaluations	27	
		1067	Posttest	10	
			ASSIGNMENTS ADDITIONAL		
			TOTAL POINTS		

√ When Assigned By Your Instructor	Study Guide Pages	Practices Required	LABORATORY ASSIGNMENTS (Procedure Number and Name)	Score*
	1074	3	**Practice for Competency** 41-1: Filing Patient Records: Alphabetic Textbook reference: p. 999	
	1075-1076		**Evaluation of Competency** 41-1: Filing Patient Records: Alphabetic	*
	1074	3	**Practice for Competency** 41-2: Filing Patient Records—Numeric Textbook reference: pp. 999-1000	
	1077-1078		**Evaluation of Competency** 41-2: Filing Patient Records—Numeric	*
	1074	3	**Practice for Competency** 41-3: Filing Reports Textbook reference: pp. 1001-1002	
	1079-1080		**Evaluation of Competency** 41-3: Filing Reports	*
			ADDITIONAL ASSIGNMENTS	

Notes

? PRETEST

True or False

_____ 1. The patient owns the original medical record.

_____ 2. The main way to enter information into an electronic medical record (EMR) is to use a scanner.

_____ 3. Medical record files or filing rooms should always be locked when the office is closed.

_____ 4. Color-coded labels are used for alphabetic filing but not for numeric file systems.

_____ 5. Outguides are placed where a paper medical record has been removed from the filing shelves.

_____ 6. If a numeric medical record system is used, the filing system is indirect.

_____ 7. In an alphabetic filing system, prefixes such as van, von, and de are the third filing unit.

_____ 8. The medical record of a married woman is filed under her last name and her husband's first name.

_____ 9. In a terminal digit numeric filing system, the last group of two digits is the first filing unit.

_____ 10. The length of time that medical records must be retained can vary depending on the age of the patient.

? POSTTEST

True or False

_____ 1. The patient controls the information in the medical record and access to it.

_____ 2. An EMR system is less expensive to initiate than a paper record system.

_____ 3. If shelving units are used to store paper medical records, folders with side tabs should be used.

_____ 4. Use of a current year label helps identify inactive paper medical records.

_____ 5. An outguide is placed in the individual medical record when removing papers to file new reports.

_____ 6. In an alphabetic medical record filing system, the patient's surname is the first filing unit.

_____ 7. If a business name includes an acronym, it is filed as if it were spelled out in full.

_____ 8. Hyphenated names are indexed as one filing unit in an alphabetic filing system.

_____ 9. A numeric terminal digit filing system is commonly used in hospitals and large clinics.

_____ 10. Medical records for minors can be destroyed 7 years after the record becomes inactive.

Directions: Match each medical term with its definition.

_____ 1. Acronym

_____ 2. Active record

_____ 3. Cross-index

_____ 4. EMR (electronic health record)

_____ 5. Filing system

_____ 6. Health information exchange (HIE)

_____ 7. Inactive record

_____ 8. Indexing units

_____ 9. Medical records management

_____ 10. Nationwide health information network (NHIN)

_____ 11. Outguide

_____ 12. Sorter

_____ 13. Surname

_____ 14. Tab

_____ 15. Terminal digit filing

A. A device that facilitates putting papers or records in alphabetic or numeric order

B. To file under one unit and use a guide or card filed under another unit that refers to the primary filing location

C. Pieces of information used to identify a correct filing location

D. The way in which records are arranged such as alphabetically or numerically

E. A cardboard or plastic card to insert in a file when a medical record is removed

F. A word formed from the first letters in a name

G. An individual patient's health record in digital format

H. The medical record of a patient who has not been seen within the past 2 to 3 years, or some other time frame specified by a given medical office

I. A projection of a folder that extends beyond the top or side of the folder

J. Activities related to the creation, management, use, and disposition of patient medical records

K. The medical record of a patient who has been seen within a time frame specified by the office (usually 2 to 3 years)

L. Last name or family name of an individual

M. Record-keeping method in which the last digits are used as the first filing unit

N. A set of standards, services, and policies to facilitate the national health information exchange

O. The electronic exchange of health care related data between different institutions.

📋 **EVALUATION OF LEARNING**

Directions: Fill in each blank with the correct answer.

1. Discuss the ownership of a paper medical record.

_____

_____

2. If an EMR is used, how is new information entered into the record? Information from a previous paper medical record?

_____

_____

3. What progress is being made in allowing for the electronic exchange of health care information between institutions that use different electronic medical record systems?

_____

_____

4. What are three challenges when a medical office changes from a paper medical record to an electronic medical record?

_____

_____

5. What equipment is used for storage of paper medical records?

_____

_____

6. What is the advantage of using color-coded labels on medical record file folders?

_____

_____

7. List seven common categories for chart dividers.

_____

_____

8. How is an outguide used when filing medical records?

_____

_____

9. What is the difference between a direct filing system and an indirect filing system?

_____

_____

10. What is the first indexing unit if an alphabetic filing system is used?

_____

11. How are names with prefixes filed if an alphabetic filing system is used?

_____

12. How are hyphenated names filed if an alphabetic filing system is used?

_____

13. What is the second filing unit if the patient's name is Mary Johnson White?

_____

14. How is the medical record of a married woman filed if an alphabetic filing system is used?

_____

15. What are two advantages of a numeric filing system for paper medical records?

_____

_____

16. Compare and contrast a terminal digit filing system with a consecutive filing system.

_____

_____

17. What are four types of documents that might be filed using a subject filing system?

_____

18. Identify two ways that documents might be arranged within a subject category.

_____

19. Describe the form and function of a tickler file.

_____

_____

20. What are three factors that influence the decision to choose an alphabetic or chronological filing system for patient records?

_____

_____

21. What is the process for removing a record from the file?

_____

_____

22. Before returning medical records to the files, what are the three things the medical assistant should do to condition the records?

_____

_____

23. How are reports and letters filed into existing medical records?

_____

_____

_____

24. What are three measures to prevent misplaced records?

_____

_____

_____

25. How is an electronic medical record updated?

_____

_____

_____

26. What conditions should be present in the storage area for active or inactive medical records?

_____

_____

_____

27. How are medical records selected to be moved to the location of inactive records?

_____

_____

28. How long should the medical records of minors be retained? Why?

_____

_____

_____

29. How long should the records of adult patients be retained? Why?

_____

_____

30. How should computerized records be stored?

_____

_____

CRITICAL THINKING ACTIVITIES

A. Filing Units: Alphabetic

Identify the filing units in the following list of names:

Name	Unit 1	Unit 2	Unit 3	Unit 4
Diane Riel				
George A. Ricker, Jr.				
Marie A. von Hayden				
Mrs. Carolyn Richenburg				
Robert T. Van Wilder				
Maria Rivera Santos				
G. A. Rickers				
James D. Smith-Richards				
The Blackburn Daily Times				
Uptown Management Corp.				

B. Alphabetic Filing

Arrange the names in the column on the left in correct filing order in the spaces on the right.

Diane Riel	1.
George A. Ricker, Jr.	2.
Marie A. von Hayden	3.
Mrs. Carolyn Richenburg	4.
Robert T. Van Wilder	5.
Maria Rivera Santos	6.
G. A. Rickers	7.
James D. Smith-Richards	8.

C. Filing Units: Terminal Digit

Identify the filing units in the following numbers assuming that a terminal digit system is used with two digits in each group.

Number	Unit 1	Unit 2	Unit 3
01-23-52			
22-19-08			
62-41-33			
00-82-99			
15-66-18			
21-19-44			
66-01-11			
21-18-08			

D. Numeric Filing

Arrange the following numbers in the column on the left in correct filing order in the spaces on the right assuming that a terminal digit filing system is used.

01-23-52	1.
22-19-08	2.
62-41-33	3.
00-82-99	4.
15-66-18	5.
21-19-44	6.
66-01-11	7.
21-18-08	8.

E. Filing Reports and Correspondence

Indicate which section of the paper medical record for each of the following reports would be filed in by writing the name of the report in the correct section of the table below.

1. Report of shoulder x-ray
2. Report of complete blood count
3. Report of laparoscopic cholecystectomy
4. Discharge summary from hospitalization
5. History and physical examination report
6. Progress note dictated at the most recent patient visit
7. Letter from consulting physician regarding a consultation visit by the patient
8. Report of MRI scan of left knee

Section of Medical Record	Reports to Be Filed in this Section
Progress notes	
History and physical examination	
Laboratory reports	
Diagnostic testing	
Hospital reports	
Immunizations/medications	
Correspondence	

Procedure 41-1: Filing Patient Records—Alphabetic. File medical records using the alphabetic system.

Procedure 41-2: Filing Medical Records—Numeric. File medical records using the terminal digit system.

Procedure 41-3: Filing Reports. File reports and correspondence in medical records.

EVALUATION OF COMPETENCY

Procedure 41-1: Filing Medical Records—Alphabetic

Name: _____   Date: _____

Evaluated by: _____   Score: _____

Performance Objective

Outcome:	File patient records using an alphabetic filing system.
Conditions:	Given the following: patient records with patient names, alphabetic sorter, file cabinet or shelves, outguides, and index cards.
Standards:	Time: 10 minutes. Student completed procedure in _____ minutes.
	Accuracy: Satisfactory score on the Performance Evaluation Checklist.

Performance Evaluation Checklist

Trial 1	Trial 2	Point Value	Performance Standards
		●	Gathered the records and removed any elastic bands or paper clips.
		●	Secured any loose sheets of paper.
		●	Sorted the records alphabetically by last name.
		✶	Found the correct location in the file for each record.
		●	Slid the record in front of the outguide and removed the outguide from the shelf or drawer.
		●	Stored the outguide with other unused outguides.
		●	Removed any index card from the outguide and discarded or stored according to office policy.
		●	Filed each record until all records were filed.
		✶	Completed the procedure within 10 minutes.
		TOTALS	

Evaluation of Student Performance

EVALUATION CRITERIA			COMMENTS
Symbol	**Category**	**Point Value**	
✶	Critical Step	16 points	
●	Essential Step	6 points	
▷	Theory Question	2 points	
Score calculation:	100 points		
	− _____ points missed		
	_____ Score		
Satisfactory score: 85 or above			

Chapter **41** **Medical Records Management**

CAAHEP Competencies Achieved

Psychomotor (Skills)

☑ V. 4. File medical records.
☑ V. 8. Maintain organization by filing.

Affective (Behavior)

☑ V. 1. Consider staff needs and limitations in establishment of a filing system.

ABHES Competencies Achieved

☑ 8. b. Prepare and maintain medical records.

Procedure 41-2: Filing Patient Records—Numeric

Name: _____ Date: _____

Evaluated by: _____ Score: _____

Performance Objective

Outcome:	File patient records using a terminal digit filing system.
Conditions:	Given the following: Patient records with terminal digit labels, file cabinet or shelves, numeric sorter, outguides, and index cards.
Standards:	Time: 10 minutes. Student completed procedure in _____ minutes.
	Accuracy: Satisfactory score on the Performance Evaluation Checklist

Performance Evaluation Checklist

Trial 1	Trial 2	Point Value	Performance Standards
		●	Gathered the records and removed any elastic bands or paper clips.
		●	Secured any loose sheets of paper.
		●	Sorted the records according to the terminal digit indexing units.
		✷	Found the correct location in the file for each record based on the final group of numbers.
		✷	Refined search based on the middle group of numbers and then the first group of numbers.
		●	Slid the record in front of the outguide and removed the outguide from the shelf or drawer.
		●	Stored the outguide with other unused outguides.
		●	Removed any index card from the outguide and discarded or stored according to office policy.
		●	Filed each record until all records were filed.
		✷	Completed the procedure within 10 minutes.
			TOTALS

Evaluation of Student Performance

EVALUATION CRITERIA			COMMENTS
Symbol	Category	Point Value	
★	Critical Step	16 points	
●	Essential Step	6 points	
▷	Theory Question	2 points	

Score calculation: 100 points

－ _____ points missed

_____ Score

Satisfactory score: 85 or above

CAAHEP Competencies Achieved

Psychomotor (Skills)

☑ V. 4. File medical records.
☑ V. 8. Maintain organization by filing.

Affective (Behavior)

☑ V. 1. Consider staff needs and limitations in establishment of a filing system.

ABHES Competencies Achieved

☑ 8. b. Prepare and maintain medical records.

Procedure 41-3: Filing Reports

Name: _____   Date: _____

Evaluated by: _____   Score: _____

Performance Objective

Outcome:	File patient records using a terminal digit filing system.
Conditions:	Given the following: Medical records, assorted reports, letters or other material to be filed, hole punch, tape, stapler, and sorter.
Standards:	Time: 10 minutes. Student completed procedure in _____ minutes.
	Accuracy: Satisfactory score on the Performance Evaluation Checklist.

Performance Evaluation Checklist

Trial 1	Trial 2	Point Value	Performance Standards
		●	Assembled materials to be filed and necessary supplies.
		●	Removed paper clips, pins, or other extraneous materials from records or materials to be filed.
		●	Mended any tears with tape.
		●	Stapled related pages together.
		●	Punched holes as needed.
		●	Verified that each report was initialed by the physician.
		●	Set aside any report without initials to be returned for physician review.
		●	Sorted reports alphabetically or numerically depending on the office filing system.
		●	Assembled all reports for a particular patient.
		●	Located the patient's medical record.
		✳	Inserted the reports into the medical record in the correct location in reverse chronological order.
		●	Inserted dividers into the medical record if necessary.
		●	Put the record back together as needed.
		●	Replaced the record in the file.
		●	Repeated until all the reports for all patients were filed.
		●	If the record could not be located in the file, placed the report back in sorter or in the pocket of the outguide according to office policy.
		✳	Completed the procedure within 10 minutes.
			TOTALS

EVALUATION CRITERIA			COMMENTS
Symbol	**Category**	**Point Value**	
✶	Critical Step	16 points	
●	Essential Step	6 points	
▷	Theory Question	2 points	

Score calculation: 100 points

            –   points missed

            ___ Score

Satisfactory score: 85 or above

CAAHEP Competencies Achieved

Psychomotor (Skills)

☑ 8. Maintain organization by filing.

ABHES Competencies Achieved

☑ 8. b. Prepare and maintain medical records.

42 Written Communications

√ After Completing	Date Due	Textbook Pages	TEXTBOOK ASSIGNMENTS	Possible Points	Points You Earned
		1007-1022	Read Chapter 42: Written Communications		
		1015 1021	Read Case Study 1 Case Study 1 questions	5	
		1017 1021	Read Case Study 2 Case Study 2 questions	5	
		1019 1021-1022	Read Case Study 3 Case Study 3 questions	5	
			TOTAL POINTS		

√ After Completing	Date Due	Study Guide Pages	STUDY GUIDE ASSIGNMENTS (CTA = Critical Thinking Activities)	Possible Points	Points You Earned
		1085	Pretest	10	
		1086	Term Key Term Assessment	18	
		1087-1088	Evaluation of Learning questions	25	
		1089	CTA A: Parts of a Letter	6	
		1089	CTA B: Letter Styles	6	
		1089	CTA C: Parts of Speech	17	
		1090	CTA D: Proofreading	10	
			Evolve Site: Quiz Show—Spelling (Record points earned)		
			Evolve Site: Comma Exercise (Record points earned)		
			Evolve Site: Hyphen Exercise (Record points earned)		
			Evolve Site: Guided Practice: Proofreading Written Correspondence	10	
			Evolve Site: Apply Your Knowledge questions	10	

√ After Completing	Date Due	Study Guide Pages	STUDY GUIDE ASSIGNMENTS (CTA = Critical Thinking Activities)	Possible Points	Points You Earned
			e Evolve Site: Video Evaluation	8	
		1085	📋 Posttest	10	
			ADDITIONAL ASSIGNMENTS		
			TOTAL POINTS		

√ When Assigned By Your Instructor	Study Guide Pages	Practices Required	LABORATORY ASSIGNMENTS (Procedure Number and Name)	Score*
	1091	2	**Practice for Competency** 42-1: Composing a Business Letter Textbook reference: pp. 1013-1014	
	1095-1096		**Evaluation of Competency** 42-1: Composing a Business Letter	*
	1091-1094	3	**Practice for Competency** 42-2: Sending a Fax Textbook reference: pp. 1019-1020	
	1097-1098		**Evaluation of Competency** 42-2: Sending a Fax	*
	1091	3	**Practice for Competency** 42-3: Preparing Copies of Multiple-Page Documents Textbook reference: p. 1020	
	1099-1100		**Evaluation of Competency** 42-3: Preparing Copies of Multiple-Page Documents	*
			ADDITIONAL ASSIGNMENTS	

Notes

Name _____   Date _____

True or False

_____ 1. Business letters are more formal than personal correspondence in form and content.

_____ 2. The body of a business letter is double spaced.

_____ 3. The name of the individual sending a business letter should always be printed below the handwritten signature.

_____ 4. If additional forms or printed material is included with a letter, this should be indicated in an end notation.

_____ 5. In the semiblock letter style, all lines of the letter are left justified.

_____ 6. An adverb modifies a verb, adjective, or other adverb.

_____ 7. Sentence fragments and comma splices are errors that should always be corrected in a business letter.

_____ 8. A comma should be used to separate two sentences that are not joined by a conjunction or separated by a period.

_____ 9. The common headings for a memo are: TO, FROM, SUBJECT, and DATE.

_____ 10. Because e-mail and fax transmissions are considered secure, they are good ways to transmit confidential information about patients.

?≡ POSTTEST

True or False

_____ 1. All business letters sent from the medical office are dictated by the physician and prepared by office staff.

_____ 2. The inside address of a business letter is placed two lines below the date line.

_____ 3. The standard closing of a business letter is "Sincerely yours."

_____ 4. If a letter has been dictated by the physician and prepared by the medical assistant (MA), a reference line should be included below the typed signature.

_____ 5. In the modified block letter style, the date line, complimentary close, and printed signature may be lined up at the center of the letter.

_____ 6. A conjunction joins words, phrases, or clauses in a sentence.

_____ 7. When two sentences are connected without punctuation, it is called a *comma splice*.

_____ 8. A comma should be used to set off information that could be omitted from a sentence without changing the meaning.

_____ 9. A memo (memorandum) may be used to inform office staff about the time and place of a staff meeting.

_____ 10. Most office photocopy machines will collate and staple documents, as well as copy on both sides of a piece of paper.

Directions: Match each medical term with its definition.

_____ 1. Clinical messaging

_____ 2. Collate

_____ 3. Complimentary closing

_____ 4. Duplex

_____ 5. E-mail

_____ 6. Fax

_____ 7. Full block style

_____ 8. Grammar

_____ 9. Left justified

_____ 10. Letterhead

_____ 11. Memo (memorandum)

_____ 12. Modified block style

_____ 13. Right-justified

_____ 14. Salutation

_____ 15. Semiblock style

_____ 16. Simplified letter style

_____ 17. Template

_____ 18. Transcription

A. A format for business letters where the date line, complimentary close, and printed signature line are aligned at the center and all other parts of the letter are left justified

B. A letter format in which all elements are left justified, the greeting is replaced by a subject line in all capital letters, and the complimentary close and typed signature are replaced by a typed signature in all capital letters

C. A form of communication within a company that is usually short and limited to one subject

D. A letter format where all parts of the letter begin at the left margin

E. To assemble the pages of a document in numerical order

F. The process of changing verbal dictation to typed or printed form

G. A standard form to which additional information can be added as needed

H. A letter format similar to modified block style, but all paragraphs are indented

I. Type that is aligned with the right margin of a document

J. Written communication sent from one computer to another using telecommunication

K. A sheet of stationery preprinted with information about a business, including name, address, telephone number, and other information.

L. The study of accepted rules used to create meaning in a language

M. To produce double-sided copies by storing images from both sides of the original in the memory of a photocopier

N. Lines of type that begin at the left margin of a document

O. Transmission of scanned, printed material by telephone

P. The greeting that begins a letter

Q. Communication between health professionals within the electronic medical record

R. Words used as a polite ending to a letter before the writer's signature

EVALUATION OF LEARNING

Directions: Fill in each blank with the correct answer.

1. What is letterhead stationery?

   _____

   _____

2. What is included in the heading of a letter?

   _____

3. Where is the inside address located on a letter?

   _____

4. What is the correct salutation for a business letter to William Masterson, MD, including punctuation?

   _____

5. What spacing is used in the body of a letter?

   _____

6. Give examples of at least two acceptable complimentary closings for a business letter.

   _____

7. How many spaces below the complimentary closing should the typed signature be placed? Why?

   _____

8. What are three examples of end notations for a letter?

   _____

9. Compare and contrast full block letter style with modified block letter style.

   _____

   _____

10. What is the advantage of using the simplified letter style?

    _____

11. Identify the eight parts of speech.

    _____

12. What type of sentence is composed of one independent clause?

    _____

13. What is a compound sentence?

    _____

14. What is a complex sentence?

_____

15. What is a sentence fragment?

_____

16. When does a comma splice occur?

_____

17. Identify at least six occasions when a comma should be used.

_____

_____

_____

_____

18. When does the spell check feature of a word processing program fail to find errors?

_____

19. What are proofreader's marks?

_____

_____

20. What is the format of a memo (memorandum)?

_____

_____

21. Give three examples of individuals that a MA might communicate with via e-mail.

_____

_____

22. Compare the tone of an e-mail with that of a business letter.

_____

23. What is clinical messaging and when is it useful?

_____

_____

24. What features on a photocopier are helpful when photocopying a multiple-page document?

_____

_____

25. What information should be included on the cover sheet for fax transmissions from a medical office?

_____

_____

CRITICAL THINKING ACTIVITIES

A. Parts of a Letter

Refer to the letter in Chapter 42, Figure 42-2. Identify the following parts of that letter.

1. Inside address: _____

_____

_____

2. Salutation: _____

_____

_____

3. First three words of the body of the letter: _____

_____

_____

4. Complimentary close: _____

_____

_____

5. Printed signature: _____

_____

_____

6. End notation(s): _____

_____

_____

B. Letter Styles

Name the letter style(s) to which each of the following apply:

1. Date line is left justified: _____

2. Instead of a salutation, a reference line is included in all caps: _____

3. The body of the letter is single spaced with two spaces between paragraphs: _____

_____

4. Paragraphs are indented: _____

5. The complimentary close is right justified or at the center: _____

6. The inside address is left justified: _____

C. Parts of Speech

Enter each word in the following sentence into the table below under the heading of the correct part of speech.
My name is Christine Walters, and I have worked continuously at a nephrology practice for the past 3 years.

Noun(s)	Pronoun(s)	Verb(s)	Adjective(s)	Adverb(s) Article(s)	Preposition(s)	Conjunction(s)

D. Proofreading

Proofread the passage on the left. In the lines on the right, correct each mistake, including spelling, punctuation, and grammar.

1. Patient instructed in *perfromance* of range of	1.
2. motion activities, especially for the *weak, right*	2.
3. *lower, extremity.* He was instructed to use both	3.
4. hands to *assisting* in extension of the knee and	4.
5. ankle, flexion of the toes, as well as *invershun*	5.
6. and eversion of the foot. The *pateint* was able	6.
7. to demonstrate all exercises, *included* those	7.
8. done as *assistave* exercises. The patient could	8.
9. *verbalized* understanding of the need to keep all	9.
10. joints mobile.	10.

Procedure 42-1: Composing a Business Letter. Practice preparing business letters and preparing envelopes using the following two letters. Assume you are using letterhead stationery. Your position: MA.

Letter 1:

Content: You received an invoice (bill) from Physicians' Medical Supply Company, 22 Birkwood Street, Western, XY 44770. It includes a charge for three boxes of extra small gloves, but you only received two boxes. The purchase order number was 12345. You need the extra box of gloves.

Format: Full block using letterhead stationery. Use 1-inch margins. Be sure the letter has at least two paragraphs and that the body of the letter is centered on the page. Prepare an envelope to accompany the letter.

Letter 2:

Content: Dr. Warner asks you to contact the following patient and ask her to schedule a physical examination. The patient's name and address are Lucille Freeman, 22 White Circle, Western, XY 44770. When you check the patient's medical record, you notice that the patient has not been seen for 2 years. Dr. Warner prefers to perform an annual physical examination.

Format: Simplified style using letterhead stationery. Prepare an envelope.

Procedure 42-2: Sending a Fax. Practice the procedure to send a fax using the following cover sheets.

Procedure 42-3: Preparing Copies of Multiple-Page Documents. Practice the procedure for preparing copies of multiple-page documents.

WESTERN MEDICAL CENTER
109 RIVER STREET
WESTERN, XY 44770

PHONE: (490) 555-6464
FAX: (490) 668-1414

To: _____

Fax: _____

Phone: _____

Re: _____

From: _____

Pages: _____

Date: _____

CC: _____

☐ URGENT   ☐ FOR REVIEW   ☐ PLEASE COMMENT   ☐ PLEASE REPLY   ☐ PLEASE RECYCLE

CONFIDENTIALITY STATEMENT:
The documents accompanying this transmission may contain confidential information that is protected under the Privacy Act of 1974. It is being faxed to you after appropriate patient authorization or under circumstances that do not require patient authorization. This information is intended only for the use of the intended recipient(s). The authorized recipient(s) of this information is/are prohibited from disclosing this information to any other party unless permitted to do so by law or regulation.

If the reader of this mess is not the intended recipient(s) or the employee or agent responsible for delivering the attached information to the intended recipient(s), please note that any dissemination, distribution, or copying of this information is strictly prohibited. **Anyone who receives this information in error should notify the sender immediately and arrange for the return or destruction of the transmitted information.**

MESSAGE:

WESTERN MEDICAL CENTER
109 RIVER STREET
WESTERN, XY 44770

PHONE: (490) 555-6464
FAX: (490) 668-1414

To: _____

From: _____

Fax: _____

Pages: _____

Phone: _____

Date: _____

Re: _____

CC: _____

☐ URGENT ☐ FOR REVIEW ☐ PLEASE COMMENT ☐ PLEASE REPLY ☐ PLEASE RECYCLE

CONFIDENTIALITY STATEMENT:
The documents accompanying this transmission may contain confidential information that is protected under the Privacy Act of 1974. It is being faxed to you after appropriate patient authorization or under circumstances that do not require patient authorization. This information is intended only for the use of the intended recipient(s). The authorized recipient(s) of this information is/are prohibited from disclosing this information to any other party unless permitted to do so by law or regulation.

If the reader of this mess is not the intended recipient(s) or the employee or agent responsible for delivering the attached information to the intended recipient(s), please note that any dissemination, distribution, or copying of this information is strictly prohibited. **Anyone who receives this information in error should notify the sender immediately and arrange for the return or destruction of the transmitted information.**

MESSAGE:

WESTERN MEDICAL CENTER
109 RIVER STREET
WESTERN, XY 44770

PHONE: (490) 555-6464
FAX: (490) 668-1414

To: _____

From: _____

Fax: _____

Pages: _____

Phone: _____

Date: _____

Re: _____

CC: _____

☐ URGENT   ☐ FOR REVIEW   ☐ PLEASE COMMENT   ☐ PLEASE REPLY   ☐ PLEASE RECYCLE

CONFIDENTIALITY STATEMENT:
The documents accompanying this transmission may contain confidential information that is protected under the Privacy Act of 1974. It is being faxed to you after appropriate patient authorization or under circumstances that do not require patient authorization. This information is intended only for the use of the intended recipient(s). The authorized recipient(s) of this information is/are prohibited from disclosing this information to any other party unless permitted to do so by law or regulation.

If the reader of this mess is not the intended recipient(s) or the employee or agent responsible for delivering the attached information to the intended recipient(s), please note that any dissemination, distribution, or copying of this information is strictly prohibited. **Anyone who receives this information in error should notify the sender immediately and arrange for the return or destruction of the transmitted information.**

MESSAGE:

Procedure 42-1: Composing a Business Letter

Name: _____   Date: _____

Evaluated by: _____   Score: _____

Performance Objective

Outcome:	Compose and key a business letter.
Conditions:	Given the following: letterhead stationery, blank stationery, and typewriter or computer and printer.
Standards:	Time: 10 minutes. Student completed procedure in _____ minutes.
	Accuracy: Satisfactory score on the Performance Evaluation Checklist.

Performance Evaluation Checklist

Trial 1	Trial 2	Point Value	Performance Standards
		●	Assembled materials.
		●	Determined the address of the recipient.
		●	Set up the letter according to selected format.
		●	Listed and organized essential content for the letter.
		●	Inserted the date on the second or third line below the letterhead.
		●	Placed the inside address 4 to 10 lines below the date at the left margin (to center the body the of the letter on the page).
		●	Placed the salutation two lines below the inside address followed by a colon.
		●	Placed a subject line two lines below the salutation, if desired.
		●	Began the body of the letter two lines below the subject line (or salutation if no subject line was used).
		●	Single-spaced the letter with double spacing between paragraphs.
		●	Began paragraphs at the left margin or indented according to the letter style being used.
		●	Summarized the contents or most important ideas in the final paragraph of the letter.
		●	Placed the complimentary close two spaces below the final paragraph of the letter followed by a comma.
		●	Placed the typed signature four lines below the complimentary close with a title on the line below if appropriate.
		●	Added reference line, enclosure notation, and/or distribution notation as needed below the typed signature.

1095

Trial 1	Trial 2	Point Value	Performance Standards
		●	Began a second page 1 inch from the top including the name of the recipient, the date, and the page number in the top left corner.
		●	Included at least two lines of the body of the letter on the second page, if one was used.
		✶	Made sure that there were no errors in the letter using the computer and manual proofreading.
		●	Printed the letter.
		●	Signed the letter or obtained the appropriate signature.
		●	Made one copy of the letter for the file and additional copies for any individuals identified in the distribution notation.
		●	Prepared an envelope (Procedure 43-3: Preparing Envelopes for Mailing).
		●	Inserted the letter in the envelope and placed in the designated area to be mailed.
		●	Filed the copy of the letter according to office policy.
		✶	Completed the procedure within 10 minutes.
			TOTALS

Evaluation of Student Performance

EVALUATION CRITERIA			COMMENTS
Symbol	**Category**	**Point Value**	
✶	Critical Step	16 points	
●	Essential Step	6 points	
▷	Theory Question	2 points	

Score calculation: 100 points

       −   points missed

         _____ Score

Satisfactory score: 85 or above

CAAHEP Competencies Achieved

Psychomotor (Skills)
☑ IV. 10. Compose Professional/Business Letters.

ABHES Competencies Achieved

☑ 7.1.(2) Typing medical correspondence and reports
☑ 7. b. (1) Efficiently maintain and understand different types of medical correspondence and medical reports.
☑ 8. ii. Recognize and respond to verbal and nonverbal communication.
☑ 8. jj. Perform fundamental writing skills including correct grammar, spelling, and formatting techniques when writing prescriptions, documenting medical records, etc.

EVALUATION OF COMPETENCY

Procedure 42-2: Sending a Fax

Name: _____ Date: _____

Evaluated by: _____ Score: _____

Performance Objective

Outcome:	Send a fax.
Conditions:	Given the following: fax machine, cover sheet, pen, and document to be faxed.
Standards:	Time: 5 minutes. Student completed procedure in _____ minutes.
	Accuracy: Satisfactory score on the Performance Evaluation Checklist.

Performance Evaluation Checklist

Trial 1	Trial 2	Point Value	Performance Standards
		●	Prepared the cover sheet including name, address, and fax and telephone number of the recipient, telephone number of the sender, and number of pages (including cover sheet).
		●	Placed any message to the sender at the bottom of the cover sheet.
		●	Organized all pages of the fax with the cover sheet first.
		●	Placed pages in the fax machine, face up or face down as required by the machine.
		●	Entered the fax number, including extra digits if required.
		●	Verified that the fax number was correct as it appeared in the window.
		●	Pressed the correct button to send the fax.
		●	Returned to remove the fax and verify that it had been sent.
		●	Filed the original document appropriately.
		✱	Completed the procedure within 5 minutes.
			TOTALS

Evaluation of Student Performance

EVALUATION CRITERIA			COMMENTS
Symbol	**Category**	**Point Value**	
✳	Critical Step	16 points	
●	Essential Step	6 points	
▷	Theory Question	2 points	

Score calculation: 100 points

−   _____ points missed

_____ Score

Satisfactory score: 85 or above

CAAHEP Competencies Achieved

Psychomotor (Skills)
☑ IX. 3. Apply HIPAA rules in regard to privacy/release of information.

ABHES Competencies Achieved

☑ 4. b. Institute federal and state guidelines when releasing medical records or information.
☑ 8. a. Perform basic clerical functions.
☑ 8. ll. Apply electronic technology.

Procedure 42-3: Preparing Copies of Multiple-Page Documents

Name: _____   Date: _____

Evaluated by: _____   Date: _____

Performance Objective

Outcome:	Copy a document with multiple pages.
Conditions:	Given the following: photocopy machine, paper, document to be copied, stapler, staples, and staple remover.
Standards:	Time: 10 minutes. Student completed procedure in _____ minutes.
	Accuracy: Satisfactory score on the Performance Evaluation Checklist.

Performance Evaluation Checklist

Trial 1	Trial 2	Point Value	Performance Standards
		●	Assembled all pages of the document and removed staples.
		●	Made sure that the copy machine was warmed up.
		●	Placed the originals in the machine according to its directions.
		●	Selected the size, number of copies, and available options to collate and/or staple the copies.
		●	Pressed the "start" button.
		●	Arranged copies in the correct order if needed, and stapled if needed.
		●	Verified number of copies, recorded as needed, and submitted for billing as needed.
		✳	Completed the procedure within 10 minutes.
			TOTALS

Evaluation of Student Performance

EVALUATION CRITERIA			COMMENTS
Symbol	Category	Point Value	
✶	Critical Step	16 points	
●	Essential Step	6 points	
▷	Theory Question	2 points	

Score calculation: 100 points

−   _____ points missed

_____ Score

Satisfactory score: 85 or above

CAAHEP Competency Achieved

Psychomotor (Skills)

☑ IX. 3. Apply HIPAA rules in regard to privacy/release of information.

ABHES Competency Achieved

☑ 8. a. Perform basic clerical functions.

43 Mail

CHAPTER ASSIGNMENTS

√ After Completing	Date Due	Textbook Pages	TEXTBOOK ASSIGNMENTS	Possible Points	Points You Earned
		1023-1038	Read Chapter 43: Mail		
		1028 1037	Read Case Study 1 Case Study 1 questions	5	
		1029 1037	Read Case Study 2 Case Study 2 questions	5	
		1035 1038	Read Case Study 3 Case Study 3 questions	5	
			TOTAL POINTS		

√ After Completing	Date Due	Study Guide Pages	STUDY GUIDE ASSIGNMENTS (CTA = Critical Thinking Activity)	Possible Points	Points You Earned
		1103	Pretest	10	
		1103	Term Key Term Assessment	7	
		1104-1106	Evaluation of Learning questions	30	
		1106	CTA A: Classifications of Mail	6	
		1106-1107	CTA B: Insurance and Delivery Confirmation Services	6	
		1107	CTA C: Determining Postage	8	
			Evolve Site: Preparing an Envelope (Record points earned)		
			Evolve Site: Apply Your Knowledge questions	10	
			Evolve Site: Video Evaluations	20	
		1103	Posttest	10	
			ADDITIONAL ASSIGNMENTS		
			TOTAL POINTS		

√ When Assigned By Your Instructor	Study Guide Pages	Practices Required	LABORATORY ASSIGNMENTS (Procedure Number and Name)	Score*
	1108	3	**Practice for Competency** 43-1: Processing Incoming Mail Textbook reference: pp. 1029-1030	
	1109-1110		**Evaluation of Competency** 43-1: Processing Incoming Mail	*
	1108	3	**Practice for Competency** 43-2: Looking Up a ZIP Code Textbook reference: p. 1033	
	1111		**Evaluation of Competency** 43-2: Looking Up a ZIP Code	*
	1108	3	**Practice for Competency** 43-3: Preparing Envelopes for Mailing Textbook reference: p. 1036	
	1113-1114		**Evaluation of Competency** 43-3: Preparing Envelopes for Mailing	*
			ADDITIONAL ASSIGNMENTS	

PRETEST

True or False

_____ 1. The ZIP + 4 gives more specific information about the destination of a letter than the 5-digit ZIP code.

_____ 2. The delivery time for Priority Mail is approximately the same as for First-Class Mail.

_____ 3. Standard Mail is used by the medical office to mail packages.

_____ 4. The post office has machines that can read barcodes but not printed addresses.

_____ 5. The attention line of the address is placed directly below the recipient line.

_____ 6. The barcode free area of an envelope is at the lower right side of the envelope.

_____ 7. If the office does not have a typewriter, a label must be prepared to place the address on an envelope.

_____ 8. A letter should be folded first in half and then in thirds to place in a number 6¾ envelope.

_____ 9. The medical office may purchase a postage meter for more efficient processing of the mail.

_____ 10. The same postage is required for a large envelope as a standard business envelope of the same weight.

POSTTEST

True or False

_____ 1. A postal barcode is often added to first-class letters by the post office to identify the letter's destination.

_____ 2. The fastest way to send an item through the USPS is Priority Mail.

_____ 3. A Return Receipt is usually combined with Certified Mail for proof of both mailing and receipt.

_____ 4. If the medical assistant (MA) opens mail for a physician, each item should be stamped with the date.

_____ 5. The attention line of the address should be placed below and to the left of the city, state, and ZIP line.

_____ 6. The address of an envelope should be printed in uppercase letters for easier optical character recognition.

_____ 7. A letter is folded exactly the same way to place in a window envelope as in a number 6¾ envelope.

_____ 8. Postage can be purchased for a postage meter by telephone, through the Internet, or from the post office.

_____ 9. Stamps can be printed in the office using an online postage service.

_____ 10. Postage meters print postage on tapes that are applied to letters but not directly on the envelope.

KEY TERM ASSESSMENT

Directions: Match each medical term with its definition.

_____ 1. Annotate

_____ 2. Barcode clear zone

_____ 3. Metered mail

_____ 4. Postage meter

_____ 5. Postal barcode

_____ 6. ZIP code

_____ 7. ZIP + 4 code

A. The area on the lower right-hand corner of a card or letter, which is left clear for the postal barcode to be printed

B. A more detailed mailing code consisting of the original 5-digit ZIP code followed by a hyphen and four additional digits

C. A 5-digit code that identifies the post office to which a given piece of mail is to be delivered

D. Mail for which the postage has been applied using a postage meter

E. To underline or highlight important words and phrases in correspondence

F. A machine that automatically stamps a piece of mail with the correct postage

G. A series of vertical bars of two lengths, which represent the delivery address of a piece of mail that facilitates automated sorting of mail

Directions: Fill in each blank with the correct answer.

1. What is a ZIP + 4 code, and how is it different from a 5-digit ZIP code?

   _____

2. How does the USPS use barcodes?

   _____

   _____

3. Describe each of the following classifications of mail:

   Express Mail: _____

   First-Class Mail: _____

   Priority Mail: _____

   Standard Mail: _____

   Parcel Post: _____

   Media Mail: _____

   Bound Printed Matter: _____

4. What is Certified Mail?

   _____

5. Why does the medical office usually use Return Receipt instead of Signature Confirmation to obtain a record of the individual who signed for receipt of a mailed item?

   _____

   _____

6. When is a Certificate of Mailing obtained?

   _____

7. What service limits delivery of an item of mail specifically to the addressee?

   _____

8. What services are included when an item of mail is sent Registered Mail?

   _____

9. What service should be purchased for an item of value sent through the mail?

   _____

10. What are the advantages of using a private delivery service instead of the USPS to deliver packages?

    _____

    _____

11. What are general guidelines for sorting mail in the medical office?

_____

_____

12. If the MA opens mail for the physician, what should he or she do as soon as each item is opened?

_____

13. How should letters regarding patients be arranged for the physician?

_____

14. Why do some physicians ask the MA to annotate their correspondence?

_____

15. How should the physician's mail be handled when he or she is on vacation?

_____

_____

16. What happens to a piece of mail that has a printed address after it has been mailed?

_____

_____

17. Name three pieces of automated equipment used by the USPS.

_____

18. If an optional attention line is used in an address, where does the USPS recommend that it be placed?

_____

19. What should be included in the bottom line of a delivery address?

_____

20. What is the recommendation regarding punctuation in the address of an envelope?

_____

21. Where should instructions such as *Personal or Confidential* be placed on an envelope?

_____

22. Where should instructions for special services such as *Certified* or *Registered* be placed on an envelope?

_____

23. What is the barcode clear zone, and where is it located on an envelope?

_____

24. How does the MA prepare an envelope with the address directly on the envelope?

_____

_____

25. How does the MA prepare envelopes for a mailing of more than 30 envelopes?

_____

_____

26. Describe how to fold a letter for a standard #10 business envelope and for a window envelope.

_____

_____

27. Describe three ways to add postage to envelopes.

_____

_____

28. What are six safety measures to keep in mind when using a postage meter?

_____

_____

_____

29. How can the MA obtain additional postage for a postage meter?

_____

30. What services are offered by online postage services?

_____

_____

CRITICAL THINKING ACTIVITIES

A. Classifications of Mail

Identify the classification of mail you would use to mail each of the following items using the USPS.

1. Patient bill: _____

2. Order form for office supplies: _____

3. Package containing two books (needs to arrive in 2 to 3 days): _____

4. Package containing two books (no rush): _____

5. Specimen for testing (weighs 9 oz): _____

6. Package of office supplies weighing 16 lb: _____

B. Insurance and Delivery Confirmation Services

For each of the following items identify whether the item should be insured, if Delivery Confirmation should be obtained, and/or if a Return Receipt should be obtained.

1. X-ray of the hip mailed to another physician: _____

2. Item of jewelry worth $12.00: _____

3. Item of jewelry worth $650.00: _____

4. Letter informing a patient that a physician is retiring: _____

1106

5. Letter informing a patient that he or she must find a new physician for failing to keep appointments:

_____

6. Official letter that must be received by a specific deadline: _____

C. Determining Postage

For each of the following, determine the correct postage (post office price) using the USPS website (www.usps.com).

First Class (rates as of 4/20/2012):

1. Letter in a #10 envelope weighing 2 oz from ZIP code 19101 to 60606: _____

2. Letter in a square envelope weighing 1 oz from ZIP code 19101 to 60606: _____

Priority Mail (from post office):

3. Package weighing 4 lb 6 oz from ZIP code 19101 to 60606: _____

4. Envelope weighing 14 oz from ZIP code 19101 to 60606: _____

Express Mail (from post office):

5. Letter weighing 2 oz (flat rate envelope) from ZIP code 02114 to 90806: _____

6. Letter weighing 2 oz (ordinary envelope) from ZIP code 02114 to 60606: _____

Parcel Post and/or Media Mail:

7. Package of 3 boxes of gloves weighing 3 lb 2 oz from ZIP code 19101 to 60606: _____

8. Package of books weighing 4 lb 8 oz from ZIP code 02114 to 90806: _____

Procedure 43-1: Processing Incoming Mail. Process incoming mail.

Procedure 43-2: Looking Up a ZIP Code. Look up ZIP codes to prepare envelopes or mailing labels for Procedure 43-3 using the USPS website (www.usps.com).

Procedure 43-3: Preparing Envelopes for Mailing. Prepare envelopes of various sizes for mailing, weigh, and look up correct postage using the USPS website. Be sure to include ZIP + 4 from Procedure 43-2.

Centers for Disease Control and Prevention
1600 Clifton Road
Atlanta, GA [ZIP + 4]

National Institutes of Health
9000 Rockville Pike
Bethesda, MD [ZIP + 4]

Centers for Medicare and Medicaid Services
7500 Security Boulevard
Baltimore, MD [ZIP + 4]

U.S. Department of Health and Human Services
200 Independence Avenue, S.W.
Washington, DC [ZIP + 4]

Procedure 43-1: Processing Incoming Mail

Name: _____   Date: _____

Evaluated by: _____   Score: _____

Performance Objective

Outcome:	Process incoming mail.
Conditions:	Given the following: letter opener, date stamp, stamp pad, paper clips, stapler, pen or highlighter, and transparent tape.
Standards:	Time: 10 minutes. Student completed procedure in _____ minutes.
	Accuracy: Satisfactory score on the Performance Evaluation Checklist.

Performance Evaluation Checklist

Trial 1	Trial 2	Point Value	Performance Standards
		●	Assembled supplies in a work area large enough to make several piles.
		●	Arranged all envelopes so they faced in the same direction.
		●	Placed any envelopes marked "personal" or "confidential" to the side.
		●	Tapped the lower edge of the first envelope on the desk so contents fell to the bottom.
		●	Used a letter opener to open the envelope along the top edge, and removed the contents of the envelope.
		●	Checked to make sure the envelope was empty.
		●	Unfolded and flattened contents of the envelope.
		●	Stamped the date on the first page, preferably in the upper right corner.
		●	Checked to be sure the letter contained an inside address.
		●	Discarded the envelope if the letter contained an inside address; if not, stapled the envelope to the letter.
		●	Fastened enclosures to the letter with a paper clip.
		●	Wrote "no" beside an enclosure notation if any enclosures were missing.
		●	Mended any tears with tape.
		●	Used a highlighter or pen to annotate important points if directed to by the physician.

1109

Trial 1	Trial 2	Point Value	Performance Standards
		●	Attached a sticky note indicating action that should be taken in response to the correspondence as needed.
		●	Opened additional envelopes in the same way until all mail was opened.
		●	Separated mail into piles of urgent mail, letters, or reports containing patient information or results, medical journals, advertising, and other categories as needed.
		●	Arranged letters and reports containing patient information in alphabetical order.
		●	Found and used a paper clip to attach the appropriate paper medical record to each letter or report containing medical information.
		●	Arranged the mail for each recipient from most important on top to least important on the bottom.
		●	Distributed each stack of mail to the appropriate individual.
		✶	Completed the procedure within 10 minutes.
			TOTALS

Evaluation of Student Performance

EVALUATION CRITERIA			COMMENTS
Symbol	Category	Point Value	
✶	Critical Step	16 points	
●	Essential Step	6 points	
▷	Theory Question	2 points	

Score calculation: 100 points
        −   points missed
        _____
        ____ Score

Satisfactory score: 85 or above

CAAHEP Competencies Achieved

Psychomotor (Skills)
☑ V. 8. Maintain organization by filing.

ABHES Competencies Achieved

☑ 8. a. Perform basic clerical functions

Procedure 43-2: Looking Up a ZIP Code

Name: _____ Date: _____

Evaluated by: _____ Score: _____

Performance Objective

Outcome:	Find the correct ZIP + 4 code for a given address.
Conditions:	Given the following: computer with Internet access, pen and pencil, address with incorrect and/or missing ZIP code.
Standards:	Time: 3 minutes. Student completed procedure in _____minutes.
	Accuracy: Satisfactory score on the Performance Evaluation Checklist

Performance Evaluation Checklist

Trial 1	Trial 2	Point Value	Performance Standards
		●	Opened the computer's web browser and entered the web address for the United States Postal Service.
		●	From the USPS home page, selected "Find a ZIP code."
		●	On the "Search by Address" tab, entered the complete delivery address.
		✶	Copied the correct ZIP + 4 code on a piece of paper or used the computer copy function to copy and past into a computer file.
		✶	Completed the procedure within 3 minutes.
			TOTALS

Evaluation of Student Performance

EVALUATION CRITERIA			COMMENTS
Symbol	**Category**	**Point Value**	
✶	Critical Step	16 points	
●	Essential Step	6 points	
▷	Theory Question	2 points	

Score calculation: 100 points

− _____ points missed

_____ Score

Satisfactory score: 85 or above

CAAHEP Competencies Achieved

Psychomotor (Skills)
☑ V. 7. Use internet to access information related to the medical office.

ABHES Competencies Achieved

☑ 8. a. Perform basic clerical functions.
☑ 8. ll. Apply electronic technology.

Notes

Procedure 43-3: Preparing Envelopes for Mailing

Name: _____ Date: _____

Evaluated by: _____ Score: _____

Performance Objective

Outcome:	Prepare envelopes for mailing.
Conditions:	Given the following: envelope, other items to be mailed, pen, typewriter, computer and printer, postal scale, postage meter (optional), and/or stamps.
Standards:	Time: 3 minutes. Student completed procedure in _____minutes.
	Accuracy: Satisfactory score on the Performance Evaluation Checklist.

Performance Evaluation Checklist

Trial 1	Trial 2	Point Value	Performance Standards
		●	Determined the exact address to be used for the envelope.
		●	Selected an envelope of the appropriate size.
		●	Decided on a means to address the envelope (e.g., typewriter, envelope wizard, label template, label program).
		✶	Keyed or typed the address correctly according to USPS guidelines including the ZIP + 4 code.
		●	Added any special notations such as "personal" or "confidential" below the return address in the upper left corner of the envelope.
		●	Added any mailing instructions on the right side of the envelope below the postage area.
		●	Folded and placed the letter or item to be mailed in the envelope and sealed it.
		●	Weighed the piece of mail if it contained more than two sheets of paper or if the envelope was larger than 6 ⅛" × 11½".
		●	Calculated and applied the correct amount of postage.
		●	If a postage meter was used, processed all envelopes to be mailed that day.
		●	Sorted envelopes and other items to be mailed according to size.
		●	Separated any items with special mailing instructions to be taken to the post office.
		●	Placed items with postage in a mailbox or requested a pickup from the postal service.
		●	Set special items aside to be taken to the post office.
		✶	Completed the procedure within 10 minutes.
			TOTALS

EVALUATION CRITERIA			COMMENTS
Symbol	Category	Point Value	
✳	Critical Step	16 points	
●	Essential Step	6 points	
▷	Theory Question	2 points	

Score calculation: 100 points

–   _____ points missed

_____ Score

Satisfactory score: 85 or above

CAAHEP Competencies Achieved

Psychomotor (Skills)

☑ IV. 10. Compose professional/business letters.

ABHES Competencies Achieved

☑ 8. a. Perform basic clerical functions.

Managing Practice Finances

√ After Completing	Date Due	Textbook Pages	TEXTBOOK ASSIGNMENTS	Possible Points	Points You Earned
		1039-1062	Read Chapter 44: Managing Practice Finances		
		1043 1060	Read Case Study 1 Case Study 1 questions	5	
		1051 1061	Read Case Study 2 Case Study 2 questions	5	
		1053 1061	Read Case Study 3 Case Study 3 questions	5	
			TOTAL POINTS		
√ After Completing	**Date Due**	**Study Guide Pages**	**STUDY GUIDE ASSIGNMENTS (CTA = Critical Thinking Activity)**	**Possible Points**	**Points You Earned**
		1119	Pretest	10	
		1120	Key Term Assessment	25	
		1121-1123	Evaluation of Learning questions	28	
		1124	CTA A: The Charge Slip	8	
		1124	CTA B: Posting Transactions	8	
		1124	CTA C: Writing Checks	6	
		1125	CTA D: Endorsing Checks	6	
			Evolve Site: Completing a Charge Slip and Posting Entries on a Day Sheet (Record points earned)		
			Evolve Site: Posting Insurance Payments and Adjustments (Record points earned)		
			Evolve Site: Guided Practice: Preparing a Bank Deposit	10	
			Evolve Site: Guided Practice: Reconciling a Bank Statement	10	
			Evolve Site: Guided Practice: Writing Checks in Payment of Bills	10	

√ After Completing	Date Due	Study Guide Pages	STUDY GUIDE ASSIGNMENTS (CTA = Critical Thinking Activity)	Possible Points	Points You Earned
			Evolve Site: Apply Your Knowledge questions	10	
			Evolve Site: Video Evaluations	15	
		1119	Posttest	10	
			ADDITIONAL ASSIGNMENTS		
			TOTAL POINTS		

√ When Assigned By Your Instructor	Study Guide Pages	Practices Required	LABORATORY ASSIGNMENTS (Procedure Number and Name)	Score*
	1127-1133	3	**Practice for Competency** 44-1: Completing a Patient Charge Slip Textbook reference: pp. 1046-1047	
	1149-1150		**Evaluation of Competency** 44-1: Completing a Patient Charge Slip	*
	1127-1133	3	**Practice for Competency** 44-2: Posting Charges Textbook reference: p. 1047	
	1151-1152		**Evaluation of Competency** 44-2: Posting Charges	*
	1127-1135	3	**Practice for Competency** 44-3: Posting Payments and/or Adjustments Textbook reference: pp. 1048-1049	
	1153-1154		**Evaluation of Competency** 44-3: Posting Payments and/or Adjustments	*
	1127-1137	3	**Practice for Competency** 44-4: Recording a Patient's Visit on the Day Sheet Textbook reference: pp. 1049-1050	
	1155-1156		**Evaluation of Competency** 44-4: Recording a Patient's Visit on the Day Sheet	*
	1127-1139	1	**Practice for Competency** 44-5: Using a Computerized Office Billing System Textbook reference: p. 1050	
	1157-1158		**Evaluation of Competency** 44-5: Using a Computerized Office Billing System	*
	1127-1141	3	**Practice for Competency** 44-6: Writing a Check Textbook reference: p. 1056	
	1159-1160		**Evaluation of Competency** 44-6: Writing a Check	*
	1127-1143	1	**Practice for Competency** 44-7: Preparing a Bank Deposit Textbook reference: p. 1057	
	1161-1162		**Evaluation of Competency** 44-7: Preparing a Bank Deposit	*
	1127-1145	1	**Practice for Competency** 44-8: Reconciling a Bank Statement Textbook reference: pp. 1057-1058	

√ When Assigned By Your Instructor	Study Guide Pages	Practices Required	LABORATORY ASSIGNMENTS (Procedure Number and Name)	Score*
	1163-1164		**Evaluation of Competency** 44-8: Reconciling a Bank Statement	*
	1127-1147	1	**Practice for Competency** 44-9: Creating and Maintaining a Petty Cash Log Textbook reference: p. 1059	
	1165-1166		**Evaluation of Competency** 44-9: Creating and Maintaining a Petty Cash Log	*
			ADDITIONAL ASSIGNMENTS	

Name _____ Date _____

True or False

_____ 1. In the cash basis of accounting, income is entered when an item is sold or a service is provided.

_____ 2. Money owed to the medical practice by patients makes up the accounts receivable.

_____ 3. Medical billing programs are usually based on the traditional pegboard system of bookkeeping.

_____ 4. A superbill contains a list of procedures commonly performed in the medical office.

_____ 5. An adjustment always reduces the balance of a patient's account.

_____ 6. If a computer billing program is used, the office will not create a manual day sheet.

_____ 7. A money market account usually has features of both a savings account and a checking account.

_____ 8. Each bank in the United States has a unique identification number.

_____ 9. Business accounting programs can often create and print checks.

_____ 10. To replenish the petty cash fund, the medical assistant can use any cash payment by a patient.

?≣ **POSTTEST**

True or False

_____ 1. If income is entered when an item is sold, the accrual basis of accounting is being used.

_____ 2. Each patient account is one of the accounts payable.

_____ 3. A daily journal is a chronological record of charges and payments for each day.

_____ 4. A superbill is an itemized charge slip.

_____ 5. The patient ledger shows only the charges and payments for a patient on a specific day.

_____ 6. The proof of posting section of a manual day sheet verifies that all columns were totaled correctly.

_____ 7. To receive interest on a checking account, it is usually necessary to maintain a minimum balance.

_____ 8. The MICR line is printed in magnetic ink across the bottom of a check.

_____ 9. If the medical assistant makes a mistake on a check, the check should be shredded or destroyed.

_____ 10. Every time money is taken from petty cash, a receipt should be completed.

Directions: Match each medical term with its definition.

_____ 1. ABA routing number

_____ 2. Accounting

_____ 3. Accounts payable

_____ 4. Accounts receivable

_____ 5. Accrual basis of accounting

_____ 6. Adjustment

_____ 7. Assets

_____ 8. Bookkeeping

_____ 9. Cash basis of accounting

_____ 10. Cashier's check

_____ 11. Certified check

_____ 12. Charge slip

_____ 13. Credit

_____ 14. Day sheet

_____ 15. Debit

_____ 16. Disbursements

_____ 17. Fee schedule

_____ 18. Ledger

_____ 19. Liabilities

_____ 20. MICR line

_____ 21. Payee

_____ 22. Petty cash

_____ 23. Proof of posting

_____ 24. Reconciling

_____ 25. Superbill

A. Accounting method where income is entered when payment is received

B. A posting that is subtracted from an account balance

C. Accounting method where income is entered at the time of sale

D. An itemized charge slip usually also containing diagnosis codes and procedure codes

E. A form used to keep track of charges and payments at the time of a patient visit

F. A nine-digit number that identifies an individual bank

G. In accounting, the amount owed by a business to creditors

H. A check on an individual account that a bank assumes responsibility for

I. The person to whom a check is made out

J. A line of numbers across the bottom of a check that are read by a magnetic character reader

K. A cash account kept in a business office to pay for incidentals

L. A change to a patient account that is neither a charge nor a payment

M. List of charges for specific procedures that may be performed in a medical office

N. In accounting, a combination of property owned and money owed to a business

O. The outstanding bills of a business such as a medical office

P. Money paid out

Q. A posting that is added to an account balance

R. Making sure that two financial records agree

S. Systematic recording and reporting of financial transactions

T. A book, card, or computer account used to record financial transactions

U. The process of posting charges and payments and balancing financial records

V. The chronological record of daily transactions

W. A process of calculation to verify that all totals on a day sheet are correct

X. Total amount owed to a business for goods and services

Y. A check drawn on a bank instead of an individual account

Directions: Fill in each blank with the correct answer.

1. What is the difference between the cash basis and the accrual basis of accounting?

   _____

   _____

2. What generates income in the medical office?

   _____

   _____

3. What are three types of financial records used in a bookkeeping system?

   _____

   _____

4. If patient charges are recorded using a computer billing program, where must the data about the charge be entered? Why is it sufficient to enter the data once?

   _____

   _____

5. Why does a charge slip (superbill) usually contain diagnosis and procedure codes?

   _____

   _____

6. How does the medical assistant (MA) know what to charge a patient for a specific procedure?

   _____

   _____

7. If the office typically charges $65.00 to perform an electrocardiogram, is this the amount paid by all patients? Why or why not?

   _____

   _____

8. How is information arranged in the patient account ledger?

   _____

9. What are four ways that payments are made to a patient account?

   _____

   _____

10. What is the difference between a credit adjustment and a debit adjustment? Give one example of each.

   _____

   _____

11. When an insurance company pays an amount that is lower than the usual charge, how is the patient's balance due returned to zero?

_____

_____

12. What information is recorded on a day sheet?

_____

13. What is the purpose of completing the proof of posting section at the bottom of a manual day sheet?

_____

_____

14. What does it mean to "close the day," and why is this important for accurate financial record-keeping?

_____

_____

15. Describe three types of bank accounts.

_____

_____

_____

16. Describe the services and function of a checking account.

_____

17. What is the advantage of maintaining a savings account or money market account compared with a checking account?

_____

_____

18. Differentiate between a cashier's check and a certified check. Which is used more often?

_____

_____

19. What is the MICR (magnetic ink character recognition) line on a check, and what information does it contain?

_____

_____

20. Identify three ways that checks can be generated or bills can be paid, and describe how information is recorded.

_____

_____

_____

_____

21. What should the MA do if he or she writes a check incorrectly?

_____

_____

22. How is the cash drawer balanced at the end of the day?

_____

_____

23. What is necessary before a check can be cashed or deposited? How is this handled in a medical office?

_____

_____

24. What is the difference between a special endorsement and a restricted endorsement?

_____

_____

25. Identify five reasons why the monthly bank statement may not agree with the medical office's calculation of the bank balance in a checking account.

_____

_____

_____

26. What steps must be taken to reconcile a bank account?

_____

_____

_____

27. What financial accounts does a medical office usually have, and what do those accounts include?

_____

_____

28. How is a petty cash fund (account) managed?

_____

_____

_____

A. The Charge Slip

Refer to the completed charge slip in your textbook (Figure 44-2), and identify the following information.

1. The name of the insured person: _____

2. The patient's insurance ID number: _____

3. The charge for the patient's office visit: _____

4. The patient's telephone number: _____

5. The name of the diagnostic test performed: _____

6. The balance owed by the patient: _____

7. The patient's birth date: _____

8. The patient's physician: _____

B. Posting Transactions

Identify whether each of the following transactions would be posted as a charge, a payment, or an adjustment in the computer billing program or on a pegboard day sheet.

1. Office visit: _____

2. Check from insurance company: _____

3. Tetanus injection: _____

4. Dipstick urinalysis: _____

5. Insurance excluded amount: _____

6. Professional courtesy discount: _____

7. Spirometry test: _____

8. Patient check: _____

C. Writing Checks

Demonstrate how to write the following amounts in words on a check.

1. $76.42 _____ DOLLARS

2. $189.28 _____ DOLLARS

3. $1,020.00 _____ DOLLARS

4. $6.40 _____ DOLLARS

5. $16.04 _____ DOLLARS

6. $382.00 _____ DOLLARS

D. Endorsing Checks

Identify if each of the following is a blank endorsement, restrictive endorsement, or special endorsement.

1. *Maria S. Sanchez* _____

2. Pay to the order of: Robert A. Wilson
   Maria S. Sanchez _____

3. *Robert A. Wilson*
   Acct. # 12345-67890 _____

4. For deposit only
   Robert A. Wilson _____

5. Pay to the order of: Diane M. Casey
   Frederick Underwood _____

6. For deposit Acct. # 3456-78901
   Edward B. Young _____

Notes

PRACTICE FOR COMPETENCY

Use the following information to practice Procedures 44-1 through 44-5. Use today's date for all work.

FEE SCHEDULE				
Office Visit, New Patient			**Office Visit, Established Patient**	
			99211 Nurse/Minimal OV	$ 40.00
99201	Problem Focused OV*	$ 55.00	99212 Problem Focused OV	$ 50.00
99202	Exp** Problem Focused OV	$ 70.00	99213 Exp Problem Focused OV	$ 65.00
OFFICE PROCEDURES				
36415	Venipuncture Collection	$ 12.00	93000 ECG*** (Global)	$ 65.00
81002	Urinalysis (Dip only)	$ 15.00	94010 Pulmonary Function (spirometry)	$ 50.00
87880	Strep test (rapid)	$ 30.00	94640 Inhalation Treatment	$ 45.00

*OV – office visit
**Exp - Expanded
***ECG - electrocardiogram

PATIENT INFORMATION

June Simmons 16 Winston Terrace Western, XY 44770 (490) 459-1000 DOB: 2/23/1962 Diagnosis: Hypertension Procedures: Problem-focused office visit Previous Balance: $45.00 Payment: $10.00 by patient check on bank #242-XX/110	Patient Number: 1010 Established Patient of Dr. Warner Name of Insured: self Insurance Plan: Standard Health HMO (490) 459-3344 Insurance ID # 10229876 Group # 45215

Robert Underwood 224 Lakeview Drive Western, XY 44770 (490) 459-1111 DOB: 1/31/1992 Diagnosis: Streptococcal sore throat Procedures: Problem-focused office visit, Strep test (rapid) Previous Balance: -0- Payment: $70.00 by check on bank # 02-XX/502 Cash Discount: - $15.00 (credit adjustment)	Patient Number: 5010 New Patient of Dr. Gomez Name of Insured: N/A Insurance Plan: None Policy #: None

<table>
<tr><td>James Winston
25 Magnolia Lane
Western, XY 44770
(490) 459-1222
DOB: 12/14/40
Diagnoses: Chest pain; Hypertension
Procedures: Expanded problem-focused office visit, ECG
Previous Balance: $15.00</td><td>Patient Number: 1020
Established Patient of Dr. Gomez
Name of Insured: self
Insurance Plan: Medicare (490) 555-2800
Policy # 000-70-7000A</td></tr>
</table>

<table>
<tr><td>Marie Richards
19 Maple Street
Western, XY 44770
(490) 459-1333
DOB: 8/22/82
Previous Balance: $39.00
Insurance Payment for Visit 9/02/XX: $26.00 by check on bank #602-XX/110
Insurance Excluded Amount: $13.00</td><td>Patient Number: 3020
Established Patient of Dr. Warner
Name of Insured: John Richards
Insurance Plan: Standard Health HMO</td></tr>
</table>

Procedure 44-1: Completing a Patient Charge Slip. Fill out charge slips for June Simmons, Robert Underwood, and James Winston using today's date and time. The forms are located on the next pages.

Procedure 44-2: Posting Charges. Post charges for June Simmons, Robert Underwood, and James Winston for the information above. Use a separate transaction entry form for each patient. For code, use the CPT code.

Transaction Entry

Date	Pt #	Patient Name	Provider	Code	Description	Amount

Transaction Entry

Date	Pt #	Patient Name	Provider	Code	Description	Amount

Transaction Entry

Date	Pt #	Patient Name	Provider	Code	Description	Amount

Western Medical Center
109 River Street
Western, XY 44770
(490) 555-6464

Richard Warner, MD   NPI # 23456781XX
Maria Gomez, MD   NPI # 34567891XX
Tax ID 52-XX63777

Patient Name and Address	Birth date	Subscriber Name	MD Name	Today's Date
	Account #	Insurance Company	Insurance Phone #	Time
Telephone No. ( )		Insurance ID #	Group/Plan #	Sex Male ☐ Female ☐

√	DESCRIPTION	CPT	FEE	√	DESCRIPTION	CPT	FEE	√	DESCRIPTION	CPT	FEE
	OFFICE VISIT				**IMMUNIZATIONS**				**PROCEDURES**		
	NEW PATIENT				Imm. admin, one	90471			EKG w/interpretation	93000	
	Problem Focused	99201			Imm. admin, each add'l	90472			Spirometry	94010	
	Exp. Prob. Focused	99202			Influenza < 3	90657			Inhalation treatment	94640	
	Detailed	99203			Influenza 3 and >	90658			Remove skin tag <15	11200	
	Comp/Mod MDM	99204			Medicare code	G0008			Cerumen removal	69210	
	Comp./High MDM	99205			Varicella	90716			Wart destruction < 14	17110	
	ESTABLISHED PATIENT				DTaP	90700			I & D abscess	10060	
	Minimal/Nurse Visit	99211			Td adult	90718					
	Problem Focused	99212			Rubella	90706					
	Exp. Problem Focused	99213			MMR	90707			**OTHER**		
	Detailed	99214			Hep B Child	90744					
	Comprehensive	99215			Hep B Adult	90746					
	Post-op Exam	99024	0.00		IPV	90713					
	WELL VISIT				**WELL VISIT**				**LABORATORY**		
	NEW PATIENT				ESTABLISHED PATIENT				Blood Collection Vein	36415	
	Infant–1 year	99381			Infant–1 year	99391			Venipuncture, Medicare	G0001	
	1 yr–4 yr	99382			1 yr–4 yr	99392			Finger stick, glucose	82948	
	5 yr – 11 yr	99383			5 yr –11 yr	99393			Hemoccult	82270	
	12 yr–17 yr	99384			12 yr–17 yr	99394			Mono Test	86308	
	18 yr –39 yr	99385			18 yr –39 yr	99395			Strep, rapid	87880	
	40 yr –64 yr	99386			40 yr –64 yr	99396			UA, dipstick (manual)	81000	
	65 yr and over	99387			65 yr and over	99397			UA, automated	81003	
									Urine pregnancy	81025	

DIAGNOSTIC CODES (ICD-10-CM)

☐ R10.9 Abdominal Pain
☐ E63.4 Allergic Reaction
☐ D64.9 Anemia
☐ D51.0 Anemia, Pernicious
☐ I12.9 Angina Pectoris
☐ I49.9 Arrhythmia, Cardiac
☐ I70.0 Atherosclerosis, Aorta
☐ J45.909 Asthma
☐ M54.9 Back Pain
☐ J20._ Bronchitis, Acute
☐ J42 Bronchitis, Chronic
☐ R07.9 Chest Pain
☐ J44.9 COPD
☐ E10.0 Diabetes I–Ins. Dep

☐ E11.9 Diabetes II–Non Ins
☐ K57.92 Diverticulitis
☐ K57.90 Diverticulosis
☐ R60.9 Edema
☐ R51 Headache
☐ R31.9 Hematuria
☐ B00.9 Herpes Zoster
☐ I10 Hypertension
☐ E03.9 Hypothyroidism
☐ H61.2_ Impacted Cerumen
☐ J10.1 Influenza
☐ K58.9 Irritable Bowel Syndrome
☐ M19.0 Osteoarthritis
☐ M19.0 Osteoarthritis

☐ H66.9_ Otitis Media
☐ J02.9 Pharyngitis
☐ M06.9 Rheumatoid Arthritis
☐ R06.02 Short of Breath
☐ J32.9 Sinusitis
☐ L19.8 Skin Tag(s)
☐ J02.0 Streptococcal Sore Throat
☐ N39.0 Urinary Tract Infection

☐ Z23 Immunization Encounter
☐ Z00.12_ Well Child Check
☐ Z00.0_ Well Adult
☐ _____
☐ _____
☐ _____
☐ _____

RETURN APPOINTMENT	**BALANCE DUE**	
_____ Days	Total Charge	$
_____ Weeks	Amount Paid	$
_____ Months	Previous Bal	$
_____ PRN	Adjustment	$
	Balance Due	$

1129

Notes

Western Medical Center
109 River Street
Western, XY 44770
(490) 555-6464

Richard Warner, MD   NPI # 23456781XX
Maria Gomez, MD   NPI # 34567891XX
Tax ID 52-XX63777

Patient Name and Address		Birth date	Subscriber Name	MD Name	Today's Date
		Account #	Insurance Company	Insurance Phone #	Time
Telephone No. ( )			Insurance ID #	Group/Plan #	Sex
					Male ☐ Female ☐

√	DESCRIPTION	CPT	FEE	√	DESCRIPTION	CPT	FEE	√	DESCRIPTION	CPT	FEE
	OFFICE VISIT				**IMMUNIZATIONS**				**PROCEDURES**		
	NEW PATIENT				Imm. admin, one	90471			EKG w/interpretation	93000	
	Problem Focused	99201			Imm. admin, each add'l	90472			Spirometry	94010	
	Exp. Prob. Focused	99202			Influenza < 3	90657			Inhalation treatment	94640	
	Detailed	99203			Influenza 3 and >	90658			Remove skin tag <15	11200	
	Comp/Mod MDM	99204			Medicare code	G0008			Cerumen removal	69210	
	Comp./High MDM	99205			Varicella	90716			Wart destruction < 14	17110	
	ESTABLISHED PATIENT				DTaP	90700			I & D abscess	10060	
	Minimal/Nurse Visit	99211			Td adult	90718					
	Problem Focused	99212			Rubella	90706					
	Exp. Problem Focused	99213			MMR	90707			**OTHER**		
	Detailed	99214			Hep B Child	90744					
	Comprehensive	99215			Hep B Adult	90746					
	Post-op Exam	99024	0.00		IPV	90713					
	WELL VISIT				**WELL VISIT**				**LABORATORY**		
	NEW PATIENT				ESTABLISHED PATIENT				Blood Collection Vein	36415	
	Infant–1 year	99381			Infant–1 year	99391			Venipuncture, Medicare	G0001	
	1 yr–4 yr	99382			1 yr–4 yr	99392			Finger stick, glucose	82948	
	5 yr – 11 yr	99383			5 yr –11 yr	99393			Hemoccult	82270	
	12 yr–17 yr	99384			12 yr–17 yr	99394			Mono Test	86308	
	18 yr –39 yr	99385			18 yr –39 yr	99395			Strep, rapid	87880	
	40 yr –64 yr	99386			40 yr –64 yr	99396			UA, dipstick (manual)	81000	
	65 yr and over	99387			65 yr and over	99397			UA, automated	81003	
									Urine pregnancy	81025	

DIAGNOSTIC CODES (ICD-10-CM)

☐ R10.9 Abdominal Pain
☐ E63.4 Allergic Reaction
☐ D64.9 Anemia
☐ D51.0 Anemia, Pernicious
☐ I12.9 Angina Pectoris
☐ I49.9 Arrhythmia, Cardiac
☐ I70.0 Atherosclerosis, Aorta
☐ J45.909 Asthma
☐ M54.9 Back Pain
☐ J20._ Bronchitis, Acute
☐ J42 Bronchitis, Chronic
☐ R07.9 Chest Pain
☐ J44.9 COPD
☐ E10.0 Diabetes I–Ins. Dep

☐ E11.9 Diabetes II–Non Ins
☐ K57.92 Diverticulitis
☐ K57.90 Diverticulosis
☐ R60.9 Edema
☐ R51 Headache
☐ R31.9 Hematuria
☐ B00.9 Herpes Zoster
☐ I10 Hypertension
☐ E03.9 Hypothyroidism
☐ H61.2_ Impacted Cerumen
☐ J10.1 Influenza
☐ K58.9 Irritable Bowel Syndrome
☐ M19.0 Osteoarthritis
☐ M19.0 Osteoarthritis

☐ H66.9_ Otitis Media
☐ J02.9 Pharyngitis
☐ M06.9 Rheumatoid Arthritis
☐ R06.02 Short of Breath
☐ J32.9 Sinusitis
☐ L19.8 Skin Tag(s)
☐ J02.0 Streptococcal Sore Throat
☐ N39.0 Urinary Tract Infection

☐ Z23 Immunization Encounter
☐ Z00.12_ Well Child Check
☐ Z00.0_ Well Adult
☐ _____
☐ _____
☐ _____
☐ _____

RETURN APPOINTMENT

_____ Days
_____ Weeks
_____ Months
_____ PRN

BALANCE DUE

Total Charge	$
Amount Paid	$
Previous Bal	$
Adjustment	$
Balance Due	$

1131

Notes

Western Medical Center
109 River Street
Western, XY 44770
(490) 555-6464

Richard Warner, MD NPI # 23456781XX
Maria Gomez, MD NPI # 34567891XX
Tax ID 52-XX63777

Patient Name and Address	Birth date	Subscriber Name	MD Name	Today's Date
	Account #	Insurance Company	Insurance Phone #	Time
Telephone No. ( )		Insurance ID #	Group/Plan #	Sex Male ☐ Female ☐

√	DESCRIPTION	CPT	FEE	√	DESCRIPTION	CPT	FEE	√	DESCRIPTION	CPT	FEE
	OFFICE VISIT				**IMMUNIZATIONS**				**PROCEDURES**		
	NEW PATIENT				Imm. admin, one	90471			EKG w/interpretation	93000	
	Problem Focused	99201			Imm. admin, each add'l	90472			Spirometry	94010	
	Exp. Prob. Focused	99202			Influenza < 3	90657			Inhalation treatment	94640	
	Detailed	99203			Influenza 3 and >	90658			Remove skin tag <15	11200	
	Comp/Mod MDM	99204			Medicare code	G0008			Cerumen removal	69210	
	Comp./High MDM	99205			Varicella	90716			Wart destruction < 14	17110	
	ESTABLISHED PATIENT				DTaP	90700			I & D abscess	10060	
	Minimal/Nurse Visit	99211			Td adult	90718					
	Problem Focused	99212			Rubella	90706					
	Exp. Problem Focused	99213			MMR	90707			**OTHER**		
	Detailed	99214			Hep B Child	90744					
	Comprehensive	99215			Hep B Adult	90746					
	Post-op Exam	99024	0.00		IPV	90713					
	WELL VISIT				**WELL VISIT**				**LABORATORY**		
	NEW PATIENT				ESTABLISHED PATIENT				Blood Collection Vein	36415	
	Infant–1 year	99381			Infant–1 year	99391			Venipuncture, Medicare	G0001	
	1 yr–4 yr	99382			1 yr–4 yr	99392			Finger stick, glucose	82948	
	5 yr – 11 yr	99383			5 yr –11 yr	99393			Hemoccult	82270	
	12 yr–17 yr	99384			12 yr–17 yr	99394			Mono Test	86308	
	18 yr –39 yr	99385			18 yr –39 yr	99395			Strep, rapid	87880	
	40 yr –64 yr	99386			40 yr –64 yr	99396			UA, dipstick (manual)	81000	
	65 yr and over	99387			65 yr and over	99397			UA, automated	81003	
									Urine pregnancy	81025	

DIAGNOSTIC CODES (ICD-10-CM)

☐ R10.9 Abdominal Pain
☐ E63.4 Allergic Reaction
☐ D64.9 Anemia
☐ D51.0 Anemia, Pernicious
☐ I12.9 Angina Pectoris
☐ I49.9 Arrhythmia, Cardiac
☐ I70.0 Atherosclerosis, Aorta
☐ J45.909 Asthma
☐ M54.9 Back Pain
☐ J20._ Bronchitis, Acute
☐ J42 Bronchitis, Chronic
☐ R07.9 Chest Pain
☐ J44.9 COPD
☐ E10.0 Diabetes I–Ins. Dep

☐ E11.9 Diabetes II–Non Ins
☐ K57.92 Diverticulitis
☐ K57.90 Diverticulosis
☐ R60.9 Edema
☐ R51 Headache
☐ R31.9 Hematuria
☐ B00.9 Herpes Zoster
☐ I10 Hypertension
☐ E03.9 Hypothyroidism
☐ H61.2_ Impacted Cerumen
☐ J10.1 Influenza
☐ K58.9 Irritable Bowel Syndrome
☐ M19.0 Osteoarthritis
☐ M19.0 Osteoarthritis

☐ H66.9_ Otitis Media
☐ J02.9 Pharyngitis
☐ M06.9 Rheumatoid Arthritis
☐ R06.02 Short of Breath
☐ J32.9 Sinusitis
☐ L19.8 Skin Tag(s)
☐ J02.0 Streptococcal Sore Throat
☐ N39.0 Urinary Tract Infection

☐ Z23 Immunization Encounter
☐ Z00.12_ Well Child Check
☐ Z00.0_ Well Adult
☐ _____
☐ _____
☐ _____
☐ _____
☐ _____

RETURN APPOINTMENT

_____ Days
_____ Weeks
_____ Months
_____ PRN

BALANCE DUE

Total Charge	$
Amount Paid	$
Previous Bal	$
Adjustment	$
Balance Due	$

1133

Notes

Procedure 44-3: Posting Payments and/or Adjustments. Post payment (CHECK) for June Simmons. Post payment (CHECK) and credit adjustment (CRADJ) for Robert Underwood. Post insurance payment (INSPAY) and insurance adjustment (INSADJ) for Marie Richards. Use a separate transaction entry form for each patient. The codes are given in parentheses.

Transaction Entry

Date	Pt #	Patient Name	Provider	Code	Description	Amount

Transaction Entry

Date	Pt #	Patient Name	Provider	Code	Description	Amount

Transaction Entry

Date	Pt #	Patient Name	Provider	Code	Description	Amount

Procedure 44-4: Recording a Patient's Visit on the Day Sheet. Record information for June Simmons, Robert Underwood, James Winston, and Marie Richards on the following day sheet.

Notes

JOURNAL OF DAILY CHARGES, PAYMENTS & DEPOSITS

	DATE	PROFESSIONAL SERVICE	FEE	PAYMENT	ADJUST-MENT	NEW BALANCE	OLD BALANCE	PATIENT'S NAME	
1									1
2									2
3									3
4									4
5									5
6									6
7									7
8									8
9									9
10									10
11									11
12									12
13									13
14									14
15									15
16									16
17									17
18									18
19									19
20									20
21									21
22									22
23									23
24									24
25									25
26									26
27									27
28									28
29									29
30									30
31								TOTALS THIS PAGE	31
32								TOTALS PREVIOUS PAGE	32
33								TOTALS MONTH TO DATE	33

COLUMN A   COLUMN B   COLUMN C   COLUMN D   COLUMN E

MEMO _____
_____
_____
_____

DAILY-FROM LINE 31

ARITHMETIC POSTING PROOF	
Column E	
Plus Column A	
Sub-Total	
Minus Column B	
Sub-Total	
Minus Column C	
Equals Column D	

Box 1

MONTH-FROM LINE 31

ARITHMETIC POSTING PROOF	
Accts. Receivable Previous Day	$
Plus Column A	
Sub-Total	
Minus Column B	
Sub-Total	
Minus Column C	
Accts. Receivable End ofDay	

Box 2

(Courtesy of Bibbero Systems, Inc., Petaluma, Calif. [800] 242-2376 fax [800] 242-9330; www.bibbero.com.)

1137

Notes

Procedure 44-5: Use Computerized Office Billing System. Create and print two patient ledgers and one patient day sheet using a computer billing system such as Medisoft.

Procedure 44-6: Writing a Check. Write checks to pay the following bills beginning with check number 1837 found on p. 1141. Use today's date. The beginning balance brought forward is $4,482.21. Complete each check stub.
a. Write a check for $822.00 to Mitchell Associates for rent.
b. Write a check for $329.62 to ABC Pharmacy for medical supplies.
c. Write a check for $219.64 to Holt Office Supply for office supplies.

Procedure 44-7: Preparing a Bank Deposit. Prepare a bank deposit slip for the checks received from June Simmons, Robert Underwood, and Standard Health HMO (for Marie Richards). Use today's date. Place the practice name (Western Medical Center) on the deposit slip found on p. 1143.

Procedure 44-8: Reconciling a Bank Deposit. Reconcile a bank statement using the form on p. 1145 based on the following information.

The new balance identified by the bank is $4,179.30. Two deposits are shown in your register but not on this statement, namely $254.00 and $48.91. There are three outstanding checks for $822.00, $329.62, and $219.64.

Procedure 44-9: Creating and Maintaining a Petty Cash Fund. Set up a petty cash fund in the petty cash log on p. 1147 assuming that the office cashed a check for $100.00 to establish the fund on 10/2/XX. Enter the following disbursements and keep a running balance:

10/3/XX	Postage due	$ 1.13
10/4/XX	AAA batteries	$ 5.98
10/6/XX	Refreshments for staff meeting	$32.50
10/10/XX	Cleaning supplies	$15.28
10/25/XX	Coffee and donuts	$16.50
10/26/XX	Parking for Dr. Green (visitor)	$ 8.00

Write receipts for the last two entries (also on p. 1147), assuming that you are the petty cash fund manager, and you bought the coffee and donuts.

On 11/2/XX, enter an amount to bring the petty cash fund to its original balance.

Notes

1837

DATE _____
TO _____
FOR _____

BALANCE BROUGHT FORWARD		
DEPOSITS		
BALANCE		
AMT THIS CK		
BALANCE CARRIED FORWARD		

BLACKBURN PRIMARY CARE ASSOCIATES, PC
1990 Turquiose Drive
Blackburn, WI 54937
608-459-8857

1837

94-72/1224

DATE _____

PAY TO THE
ORDER OF _____ $ _____

_____ DOLLARS

DERBYSHIRE SAVINGS Member FDIC
P.O. BOX 8923
Blackburn, WI 54937

FOR _____

⑈055003⑈ ⑊44678201⑊⑈ 678800470

1838

DATE _____
TO _____
FOR _____

BALANCE BROUGHT FORWARD		
DEPOSITS		
BALANCE		
AMT THIS CK		
BALANCE CARRIED FORWARD		

BLACKBURN PRIMARY CARE ASSOCIATES, PC
1990 Turquiose Drive
Blackburn, WI 54937
608-459-8857

1838

94-72/1224

DATE _____

PAY TO THE
ORDER OF _____ $ _____

_____ DOLLARS

DERBYSHIRE SAVINGS Member FDIC
P.O. BOX 8923
Blackburn, WI 54937

FOR _____

⑈055003⑈ ⑊44678201⑊⑈ 678800470

1839

DATE _____
TO _____
FOR _____

BALANCE BROUGHT FORWARD		
DEPOSITS		
BALANCE		
AMT THIS CK		
BALANCE CARRIED FORWARD		

BLACKBURN PRIMARY CARE ASSOCIATES, PC
1990 Turquiose Drive
Blackburn, WI 54937
608-459-8857

1839

94-72/1224

DATE _____

PAY TO THE
ORDER OF _____ $ _____

_____ DOLLARS

DERBYSHIRE SAVINGS Member FDIC
P.O. BOX 8923
Blackburn, WI 54937

FOR _____

⑈055003⑈ ⑊44678201⑊⑈ 678800470

(From Hunt SA: *Saunders fundamentals of medical assisting student mastery manual,* St. Louis, 2007, Saunders.)

Notes

DEPOSIT TICKET

BANK OF OHIO
223 MAIN STREET
WESTERN, OH 44770

DATE: _____

	DOLLARS	CENTS
CURRENCY		
COIN		
CHECKS (LIST SEPARATELY)		
1		
2		
3		
4		
5		
6		
7		
8		
9		
10		
11		
12		
13		
14		
15		
16		
17		
18		
19		
20		
TOTAL FROM ATTACHED LIST:		
TOTAL		

Total Deposit

Total Items

⑈50 ⅎ0000001⑈: 007387720⑆9⑆"

Notes

THIS WORKSHEET IS PROVIDED TO HELP YOU BALANCE YOUR ACCOUNT

1. Go through your register and mark each check, withdrawal, Express ATM transaction, payment, deposit or other credit listed on this statement. Be sure that your register shows any interest paid into your account, and any service charges, automatic payments, or Express Transfers withdrawn from your account during this statement period.

2. Using the chart below, list any outstanding checks, Express ATM withdrawals, payments or any other withdrawals (including any from previous months) that are listed in your register but are not shown on this statement.

3. Balance your account by filling in the spaces below.

ITEMS OUTSTANDING		
NUMBER	**AMOUNT**	
TOTAL	**$**	

ENTER

The NEW BALANCE shown on
this statement_____$

ADD

Any deposits listed in your register $
or transfers into your account $
which are not shown on this $
statement.   +$ _____

           TOTAL

CALCULATE THE SUBTOTAL_____$

SUBTRACT

The total outstanding checks and
withdrawals from the chart at left_____-$

CALCULATE THE ENDING BALANCE

This amount should be the same
as the current balance shown in
your check register_____$

(From Hunt SA: *Saunders fundamentals of medical assisting student mastery manual,* St. Louis, 2007, Saunders.)

Notes

Chapter **44** **Managing Practice Finances**

Petty Cash Log

Date	Description	Cash In	Cash Out	Balance

Petty Cash Receipt   Date: _____ No. 5

Description:	
Received By:	
Approved By:	
Amount:	

Petty Cash Receipt   Date: _____ No. 6

Description:	
Received By:	
Approved By:	

Notes

Procedure 44-1: Completing a Patient Charge Slip

Name: _____ Date: _____

Evaluated by: _____ Score: _____

Performance Objective

Outcome:	Complete a patient charge slip.
Conditions:	Given the following: blank charge slip, patient information form or computer data, daily patient schedule, calculator, and fee schedule.
Standards:	Time: 5 minutes. Student completed procedure in _____ minutes.
	Accuracy: Satisfactory score on the Performance Evaluation Checklist.

Performance Evaluation Checklist

Trial 1	Trial 2	Point Value	Performance Standards
		●	Completed the top part of a patient charge slip manually, using a computer, or by printing a label from the computer.
		●	Verified that the patient's name, date of birth, insurance, insurance group and ID numbers, and name of the subscriber have been entered or have printed correctly.
		●	Entered the patient's previous balance on the bottom of the charge slip.
		●	Used the fee schedule to fill in the fee in the box beside the code and name of each procedure performed during the office visit.
		●	Completed the bottom of the charge slip by entering the total charges, payments, and any adjustments.
		●	Totaled the new balance at the bottom of the charge slip correctly.
		●	Completed any other information requested on the charge slip.
		✶	Completed the entire charge slip accurately.
		✶	Completed the procedure within 5 minutes.
			TOTALS

Evaluation of Student Performance

EVALUATION CRITERIA			COMMENTS
Symbol	Category	Point Value	
✶	Critical Step	16 points	
●	Essential Step	6 points	
▷	Theory Question	2 points	

Score calculation: 100 points

      −   points missed

         Score

Satisfactory score: 85 or above

CAAHEP Competencies Achieved

Psychomotor (Skills)
☑ VI. 2. b. Perform billing procedures.

ABHES Competencies Achieved

☑ 8. i. Perform billing and collection procedures.
☑ 8. v. Use physician fee schedule.
☑ 8. w. Use manual or computerized bookkeeping systems.

Procedure 44-2: Posting Charges

Name: _____   Date: _____

Evaluated by: _____   Score: _____

Performance Objective

Outcome:	Post charges to the patient account.
Conditions:	Given the following: patient charge slip, patient ledger card or computer account, fee schedule, and pen and/or computer.
Standards:	Time: 5 minutes. Student completed procedure in _____ minutes.
	Accuracy: Satisfactory score on the Performance Evaluation Checklist.

Performance Evaluation Checklist

Trial 1	Trial 2	Point Value	Performance Standards
		●	Posted total charges in the column labeled "charges" of a manual ledger card or the first charge on the first line of a transaction entry screen in a computer program.
		●	If using a computer system, posted each additional charge on a new line.
		●	If using a manual system, entered the total charge in the balance column. If using a computer system, saved work after all charges were posted.
		✳	Entered the charges and calculated the new balance accurately.
		✳	Completed the procedure within 5 minutes.
			TOTALS

Evaluation of Student Performance

EVALUATION CRITERIA			COMMENTS
Symbol	Category	Point Value	
✶	Critical Step	16 points	
●	Essential Step	6 points	
▷	Theory Question	2 points	

Score calculation: 100 points

− _____ points missed

_____ Score

Satisfactory score: 85 or above

CAAHEP Competencies Achieved

Psychomotor (Skills)

☑ VI. 2. b. Perform billing procedures.

ABHES Competencies Achieved

☑ 8. i. Perform billing and collection procedures.

☑ 8. k. Perform accounts receivable procedures.

☑ 8. w. Use manual or computerized bookkeeping systems.

Procedure 44-3: Posting Charges

Name: _____   Date: _____

Evaluated by: _____   Score: _____

Performance Objective

Outcome:	Post payments and/or adjustments.
Conditions:	Given the following: Patient ledger card or computer account, cash or check from the patient or check from the insurance carrier, calculator, stamp with a restrictive endorsement, stamp pad, and pen.
Standards:	Time: 5 minutes. Student completed procedure in _____ minutes.
	Accuracy: Satisfactory score on the Performance Evaluation Checklist.

Performance Evaluation Checklist

Trial 1	Trial 2	Point Value	Performance Standards
		●	Located the patient account in the computer or selected the patient ledger card.
		●	Posted a payment from a completed patient charge slip to the patient account accurately using the same line or screen as the charges for that day.
		●	Included the check number in a manual system or used the correct code for a patient payment in a computer system.
		●	Posted an insurance payment under the date the payment was received.
		●	Used a new line for an insurance payment in a manual system and a new transaction entry screen or a payment screen in a computer system.
		●	Used the correct code or designation for an insurance payment.
		●	Entered the amount excluded by the insurance carrier as a credit adjustment in the adjustment column of a manual system and using the code for insurance write off in a computer system.
		●	Calculated or verified the patient balance and saved work in a computer system.
		✱	Posted payment and any adjustment accurately, and calculated correct new patient balance.
		●	Endorsed a check using a stamp with the restrictive endorsement "For deposit only" and the number of the checking account.
		●	Placed a processed check or cash in the designated drawer or money box.
		✱	Completed the procedure within 5 minutes.
		TOTALS	

EVALUATION CRITERIA			COMMENTS
Symbol	**Category**	**Point Value**	
✶	Critical Step	16 points	
●	Essential Step	6 points	
▷	Theory Question	2 points	

Score calculation: 100 points

− _____ points missed

_____ Score

Satisfactory score: 85 or above

CAAHEP Competencies Achieved

Psychomotor (Skills)

☑ VI. 2. b. Perform billing procedures.
☑ VI. 2. d. Post adjustments.

ABHES Competencies Achieved

☑ 8. i. Perform billing and collection procedures.
☑ 8. k. Perform accounts receivable procedures.
☑ 8. m. Post adjustments.
☑ 8. w. Use manual or computerized bookkeeping systems.

Procedure 44-4: Recording a Patient's Visit on the Day Sheet

Name: _____   Date: _____

Evaluated by: _____   Score: _____

Performance Objective

Outcome:	Post charges, payments and adjustments on a day sheet.
Conditions:	Given the following: day sheet, day sheet from the previous day, charge slips, ledger cards (optional), checks, and pen.
Standards:	Time: 10 minutes. Student completed procedure in _____ minutes.
	Accuracy: Satisfactory score on the Performance Evaluation Checklist.

Performance Evaluation Checklist

Trial 1	Trial 2	Point Value	Performance Standards
		●	Placed the day sheet on the pegboard and dated the day sheet and deposit itemization.
		●	If using pegboard receipts, laid a bank of patient receipts on the pegs so that the top receipt lined up with the first line of the day sheet.
		●	Entered information for a patient appointment on the first blank line in ink including the name of the patient, code(s) for professional services, total charge, payment, any adjustment, new balance, and old balance.
		●	Completed columns on the right side of the day sheet according to office policy (such as tracking for individual physicians).
		●	Entered information for the charges for each patient in the order that the patient was seen.
		●	Recorded each payment received in the mail on a separate line on the day sheet and in the patient computer account when the mail was processed.
		●	Recorded insurance adjustments with insurance payments as needed.
		●	Recorded payments made at the time of an office visit and payments received in the mail on the corresponding line of the deposit itemization at the far right of the day sheet.
		✳	Completed all entries on the day sheet accurately.
		✳	Completed the procedure within 10 minutes.
			TOTALS

Evaluation of Student Performance

EVALUATION CRITERIA			COMMENTS
Symbol	**Category**	**Point Value**	
✱	Critical Step	16 points	
●	Essential Step	6 points	
▷	Theory Question	2 points	

Score calculation: 100 points

−   _____ points missed

_____ Score

Satisfactory score: 85 or above

CAAHEP Competencies Achieved

Psychomotor (Skills)

☑ VI. 2. a. Post entries on a day sheet.

ABHES Competencies Achieved

☑ 8. h. Post entries on a day sheet.

Procedure 44-5: Using a Computerized Office Billing System

Name: _____   Date: _____

Evaluated by: _____   Score: _____

Performance Objective

Outcome:	Utilize a computerized office billing system to view and print reports such as a patient ledger and/or a day sheet.
Conditions:	Given the following: computer, computer billing program.
Standards:	Time: 10 minutes. Student completed procedure in _____ minutes.
	Accuracy: Satisfactory score on the Performance Evaluation Checklist.

Performance Evaluation Checklist

Trial 1	Trial 2	Point Value	Performance Standards
		●	Made sure the computer billing system was open or opened the computer billing program.
		●	To view or print a patient ledger, selected the patient leger function from the reports menu.
		●	Selected the desired range of patients, range of dates, range of providers or other criteria to create a report with the desired information.
		●	Reviewed the report for completeness, using arrows as needed to view all pages.
		●	Printed a hard copy by clicking the printer icon.
		●	To create a computer day sheet, selected patient day sheet or daily journal from the reports menu.
		●	Selected the desired range and previewed the report.
		●	Printed a hard copy by clicking the printer icon.
		●	Created additional reports as needed.
		★	Completed the procedure within 10 minutes.
			TOTALS

Evaluation of Student Performance

EVALUATION CRITERIA			COMMENTS
Symbol	**Category**	**Point Value**	
✸	Critical Step	16 points	
●	Essential Step	6 points	
▷	Theory Question	2 points	

Score calculation: 100 points
  − _____ points missed
    _____
    ___ Score

Satisfactory score: 85 or above

CAAHEP Competencies Achieved

Psychomotor (Skills)
☑ VI. 3. Utilize computerized office billing system.

ABHES Competencies Achieved

☑ 8. w. Use manual or computerized bookkeeping systems.

Procedure 44-6: Writing a Check

Name: _____   Date: _____

Evaluated by: _____   Score: _____

Performance Objective

Outcome:	Write a check, and record and calculate new account balance.
Conditions:	Given the following: checks, check register or check stubs, bill to be paid, and pen.
Standards:	Time: 5 minutes. Student completed procedure in _____ minutes.
	Accuracy: Satisfactory score on the Performance Evaluation Checklist.

Performance Evaluation Checklist

Trial 1	Trial 2	Point Value	Performance Standards
		●	Selected a bill to be paid.
		●	Using a pen, wrote the date on the date line.
		●	Wrote the name of the payee on the correct line.
		●	Wrote the amount of the check in numbers in the box next to the dollar sign.
		●	Used a decimal between the number of dollars and the number of cents.
		●	Wrote the amount of the check in words on the line below the name of the payee correctly.
		●	Expressed the number of cents as a fraction over 100.
		●	Drew a line from the end of the fraction to the word "dollars."
		●	Wrote the invoice number, account number, and/or purpose of the check on the memo line.
		●	Completed the checkbook stub or register including the date, check number, payee, amount of the check, and reason for the check.
		●	Added any deposits since the previous check and entered the new balance.
		●	Subtracted the amount of the check from the previous balance and entered the balance carried forward.
		●	Drew a single line through a minor mistake, corrected the error, and initialed the correction.

1159

Trial 1	Trial 2	Point Value	Performance Standards
		✶	Wrote the check for the correct amount using the correct format with minor corrections as necessary.
		●	Wrote "void" across the any check with a major mistake and entered "void" on the check stub or in the check register.
		●	Placed a voided check in the folder with accounts payable records.
		●	Prepared an envelope to mail the payment (or used the envelope supplied by the vendor).
		●	Clipped the prepared check to the envelope with the payment slip and placed in the designated place for review and signature by the physician authorized to sign office checks.
		✶	Completed the procedure within 5 minutes.
			TOTALS

Evaluation of Student Performance

EVALUATION CRITERIA			COMMENTS
Symbol	**Category**	**Point Value**	
✶	Critical Step	16 points	
●	Essential Step	6 points	
▷	Theory Question	2 points	

Score calculation: 100 points

     −   _____ points missed

         _____ Score

Satisfactory score: 85 or above

ABHES Competencies Achieved

☑ 8. j. Perform accounts payable procedures.

EVALUATION OF COMPETENCY

Procedure 44-7: Preparing a Bank Deposit

Name: _____   Date: _____

Evaluated by: _____   Score: _____

Performance objective

Outcome:	Prepare a bank deposit.
Conditions:	Given the following: account deposit slip, deposit itemization record from a day sheet (optional), cash and checks received as payments, calculator, and bank deposit envelope or bag.
Standards:	Time: 10 minutes. Student completed procedure in _____ minutes.
	Accuracy: Satisfactory score on the Performance Evaluation Checklist.

Performance Evaluation Checklist

Trial 1	Trial 2	Point Value	Performance Standards
		●	Obtained an account deposit slip and placed a date on it. If using the deposit itemization from a day sheet, wrote the name of the medical practice and the account number.
		●	Counted any currency and coins, and entered the totals on the correct line of the deposit slip.
		●	Stamped each check with a restrictive endorsement (if not already done).
		●	Wrote the amount of each check on a separate line of the bank deposit detail, or verified that each check was entered on the daysheet deposit itemization record.
		●	Used the numerator of the fractional ABA number, check number or name on the checking account to identify each check on the itemization.
		●	Totaled all checks and entered the total correctly.
		✱	Totaled the cash and check amounts and entered as the total amount of the bank deposit.
		●	Verified that the total deposit was equal to the amount in the payments column on the day sheet (minus any credit card payments).
		●	Made a copy of the deposit slip and deposit itemization.
		●	Placed the cash, checks, deposit slip, and deposit itemization (if separate) in a bank envelope or bank deposit bag.
		●	Recorded the amount of the deposit in the check register or on the check stub nearest to the date of deposit.
		●	Recorded the amount of the deposit in the accounts payable record according to office policy.

1161

Trial 1	Trial 2	Point Value	Performance Standards
		●	Filed the copy of the bank deposit and bank deposit itemization as well as the bank deposit receipt after making the deposit.
		✶	Completed the procedure within 10 minutes.
			TOTALS

Evaluation of Student Performance

EVALUATION CRITERIA			COMMENTS
Symbol	**Category**	**Point Value**	
✶	Critical Step	16 points	
●	Essential Step	6 points	
▷	Theory Question	2 points	

Score calculation: 100 points

−   points missed
_____
____ Score

Satisfactory score: 85 or above

CAAHEP Competencies Achieved

Psychomotor (Skills)
☑ VI. 1. Prepare a bank deposit.

ABHES Competencies Achieved

☑ 8. k. Perform accounts receivable procedures.

Procedure 44-8: Reconciling a Bank Statement

Name: _____   Date: _____

Evaluated by: _____   Score: _____

Performance Objective

Outcome:	Reconcile a bank statement.
Conditions:	Given the following: monthly bank statement, checkbook, check stubs or check register, calculator, and pen.
Standards:	Time: 15 minutes. Student completed procedure in _____ minutes.
	Accuracy: Satisfactory score on the Performance Evaluation Checklist.

Performance Evaluation Checklist

Trial 1	Trial 2	Point Value	Performance Standards
		●	Located the ending balance and the list of checks and deposits on the current bank statement.
		●	Located the same time period in the checkbook register or check stubs.
		●	Checked the checkbook register against the bank statement, placing a check mark against each check and deposit recorded on the bank statement.
		●	Noted any checks or deposits in the check register that did not appear on the bank statement.
		●	Recorded any service charges, ATM charges, or other additional charges on the bank statements in the checkbook register or on a check stub and subtracted it from the account balance.
		●	Entered any credit such as interest in the checkbook register or on a check stub and added it to the account balance.
		●	Used the bank reconciliation form to balance the account.
		●	Entered the bank's ending balance.
		●	Added any deposits listed on the check register that were not listed on the bank statement.
		●	Subtracted any outstanding checks from the subtotal.
		●	Compared to the checkbook register or last check stub.
		✳	If the total did not equal the account balance in the checkbook register, recalculated until the error was found.
		✳	Completed the procedure within 15 minutes.
			TOTALS

Chapter **44** **Managing Practice Finances**

Evaluation of Student Performance

EVALUATION CRITERIA			COMMENTS
Symbol	**Category**	**Point Value**	
★	Critical Step	16 points	
●	Essential Step	6 points	
▷	Theory Question	2 points	

Score calculation: 100 points

            −   points missed

            _____

            ___ Score

Satisfactory score: 85 or above

ABHES Competencies Achieved

☑ 8. g. Prepare and reconcile a bank statement and deposit record.

Procedure 44-9: Creating and Maintaining a Petty Cash Fund

Name: _____ Date: _____

Evaluated by: _____ Score: _____

Performance Objective

Outcome:	Create and maintain a petty cash log
Conditions:	Given the following: bag or box with a lock, receipt slips, pen, petty cash log sheet, computer (optional).
Standards:	Time: 15 minutes. Student completed procedure in _____ minutes.
	Accuracy: Satisfactory score on the Performance Evaluation Checklist.

Performance Evaluation Checklist

Trial 1	Trial 2	Point Value	Performance Standards
		●	Set aside a predetermined amount such as $100.00 in a locked bag or box.
		●	Designated a petty cash fund manager to hold the key to the petty cash bag or box.
		●	Approved and completed all petty cash requests, including the date, amount, and reason for the request.
		●	Recorded all transactions on the petty cash log.
		●	Replenished the fund to its designated amount weekly or monthly according to office policy.
		●	Counted the cash to be sure it contained the correct amount and gave the old log and receipts to the accountant when starting a new log.
		★	Completed the procedure within 15 minutes.
			TOTALS

Evaluation of Student Performance

EVALUATION CRITERIA			COMMENTS
Symbol	**Category**	**Point Value**	
★	Critical Step	16 points	
●	Essential Step	6 points	
▷	Theory Question	2 points	

Score calculation: 100 points

      −   _____ points missed

             ___ Score

Satisfactory score: 85 or above

ABHES Competencies Achieved

☑ 8. 1. Establish and maintain a petty cash fund.

45 Medical Coding

CHAPTER ASSIGNMENTS

√ After Completing	Date Due	Textbook Pages	TEXTBOOK ASSIGNMENTS	Possible Points	Points You Earned
		1063-1082	Read Chapter 45: Medical Coding		
		1072 1080	Read Case Study 1 Case Study 1 questions	5	
		1072 1081	Read Case Study 2 Case Study 2 questions	5	
		1079 1081	Read Case Study 3 Case Study 3 questions	5	
			TOTAL POINTS		

√ After Completing	Date Due	Study Guide Pages	STUDY GUIDE ASSIGNMENTS (CTA = Critical Thinking Activity)	Possible Points	Points You Earned
		1171	Pretest	10	
		1172	Term Key Term Assessment	11	
		1172-1175	Evaluation of Learning questions	33	
		1175-1176	CTA A: Evaluation and Management Codes	10	
		1176-1178	CTA B: CPT Codes	40	
		1178	CTA C: HCPCS Codes	10	
		1179-1180	CTA D: Diagnosis Codes	100	
		1181	CTA E: Code Format	8	
			Evolve Site: Guided Practice: Assigning CPT Codes	10	
			Evolve Site: Guided Practice: Assigning ICD-9 Codes	10	
			Evolve Site: Apply Your Knowledge questions	10	
		1171	Posttest	10	

√ After Completing	Date Due	Study Guide Pages	STUDY GUIDE ASSIGNMENTS (CTA = Critical Thinking Activity)	Possible Points	Points You Earned
			ADDITIONAL ASSIGNMENTS		
			TOTAL POINTS		

√ When Assigned By Your Instructor	Study Guide Pages	Practices Required	LABORATORY ASSIGNMENTS (Procedure Number and Name)	Score*
	1183	3	**Practice for Competency** 45-1: Performing CPT Coding Textbook reference: pp. 1070-1071	
	1185-1186		**Evaluation of Competency** 45-1: Performing CPT Coding	*
	1183	3	**Practice for Competency** 45-2: Performing HCPCS Coding Textbook reference: p. 1072	
	1187-1188		**Evaluation of Competency** 45-2: Performing CPT Coding	*
	1183	3	**Practice for Competency** 45-3: Performing ICD Coding Textbook reference: pp. 1079-1080	
	1189-1190		**Evaluation of Competency** 45-3: Performing ICD Coding	*
			ADDITIONAL ASSIGNMENTS	

Notes

Procedure 45-1: Performing CPT Coding

Name: _____ Date: _____

Evaluated by: _____ Score: _____

Performance Objective

Outcome:	Perform CPT coding for procedures
Conditions:	Given the following: charge slip or procedure to look up code for, medical record, and CPT manual.
Standards:	Time: 5 minutes. Student completed procedure in _____ minutes.
	Accuracy: Satisfactory score on the Performance Evaluation Checklist.

Performance Evaluation Checklist

Trial 1	Trial 2	Point Value	Performance Standards
		●	Found name of procedure to look up from charge slip or other document.
		●	Determined any necessary additional information from the patient's medical record.
		●	For evaluation and management services, identified if the patient is a new patient or an established patient.
		●	For evaluation and management services, identified the location where the patient was seen.
		●	Located the name of the procedure in the index.
		●	From the information in the index, located the correct range of codes in the list of codes.
		▷	Stated the reason for coding from the list of codes instead of the index.
		✶	Selected the correct code from the list of codes
		●	If the service was unusual, decided if a modifier was needed.
		✶	Selected the correct modifier, if one was needed
		●	Entered the correct code on the charge slip, on any other document, and in the computer as needed.
		✶	Completed the procedure within 5 minutes.
			TOTALS

Evaluation of Student Performance

EVALUATION CRITERIA			COMMENTS
Symbol	**Category**	**Point Value**	
✶	Critical Step	16 points	
●	Essential Step	6 points	
▷	Theory Question	2 points	

Score calculation: 100 points

− _____ points missed

_____

____ Score

Satisfactory score: 85 or above

CAAHEP Competencies Achieved

Psychomotor (Skills)

☑ VIII. 1. Perform procedural coding.

ABHES Competencies Achieved

☑ 8. t. Perform diagnostic and procedural coding.

EVALUATION OF COMPETENCY

Procedure 45-2: Performing HCPCS Coding

Name: _____   Date: _____

Evaluated by: _____   Score: _____

Performance Objective

Outcome:	Perform HCPCS coding for services or equipment
Conditions:	Given the following: charge slip or procedure to look up code for, medical record, and HCPCS manual.
Standards:	Time: 5 minutes. Student completed procedure in _____ minutes.
	Accuracy: Satisfactory score on the performance Evaluation Checklist

Performance Evaluation Checklist

Trial 1	Trial 2	Point Value	Performance Standards
		●	Found name of service or item to look up from charge slip or other document.
		●	Determined any necessary additional information from the patient's medical record.
		●	Located the name of the service or item in the index. Found name of medication in the Table of Drugs.
		●	From the information in the index, located the correct code or range of codes in the list of codes.
		▷	Stated the reason for coding from the list of codes instead of the index.
		★	Selected the correct code from the list of codes
		●	Validated that the code was appropriate for the patient's insurance.
		●	Entered the correct code on the charge slip, on any other document, and in the computer as needed.
		★	Completed the procedure within 5 minutes.
			TOTALS

EVALUATION CRITERIA			COMMENTS
Symbol	Category	Point Value	
✱	Critical Step	16 points	
●	Essential Step	6 points	
▷	Theory Question	2 points	

Score calculation: 100 points

     −   points missed

         Score

Satisfactory score: 85 or above

CAAHEP Competencies Achieved

Psychomotor (Skills)

☑ III. C. 3. c. (3) (c): Perform procedural coding.

ABHES Competencies Achieved

☑ 8. t. Perform diagnostic and procedure coding.

Procedure 45-3: Performing ICD Coding

Name: _____ Date: _____

Evaluated by: _____ Score: _____

Performance Objective

Outcome:	Perform ICD-10-CM coding for a patient's diagnosis
Conditions:	Given the following: charge slip or diagnosis to look up code for, medical record, and an ICD-9-CM or ICD-10-CM manual.
Standards:	Time: 5 minutes. Student completed procedure in _____ minutes.
	Accuracy: Satisfactory score on the Performance Evaluation Checklist.

Performance Evaluation Checklist

Trial 1	Trial 2	Point Value	Performance Standards
		●	Found diagnosis to look up from charge slip or other document.
		●	Determined any necessary additional information from the patient's medical record.
		●	Decided on the key word or phrase to look for in the alphabetic index.
		●	Looked under as many terms as necessary to locate the diagnosis in the alphabetic index.
		●	From the information in the index, located the correct range of codes to look under in the tabular list.
		▷	Stated the reason for coding from the tabular list instead of the index.
		●	Checked all potential codes against the diagnosis to identify the most specific code.
		●	If there was a list of possible fifth (ICD-9-CM) or seven (ICD-10-CM) characters, selected the most specific letter to use as a final character
		✶	Selected the correct code from the list of codes.
		●	Entered the correct code on the charge slip, on any other document, and in the computer as needed.
		✶	Completed the procedure within 5 minutes.
			TOTALS

EVALUATION CRITERIA			COMMENTS
Symbol	Category	Point Value	
✱	Critical Step	16 points	
●	Essential Step	6 points	
▷	Theory Question	2 points	

Score calculation: 100 points

     –   _____ points missed

          ___ Score

Satisfactory score: 85 or above

CAAHEP Competencies Achieved

Psychomotor (Skills)

☑ VIII. 2. Perform diagnostic coding.

ABHES Competencies Achieved

☑ 8. t. Perform diagnostic and procedure coding.

46 Medical Insurance

√ After Completing	Date Due	Textbook Pages	TEXTBOOK ASSIGNMENTS	Possible Points	Points You Earned
		1083-1106	Read Chapter 46: Medical Insurance		
		1088 1103	Read Case Study 1 Case Study 1 questions	5	
		1100 1103	Read Case Study 2 Case Study 2 questions	5	
		1101 1104	Read Case Study 3 Case Study 3 questions	5	
			TOTAL POINTS		

√ After Completing	Date Due	Study Guide Pages	STUDY GUIDE ASSIGNMENTS (CTA = Critical Thinking Activity)	Possible Points	Points You Earned
		1195	Pretest	10	
		1196 1197	Key Term Assessment: A. General Insurance Terms B. Insurance Plans and Methods of Reimbursement	25 10	
		1198-1201	Evaluation of Learning questions	33	
		1202	CTA A: Primary and Secondary Insurance	10	
		1203	CTA B: Managed Care Plans	5	
		1203	CTA C: The Insurance Claim Form	10	
			Evolve Site: Guided Practice: Obtaining a Managed Care Referral	10	
			Evolve Site: Guided Practice: Completing a Health Insurance Claim Form: Patient/Insured Section	10	
			Evolve Site: Guided Practice: Completing a Health Insurance Claim Form: Physician/Supplier Portion	10	

√ After Completing	Date Due	Textbook Pages	TEXTBOOK ASSIGNMENTS	Possible Points	Points You Earned
			Evolve Site: Apply Your Knowledge questions	10	
			Evolve Site: Video Evaluation	12	
		1195	Posttest	10	
			ADDITIONAL ASSIGNMENTS		
			TOTAL POINTS		

1192

√ When Assigned By Your Instructor	Study Guide Pages	Practices Required	LABORATORY ASSIGNMENTS (Procedure Number and Name)	Score*
	1205	1	**Practice for Competency** 46-1: Applying Managed Care Policies and Procedures Textbook reference: p. 1092	
	1211-1212		**Evaluation of Competency** 46-1: Applying Managed Care Policies and Procedures	*
	1205-1207	3	**Practice for Competency** 46-2: Obtaining Insurance Preauthorization (Precertification) Textbook reference: p. 1094	
	1213-1214		**Evaluation of Competency** 46-2: Obtaining Insurance Preauthorization (Precertification)	*
	1207-1210	3	**Practice for Competency** 46-3: Completing/Reviewing the CMS-1500 Insurance Claim Form Textbook reference: pp. 1097-1099	
	1215-1217		**Evaluation of Competency** 46-3: Completing/Reviewing the CMS-1500 Insurance Claim Form	*
			ADDITIONAL ASSIGNMENTS	

Notes

Procedure 46-1 Applying Managed Care Policies and Procedures

Name: _____ Date: _____

Evaluated by: _____ Score: _____

Performance Objective

Outcome:	Apply managed care policies and procedures
Conditions:	Given the following: managed care handbooks, managed care contract, username and password for managed care web site.
Standards:	Time: 30 minutes. Student completed procedure in _____ minutes.
	Accuracy: Satisfactory score on the Performance Evaluation Checklist.

Performance Evaluation Checklist

Trial 1	Trial 2	Point Value	Performance Standards
		●	Assembled information to review policies and procedures for a specific managed care organization
		●	Signed in to the managed care organization's web site and/or used the contract and handbooks to read about requirements for the managed care organization.
		●	Became familiar with different plans offered by a managed care organization.
		▷	Simulated instructing a patient about laboratories that could be used for a specfic insurance plan.
		●	Became familiar with the preferred method to verify eligibility, notify the plan about procedures or treatments and obtain preauthorization or precertification.
		▷	Described the preferred method to notify a specific plan about surgery and obtain preauthorization or precertifiction.
		●	Reviewed forms used by the managed care organization.
		▷	Explained the importance of following the same process to become familiar with the guidelines of each managed care organization that a practice is affiliated with
		●	Made a note of the process for obtaining additional information if questions should arise.
		●	Followed the guidelines for each managed care organization before providing services that require notification or authorization, when submitting insurance claims and when answering patient questions about insurance.
		●	Demonstrated sensitivity when communicating with both providers and patients.
		●	Communicated with patients about their managed care plans in terms the patient could understand.
		★	Completed the procedure within 30 minutes.
			TOTALS

EVALUATION CRITERIA			COMMENTS
Symbol	Category	Point Value	
✶	Critical Step	16 points	
●	Essential Step	6 points	
▷	Theory Question	2 points	

Score calculation: 100 points

      − _____ points missed

      _____ Score

Satisfactory score: 85 or above

CAAHEP Competencies Achieved

Psychomotor (Skills)

☑ VII. 1. Apply both managed care policies and procedures.

Affective (Behavior)

☑ VII. 2. Demonstrate sensitivity in communicating with both providers and patients.
☑ VII. 3. Communicate in language the patient can understand regarding managed care and insurance plans.

ABHES Competencies Achieved

☑ 8. r. Apply third party guidelines.

Procedure 46-2: Obtaining Insurance Preauthorization (Precertification)

Name: _____   Date: _____

Evaluated by: _____   Score: _____

Performance Objective

Outcome:	Obtain insurance preauthorization (precertification).
Conditions:	Given the following: patient medical record, patient insurance information, physician's directions about the service to be provided, electronic or paper preauthorization (precertification) request form, pen, telephone
Standards:	Time: 15 minutes. Student completed procedure in _____ minutes.
	Accuracy: Satisfactory score on the Performance Evaluation Checklist

Performance Evaluation Checklist

Trial 1	Trial 2	Point Value	Performance Standards
		●	Assembled information to request preauthorization (precertification) • Patient demographic information • Patient insurance information • Information about service to be provided including diagnosis code(s) and procedure code(s) • Forms as needed • Pen, computer • Telephone (optional)
		●	Assembled additional information including physician's NPI number.
		●	Completed preauthorization or precerification form, or called the patient's insurance carrier and provided all information requested.
		●	Submitted from electronically or by mail as appropriate.
		●	Informed the patient that he or she could not obtain service until the preauthorization/precertification was approved by the insurance company.
		●	When approval was received, notified the patient, instructed the patient to schedule the service, and sent a copy as needed to any other physician or provider of service.
		●	Filed a copy of the approval form in the patient's medical record.
		✶	Completed the procedure within 15 minutes.
			TOTALS

EVALUATION CRITERIA			COMMENTS
Symbol	**Category**	**Point Value**	
✱	Critical Step	16 points	
●	Essential Step	6 points	
▷	Theory Question	2 points	

Score calculation: 100 points

            −   points missed
            _____
            ____ Score

Satisfactory score: 85 or above

CAAHEP Competencies Achieved

Psychomotor (Skills)
☑ VII. 4. Obtain precertification including documentation.
☑ VII. 5. Obtain preauthorization including documentation.
☑ VII. 6. Verify eligibility for managed care services.

Affective (Behavior)
☑ VII. 1. Demonstrate assertive communication with managed care and/or insurance providers.
☑ VII. 2. Demonstrate sensitivity in communicating with both providers and patients.
☑ VII. 3. Communicate in language the patient can understand regarding managed care and insurance plans.

ABHES Competencies Achieved

☑ 8. s. Obtain managed care referrals and precertification.

EVALUATION OF COMPETENCY

Procedure 46-3: Completing/Reviewing the CMS-1500 Insurance Claim Form

Name: _____   Date: _____

Evaluated by: _____   Score: _____

Performance Objective

Outcome:	Complete (or review) a CMS-1500 insurance claim form.
Conditions:	Given the following: patient information form or computer screen, patient account or ledger, photocopy of patient's insurance card, insurance claim form, computer with medical billing program, printer, and pen.
Standards:	Time: 15 minutes. Student completed procedure in _____ minutes. Accuracy: Satisfactory score on the Performance Evaluation Checklist.

Performance Evaluation Checklist

Trial 1	Trial 2	Point Value	Performance Standards
		●	Assembled information and supplies.
		●	If creating a paper claim, used only capital letters without commas, dollar signs, or other punctuation.
		●	In the carrier section entered the name and address of the insurance company using correct address format.
		●	Entered the type of insurance.
		●	Entered the ID number and group number of the insured individual as shown on photocopy of the insurance card.
		●	Entered patient information accurately.
		●	Identified the patient's relationship to the insured.
		●	If the insured was not the patient, entered the required information about the insured.
		●	Entered the patient's marital status and employment status.
		●	Entered complete information about any secondary insurance as needed.
		●	Entered information related to the cause of the patient's condition(s).
		●	Identified if the patient did or did not have other insurance.
		●	Validated the patient signature on the form to allow insurance billing and assignment of benefits.
		●	Entered Signature on File (SOF) in boxes authorizing permission.
		▷	Explained how to obtain signatures if they were not on file.

1215

Trial 1	Trial 2	Point Value	Performance Standards
		★	Completed the patient and insured information section accurately and completely.
		●	Entered any special information required by a specific insurance carrier as needed.
		●	Entered the name and identifying number of the referring physician, if any.
		●	Entered dates of hospitalization if services were provided in the hospital.
		●	Checked the correct box to identify if outside laboratory services were provided.
		●	Entered up to four ICD codes.
		●	Entered reference numbers for a Medicaid resubmission, referral, preauthorization, and/or precertification.
		●	Entered information about the first procedure including date(s) of service, place of service, CPT or HCPCS Level II code and modifiers, number to point to the appropriate diagnosis, charges, number of units, and the NPI number or other ID number.
		●	Entered complete information about each additional procedure.
		●	Entered the tax identification number and checked if the Social Security number or employer identification number was used.
		●	Entered the patient account number, if any.
		●	Checked the correct box to indicate acceptance of assignment of benefits.
		●	Entered the total charges, total amount paid, and total balance due.
		●	Entered SOF or the physician's legal signature including credentials and date.
		●	Entered the name, address, and telephone number of the billing facility, and the name of the facility where services were provided, if different.
		●	Entered the NPI number or other ID number for the billing facility and facility where services were provided, if different.
		●	Made a copy of a paper claim and filed in an insurance claims file.
		●	Reviewed the claim for accuracy before submission.
		★	Completed the physician or supplier section accurately and completely.
		★	Completed the procedure within 15 minutes.
			TOTALS

Evaluation of Student Performance

EVALUATION CRITERIA			COMMENTS
Symbol	Category	Point Value	
✳	Critical Step	16 points	
●	Essential Step	6 points	
▷	Theory Question	2 points	

Score calculation: 100 points

–_____ points missed

_____ Score

Satisfactory score: 85 or above

CAAHEP Competencies Achieved

Psychomotor (Skills)
☑ VII. 3. Complete insurance claim forms.

Affective (Behavior)
☑ VIII. 1. Work with physician to achieve the maximum reimbursement.

ABHES Competencies Achieved

☑ 8. u. Prepare and submit insurance claims.

Notes

47 Billing and Collections

√ After Completing	Date Due	Textbook Pages	TEXTBOOK ASSIGNMENTS	Possible Points	Points You Earned
		1107-1123	Read Chapter 47: Billing and Collections		
		1111 1122	Read Case Study 1 Case Study 1 questions	5	
		1113 1122	Read Case Study 2 Case Study 2 questions	5	
		1121 1123	Read Case Study 3 Case Study 3 questions	5	
			TOTAL POINTS		
√ After Completing	**Date Due**	**Study Guide Pages**	**STUDY GUIDE ASSIGNMENTS (CTA = Critical Thinking Activity)**	**Possible Points**	**Points You Earned**
		1223	Pretest	10	
		1224	Term Key Term Assessment	9	
		1225-1227	Evaluation of Learning questions	23	
		1227	CTA A: Cycle Billing	10	
		1228	CTA B: Adjustments	8	
		1228	CTA C: Aging Accounts	8	
			Evolve Site: Guided Practice: Preparing Monthly Billing Statements	10	
			Evolve Site: Apply Your Knowledge questions	10	
			Evolve Site: Video Evaluation	5	
		1223	Posttest	10	

√ After Completing	Date Due	Study Guide Pages	STUDY GUIDE ASSIGNMENTS (CTA = Critical Thinking Activity)	Possible Points	Points You Earned
			ADDITIONAL ASSIGNMENTS		
			TOTAL POINTS		

√ When Assigned By Your Instructor	Study Guide Pages	Practices Required	LABORATORY ASSIGNMENTS (Procedure Number and Name)	Score*
	1229	3	**Practice for Competency** 47-1: Processing Patient Bills Textbook reference: pp. 1108-1109	
	1237-1238		**Evaluation of Competency** 47-1: Processing Patient Bills	*
	1229-1230	1	**Practice for Competency** 47-2: Posting an NSF Check Textbook reference: p. 1111	
	1239-1240		**Evaluation of Competency** 47-2: Posting an NSF Check	*
	1230-1231	1	**Practice for Competency** 47-3: Processing a Credit Balance Textbook reference: p. 1112	
	1241-1242		**Evaluation of Competency** 47-3: Processing a Credit Balance	*
	1231-1232	1	**Practice for Competency** 47-4: Processing a Refund Textbook reference: pp. 1112-1113	
	1243-1244		**Evaluation of Competency** 47-4: Processing a Refund	*
	1233-1234	1	**Practice for Competency** 47-5: Creating an Accounts Receivable Aging Record Textbook reference: pp. 1113-1114	
	1245-1246		**Evaluation of Competency** 47-5: Creating an Accounts Receivable Aging Record	*
	1235	1	**Practice for Competency** 47-6: Writing a Collection Letter Textbook reference: pp. 1118-1119	
	1247-1248		**Evaluation of Competency** 47-6: Writing a Collection Letter	*
	1235	1	**Practice for Competency** 47-7: Posting a Collection Agency Payment Textbook reference: pp. 1118-1119	
	1249-1250		**Evaluation of Competency** 47-7: Posting a Collection Agency Payment	*
			ADDITIONAL ASSIGNMENTS	

1221

Notes

Name _____   Date _____

True or False

_____ 1. The first bill is usually sent to the patient the day after a patient visit.

_____ 2. Almost all medical offices do monthly billing from the office.

_____ 3. Credit agreements with patients must be in writing even if the patient is not charged interest.

_____ 4. A check written on an account that does not have sufficient funds is called an *overdraft*.

_____ 5. When a check is reported lost, the bank should be notified to stop payment on the check.

_____ 6. If a patient overpays his or her account, the office usually issues a refund to the patient.

_____ 7. The medical assistant must create an accounts receivable aging report manually at least once a month.

_____ 8. Overdue accounts older than 120 days are definitely subject to collection activity.

_____ 9. The first time a claim message is used on a patient's bill is when the bill is older than 120 days.

_____ 10. It is illegal to call a patient at his or her place of employment about an overdue bill.

?≣ **POSTTEST**

True or False

_____ 1. Medical offices usually send a bill to patients to collect copayments.

_____ 2. The *billing cycle* is a term used to describe how long it takes to prepare bills for mailing.

_____ 3. Sending some patient bills every week is usually more efficient than sending all bills at the end of the month.

_____ 4. The bank only charges a fee to the account a nonsufficient funds (NSF) check is written on.

_____ 5. An NSF check is entered to the patient's account as a positive adjustment to increase the balance.

_____ 6. If a patient has a credit balance, it means that the office owes the patient money.

_____ 7. Accounts are first considered overdue at 90 days after the date billed.

_____ 8. The medical office can sue patients for overdue accounts in small claims court.

_____ 9. The best time to call a patient about an overdue bill is after 9:00 PM.

_____ 10. A written truth in lending statement is required if the medical office makes an agreement for monthly payments.

Directions: Match each medical term with its definition.

_____ 1. Account aging

_____ 2. Balance due

_____ 3. Bankruptcy

_____ 4. Claim message

_____ 5. Credit balance

_____ 6. Collection agency

_____ 7. Overdraft

_____ 8. Skip

_____ 9. Truth in lending

A. Money owed by the medical office to a patient, usually due to an overpayment

B. A check (or draft) that exceeds the amount of funds in a bank account

C. Total amount owed

D. A firm that is in the business of collecting overdue accounts

E. The process of finding out how long specific account balances have been outstanding

F. Legal requirement to provide written terms of a loan in language that can be easily understood

G. The legal process by which the debts of an individual or business are resolved if they cannot be paid

H. Messages encouraging payment of a bill, usually attached to or printed on the monthly statement

I. Account for which no billing information is available

Directions: Fill in each blank with the correct answer.

1. What is the advantage to the office of a weekly billing cycle?

   _____

   _____

2. If the medical office bills every week, how are patient accounts usually divided?

   _____

   _____

3. What are three ways that bills can be produced?

   _____

   _____

4. Give examples of two special situations that may affect billing.

   _____

   _____

5. What is overdraft protection?

   _____

   _____

6. When should the medical office stop payment on a check?

   _____

   _____

7. How should the medical assistant (MA) handle a check that is returned for insufficient funds?

   _____

   _____

8. When does a credit balance occur in a patient account, and how is a credit balance handled?

   _____

   _____

9. When is a patient account considered overdue?

   _____

10. What are the usual categories of overdue accounts when an accounts receivable aging record is created?

   _____

   _____

11. What is the usual progression in collection activity when a patient's account is overdue?

_____

_____

12. Why is it recommended to place a telephone call regarding an overdue account in addition to placing claim messages on the bill?

_____

_____

13. When does the office need to have a written credit arrangement with a patient?

_____

_____

14. What does a truth in lending statement include, and when should it be sent to a patient?

_____

_____

15. Identify three methods to try to trace a patient whose bill is returned with the notation "address unknown."

_____

_____

16. If the three methods identified in the previous question fail to locate a "skip," what should the medical office do to try to collect a bill?

_____

_____

17. What is the process for sending a patient account to a collection agency?

_____

_____

18. How should a collection agency payment be entered on the patient's ledger card and on the day sheet?

_____

_____

19. What is small claims court, and how might it be used by the medical office?

_____

_____

20. If a patient has died, how and when should the bill for services rendered before death be sent?

_____

_____

21. If the bill of a deceased individual is not paid promptly, how should the MA follow up?

_____

_____

1226

22. What is the status of outstanding medical bills if a person declares bankruptcy under Chapter 7? Under Chapter 13?

_____

_____

23. Describe briefly how each of the following laws affects credit and collection activities in the medical office:

a. Equal Credit Opportunity Act: _____

_____

b. Fair Debt Collection Practices Act: _____

_____

c. Federal Truth in Lending Act: _____

_____

d. Fair Credit Reporting Act: _____

_____

e. Bankruptcy Abuse and Consumer Protection Act of 2005: _____

_____

CRITICAL THINKING ACTIVITIES

A. Cycle Billing

Assume that a billing cycle is used in which patients with a last name beginning with the letters A-E are billed the first week of the month; the second week, F-L; the third week, M-S; and the fourth week, T-Z. Identify which week each of the following patients would be billed.

1. John T. Sanders _____

2. Eileen McDonald _____

3. Winston A. Robertson _____

4. Tracy Marie Jordan _____

5. Julian W. Allen _____

6. Edward Elliot Hubbard _____

7. Joanne Mason-Taylor _____

8. Diane von Bohlen _____

9. Carolyn Ann Oppenheimer _____

10. Douglas P. Benson _____

B. Adjustments

For each of the following situations identify whether the MA will post the transaction to the patient account as a credit adjustment (reduces the patient balance), a payment, or a debit adjustment (increases the patient balance).

1. Patient pays $50.00 by check, which is an overpayment of $25.00: _____

2. Patient's check for $25.00 is returned by the bank marked "Not sufficient funds:" _____

3. A collection agency payment is received, and the patient balance is zero: _____

4. A check from an insurance company is received for a patient account: _____

5. A patient pays a copayment of $10.00 at the time of the visit: _____

6. A patient is given a discount of $15.00 for paying the bill in cash: _____

7. A check is issued as a refund for a patient overpayment: _____

8. The insurance company identifies $12.00 of the patient charge as an excluded amount: _____

C. Aging Accounts

Assume that accounts are aged from the date of billing. If you are aging accounts on 10/30/XX, select the letter of the correct length of time that each of the following accounts has been outstanding.

   a. Current (0 to 30 days)
   b. 31 to 60 days
   c. 61 to 90 days
   d. 91 to 120 days
   e. Older than 120 days

_____ 1. Service provided on 7/4/XX, billed on 8/1/XX

_____ 2. Service provided on 9/22/XX, billed on 10/3/XX

_____ 3. Service provided on 8/13/XX, billed on 8/22/XX

_____ 4. Service provided on 4/18/XX, billed on 4/25/XX

_____ 5. Service provided on 5/13/XX, billed on 6/6/XX

_____ 6. Service provided on 6/19/XX, billed on 7/12/XX

_____ 7. Service provided on 6/25/XX, billed on 7/18/XX

_____ 8. Service provided on 7/18/XX, billed on 8/15/XX

PRACTICE FOR COMPETENCY

Procedure 47-1: Processing Patient Bills. Using a computer billing program, practice printing selected patient bills and placing them in window envelopes.

Create a manual statement using a statement template for Darla Sissle (see textbook Figure 47-1) on 8/15/XX assuming that she paid $20.00 on 8/1/XX.

Procedure 47-2: Posting an NSF Check. The bank has returned Marie Ryan's check No. 938 for $10.00 marked NSF (not sufficient funds). Your bank charges $15.00 for each returned check. Using today's date, enter the returned check as an adjustment as well as the bank fee on the day sheet. Her old balance was zero.

JOURNAL OF DAILY CHARGES, PAYMENTS & DEPOSITS

PLACE FIRST PEG HERE

	DATE	PROFESSIONAL SERVICE	FEE	PAYMENT	ADJUST-MENT	NEW BALANCE	OLD BALANCE	PATIENT'S NAME	
1									1
2									2
3									3
4									4
5									5
6									6
7									7
8									8
9									9
10									10
11									11
12									12
13									13
14									14
15									15
16									16
17									17
18									18
19									19
20									20
21									21
22									22
23									23
24									24
25									25
26									26
27									27
28									28
29									29
30									30
31								TOTALS THIS PAGE	31
32								TOTALS PREVIOUS PAGE	32
33								TOTALS MONTH TO DATE	33

COLUMN A   COLUMN B   COLUMN C   COLUMN D   COLUMN E

MEMO _____
_____
_____
_____

DAILY-FROM LINE 31

ACCOUNTS RECEIVABLE PROOF	
Column E	
Plus Column A	
Sub-Total	
Minus Column B	
Sub-Total	
Minus Column C	
Equals Column D	

Box 1

MONTH-FROM LINE 31

ACCOUNTS RECEIVABLE PROOF	
Accts. Receivable Previous Day	$
Plus Column A	
Sub-Total	
Minus Column B	
Sub-Total	
Minus Column C	
Accts. Receivable End ofDay	

Box 2

(Courtesy of Bibbero Systems, Inc., Petaluma, Calif. [800] 242-2376 fax [800] 242-9330; www.bibbero.com)

1230

Procedure 47-3: Processing a Credit Balance. You receive check No. 332 in the amount of $70.00 from James Winston for payment of charges for an office visit 1 month ago. Using today's date, enter the payment on the day sheet used for Procedure 47-2. Mr. Winston's previous balance was $10.00. Remember to post negative amounts in parentheses.

Procedure 47-4: Processing a Refund. Prepare a refund for James Winston to bring the balance of his account to zero. Post the refund on the third line of the day sheet used for Procedure 47-2 as a credit adjustment. Write a check to James Winston for the refund amount using the first check form below. Leave the signature line blank, because you are not authorized to sign checks. The old balance of the checking account is $4,166.82. Complete the check stub. Prepare a letter to James Winston informing him that you are enclosing a check for the amount of his overpayment. His address is James Winston, 25 Magnolia Lane, Western, XY 44770. Inform him that he can call you at extension 24 if he has any questions. Assume that you will print the letter on office letterhead, and sign the letter using your own name and the title Medical Assistant on the next line. This means that a reference line is not necessary. Specify the check on the enclosure line. (Enc: Check #1837)

1837

DATE _____

TO _____

FOR _____

BALANCE BROUGHT FORWARD	
DEPOSITS	
BALANCE	
AMT THIS CK	
BALANCE CARRIED FORWARD	

1837

BLACKBURN PRIMARY CARE ASSOCIATES, PC
1990 Turquiose Drive
Blackburn, WI 54937
608-459-8857

94-72/1224

DATE _____

PAY TO THE
ORDER OF _____ $ [   ]

_____ DOLLARS

DERBYSHIRE SAVINGS
Member FDIC
P.O. BOX 8923
Blackburn, WI 54937

FOR _____

⑈055003⑈ 446782011⑈ 678800470

SAMPLE

1838

DATE _____

TO _____

FOR _____

BALANCE BROUGHT FORWARD	
DEPOSITS	
BALANCE	
AMT THIS CK	
BALANCE CARRIED FORWARD	

1838

BLACKBURN PRIMARY CARE ASSOCIATES, PC
1990 Turquiose Drive
Blackburn, WI 54937
608-459-8857

94-72/1224

DATE _____

PAY TO THE
ORDER OF _____ $ [   ]

_____ DOLLARS

DERBYSHIRE SAVINGS
Member FDIC
P.O. BOX 8923
Blackburn, WI 54937

FOR _____

⑈055003⑈ 446782011⑈ 678800470

SAMPLE

1839

DATE _____

TO _____

FOR _____

BALANCE BROUGHT FORWARD	
DEPOSITS	
BALANCE	
AMT THIS CK	
BALANCE CARRIED FORWARD	

1839

BLACKBURN PRIMARY CARE ASSOCIATES, PC
1990 Turquiose Drive
Blackburn, WI 54937
608-459-8857

94-72/1224

DATE _____

PAY TO THE
ORDER OF _____ $ [   ]

_____ DOLLARS

DERBYSHIRE SAVINGS
Member FDIC
P.O. BOX 8923
Blackburn, WI 54937

FOR _____

⑈055003⑈ 446782011⑈ 678800470

SAMPLE

(From Hunt SA: *Saunders fundamentals of medical assisting student mastery manual,* St. Louis, 2007, Saunders.)

Procedure 47-5: Creating an Accounts Receivable Aging Record. Create a patient aging report based on information from the accounts of the following patients. Assume that you are creating the report on 11/30. Bills were sent on the first day of the month after an insurance payment was received: 8/1, 9/1, 10/1, or 11/1. Beside each account on the report, mark the action that should be taken according to Procedure 47-5.

Daryl P. Sanders
24 Lakeview Drive
Western, XY 44770

Date	Professional Service	Fee	Payment	Adjustment	New Balance
6/4/XX	99202, cash payment	55.00	20.00		35.00
6/28/XX	Ins. ck #219		20.00		15.00

Lloyd Hanson
10 High Street
Western, XY 44770

Date	Professional Service	Fee	Payment	Adjustment	New Balance
7/15/XX	99204, 93000, ck #664	150.00	15.00		135.00
7/28/XX	Ins ck #604 (for 6/15)		128.00	7.00	0.00
8/25/XX	99212	48.00	15.00		33.00

Maria Rivera Santos
160 Underwood Street
Western, XY 44770

Date	Professional Service	Fee	Payment	Adjustment	New Balance
9/28/XX	99204, ck #259	135.00	27.00		108.00

Thomas Maxwell
1100 Main Street
Western, XY 44770

Date	Professional Service	Fee	Payment	Adjustment	New Balance
9/1/XX	99213, 81002, 98000, ck #22	122.00	50.00		72.00
10/12/XX	99212, ck #602	48.00	15.00		105.00
10/15/XX	Ins ck #2298 (for 9/1)		56.00	16.00	33.00

Account Aging Report

Patient Name	Last Payment	Current 0 - 30	Past 31 - 60	Past 61 - 90	Past 91 - 120	Past 121+	Total Balance

(From Hunt SA: *Saunders fundamentals of medical assisting student mastery manual,* St. Louis, 2007, Saunders.)

Procedure 47-6: Writing a Collection Letter. Write a collection letter to each individual on the aging report above if you marked the account: "Payment is now overdue." Instruct the recipient to pay the bill or contact the office to make other arrangements. Use the date of 11/30/XX and assume that the letters will be printed on office letterhead. Sign any letter using your own name and use the title, Medical Assistant, on the next line.

Procedure 47-7: Posting a Collection Agency Payment. You received a payment from a collection agency of $50.00 (check No. 554) for the account of Helen McDonald. The current balance of her account is zero. Using line four on the day sheet, post a credit adjustment as a reverse collection. Using line five, post the collection agency payment. Total all columns of the day sheet.

Notes

Name: _____   Date: _____

Evaluated by: _____   Score: _____

Performance Objective

Outcome:	Process patient bill.
Conditions:	Given the following: computer, patient accounts, paper or statement forms, window envelopes with two windows, statement template for word processing program (optional) and postage.
Standards:	Time: 10 minutes. Student completed procedure in _____ minutes.
	Accuracy: Satisfactory score on the Performance Evaluation Checklist.

Performance Evaluation Checklist

Trial 1	Trial 2	Point Value	Performance Standards
		●	Located patient accounts with outstanding balances after insurance payments in the computer database.
		●	Selected accounts to be billed.
		●	Printed patient statements using paper forms or forms generated by the computer program or created one or more patient bills manually using a statement template and word processing program.
		●	Verified that statements printed correctly.
		●	Folded statements so that the practice and patient name and address would be facing outward.
		●	Inserted statements in window envelopes.
		●	Verified that name and address were visible through the window.
		●	Placed postage on envelopes and set aside for mailing.
		✱	Prepared statements correctly for mailing.
		✱	Completed the procedure within 10 minutes.
			TOTALS

EVALUATION CRITERIA			COMMENTS
Symbol	**Category**	**Point Value**	
✱	Critical Step	16 points	
●	Essential Step	6 points	
▷	Theory Question	2 points	

Score calculation: 100 points

−   points missed

_____

___ Score

Satisfactory score: 85 or above

CAAHEP Competencies Achieved

Psychomotor (Skills)

☑ VI. 2. b. Perform billing procedures.
☑ VI. 3. Use computerized office billing systems.

ABHES Competencies Achieved

☑ 8. i. Perform billing and collection procedures.
☑ 8. w. Use manual or computerized bookkeeping systems.

EVALUATION OF COMPETENCY

Procedure 47-2: Posting an NSF Check

Name: _____   Date: _____

Evaluated by: _____   Score: _____

Performance Objective

Outcome:	Post an NSF check.
Conditions:	Given the following: computer, patient accounts, returned check, day sheet, pen, and calculator.
Standards:	Time: 10 minutes. Student completed procedure in _____ minutes.
	Accuracy: Satisfactory score on the Performance Evaluation Checklist.

Performance Evaluation Checklist

Trial 1	Trial 2	Point Value	Performance Standards
		●	Located the patient account for the patient whose check was returned.
		●	Wrote the patient's name and old balance on the first open line of the day sheet.
		●	Created a new transaction for the patient in the computer account, and posted the returned check using the code for "NSF check" or "adjustment charge" depending on office policy.
		●	Entered the returned check fee in the computer account using the code for "returned check fee," verifying that insurance would not be billed.
		●	Wrote "NSF check," the check number, and "returned check fee" in the professional service column of the day sheet.
		●	Placed the amount of the check in the adjustment column in parentheses.
		▷	Explained the difference between the notation for a credit adjustment and a debit adjustment.
		●	Entered the returned check fee on the day sheet in the fee column.
		●	Entered the sum of the NSF check, the returned check fee, and the old balance in the new balance column.
		✷	When totaling the adjustment column of the day sheet, subtracted the adjustment from the total of other adjustments.
		●	Notified the patient by telephone or letter that the check was returned and a fee was charged.
		●	Enclosed an updated patient statement with a letter.
		✷	Completed the procedure within 10 minutes.
			TOTALS

1239

Evaluation of Student Performance

EVALUATION CRITERIA			COMMENTS
Symbol	**Category**	**Point Value**	
★	Critical Step	16 points	
●	Essential Step	6 points	
▷	Theory Question	2 points	

Score calculation: 100 points

      −   _____ points missed

           ___ Score

Satisfactory score: 85 or above

CAAHEP Competencies Achieved

Psychomotor (Skills)

☑ VI. 2. g. Post nonsufficient fund (NSF) checks.

Affective (Behavior)

☑ VI. 1. Demonstrate sensitivity and professionalism in handling accounts receivable activities with patients.

ABHES Competencies Achieved

☑ 8. p. Post nonsufficient funds (NSF).

Procedure 47-3: Processing a Credit Balance

Name: _____   Date: _____

Evaluated by: _____   Score: _____

Performance Objective

Outcome:	Post an overpayment.
Conditions:	Given the following: computer, patient accounts, payment check(s), day sheet, pen, and calculator.
Standards:	Time: 5 minutes. Student completed procedure in _____ minutes.
	Accuracy: Satisfactory score on the Performance Evaluation Checklist.

Performance Evaluation Checklist

Trial 1	Trial 2	Point Value	Performance Standards
		●	Located the patient account after receiving payment. If using a manual day sheet, entered the patient name and old balance on the first blank line of the day sheet.
		●	Created a new transaction for the patient in the computer account, and posted the payment using the correct code (patient check or insurance check) linked to the charges being paid.
		●	Noted that the balance due is a negative number.
		▷	Explained the meaning of a negative number as a balance in the accounts receivable.
		●	Entered the type of payment and check number in the professional service column of the day sheet.
		●	Entered the amount of the payment in the payment column of the day sheet.
		●	Entered the sum of the payment and the old balance in the new balance column in parentheses.
		✶	When totaling the new balance column of the day sheet, subtracted the negative balance from the total.
		●	Arranged to clear the negative balance from the system according to office policy.
		✶	Completed the procedure within 5 minutes.
			TOTALS

Evaluation of Student Performance

EVALUATION CRITERIA			COMMENTS
Symbol	**Category**	**Point Value**	
✶	Critical Step	16 points	
●	Essential Step	6 points	
▷	Theory Question	2 points	

Score calculation: 100 points

            −   points missed

                      ___ Score

Satisfactory score: 85 or above

CAAHEP Competencies Achieved

Psychomotor (Skills)
☑ VI. 2. e. Process a credit balance.

Affective (Behavior)
☑ VI. 1. Demonstrate sensitivity and professionalism in handling accounts receivable activities with patients.

ABHES Competencies Achieved

☑ 8. n. Process credit balances.

Procedure 47-4: Processing a Refund

Name: _____ Date: _____

Evaluated by: _____ Score: _____

Performance Objective

Outcome:	Process a refund.
Conditions:	Given the following: computer, patient accounts, payment check(s), day sheet, pen, calculator, and printer.
Standards:	Time: 10 minutes. Student completed procedure in _____ minutes.
	Accuracy: Satisfactory score on the Performance Evaluation Checklist

Performance Evaluation Checklist

Trial 1	Trial 2	Point Value	Performance Standards
		●	Located the patient account in the computer.
		●	Entered the patient's name and old balance on the first open line of the day sheet.
		●	Calculated the amount to be refunded.
		●	Created a new transaction in the computer and entered the amount of the refund using the code for a refund.
		●	Verified that the patient's balance was zero after the transaction was entered.
		●	Wrote "Refund for Overpayment" *in the professional services* column of the day sheet.
		●	Entered the amount of the refund in the *adjustment* column.
		●	Subtracted the amount of the refund from the old balance, and entered zero in the new balance column.
		●	Wrote a check for the amount of the refund leaving the signature line blank.
		●	Recorded the check number, date, payee, and reason for the check on the check stub or in the check register.
		●	Subtracted the amount of the check from the checking account balance and entered the balance carried forward.
		●	Wrote a letter to the patient explaining the refund and prepared an envelope.
		●	Signed the letter and clipped the check to the letter and envelope.
		●	Left the check, letter, and envelope in the designated location to obtain a physician signature on the check.
		✱	Posted transaction correctly and prepared a letter without errors.
		✱	Completed the procedure within 10 minutes.
			TOTALS

1243

EVALUATION CRITERIA			COMMENTS
Symbol	**Category**	**Point Value**	
★	Critical Step	16 points	
●	Essential Step	6 points	
▷	Theory Question	2 points	

Score calculation: 100 points

− _____ points missed

___ Score

Satisfactory score: 85 or above

CAAHEP Competencies Achieved

Psychomotor (Skills)

☑ VI. 2. f. Process refunds.

Affective (Behavior)

☑ VI. 1. Demonstrate sensitivity and professionalism in handling accounts receivable activities with patients.

ABHES Competencies Achieved

☑ 8. o. Process refunds.

1244

Procedure 47-5: Creating an Accounts Receivable Aging Record

Name: _____   Date: _____

Evaluated by: _____   Score: _____

Performance Objective

Outcome:	Create an accounts receivable aging record.
Conditions:	Given the following: computer, patient accounts, accounts receivable aging record analysis form (optional), office policy or procedure manual, and pen.
Standards:	Time: 15 minutes. Student completed procedure in _____ minutes.
	Accuracy: Satisfactory score on the Performance Evaluation Checklist.

Performance Evaluation Checklist

Trial 1	Trial 2	Point Value	Performance Standards
		●	Used the reports function of the computer billing program to print an aging report for patients and insurance companies, or created the report manually from individual patient accounts.
		●	Reviewed the accounts on the report and marked the appropriate action for each account according to office policy.
		●	Marked all accounts less than 31 days old: "No action needed."
		●	Marked accounts with unpaid insurance claims older than 31 days: "Follow up with insurance."
		●	Marked accounts 31 to 60 days old with paid insurance claims according to office policy (e.g., "Attach first claim note to statement").
		●	Marked accounts 61 to 90 days old with paid insurance claims according to office policy (e.g., "Attach second claim note to statement").
		●	Marked accounts 91 to 120 days old with paid insurance claims according to office policy (e.g., "Telephone patient").
		●	Reviewed previous collection attempts for accounts over 120 days.
		●	Prepared a collection letter for each account over 120 days informing the patient of a specific deadline and intended action if payment is not received.
		●	Filed a copy of any collection letter in the patient's medical record.
		●	Recorded all action taken beside each account on the report.
		●	Documented any telephone calls and/or collection letter in the progress notes of the patient's medical record.
		✶	Analyzed outstanding accounts accurately, and indicated appropriate follow-up.
		✶	Completed the procedure within 15 minutes.
			TOTALS

1245

	CHART	
Date		

Evaluation of Student Performance

EVALUATION CRITERIA			COMMENTS
Symbol	**Category**	**Point Value**	
★	Critical Step	16 points	
●	Essential Step	6 points	
▷	Theory Question	2 points	

Score calculation: 100 points

−   points missed

_____

____ Score

Satisfactory score: 85 or above

CAAHEP Competencies Achieved

Psychomotor (Skills)

☑ VI. 2. c. Perform collection procedures.

ABHES Competencies Achieved

☑ 8. i. Perform billing and collection procedures.

Procedure 47-6: Writing a Collection Letter

Name: _____ Date: _____

Evaluated by: _____ Score: _____

Performance Objective

Outcome:	Write a collection letter.
Conditions:	Given the following: accounts receivable aging report, computer, patient accounts, letterhead stationery, envelope, and printer.
Standards:	Time: 10 minutes. Student completed procedure in _____ minutes.
	Accuracy: Satisfactory score on the Performance Evaluation Checklist

Performance Evaluation Checklist

Trial 1	Trial 2	Point Value	Performance Standards
		●	Determined which accounts were over 120 days old from an accounts receivable aging report.
		●	Reviewed accounts over 120 days to be sure that there are no extenuating circumstances for which the patient might be given more time to pay.
		●	Set up a letter for the first account over 120 days using the format preferred by the office.
		●	Identified the patient's address from the patient information sheet or computer screen.
		●	Included the outstanding balance, the date charges were incurred, the service provided, and the amount paid by insurance in the letter.
		●	Described any previous telephone conversations and/or agreements in the letter.
		●	Stated the amount of the outstanding balance and the date by which it must be paid.
		●	Entered the typed signature of the individual designated by office policy to write collection letters. Used a reference line if another staff member will sign the letter.
		●	Signed the letter or placed it in the designated location to obtain a signature.
		●	Prepared an envelope.
		●	Copied the letter and filed the copy in the patient's medical record and/or a collection follow-up file.
		●	Placed a notation on the aging report and in the computer account that the letter was sent to the patient.

1247

Trial 1	Trial 2	Point Value	Performance Standards
		●	Placed the letter in the envelope and mailed the letter.
		✶	Created error-free letter and envelope.
		✶	Completed the procedure within 10 minutes.
			TOTALS

Evaluation of Student Performance

EVALUATION CRITERIA			COMMENTS
Symbol	**Category**	**Point Value**	
✶	Critical Step	16 points	
●	Essential Step	6 points	
▷	Theory Question	2 points	

Score calculation: 100 points

−   _____ points missed

_____ Score

Satisfactory score: 85 or above

CAAHEP Competencies Achieved

Psychomotor (Skills)

☑ IV. 10. Compose professional/business letters.
☑ VI. 2. c. Perform collection procedures.
☑ IX. 8. Apply local, state, and federal health care legislation and regulation appropriate to the medical assisting practice setting.

Affective (Behavior)

☑ VI. 1. Demonstrate sensitivity and professionalism in handling accounts receivable activities with patients.
☑ IX. 3. Recognize the importance of local, state, and federal legislation and regulations in the practice setting.

ABHES Competencies Achieved

☑ 8. i. Perform billing and collection procedures.
☑ 8. dd. Serve as liaison between physician and others.
☑ 8. jj. Perform fundamental writing skills including correct grammar, spelling, and formatting techniques when writing prescriptions, documenting medical records, etc.

Procedure 47-7: Posting a Collection Agency Payment

Name: _____   Date: _____

Evaluated by: _____   Score: _____

Performance Objective

Outcome:	Post a collection agency payment.
Conditions:	Given the following: computer, patient account, payment check, day sheet, calculator, and pen.
Standards:	Time: 5 minutes. Student completed procedure in _____ minutes.
	Accuracy: Satisfactory score on the Performance Evaluation Checklist.

Performance Evaluation Checklist

Trial 1	Trial 2	Point Value	Performance Standards
		●	Located the account of the patient for whom a check has been received from the collection agency.
		●	Wrote the patient's name and old balance on the first open line of the day sheet.
			Explained why the account balance was adjusted to zero when the account was sent for collection.
		●	Created a new transaction for the patient, selected the code for "Reverse collection," and entered the amount of the check.
		●	Verified that the computer showed a positive balance after this entry.
		●	Wrote "Reverse collection" in the professional service column of the day sheet.
		●	Entered the amount of the check in the adjustment column of the day sheet in parentheses as a debit adjustment.
		▷	Explained the difference between the notation for a credit adjustment and a debit adjustment.
		✳	When totaling the adjustment column of the day sheet, subtracted the debit adjustment from the total of the credit adjustments.
		●	Entered the amount of the check in the new balance column.
		●	In the computer, on a new line, selected the code for "Collection agency payment," and entered the amount of the check.
		●	Verified that the patient balance returned to zero.
		●	On the next line of the day sheet entered the patient's name again, and wrote the amount of the collection agency check as the old balance.

Trial 1	Trial 2	Point Value	Performance Standards
		●	Wrote "Collection agency payment" and the check number in the professional service column of the day sheet.
		●	Entered the amount of the check in the payment column.
		●	Performance Standards
		●	Entered zero in the new balance column.
		★	Completed the procedure within 5 minutes.
			TOTALS

Evaluation of Student Performance

EVALUATION CRITERIA			COMMENTS
Symbol	**Category**	**Point Value**	
★	Critical Step	16 points	
●	Essential Step	6 points	
▷	Theory Question	2 points	

Score calculation: 100 points

– _____ points missed

___ Score

Satisfactory score: 85 or above

CAAHEP Competencies Achieved

Psychomotor (Skills)

☑ VI. 2. h. Post collection agency payments.

ABHES Competencies Achieved

☑ 8. q. Post collection agency payments.

The Medical Assistant as Office Manager

CHAPTER ASSIGNMENTS

√ After Completing	Date Due	Textbook Pages	TEXTBOOK ASSIGNMENTS	Possible Points	Points You Earned
		1124-1143	Read Chapter 48: The Medical Assistant as Office Manager		
		1128 1141-1142	Read Case Study 1 Case Study 1 questions	5	
		1135 1142	Read Case Study 2 Case Study 2 questions	5	
		1140 1142	Read Case Study 3 Case Study 3 questions	5	
			TOTAL POINTS		
√ After Completing	**Date Due**	**Study Guide Pages**	**STUDY GUIDE ASSIGNMENTS (CTA = Critical Thinking Activity)**	**Possible Points**	**Points You Earned**
		1255	Pretest	10	
		1256	Term Key Term Assessment	18	
		1257-1260	Evaluation of Learning questions	32	
		1260	CTA A: Equipment Inventory List	10	
		1260	CTA B: Supply Inventory List	10	
		1261	CTA C: Community Resources	5	
		1261	CTA D: Incident Report	7	
			Evolve Site: Guided Practice: Establishing and Maintaining a Supply Inventory and Ordering System	10	
			Evolve Site: Apply Your Knowledge questions	10	
			Evolve Site: Video Evaluations	12	
		1255	Posttest	10	

√ After Completing	Date Due	Study Guide Pages	STUDY GUIDE ASSIGNMENTS (CTA = Critical Thinking Activity)	Possible Points	Points You Earned
			ADDITIONAL ASSIGNMENTS		
			TOTAL POINTS		

√ When Assigned By Your Instructor	Study Guide Pages	Practices Required	LABORATORY ASSIGNMENTS (Procedure Number and Name)	Score*
	1263	5	**Practice for Competency** 48-1: Creating an Environmental Checklist and Performing a Safety Inspection Textbook Reference: p. 1130	
	1267-1269		**Evaluation of Competency** 48-1: Creating an Environmental Checklist and Performing a Safety Inspection	*
	1264	2	**Practice for Competency** 48-2: Performing Routine Maintenance of Equipment Textbook reference: p. 1132	
	1271-1272		**Evaluation of Competency** 48-2: Performing Routine Maintenance of Equipment	*
	1265	1	**Practice for Competency** 48-3: Taking a Supply or Equipment Inventory Textbook reference: p. 1134	
	1273-1274		**Evaluation of Competency** 48-3: Taking a Supply or Equipment Inventory	*
	1265	1	**Practice for Competency** 48-4: Locating Community Resources Textbook reference: p. 1139	
	1275-1276		**Evaluation of Competency** 48-4: Locating Community Resources	*
	1265-1266	1	**Practice for Competency** 48-5: Completing an Incident Report Textbook reference: p. 1141	
	1277-1278		**Evaluation of Competency** 48-5: Completing an Incident Report	*
			ADDITIONAL ASSIGNMENTS	

Chapter **48**   **The Medical Assistant as Office Manager**

Notes

Name _____   Date _____

True or False

_____ 1. Stationery, envelopes, and billing forms should be located in the administrative area of the medical office.

_____ 2. Old telephone logs should be shredded if they are discarded.

_____ 3. Rigid biohazard waste containers are usually stored under the sink in an examination room.

_____ 4. The waiting room often has a sign requesting that patients pay copayments at the time of the visit.

_____ 5. Falls are a common cause of workplace injury.

_____ 6. Treatment rooms or special procedure rooms are usually kept a little warmer than examination rooms.

_____ 7. The medical assistant (MA) is usually responsible for changing the plastic liners in biohazard waste containers.

_____ 8. The doors to the laboratory and medical records shelves or area may have additional locks.

_____ 9. Areas where x-ray is used should be marked with signs.

_____ 10. An equipment inventory includes the date of purchase, cost, and serial number of each piece of equipment.

? POSTTEST

True or False

_____ 1. Business operations may be performed at the front desk or separate area of the medical office.

_____ 2. Each examination room should have a sink and wall-mounted paper towel dispenser.

_____ 3. Biohazard waste containers with a plastic liner only need to be covered at night.

_____ 4. The medical office may have a display rack with informational brochures in the waiting room.

_____ 5. Tripping or slipping without falling may still cause workplace injuries.

_____ 6. A good temperature for the office waiting room is 70°F to 72°F.

_____ 7. All cleaning is done at night in the medical office by an outside cleaning company.

_____ 8. Controlled substances should always be stored in an area with two locks and two separate keys.

_____ 9. Exit signs should be yellow with black lettering.

_____ 10. A supply inventory is used to keep records for tax purposes.

Directions: Match each medical term with its definition.

_____ 1. Back order

_____ 2. Depreciation

_____ 3. Gross pay

_____ 4. Inventory

_____ 5. Invoice

_____ 6. Minutes

_____ 7. Net pay

_____ 8. Per diem

_____ 9. Policy

_____ 10. Procedure

_____ 11. Reorder point

_____ 12. Risk management

_____ 13. Salary

_____ 14. Service contract

_____ 15. Social Security tax (FICA)

_____ 16. Vendor

_____ 17. Warranty

_____ 18. W-4 form

A. A written record of the proceedings of a meeting

B. The form used to claim allowances for federal income tax reporting

C. The total amount earned in a time period by an employee before any deductions

D. A guiding principle for the management of a medical office or business

E. A tax collected from employees to fund the Social Security program

F. A fixed amount of wages that does not depend on the number of hours worked

G. A detailed list of items in stock or in possession of an individual or business

H. A promise by the manufacturer to repair or replace defective parts in an item during a specific time period

I. A term used for items ordered that cannot be shipped immediately, usually because they are out of stock

J. A number on a supply inventory that indicates when a specific item should be reordered

K. A list of the steps to handle a certain situation or perform a certain task

L. The actual amount of money paid directly to an employee after taxes and other deductions

M. An agreement that provides for service for a piece of equipment after the warranty expires

N. An itemized bill for items that have not been prepaid

O. Employees who are scheduled by the day according to office needs

P. Accounting methods to record the loss of value of a property or piece of equipment over time

Q. The process of assessing risk and putting policies and procedures in place to minimize it

R. A company from whom supplies or equipment is purchased

Directions: Fill in each blank with the correct answer.

1. Write a general statement identifying the type of equipment and supplies needed in the administrative area of the medical office.

    a. Equipment: _____

    _____

    b. Supplies: _____

    _____

2. Write a general statement identifying the type of equipment and supplies needed for examination rooms and treatment rooms.

    a. Equipment: _____

    _____

    b. Supplies: _____

    _____

3. What are four common signs that might be found in a medical office waiting room?

    _____

    _____

4. What are areas within the medical office that can often be locked separately and are often kept locked at night?

    _____

    _____

5. List five activities that are considered part of routine maintenance.

    _____

    _____

    _____

6. Identify two important components for controlling the air in the medical office.

    _____

    _____

7. What parts of the medical office are MAs usually responsible for cleaning and/or tidying?

    _____

    _____

    _____

8. What are five general guidelines recommended by the Occupational Safety and Health Administration (OSHA) to maintain workplace safety?

_____

_____

_____

9. What should be included in a safety plan for a medical office?

_____

_____

_____

10. What are five examples of signs that should be present in the medical office?

_____

_____

_____

11. Identify two reasons why it is important to maintain an accurate inventory of equipment.

_____

_____

12. Describe how service contracts work. When do they go into effect?

_____

_____

13. What are some helpful things to do when a new piece of equipment is placed into service?

_____

_____

14. Name five types of information that should be included on a supply inventory list.

_____

_____

_____

15. What is the reorder point on a supply inventory list? How is it used?

_____

_____

16. What is the MA's responsibility for restocking administrative and clinical areas?

_____

_____

17. Why is a tracking number or purchase order number useful when ordering supplies?

_____

_____

18. Identify three steps the MA should take when supplies are delivered.

_____

_____

_____

19. How can staff meetings help create an environment for teamwork?

_____

_____

_____

20. Describe two methods to prepare meeting participants, keep a meeting running smoothly, and keep track of decisions made during the meeting.

_____

_____

21. What paperwork is required for a new employee?

_____

_____

22. What are five things that must be documented in an employee's payroll record?

_____

_____

_____

23. Identify three types of deductions that the employer must withhold from an employee paycheck.

_____

24. What is unemployment tax, and how is it paid?

_____

_____

25. When preparing payroll checks for employees, what five items of information must be recorded in the payroll record for each employee?

_____

_____

_____

26. What is the MA's responsibility in relation to the physician and office schedule?

_____

_____

_____

27. Differentiate between a policy and a procedure.

_____

28. Identify three reasons why it is valuable for organizations to have procedure manuals available.

_____

_____

29. Identify eight types of community resources to which patients might be referred for information or services.

_____

_____

_____

_____

30. Describe when incident reports are completed and how they fit into the risk management plan of an organization.

_____

_____

31. Give four examples of damage or injury that should be covered by the medical office's general property and/or liability insurance.

_____

_____

32. What kind of protection is provided by professional liability insurance?

_____

_____

CRITICAL THINKING ACTIVITIES

A. Equipment Inventory List

Create an inventory list of equipment in the clinical laboratory of your medical assisting program. Include the name of each piece of equipment, a description, and a serial number or school ID number. Set up your list with columns for at least three dates to check off items when you take inventory.

B. Supply Inventory List

Working with at least one classmate, set up a supply inventory list for at least 15 supply items that might be used during the physical examination. The categories should include the following: item name, quantity in stock, reorder point, and quantity to reorder. For this assignment, a supply meets one or more of the following conditions:

• It is consumed in use.
• It is expendable, and if it is damaged, it will be replaced rather than repaired.
• It costs less than $250.00.

Assume that your office wants to keep a 3-month supply of each item on hand. Assume that 100 patients are seen in the office each day, 5 days a week. Assume that there will be a 2-week delay between the time the order is placed and the time the order is received.

1260

C. Community Resources

Describe the types of community services that might be appropriate for each of the following patients:

1. Patient discharged from the hospital after hip replacement surgery.

_____

2. Elderly patient who lives alone with limited mobility and no family members living in the community.

_____

3. Male patient (65 years old) diagnosed with inoperable lung cancer with planned radiation treatments. Wife does not drive.

_____

_____

4. Family with a 6-year-old child who sustains an injury resulting in permanent paralysis from the waist down.

_____

_____

5. Elderly couple with the wife diagnosed with Alzheimer disease's and who cannot be left alone. Husband still drives. Daughter lives in the community.

_____

_____

D. Incident Report

You are working in a medical office, and a patient slips and falls in the corridor when being taken back to an examination room. The physician is called, assists the patient to get up, and finds a bruise on the right hip but no other apparent injury. The physician instructs the patient to telephone if any problems arise later and documents the examination and findings in the patient's medical record. It is office policy to fill out an incident report for any fall that occurs in the office. Make a list of all information that you would have to include on the incident report.

_____

_____

_____

_____

_____

_____

_____

_____

_____

_____

_____

_____

Chapter **48**   **The Medical Assistant as Office Manager**

Notes

PRACTICE FOR COMPETENCY

Procedure 48-1: Creating an Environmental Checklist and Performing a Safety Inspection. Expand the following checklist adhering to the guidelines outlined in Procedure 48-1. Make three copies of your revised checklist. Use it to inspect at least two rooms in your own home, and use it to inspect a medical office environment. After completing the inspections, write down any problems that could not be fixed during the inspection. Discuss with your classmates the difference between safety hazards in the home and safety hazards in the medical office.

Safety Inspection Checklist

Date: _____ Person Making Inspection: _____

Label as **C** if there are no problems; label as **NC** if a problem is found.

	C or NC	Problem/Action Taken
General Visual Inspection		
Walkways		
Electrical Cords and Plugs		
Storage Areas		
Lighting		
Storage and Labeling of Chemicals/Biohazards		

Plan to Correct Items that Could not be Corrected During Inspection:

1.
2.
3.
4.
5.

Procedure 48-2: Performing Routine Maintenance of Equipment. Perform routine maintenance of both administrative and clinical equipment such as the autoclave, electrocardiograph, photocopier, and/or fax machine. Complete an equipment maintenance log for each item.

Equipment Maintenance Log			
Equipment Description:			
Serial Number:	**Model Number:**		
			Initials
Date:	**Action Taken/Comments:**		

Equipment Maintenance Log			
Equipment Description:			
Serial Number:	**Model Number:**		
			Initials
Date:	**Action Taken/Comments:**		

Procedure 48-3: Taking a Supply or Equipment Inventory. Take a supply and equipment inventory using the lists you prepared for Critical Thinking Activities B and C. Prepare a list of supplies to be ordered.

Procedure 48-4: Locating Community Resources. Make a list of community resources to which patients may be referred including visiting nurse services, homemaker services, meal delivery, senior services, etc.

Procedure 48-5: Completing an Incident Report
Use the following information to complete an incident report. Role play the situation with a classmate, and take turns playing the file clerk who is injured and the MA completing the report.
You are working in a medical office, and another employee (file clerk) slips and falls in the corridor when walking to the break room. She has been at work since 8:30 AM. The floor appears to have a wet area. The physician is called, assists the injured employee to get up, and finds a large tender area on the right hip but no other apparent injury. An x-ray is done in the office which is normal. The physician instructs the patient to telephone if any problems arise later and documents the examination and findings in the injury log. It is office policy to fill out an incident report for any fall that occurs in the office and the physician asks you (MA) to fill out the incident report.

OSHA's Form 301
Injury and Illness Incident Report

U.S. Department of Labor

Occupational Safety and Health Administration

Form approved OMB no. 1218-0176

Attention: This form contains information relating to employee health and must be used in a manner that protects the confidentiality of employees to the extent possible while the information is being used for occupational safety and health purposes.

This *Injury and Illness Incident Report* is one of the first forms you must fill out when a recordable work-related injury or illness has occurred. Together with the *Log of Work-Related Injuries and Illnesses* and the accompanying *Summary*, these forms help the employer and OSHA develop a picture of the extent and severity of work-related incidents.

Within 7 calendar days after you receive information that a recordable work-related injury or illness has occurred, you must fill out this form or an equivalent. Some state workers' compensation, insurance, or other reports may be acceptable substitutes. To be considered an equivalent form, any substitute must contain all the information asked for on this form.

According to Public Law 91-596 and 29 CFR 1904, OSHA's recordkeeping rule, you must keep this form on file for 5 years following the year to which it pertains.

If you need additional copies of this form, you may photocopy and use as many as you need.

Information about the employee

1) Full name _____

2) Street _____

City _____ State _____ ZIP _____

3) Date of birth ____ / ____ / ____

4) Date hired ____ / ____ / ____

5) ☐ Male
   ☐ Female

Information about the physician or other health care professional

6) Name of physician or other health care professional _____

7) If treatment was given away from the worksite, where was it given?

Facility _____

Street _____

City _____ State _____ ZIP _____

8) Was employee treated in an emergency room?
   ☐ Yes
   ☐ No

9) Was employee hospitalized overnight as an in-patient?
   ☐ Yes
   ☐ No

Information about the case

10) Case number from the *Log* _____
    (Transfer the case number from the *Log* after you record the case.)

11) Date of injury or illness ____ / ____ / ____

12) Time employee began work _____ AM / PM

13) Time of event _____ AM / PM
    ☐ Check if time cannot be determined

14) **What was the employee doing just before the incident occurred?** Describe the activity, as well as the tools, equipment, or material the employee was using. Be specific. *Examples:* "climbing a ladder while carrying roofing materials"; "spraying chlorine from hand sprayer"; "daily computer key-entry."

15) **What happened?** Tell us how the injury occurred. *Examples:* "When ladder slipped on wet floor, worker fell 20 feet"; "Worker was sprayed with chlorine when gasket broke during replacement"; "Worker developed soreness in wrist over time."

16) **What was the injury or illness?** Tell us the part of the body that was affected and how it was affected; be more specific than "hurt," "pain," or "sore." *Examples:* "strained back"; "chemical burn, hand"; "carpal tunnel syndrome."

17) **What object or substance directly harmed the employee?** *Examples:* "concrete floor"; "chlorine"; "radial arm saw." *If this question does not apply to the incident, leave it blank.*

18) **If the employee died, when did death occur?** Date of death ____ / ____ / ____

Completed by _____

Title _____

Phone (_____) _____ - _____ Date _____

Public reporting burden for this collection of information is estimated to average 22 minutes per response, including time for reviewing instructions, searching existing data sources, gathering and maintaining the data needed, and completing and reviewing the collection of information. Persons are not required to respond to the collection of information unless it displays a current valid OMB control number. If you have any comments about this estimate or any other aspects of this data collection, including suggestions for reducing this burden, contact: US Department of Labor, OSHA Office of Statistics, Room N-3644, 200 Constitution Avenue, NW, Washington, DC 20210. Do not send the completed forms to this office.

Procedure 48-1: Creating an Environmental Checklist and Performing a Safety Inspection

Name: _____   Date: _____

Evaluated by: _____   Score: _____

Performance Objective

Outcome: Create an environmental checklist and perform a safety inspection.

Conditions: Given the following: area to be inspected, pen and paper (or computer and word processing file) to create an environmental checklist

Standards: Time: 1 hour.   Student completed procedure in _____ minutes.

Accuracy: Satisfactory score on the Performance Evaluation Checklist.

Performance Evaluation Checklist

Trial 1	Trial 2	Point Value	Performance Standards
		●	Using the form below, added specific items to inspect to create a checklist of hazards to be inspected for including: clear walkways and tripping hazards; electrical hazards; proper storage of boxes; adequate lighting; dry floors; and proper labels and storage of biohazards, medications and chemicals.
		●	Made a general inspection to be sure that all floors were dry and all furniture and fixtures in good repair. Then filled out the appropriate parts of the checklist.
		●	Made a detailed inspection as required for each section on the checklist and filled out the checklist.
		●	Noted any problems and either fixed the problem or removed a potential hazard. Recorded any action performed and/or needed action on the checklist.
		●	Checked for walkways that were wide enough for usual traffic without anything to obstruct the walkway or cause a tripping hazard.
		●	Checked all electrical cords and plugs to ensure that there was no fraying or malfunction.
		●	Checked all storage areas for clear tops of cabinets and proper storage of supplies without potential to fall.
		●	Made sure all light bulbs worked. Either changed burned out bulbs or made a note to have them changed.
		●	Noted any areas with inadequate lighting.
		●	Made sure that all biohazards, chemicals or other potentially hazardous materials were labeled correctly and stored in secure areas away from patients.
		✶	Filled out the checklist completely.
		●	After filling out the checklist, made a written plan to respond to any areas that could not be corrected during the inspection.
		✶	Completed the procedure within 1 hour.
			TOTALS

Safety Inspection Checklist

Date: _____ Person Making Inspection: _____

Label as **C** if there are no problems; label as **NC** if a problem is found.

	C or NC	Problem/Action Taken
General Visual Inspection		
Walkways		
Electrical Cords and Plugs		
Storage Areas		
Lighting		
Storage and Labeling of Chemicals/Biohazards		

Plan to Correct Items that Could not be Corrected During Inspection:

1.

2.

3.

4.

5.

Evaluation of Student Performance

EVALUATION CRITERIA			COMMENTS
Symbol	**Category**	**Point Value**	
✶	Critical Step	16 points	
●	Essential Step	6 points	
▷	Theory Question	2 points	

Score calculation: 100 points

       −   points missed

                 ___ Score

Satisfactory score: 85 or above

CAAHEP Competencies Achieved

Psychomotor (Skills)

☑ XI. 2. Evaluate the work environment to identify safe vs. unsafe working conditions.

☑ XI. 3. Develop a personal (patient and employee) safety plan.

☑ XI. 4. Develop an environmental safety plan.

ABHES Competencies Achieved

☑ 8. x. Maintain medical facility.

Notes

Procedure 48-2: Performing Routine Maintenance of Equipment

Name: _____ Date: _____

Evaluated by: _____ Score: _____

Performance Objective

Outcome:	Perform equipment maintenance and document on equipment maintenance log.
Conditions:	Given the following: piece of equipment to be maintained, cloth for dusting, maintenance log sheet, and supplies necessary for the piece or equipment (such as paper, batteries, toner, fluids, etc).
Standards:	Time: 10 minutes. Student completed procedure in _____ minutes.
	Accuracy: Satisfactory score on the Performance Evaluation Checklist.

Performance Evaluation Checklist

Trial 1	Trial 2	Point Value	Performance Standards
		●	Located the piece of equipment to be maintained.
		●	Checked all electrical cords to be sure there is no fraying or malfunction.
		●	Checked the piece of equipment for cracks, dents, or other damage, obvious impairment or malfunction.
		●	Checked any keyboard or keypad for cracks, faded numbers, or other impairment.
		▷	Explained what to do if the piece of equipment was damaged.
		●	Dusted or cleaned the outside or case of the piece of equipment according to manufacturer's directions.
		●	Checked leads and other wires, or other tubing.
		●	Checked or changed batteries, fluid, toner, or other essential components.
		●	Scheduled any required maintenance if appropriate.
		✶	Filled out the equipment maintenance log correctly.
		✶	Completed the procedure within 10 minutes.
			TOTALS

Equipment Maintenance Log

Equipment Description:			
Serial Number:	Model Number:		
			Initials
Date:	Action Taken/Comments:		

Evaluation of Student Performance

EVALUATION CRITERIA			COMMENTS
Symbol	Category	Point Value	
✱	Critical Step	16 points	
●	Essential Step	6 points	
▷	Theory Question	2 points	

Score calculation: 100 points

− _____ points missed

_____ Score

Satisfactory score: 85 or above

CAAHEP Competencies Achieved

Psychomotor (Skills)

☑ V. 9. Perform routine maintenance of office equipment with documentation.
☑ XI. 2. Evaluate the work environment to identify safe vs. unsafe working conditions.

ABHES Competencies Achieved

☑ 8. y. Perform routine maintenance of administrative and clinical equipment.

Procedure 48-3: Taking a Supply or Equipment Inventory

Name: _____   Date: _____

Evaluated by: _____   Score: _____

Performance Objective

Outcome:	Take a supply and equipment inventory.
Conditions:	Given the following: inventory list, notebook or cards, items to inventory, and pen.
Standards:	Time: 15 minutes. Student completed procedure in _____ minutes.
	Accuracy: Satisfactory score on the Performance Evaluation Checklist.

Performance Evaluation Checklist

Trial 1	Trial 2	Point Value	Performance Standards
		●	Obtained list of items in inventory, inventory notebook, or box of inventory cards.
		●	Checked each item in the inventory record against items present in the area being inventoried.
		●	Validated serial numbers or equipment and checked the expiration date of supplies.
		●	Discarded any expired supplies and did not include in the inventory count.
		●	Documented any missing piece of equipment after making an effort to locate.
		●	Documented any item that needed repair.
		●	Flagged any supplies close to or below the reorder point as needing to be reordered.
		●	Checked that information on the inventory card or list was correct and complete.
		●	Made sure that the storage space was tidy and arranged so that items with the oldest expiration date were at the front of the storage area.
		●	Placed inventory cards, list, or book in the proper location for follow-up.
		✱	Completed the procedure within 15 minutes.
		TOTALS	

Evaluation of Student Performance

EVALUATION CRITERIA			COMMENTS
Symbol	Category	Point Value	
✶	Critical Step	16 points	
●	Essential Step	6 points	
▷	Theory Question	2 points	

Score calculation: 100 points

− _____ points missed

_____ Score

Satisfactory score: 85 or above

CAAHEP Competencies Achieved

Psychomotor (Skills)

☑ V. 10. Perform an office inventory.

ABHES Competencies Achieved

☑ 8. z. Maintain inventory equipment and supplies.

Procedure 48-4: Locating Community Resources

Name: _____   Date: _____

Evaluated by: _____   Score: _____

Performance Objective

Outcome:	Locate community resources.
Conditions:	Given the following: local telephone book, office list of community resources, computer, local hospital newsletter(s), library access, local newspapers, pen, and notepad.
Standards:	Time: 30 minutes. Student completed procedure in _____ minutes.
	Accuracy: Satisfactory score on the Performance Evaluation Checklist.

Performance Evaluation Checklist

Trial 1	Trial 2	Point Value	Performance Standards
		●	Researched local sources to identify community agencies.
		●	As resources were identified, created a list.
		●	Included pertinent information such as name, services available, address, telephone number, web address, contact information, and other useful information.
		●	Transferred handwritten list to a computer document.
		●	Grouped resources by category and alphabetized within each group.
		●	Obtained physician approval of finished list.
		●	Updated the list when information changed, new resources were identified.
		●	Used a list of community resources for patients to make recommendations to patients and families.
		★	Completed the procedure within 30 minutes.
			TOTALS

Evaluation of Student Performance

EVALUATION CRITERIA			COMMENTS
Symbol	Category	Point Value	
✶	Critical Step	16 points	
●	Essential Step	6 points	
▷	Theory Question	2 points	

Score calculation: 100 points

        −   _____ points missed

              ____ Score

Satisfactory score: 85 or above

CAAHEP Competencies Achieved

Psychomotor (Skills)

☑ IV. 12. Develop and maintain a current list of community resources related to patients' health care needs.

ABHES Competencies Achieved

☑ 8. e. Locate resources and information for patients and employers.

Procedure 48-5: Completing an Incident Report

Name: _____ Date: _____

Evaluated by: _____ Score: _____

Performance Objective

Outcome:	Locate community resources.
Conditions:	Given the following: incident report form (such as OSHA form 301), pen, notes from witnesses to the incident
Standards:	Time: 20 minutes. Student completed procedure in _____ minutes.
	Accuracy: Satisfactory score on the Performance Evaluation Checklist.

Performance Evaluation Checklist

Trial 1	Trial 2	Point Value	Performance Standards
		●	Interviewed all individuals involved in the incident and all witnesses and make notes as needed to complete the written incident report.
		●	Obtained an incident report form and fill in information about the person (or persons) who are the main subject of the incident including name, date of birth, and address.
		●	Completed any information about health care provided, including the names and identifying formation for physicians or health care professionals who provided treatment.
		●	Included pertinent information to describe the incident in detail including time, location (address, building, room number), what happened, and any injury or illness that resulted from the incident.
		●	Included the name and contact information of the individual to whom the incident was reported.
		●	Reviewed the report with the subject of the incident if possible before signing the report and obtaining the signature of the subject of the report if possible. Also obtained a supervisor's signature.
		●	Obtained physician approval of finished list.
		✱	Completed the procedure within 20 minutes.
			TOTALS

EVALUATION CRITERIA			COMMENTS
Symbol	**Category**	**Point Value**	
✱	Critical Step	16 points	
●	Essential Step	6 points	
▷	Theory Question	2 points	

Score calculation: 100 points

       −   points missed

                ___ Score

Satisfactory score: 85 or above

CAAHEP Competencies Achieved

Psychomotor (Skills)

☑ IX. 6. Complete an incident report.

ABHES Competencies Achieved

☑ 4. e. Perform risk management procedures.

49 Emergency Protective Practices for the Medical Office

CHAPTER ASSIGNMENTS

√ After Completing	Date Due	Textbook Pages	TEXTBOOK ASSIGNMENTS	Possible Points	Points You Earned
		1144-1156	Read Chapter 49: Emergency Protective Practices for the Medical Office		
		1149 1154	Read Case Study 1 Case Study 1 questions	5	
		1152 1154-1155	Read Case Study 2 Case Study 2 questions	5	
		1153 1155	Read Case Study 3 Case Study 3 questions	5	
			TOTAL POINTS		
√ After Completing	**Date Due**	**Study Guide Pages**	**STUDY GUIDE ASSIGNMENTS (CTA = Critical Thinking Activity)**	**Possible Points**	**Points You Earned**
		1283	Pretest	10	
		1284	Term Key Term Assessment	8	
		1284-1287	Evaluation of Learning questions	39	
		1288	CTA A: Disasters	20	
		1288	CTA B: Personal Safety Plan	30	
		1288-1289	CTA C: Disaster Planning in the Medical Office	30	
		1289	CTA D: Fire Hazards	20	
		1289	CTA E: Fire Protection and Prevention Methods	20	
		1289	CTA F: Use of Fire Extinguisher	20	
		1289	CTA G: Evacuation Floor Plan	40	
		1290	CTA H: Mock Environmental Exposure Event	40	
		1290	CTA I: Disaster Evacuation of a Medical Office	40	
		1290-1291	CTA J: Community Resources	8	
		1291	CTA K: Crossword Puzzle	19	

√ After Completing	Date Due	Study Guide Pages	STUDY GUIDE ASSIGNMENTS (CTA = Critical Thinking Activity)	Possible Points	Points You Earned
			e Evolve Site: Apply Your Knowledge questions	10	
		1283	[?] Posttest	10	
			ADDITIONAL ASSIGNMENTS		
			TOTAL POINTS		

1280

√ When Assigned By Your Instructor	Study Guide Pages	Practices Required	LABORATORY ASSIGNMENTS (Procedure Number and Name)	Score*
	1292	5	**Practice for Competency** 49-1: Demonstrating Proper Use of a Fire Extinguisher Textbook reference: p. 1149	
	1293-1294		**Evaluation of Competency** 49-1: Demonstrating Proper Use of a Fire Extinguisher	*
	1292	4	**Practice for Competency** 49-2: Participating in a Mock Environmental Exposure Event Textbook reference: pp. 1151-1152	
	1295-1296		**Evaluation of Competency** 49-2: Participating in a Mock Environmental Exposure Event	*
	1292	5	**Practice for Competency** 49-3: Maintaining a List of Community Resources for Emergency Preparedness Textbook reference: p. 1154	
	1297-1298		**Evaluation of Competency** 49-3: Maintaining a List of Community Resources for Emergency Preparedness	*
			ADDITIONAL ASSIGNMENTS	

Notes

Name _____   Date _____

?≡ **PRETEST**

True or False

_____ 1. A flood is an example of a man-made disaster.

_____ 2. A positive reaction to a disaster involves the triggering of resources to meet the challenge.

_____ 3. During the alarm reaction of the general adaptation syndrome (GAS), the body prepares for fight or flight.

_____ 4. During the recovery phase of the GAS, epinephrine is released into the bloodstream.

_____ 5. Hyperventilation may occur during an anxiety attack.

_____ 6. The local fire marshal is responsible for the fire protection of the contents of a medical office.

_____ 7. The number and locations of smoke detectors in a medical office are governed by federal law.

_____ 8. The sequence of events that should be included in responding to a fire include: rescue, activate, confine, extinguish.

_____ 9. A medical assistant might be required to rappel down the side of a cliff in an emergency.

_____ 10. Citizen Corps is responsible for coordinating volunteer activities to prevent crime and respond to emergencies.

POSTTEST

True or False

_____ 1. A fire is an example of a man-made disaster.

_____ 2. Stress is the body's response to threat or change.

_____ 3. Epinephrine causes a decrease in the blood pressure.

_____ 4. Anxiety is a feeling of worry or uneasiness.

_____ 5. Posttraumatic stress disorder is the term for the psychiatric condition that may occur after a catastrophic life disturbance.

_____ 6. A fire extinguisher should be located near the exit of each room of a medical office.

_____ 7. A written Emergency Action Plan is required for almost all businesses by the U.S. Environmental Protection Agency (EPA).

_____ 8. An Emergency Action Plan should include a way to account for all employees after an evacuation.

_____ 9. A gas leak is an example of environmental exposure.

_____ 10. The American Red Cross is responsible for coordinating a response to any disaster that overwhelms the resources of state and local authorities.

Chapter **49** **Emergency Protective Practices for the Medical Office**

Directions: Match each medical term with its definition.

_____ 1. Anxiety

_____ 2. Environmental exposure

_____ 3. Evacuation plan

_____ 4. Fire extinguisher

_____ 5. Man-made disaster

_____ 6. Natural disaster

_____ 7. Posttraumatic stress disorder

_____ 8. Stress

A. A portable device that discharges foam or another material to extinguish a fire

B. Serious damage to the environment resulting from a natural hazard that leads to environmental, financial, and human losses

C. A feeling of worry or uneasiness, often triggered by an event with an uncertain outcome

D. A psychiatric condition that develops months or years after a traumatic catastrophic life experience

E. A plan that includes escape routes for all locations in a building or other facility

F. Employee's exposure to hazardous substances in their workplace

G. Serious damage either directly or indirectly caused by intentional or negligent human actions or the failure of a man-made system.

H. The body's response to threat or change

EVALUATION OF LEARNING

1. Why is it important to plan ahead for a disaster or serious emergency?

_____

_____

2. What is a natural disaster?

_____

_____

3. What is a man-made disaster?

_____

_____

4. What are some examples of natural disasters.

_____

5. What are some examples of man-made disasters?

_____

_____

6. What is a positive reaction to a disaster?

_____

_____

7. When do individuals usually react negatively to a disaster?

_____

1284

8. What characteristics of a disaster tend to cause the most serious psychological effects?

_____

_____

_____

9. What occurs during the alarm reaction of the GAS?

_____

10. What signs/symptoms occur when epinephrine stimulates the sympathetic nervous system?

_____

_____

11. What occurs during the stage of resistance?

_____

12. What occurs during the recovery phase?

_____

13. What happens to a person who is subjected to chronic stress?

_____

14. What is anxiety?

_____

_____

15. Why is it important to learn and practice emergency procedures?

_____

_____

16. What are the symptoms of a full-blown anxiety attack?

_____

_____

17. What should the medical assistant do if an emergency occurs at his or her workplace?

_____

_____

18. What symptoms may occur following a disaster or serious emergency?

_____

_____

19. What is posttraumatic stress disorder and what are the symptoms?

_____

_____

_____

20. What are examples of common fire hazards in the medical office?

_____

_____

_____

_____

21. What guidelines should be followed regarding exits in the medical office?

_____

_____

_____

22. Where should fire extinguishers be located and why?

_____

_____

23. What does the acronym PASS stand for in terms of the use of a fire extinguisher?

_____

24. What is the preferred method for storing a backup copy of computer files?

_____

25. Who sets the standard for the number of detectors and locations of the detectors in the medical office?

_____

26. List and describe the steps that should be taken in responding to a fire following the RACE format.

1. _____

2. _____

3. _____

4. _____

27. What elements must be included in an OSHA Emergency Action Plan?

_____

_____

_____

_____

28. What is an evacuation plan?

_____

_____

_____

29. What information should be included in an evacuation plan for individuals with disabilities?

_____

_____

30. What information should be included in the evacuation plan regarding what employees should do after evacuating?

_____

_____

31. What information should be included in the training of employees under the Emergency Action Plan?

_____

_____

32. Who determines whether or not fire drills must be held at a facility?

_____

33. What tasks might be performed by a medical assistant in a disaster?

_____

_____

34. What are some examples of disasters that have occurred in the past 20 years.

_____

_____

35. What agencies must be coordinated in a community or state emergency preparedness plan?

_____

_____

36. What typically occurs if the state's resources are inadequate to handle a disaster?

_____

_____

37. What is the responsibility of the Federal Emergency Management Agency (FEMA)?

_____

_____

38. What is the Citizen Corps?

_____

_____

39. What specific functions are provided by local chapters of the American Red Cross?

_____

_____

Chapter **49** **Emergency Protective Practices for the Medical Office**

CRITICAL THINKING ACTIVITIES

A. Disasters

Indicate a major natural disaster and a man-made disaster that has occurred in your community and/or state. Provide a brief description and damage caused by each of these disasters. (*Note:* An Internet search using the terms: "Disasters in (name of your state)" will assist you in completing this activity.

1. Natural disaster:

_____

_____

_____

_____

_____

2. Man-made disaster:

_____

_____

_____

_____

_____

B. Personal Safety Plan

Choose a natural disaster (e.g., tornado, hurricane, flood, blizzard) or man-made disaster (e.g., fire, power outage, burglary) that might occur in your locale, and develop and outline a personal safety plan for responding to the disaster in your home environment. Include information on what you would do before, during, and after the disaster occurred. The following website can assist you in locating information to complete this activity: www.redcross.org.

1. Before: _____

_____

_____

2. During: _____

_____

_____

3. After: _____

_____

C. Disaster Planning in the Medical Office

Choose a natural disaster or man-made disaster that might occur in your locale, and develop and outline an emergency action plan for responding to the disaster in a medical office setting. Include information on what you would do before, during, and after the disaster occurred. The following websites can assist you in locating information to complete this activity:
www.redcross.org
http://www.osha.gov/Publications/osha3088.pdf
http://www.osha.gov/SLTC/emergencypreparedness

1. Before: _____

_____

1288

2. During: _____

_____

_____

3. After: _____

_____

_____

D. Fire Hazards

Perform a survey of your home to determine if there are any fire hazards. If so, list these hazards and what steps should be taken to correct them. Your textbook and the following websites will assist you in completing this activity: www. fire-extinguisher101.com/hazards.html, www.usfa.fema.gov/citizens/home_fire_prev/cooking.shtm, hartfordauto.the hartford.com/Safe-Driving/Home-Safety/Fire-Safety.

Fire Hazard: **Steps Needed to Correct:**

_____

_____

_____

_____

E. Fire Protection and Prevention Methods

Survey the interior of a health care facility in your community and indicate the fire protection and prevention methods in place at this facility. List these below:

_____

_____

_____

_____

F. Use of Fire Extinguisher

Perform an Internet search for a video of the operation of a fire extinguisher. Write a short paragraph below describing the video.

_____

_____

_____

_____

G. Evacuation Floor Plan

On a blank piece of paper, draw a floor plan for a medical office and indicate the evacuation route for each room on the floor plan. Include the following in your floor plan: primary and secondary escape routes for each room and exits. You can use an existing evacuation floor plan from a medical office in your community and/or the information presented in your textbook to assist you in completing this activity.

Chapter **49** **Emergency Protective Practices for the Medical Office**

H. Mock Environmental Exposure Event

Create a small "paper-doll" figure out of cardboard or other materials (e.g., a tongue blade or popsicle stick). Form a group of students and choose an evacuation coordinator. Using the information presented in Procedure 49-2, participate in the mock environmental exposure event outlined in this procedure.

The evacuation coordinator's responsibilities are to:

1. Select an evacuation floor plan developed by one of the group members (Refer to CTA G).

2. Assign roles to each individual's "paper-doll" figure. These roles should include staff and patients. The patients should be of various ages/genders and with various types of conditions, disabilities, and emotional states (e.g., fear, anxiety, immobilization, calmness). If possible, attach masking tape labeled with identifying information on each figure.

3. Assign two staff members with the responsibility of assisting patients to leave the office.

4. Assign one staff member to do a final check before leaving the office.

5. Designate a meeting place on the floor plan following the evacuation.

6. Account for everyone in the group following the evacuation.

7. Lead a discussion to evaluate the timeliness and effectiveness of the evacuation process. Record the key points of this discussion below:

_____

_____

_____

_____

_____

I. Disaster Evacuation of a Medical Office

Repeat the activity described above (CTA H) using an emergency action plan developed by a group member as outlined in CTA C. The group member who created the emergency action plan should take the role of the evacuation coordinator. If time permits, participate in as many mock disaster evacuations as possible using an emergency action plans developed by other members of your group. Evaluate the timeliness and effectiveness of each evacuation process and record the key points below:

_____

_____

_____

_____

J. Community Resources

Look up and indicate below the name and telephone number of the following:

1. Emergency Management Services (will usually be 911): _____

2. Poison Control Center: _____

3. Local hospital(s): _____

4. Local health department: _____

5. State health department: _____

1290

6. State HAZMAT response team: _____

7. Local area emergency management (LEMA) office: _____

8. Local chapter of the American Red Cross: _____

9. Citizen Corps Council or Citizen Emergency Response Team (if any): _____

K. Crossword Puzzle: Emergency Protective Practices for the Medical Office
Directions: Complete the crossword puzzle using the clues provided.

Across
1 Alarm reaction response
6 Stimulates sympathetic NS
8 How to respond to a fire
10 Caused by threat or change
12 Releases epinephrine
15 Gas leak (ex)
16 Fire extinguisher procedure
17 Volunteer disaster agency
18 Reaction to stress
19 PTSD symptom

Down
2 Anxiety attack symptom
3 Overloaded electrical circuit (ex)
4 Man-made disaster (ex)
5 Private disaster agency
7 Natural disaster (ex)
9 Helps to control anxiety
11 Fire alerter
13 Worry or uneasiness
14 Federal disaster agency

Procedure 49-1: Demonstrating Proper Use of a Fire Extinguisher: Demonstrate the proper use of a fire extinguisher. This can be accomplished in one of the following ways:

A. Role playing using a discharged fire extinguisher.

B. Using a new fire extinguisher in an outdoor location

Using the information printed on the label of the fire extinguisher (or owner's manual), complete the information requested below:

1. What is the brand name of the extinguisher? _____

2. What type of agent (expellant) is contained in the extinguisher (e.g., dry chemical, water, foam)?

_____

3. What types of fires is this extinguisher capable of extinguishing (e.g., grease, wood, paper)? _____

_____

4. How far away should you stand when operating this extinguisher? _____

5. What type of precautions should be observed with this extinguisher (e.g., Keep away from children)? _____

_____

_____

6. What type of care and maintenance is required for this extinguisher?

_____

_____

_____

Procedure 49-2: Participating in a Mock Environmental Exposure Event: Prepare for participating in a mock environmental exposure event by first completing Critical Thinking Activity H.

Procedure 49-3: Maintaining a Current List of Community Resources for Emergency Preparedness: Prepare for this procedure by first completing Critical Thinking Activity J.

Procedure 49-1: Demonstrating Proper Use of a Fire Extinguisher

Name: _____   Date: _____

Evaluated by: _____   Score: _____

Performance Objective

Outcome:	Demonstrate Use of a Fire Extinguisher.
Conditions:	Given the following: Portable ABC fire extinguisher
Standards:	Time: 5 minutes. Student completed procedure in _____ minutes.
	Accuracy: Satisfactory score on the Performance Evaluation Checklist.

Performance Evaluation Checklist

Trial 1	Trial 2	Point Value	Performance Standards
			Perform the following through one of the following methods: A. Role playing using a discharged fire extinguisher. B. Using a new fire extinguisher in an outdoor setting.
		●	Pulled the safety pin from the handle of the fire extinguisher.
		▷	Stated the purpose of the safety pin.
		●	Aimed the nozzle or hose at the base of the fire.
		▷	Stated why the nozzle should be directed to the base of the fire.
		●	Stood at the recommended distance from the fire.
		▷	Stated how to determine the recommended standing distance.
		●	Squeezed the moveable top handle against the bottom handle until the extinguisher discharges.
		●	Swept the extinguisher from side to side until the flames are extinguished.
		●	Gradually moved closer to the flames and continued to sweep the extinguisher from side to side.
		▷	Stated why the extinguisher should be swept from side to side.
		●	Continued to watch the area.
		▷	Stated the reason for continuing to watch the area.
		▷	Stated the meaning of the following acronym: PASS (Pull, Aim, Squeeze, Sweep)
		✱	Completed the procedure within 5 minutes.
			TOTALS

Evaluation of Student Performance

EVALUATION CRITERIA			COMMENTS
Symbol	Category	Point Value	
✶	Critical Step	16 points	
●	Essential Step	6 points	
▷	Theory Question	2 points	

Score calculation: 100 points

− _____ points missed

_____ Score

Satisfactory score: 85 or above

CAAHEP Competencies Achieved

Psychomotor (Skills)
☑ XI. 1. Comply with safety signs, symbols, and labels.
☑ XI. 5. b. Demonstrate proper use of the following equipment: Fire extinguisher.

Affective (Behavior)
☑ IX. 2. Demonstrate self awareness in responding to emergency situations
and care.

ABHES Competencies Achieved

☑ 9. e. Recognize emergencies and treatments and minor office surgical procedures.

Procedure 49-2: Participating in a Mock Environmental Exposure Event

Name: _____ Date: _____

Evaluated by: _____ Score: _____

Performance Objective

Outcome:	Participate in a mock environmental exposure event.
Conditions:	Given the following: scenario, evacuation plan, building evacuation route map, pen, and paper.
Standards:	Time: 20 minutes. Student completed procedure in _____ minutes.
	Accuracy: Satisfactory score on the Performance Evaluation Checklist.

Performance Evaluation Checklist

Trial 1	Trial 2	Point Value	Performance Standards
			Prepare for the disaster simulation by performing the following:
		●	Obtaining the building evacuation plan and floor map.
		●	Reading the scenario.
		●	Making a list of group members.
		●	Assigning group members to be staff or patients.
		●	Designating a meeting place.
		▷	Stated the purpose of an evacuation plan.
		●	Selected an evacuation coordinator.
			Began the simulation as follows:
		●	Assume your medical office has been notified to evacuate due to the possibility of a natural gas leak.
		●	The coordinator assigns two staff members to assist patients in leaving the building.
		●	The coordinator assigns one staff member to check that there is no open flame and be the last to leave the office area.
		●	The last staff member to leave should also make sure that all staff and patients have left each room in the office.
		●	Left the building using the primary escape route designated on the evacuation floor plan.
		▷	Stated why the primary escape route should be used.
		●	Met at the designated meeting area.
		●	The coordinator checked the list to ensure everyone is present.

    Chapter **49** **Emergency Protective Practices for the Medical Office**

Trial 1	Trial 2	Point Value	Performance Standards
		●	Discussed the evacuation process.
		●	Documented the evacuation process.
		▷	Stated the purpose of the evacuation process.
		✱	Completed the procedure within 5 minutes.
			TOTALS
		DOCUMENTATION	
Date			

Evaluation of Student Performance

EVALUATION CRITERIA			COMMENTS
Symbol	**Category**	**Point Value**	
✱	Critical Step	16 points	
●	Essential Step	6 points	
▷	Theory Question	2 points	

Score calculation: 100 points

—   _____ points missed

_____

_____ Score

Satisfactory score: 85 or above

CAAHEP Competencies Achieved

Psychomotor (Skills)
☑ XI. 2. Evaluate the work environment to identify safe vs. unsafe working conditions.
☑ XI. 3. Develop a personal (patient and employee) safety plan.
☑ XI. 2. XI. 4. Develop an environmental safety plan.
☑ XI. 6. Participate in a mock environmental exposure event with documentation of steps taken.
☑ XI. 7. Explain an evacuation plan for a physician's office.

Affective (Behavior)
☑ I. 1. Apply critical thinking skills in performing patient assessment and care.
☑ 1.2. Use language/verbal skills that enable patients' understanding.
☑ XI. 1. Recognize the effects of stress on all persons involved in emergency situations.
☑ XI. 2. Demonstrate self awareness in responding to emergency situations.

ABHES Competencies Achieved

☑ 5. b. Identify and respond appropriately when working/caring for patients with special needs.
☑ 9. e. Recognize emergencies and treatments and minor office surgical procedures.

Procedure 49-3: Maintaining a List of Community Resources for Emergency Preparedness

Name: _____   Date: _____

Evaluated by: _____   Score: _____

Performance Objective

Outcome:	Maintain a list of community resources for emergency preparedness.
Conditions:	Given the following: local telephone book, computer and Internet, telephone, pen and paper.
Standards:	Time: 30 minutes. Student completed procedure in _____ minutes.
	Accuracy: Satisfactory score on the Performance Evaluation Checklist.

Performance Evaluation Checklist

Trial 1	Trial 2	Point Value	Performance Standards
		●	Prepared a list of community agencies for emergency response.
			The list included the following agencies:
		●	EMS (911)
		●	Poison Control Center
		●	Local hospitals
		●	Local and state health departments
		●	State HAZMAT response team
		●	Posted the list by every telephone in the medical office.
		▷	Stated the reason for posting the emergency response numbers by every telephone.
		●	Researched and created a more detailed list of agencies to respond to a widespread disaster or emergency affecting the community.
			The list included the following agencies:
		●	Local area emergency management (LEMA) office
		●	Local chapter of the American Red Cross
		●	Citizen Corps Council or Citizen Emergency Response Team
		●	Transferred the list to a word processing file for ease of duplication.
		●	Grouped resources by subject and/or age group served.
		●	Alphabetized resources within each group.

Trial 1	Trial 2	Point Value	Performance Standards
		●	Saved and printed copies of the list as needed.
		●	Updated the list when information changes, when a new resource is identified, and on a periodic basis.
		✶	Completed the procedure within 5 minutes.
			TOTALS

Evaluation of Student Performance

EVALUATION CRITERIA			COMMENTS
Symbol	**Category**	**Point Value**	
✶	Critical Step	16 points	
●	Essential Step	6 points	
▷	Theory Question	2 points	

Score calculation: 100 points

− _____ points missed

_____ Score

Satisfactory score: 85 or above

CAAHEP Competencies Achieved

Psychomotor (Skills)
☑ XI. 12. Maintain a current list of community resources for emergency preparedness.

ABHES Competencies Achieved

☑ 4.e. Perform risk management procedures.
☑ 8. e. Locate resources and information for patients and employers.
☑ 9. e. Recognize emergencies and treatments and minor office surgical procedures.

50 Obtaining Employment

CHAPTER ASSIGNMENTS

√ After Completing	Date Due	Textbook Pages	TEXTBOOK ASSIGNMENTS	Possible Points	Points You Earned
		1157-1171	Read Chapter 50: Obtaining Employment		
		1164 1170	Read Case Study 1 Case Study 1 questions	5	
		1165 1170-1171	Read Case Study 2 Case Study 2 questions	5	
		1168 1171	Read Case Study 3 Case Study 3 questions	5	
			TOTAL POINTS		

√ After Completing	Date Due	Study Guide Pages	STUDY GUIDE ASSIGNMENTS (CTA = Critical Thinking Activity)	Possible Points	Points You Earned
		1301	Pretest	10	
		1301	Term Key Term Assessment	5	
		1302-1304	Evaluation of Learning questions	24	
		1304-1309	CTA A: Preparing a Résumé	15	
		1309	CTA B: Preparing a Cover Letter	10	
		1309-1310	CTA C: References	10	
		1310	CTA D: Interview Questions	10	
			Evolve Site: Apply Your Knowledge questions	10	
		1301	Posttest	10	
			ADDITIONAL ASSIGNMENTS		
			TOTAL POINTS		

Notes

Name _____   Date _____

True or False

_____ 1. Networking to find employment means applying for jobs using the Internet.

_____ 2. It is recommended to limit a résumé to one page.

_____ 3. Hobbies and other personal information are included in the last section of a résumé.

_____ 4. A functional résumé is recommended when an individual wants to change to a different type of work.

_____ 5. Begin a résumé with your name, address, telephone number, and e-mail address.

_____ 6. The medical assisting externship and volunteer work should not be included under Work Experience.

_____ 7. When describing job duties, use all past tense or all participle forms of verbs.

_____ 8. It is assumed that a medical assistant (MA) has a valid CPR (cardiopulmonary resuscitation) certification, and it is not necessary to put on the résumé.

_____ 9. The MA should always ask permission before using a supervisor's name as a reference.

_____ 10. The MA may ask about a salary range during the interview.

📋 **POSTTEST**

True or False

_____ 1. Using several methods to identify potential employers is an important step to find a job.

_____ 2. If a résumé is submitted to an employer, it is not necessary to complete a job application.

_____ 3. A résumé that categorizes experience according to skills is called a chronological résumé.

_____ 4. When including information about education, it should be listed with the most recent first.

_____ 5. The high school and date diploma was received should always be included on a résumé.

_____ 6. It is important not to leave gaps of time unaccounted for on a chronological résumé.

_____ 7. Job duties may be summarized in bullet form on a résumé.

_____ 8. The names and addresses of three personal references should be listed on the résumé.

_____ 9. Résumés can be sent through the mail, attached to e-mail, by fax, or attached to an online application.

_____ 10. The interviewer should not ask about marital status or number of children during a job interview.

🔑 **KEY TERM ASSESSMENT**

Directions: Match each medical term with its definition.

_____ 1. Burnout

_____ 2. Continuing education unit (CEU)

_____ 3. Cover letter

_____ 4. Networking

_____ 5. Résumé

A. A summary of information about a person that describes education, work experience, and other information

B. A letter sent with one or more documents (such as a résumé) to provide an explanation

C. Contacting acquaintances and their contacts who may know of potential jobs

D. Disillusionment with work and physical or emotional exhaustion

E. A standard measure of qualified instruction or contact hours as defined by a specific profession

Directions: Fill in each blank with the correct answer.

1. What are the two parts of successful job hunting?

   _____

   _____

2. What are three questions the MA might ask himself or herself when setting goals for job hunting?

   _____

   _____

   _____

3. Identify three resources to identify potential employers other than newspaper or Internet advertisements.

   _____

   _____

   _____

4. Describe what a résumé is and identify its function.

   _____

   _____

   _____

5. Should an MA include personal information on a résumé? Why or why not?

   _____

   _____

6. Describe three styles of résumés.

   _____

   _____

   _____

7. What information should be included on a résumé?

   _____

   _____

8. What specific information should be included in the education section of a résumé?

   _____

   _____

   _____

1302

9. Discuss two ways that previous experience can be presented, and give the advantages and disadvantages of each.

_____

_____

_____

10. In a previous job at a supermarket, the MA often helped put price tags on new items and arrange them in the store. Describe this using the past tense as she might include it on a résumé.

_____

_____

11. In a previous job at a retail store, the MA worked at the cash register. Describe this using the participle form of the verb as it would appear in a bulleted list.

_____

_____

12. What are three types of information that might be included in the "Special Skills" section of a résumé?

_____

_____

13. How should the MA prepare a list of references?

_____

_____

14. What format should be used for the final version of a résumé?

_____

_____

15. What is the purpose of a cover letter when sending out résumés?

_____

16. What are the advantages and disadvantages of faxing a résumé?

_____

_____

17. In addition to a résumé, what information should the MA bring when applying for a job?

_____

_____

18. Identify six specific ways that the MA can make a favorable impression during a job interview.

_____

_____

_____

_____

19. What kinds of questions might an MA ask during a job interview?

_____

_____

20. What kind of follow-up is appropriate after a job interview?

_____

_____

21. After obtaining employment, how can the MA keep his or her administrative and clinical skills current?

_____

_____

22. Identify three specific actions an MA can take to avoid or respond to job burnout.

_____

_____

23. Identify four benefits for members of a national professional organization.

_____

_____

24. Identify four routes that an MA may take to advance his or her career.

_____

_____

CRITICAL THINKING ACTIVITIES

A. Preparing a Résumé

Complete the following information as a basis for preparing your résumé. Then create a professional résumé.

1. Identify the kind of job(s) you are looking for:

First choice

Second choice

2. Summarize your education beginning with your most recent:

Name of school _____

City _____ State _____

Dates attended: _____/_____/_____ to _____/_____/_____

Degree: _____ Date: _____/_____/_____

Major (or courses completed if you did not graduate):

Awards, GPA (if higher than 3.0), Dean's list (dates):

Previous education (beyond high school)

Name of school _____

City _____ State _____

Dates attended: _____/_____/_____ to _____/_____/_____

Degree: _____ Date: _____/_____/_____

Major (or courses completed if you did not graduate):

_____

_____

Awards, GPA (if higher than 3.0), Dean's list (dates):

_____

Provide information for other educational experience.

_____

_____

Other relevant training and dates of completion including first-aid training, CPR training, and computer training.

Other skills including foreign languages spoken and skills you have learned but never practiced in an externship or work setting.

3. Summarize your experience in the health care field beginning with your most recent. Include your medical assisting externship.

Name of organization or physician: _____

City _____ State _____

Dates of experience: _____/_____/_____ to _____/_____/_____

Type of experience or job title: _____

Indicate if the following apply: Externship/Practicum _____ Volunteer _____ Part-time _____

Summer _____

Identify your duties and responsibilities, one per line. Use a consistent form (e.g., "prepared patients for examinations," "responsible for preparing patients for examinations").

_____

_____

_____

_____

Identify any special accomplishments, promotions, or other positive outcomes from this position.

_____

_____

Next most recent health-related experience:

Name of organization or physician: _____

City _____ State _____

Dates of experience: _____/_____/_____to _____/_____/_____

Type of experience or job title: _____

Indicate if the following apply: Externship/Practicum _____ Volunteer _____ Part-time _____

Summer _____

Identify your duties and responsibilities, one per line. Use a consistent form (e.g., "prepared patients for examinations," or "responsible for preparing patients for examinations").

_____

_____

_____

_____

Identify any special accomplishments, promotions, or other positive outcomes from this position.

_____

_____

Next most recent health-related experience:

Name of organization or physician: _____

City _____ State _____

Dates of experience: _____/_____/_____to _____/_____/_____

Type of experience or job title: _____

Indicate if the following apply: Externship/Practicum _____ Volunteer _____ Part-time _____

Summer _____

Identify your duties and responsibilities, one per line. Use a consistent form (e.g., "prepared patients for examinations," or "responsible for preparing patients for examinations").

_____

_____

_____

_____

Identify any special accomplishments, promotions, or other positive outcomes from this position.

_____

_____

Provide information for other experience in the health care field.

_____

_____

4. Identify work experience that is not related to health care. Include all full-time jobs, but if you have not been employed consistently, include part-time and/or summer employment, volunteer experience, or time spent as a homemaker.

Employer (or organization): _____

City _____ State _____

Dates of experience: _____/_____/_____to _____/_____/_____

Type of experience or job title: _____

Indicate if the following apply: Externship/Practicum _____ Volunteer _____ Part-time _____

Summer _____

Identify your duties and responsibilities, one per line. Use a consistent form (e.g., "prepared patients for examinations," or "responsible for preparing patients for examinations").

_____

_____

_____

_____

Identify any special accomplishments, promotions, or other positive outcomes from this position.

_____

_____

Provide information for other work experience.

_____

_____

Next most recent experience:

Employer (or organization): _____

City _____ State _____

1307

Dates of experience: _____/_____/_____to _____/_____/_____

Type of experience or job title: _____

Indicate if the following apply: Externship/Practicum _____ Volunteer _____ Part-time _____

Summer _____

Identify your duties and responsibilities, one per line. Use a consistent form (e.g., "prepared patients for examinations," or "responsible for preparing patients for examinations").

_____

_____

_____

_____

Identify any special accomplishments, promotions, or other positive outcomes from this position.

_____

_____

Provide information for other work experience.

_____

_____

Next most recent experience:

Employer (or organization): _____

City _____ State _____

Dates of experience: _____/_____/_____ to _____/_____/_____

Type of experience or job title: _____

Indicate if the following apply: Externship/Practicum _____ Volunteer _____ Part-time _____

Summer _____

Identify your duties and responsibilities, one per line. Use a consistent form (e.g., "prepared patients for examinations," or "responsible for preparing patients for examinations").

_____

_____

_____

_____

Identify any special accomplishments, promotions, or other positive outcomes from this position.

_____

_____

Provide information for other work experience.

_____

_____

1308

B. Preparing a Cover Letter

Complete the following information to help you prepare a cover letter to accompany your résumé when you look for a job.

1. Describe in one sentence the reason that you are currently seeking a job.

   _____

   _____

2. Describe the type of position you seek (job title, full-time, and/or part-time) and when you will be available to begin working.

   _____

   _____

3. Describe your personal qualifications in a few sentences focusing on your strengths as a person, as well as your skills.

   _____

   _____

C. References

Complete the following information to help you prepare a list of at least three references. If possible, include a supervisor from employment and/or externship and an instructor or coach from your educational program. Indicate if you have already obtained permission from the person to use him or her as a reference.

Name: _____ Permission Requested: _____

This person's relationship to you: _____

Contact information:

Employer: _____ Job Title: _____

Address: _____

Telephone Number: _____

Name: _____ Permission Requested: _____

This person's relationship to you: _____

Contact information:

Employer: _____ Job Title: _____

Address: _____

_____

Telephone Number: _____

Name: _____ Permission Requested: _____

This person's relationship to you: _____

Contact information:

Employer: _____ Job Title: _____

Address: _____

Telephone Number: _____

Provide information for two other references.

_____

_____

1309

D. Interview Questions

Prepare a personalized and thoughtful response to each of the following questions you might be asked during a job interview.

1. Where do you see yourself in 5 years?

   _____

   _____

   _____

2. Describe a difficult situation you have had at work and how you handled it.

   _____

   _____

   _____

3. What could you contribute to our office?

   _____

   _____

   _____

4. What are some of your weaknesses or areas you need to work on?

   _____

   _____

   _____

5. What would your medical assisting instructor say about you if I were to call her for a reference?

   _____

   _____

   _____